Healthy Aging

Principles and Clinical Practice for Clinicians

Healthy Aging

Principles and Clinical Practice for Clinicians

Virginia Burggraf, RN, DNS, FAAN

Marcella J. Griggs Endowed Chair
Gerontological Nursing Coordinator Graduate Program
Radford University
Radford, Virginia

Kye Y. Kim, MD

Professor and Director, Academic Affairs
Department of Psychiatry and Behavioral Medicine
Virginia Tech Carilion School of Medicine
Roanoke, Virginia

Aubrey L. Knight, MD

Associate Dean for Student Affairs
Professor of Medicine and Family & Community Medicine
Virginia Tech Carilion School of Medicine
Roanoke, Virginia

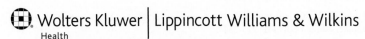

Wolters Kluwer | Lippincott Williams & Wilkins
Health

Philadelphia · Baltimore · New York · London
Buenos Aires · Hong Kong · Sydney · Tokyo

Senior Acquisitions Editor: Shannon Magee
Product Manager: Ashley Fischer
Production Project Manager: Marian Bellus
Manufacturing Manager: Kathleen Brown
Marketing Manager: Mark Wiragh
Design Coordinator: Stephen Druding
Production Service: S4Carlisle Publishing Services

Printed in China

Library of Congress Cataloging-in-Publication Data

Healthy aging (Burggraf)
Healthy aging: principles and clinical practice for clinicians/[edited by] Virginia Burggraf, Kye Y. Kim,
 Aubrey L. Knight.—First edition.
  p.; cm.
 Includes bibliographical references.
 ISBN 978-1-4511-9104-2
 I. Burggraf, Virginia, editor of compilation.   II. Kim, Kye Y., editor of compilation.   III. Knight,
Aubrey L., editor of compilation.   IV. Title.
 [DNLM: 1. Aging. 2. Aged. 3. Clinical Medicine—Methods. 4. Health Behavior. 5. Health Services for
the Aged. 6. Longevity. WT 104]
 RA776.75
 613.2—dc23

2013033817

Care has been taken to confirm the accuracy of the information presented and to describe generally accepted practices. However, the authors, editors, and publisher are not responsible for errors or omissions or for any consequences from application of the information in this book and make no warranty, expressed or implied, with respect to the currency, completeness, or accuracy of the contents of the publication. Application of the information in a particular situation remains the professional responsibility of the practitioner.

The authors, editors, and publisher have exerted every effort to ensure that drug selection and dosage set forth in this text are in accordance with current recommendations and practice at the time of publication. However, in view of ongoing research, changes in government regulations, and the constant flow of information relating to drug therapy and drug reactions, the reader is urged to check the package insert for each drug for any change in indications and dosage and for added warnings and precautions. This is particularly important when the recommended agent is a new or infrequently employed drug.

Some drugs and medical devices presented in the publication have Food and Drug Administration (FDA) clearance for limited use in restricted research settings. It is the responsibility of the health care provider to ascertain the FDA status of each drug or device planned for use in their clinical practice.

To purchase additional copies of this book, call our customer service department at (800) 638-3030 or fax orders to (301) 223-2320. International customers should call (301) 223-2300.

Visit Lippincott Williams & Wilkins on the Internet: at LWW.com. Lippincott Williams & Wilkins customer service representatives are available from 8:30 am to 6 pm, EST.

10 9 8 7 6 5 4 3 2 1

RRS1401

"When we talk about old age, each of us is talking about his or her own future. We must ask ourselves if we are willing to settle for mere survival when so much is possible." Robert Butler, 1975

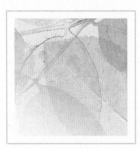

I dedicate this book to Tom, my husband, who never had a chance to grow old, and to my mentors Mary Opal Wolanin and Priscilla Ebersole, who taught me who I was and who I could become.
VB

To my wife and inspiration, Esther, for doing the nearly impossible, that of keeping me grounded while giving me wings to fly.
AK

I dedicate this book to all of my patients who gave me the opportunity to be their physician and taught me the true meaning of healing.
KYK

Rizwan Ali, MD, DFAPA
Assistant Professor
Department of Psychiatry and Behavioral
  Medicine
Virginia Tech Carilion School of Medicine
Staff Psychiatrist
Veterans Affair Medical Center
Salem, Virginia

Martha Smith Anderson, DNP, CNS, FNGNA
Associate Professor
Jefferson College of Health Sciences
Roanoke, Virginia

Adegbenga A. Bankole, MD
Rheumatology, Assistant Professor
Virginia Tech Carilion School of Medicine
Department of Internal Medicine,
  Rheumatology
Roanoke, Virginia

Azziza Bankole, MD
Assistant Professor, Virginia Tech Carilion School
  of Medicine
Assistant Program Director, Geriatric Psychiatry
  Fellowship Program Virginia Tech Carilion
  School of Medicine
Roanoke, Virginia

Jill Bass, RN, DNP, GCNS-BC
Gerontological Clinical Nurse Specialist
Carilion Clinic Center for Healthy Aging
Roanoke, Virginia

Melissa Bernstein, PhD, RD, LD
Assistant Professor, Department of Nutrition
Rosalind Franklin University of Medicine
  and Science
North Chicago, Illinois

Victoria Bierman, PhD, LCSW, FNP-BC
Psychiatric Mental Health Nurse Practitioner
  Program Coordinator
Assistant Professor of Nursing at Radford
  University, Radford, Virginia
Psychiatric Nurse Practitioner for Carilion Clinic
St. Alban's Psychiatric and Behavioral Health
  Outpatient Clinic
Christiansburg, Virginia

Soheir S. Boshra, MD, FAAFP, CMD
Program Director—Geriatric Medicine Fellowship
VTC Carilion
Associate Professor VTC Carilion School
  of Medicine
Associate Professor University of Virginia
Associate Professor Edward Vis Osteopathic School
Roanoke, Virginia

Nancy Brossoie, PhD
Senior Research Associate, Center for Gerontology
Virginia Polytechnic Institute and State University
Blacksburg, Virginia

Virginia Burggraf, RN, DNS, FAAN
Marcella J. Griggs Endowed Chair
Gerontological Nursing Coordinator Graduate
  Program
Radford University
Radford, Virginia

Lisa Campo, DNP, ANP-BC
Assistant Professor, NP Program
George Mason University
Fairfax, Virginia

Carey A. Cole, RN, FNP-BC, DNP
Family Nurse Practitioner
Adjunct Faculty, Radford University
Radford, Virginia

DeEtta Compton, DNP, FNP-BC
Carilion Clinic Cardiology
Christiansburg, Virginia

Deborah D. Cox, FNP-C
Nurse Practitioner, Center for Healthy Aging
Carilion Clinic
Roanoke, Virginia

Julia D'Amora, DO
Assistant Professor of Medicine
Virginia Tech Carilion School of Medicine
Board Certified Physician in Family Medicine and
    Geriatric Medicine
Carilion Clinic
Roanoke, Virginia

Shravan Kumar R. Gaddam, MD, CMD
Assistant Professor in Medicine VTC School of
    Medicine, VCOM
Consultant Geriatrician Carilion Roanoke
    Memorial Hospital
Medical Director of ACE Unit CRMH
Medical Director Berkshire Health & Rehabilitation
Roanoke, Virginia

Deborah T. Gold, PhD
Associate Professor, Departments of Psychiatry
    and Behavioral Sciences, Sociology, and
    Psychology and Neuroscience
Senior Fellow, Duke Center for the Study of Aging
    and Human Development
Director, Postdoctoral Research Training
    Program in Aging, the Undergraduate Human
    Development Program, and the Leadership in
    an Aging Society Program
Duke University Medical Center
Durham, North Carolina

Joni Goldwasser, RN, DNP, FNP-BC
Primary Care
Veterans Administration Medical Center
Salem, Virginia

Andrea D. Harrelson, FNP-BC
Carilion Center for Healthy Aging
Roanoke, Virginia

David W. Hartman, MD
Section Chief Adult Outpatient Department
Department of Psychiatry and Behavioral
    Medicine
Associate Professor VTC Medical School
Carilion Clinic
Roanoke, Virginia

Katie R. Katz, DNP, RN, FNP-BC
Instructor
Radford University
School of Nursing
Radford, Virginia

Bush Kavuru, MD
Section Chief, Consultation Liaison Psychiatry
Department of Psychiatry and Behavioral
    Medicine
Virginia Tech Carilion School of Medicine
Roanoke, Virginia

Kye Y. Kim, MD
Professor and Director, Academic Affairs
Department of Psychiatry and Behavioral
    Medicine
Virginia Tech Carilion School of Medicine
Roanoke, Virginia

Kathy Kleppin, BS, MS Ed
Instructional Technologist
Radford University
School of Nursing
Radford, VA

Aubrey L. Knight, MD
Associate Dean for Student Affairs
Professor of Medicine and Family & Community
    Medicine
Virginia Tech Carilion School of Medicine
Roanoke, Virginia

Eunyoung Lee, RN, PhD, ANP, ACNP,
    FAHA, FNP
Assistant Professor
Radford University
Radford, Virginia

Faye Lyons, RN, DNP-C
Dermatology Nurse Certified
Manager/Provider of The Pain Center of
  Christiansburg, Virginia
Adjunct Instructor, Jefferson College of Health
  Science
Roanoke, Virginia

Mazen Madhoun, MD
Medical Director of Springtree Health and
  Rehabilitation
Family Medicine/Geriatric Medicine
Palliative Care
Roanoke, Virginia

Marya C. McPherson, MS
Research Associate, Center for Gerontology
Virginia Polytechnic Institute and State
  University
Blacksburg, Virginia

David M. Mercer, ACNP-BC, CWOCN, CFCN
Advanced Practice Nurse 2 University of Virginia
  Health System
Department of Wound, Ostomy, and Continence
  Services
Charlottesville, Virginia

Thomas R. Milam, MD, MDiv
Associate Program Director & Assistant
  Professor
Department of Psychiatry and Behavioral
  Medicine
Virginia Tech Carilion School of Medicine and
  Research Institute
Roanoke, Virginia

Nancy Munoz, DCN, MHA, RD, LDN
Lecturer University of Massachusetts Amherst
  Nutrition Department
Instructor University of Phoenix College of
  Nursing and HealthCare Program
Clinical Nutrition Manager for Genesis
  HealthCare Corporation
Kennett Square, Pennsylvania

Karen A. Roberto, PhD
Professor & Director, Center
  for Gerontology
Director, Institute for Society, Culture &
  Environment
Virginia Polytechnic Institute & State University,
  Blacksburg, Virginia
Adjunct Professor, Departments of Internal
  Medicine and Psychiatry and Behavioral
  Medicine
Virginia Tech Carilion School
  of Medicine
Roanoke, Virginia

Susan Russell, MSN, FNP-BC
Adult and Pediatric Outpatient Department
Department of Psychiatry and Behavioral
  Medicine
Carilion Clinic
Roanoke, Virginia

Mamta Sapra, MD
Geriatric Psychiatrist
Salem Veteran Affairs Medical Center
Assistant Professor, Department
  of Psychiatry
Virginia Tech Carilion School
  of Medicine
Roanoke, Virginia

Tanya Sigmon, MPAS, PA-C
Physician Assistant
Carilion Clinic, Center for Healthy Aging
Roanoke, Virginia

Harini Singireddy, MBBS
Research Assistant
Department of Psychiatry
Carilion Clinic
Roanoke, Virginia

Margaret B. Sproule, PhD, CHES
Department of Exercise, Sport, & Health
  Education
Radford University
Radford, Virginia

Anjali Varma, MD
Staff Psychiatrist
Salem Veteran Affairs Medical Center
Assistant Professor, Virginia Tech Carilion School
  of Medicine
Roanoke, Virginia

Phyllis Brown Whitehead, PhD, MSN, BSN,
  APRN, ACHPN
Clinical Nurse Specialist
Carilion Roanoke Memorial Hospital
Roanoke, Virginia

Brent S. Williams, MD
Diplomate—American Board of Family
  Medicine
Geriatric Fellow
Carilion Clinic—Virginia Tech
Roanoke, Virginia

Christopher D. Wood, DO
Assistant Professor
Department of Internal Medicine
Virginia Tech Carilion School of Medicine
Roanoke, Virginia

This newly published book, *Healthy Aging: Principles and Clinical Practice for Clinicians*, coedited by Dr. Virginia Burggraf, Dr. Aubrey Knight, and Dr. Kye Kim, is most definitely a must-have for bookshelves, Ipads, tablets, phones, or other types of resource media! The book, written for health care providers, is relevant for advanced practice nurses, physicians, and physician assistants that provide care to older adults across any setting. It would certainly be a valuable addition to nursing staff and others in long-term care settings. The book covers an amazing array of clinical and psychosocial issues in the management of older adults and does so in a wonderfully eclectic manner. The chapters cover every imaginable issue one would anticipate when doing geriatrics, and each chapter can be read and utilized independently of the other.

The book starts with an overview of geriatrics and provides an extremely useful review of the different types of providers, education, skill set, and scope. It then addresses health promotion in older adults and moves to evaluation of the patient through physical assessment. The physical assessment chapter nicely addresses the differences between what is normal and abnormal and provides forms to help guide the clinician in the assessment process.

Following a focus on health and health promotion the chapters review systems and address normal age changes as well as the most prevalent disease states. For example, there is a chapter on cardiovascular disease and common clinical concerns such as congestive heart failure and hypertension. Up-to-date and evidence-based information on management is provided as well. Other systems reviewed include skin, with very useful pictures of common skin malignancies; gastrointestinal system, specifically common problems, including gastroesophageal reflux disease and diverticulitis; neurological diseases and prevalent problems such as stroke and Parkinson Disease; pulmonary disorders and common problems including pneumonia, influenza, and chronic obstructive pulmonary disease. Following systems, there are numerous chapters on a variety of health-related issues and problems that are common in older adults.

There is a chapter covering the nutrition needs of older adults, followed by a very practical chapter on inactivity and exercise that includes screening and motivational recommendations to engage older adults in a more active lifestyle. Exercise is followed by chapters on other disease states and clinical problems such as osteoporosis, degenerative joint disease, and associated joint problems, and pain and pain management, kidney disease, septicemia, anemia, and pressure ulcers.

Following a focus on disease, the remainder of the book addresses more of the psychosocial problems encountered in aging and in the management of older adults. There is a chapter on medication safety that reviews current guidance on this topic, the use of the Beers criteria, and other ways to look for and prevent critical errors related to medication prescribing and use in older adults. The remaining chapters cover ways in which to assess psychosocial health of older individuals, the psychosocial challenges that are encountered, with consideration here given to cultural issues and diversity, and the use and abuse of alcohol and other substances. The need for increased appreciation of drug use and abuse is stressed in light of the current and aging population and in preparation for the aging of the baby boomers. The book ends with a series of important chapters that include the assessment and management of dementia, bipolar depression, schizophrenia, depression, suicide, anxiety, and finally a chapter on end-of-life care.

One of the features I found particularly fun and exciting about this book was related to how different each chapter was. One chapter had a case study, while others included numerous tools and practical guidelines for disease assessment and management. This was a refreshing change from books in which the format stays consistent across each chapter. In addition to the text within the chapters, each chapter has an amazing section of Internet-based resources, which include webpages, videos, measures, and other relevant resources.

Kudos to the editor and numerous authors involved in the development of this resource; I strongly recommend it for all types of providers at any stage in their careers.

Barbara Resnick, PhD, CRNP, FAAN, FAANP
Professor, OSAH
Sonya Ziporkin Gershowitz Chair in Gerontology
University of Maryland School of Nursing
Baltimore, Maryland

Recently, the words *Silver Tsunami* were used in reference to the growth of older adults in the United States. The Alliance for Aging Research (http://www.agingresearch .org/contnet/article/detail/826) states that "when the aging baby boomers turned 65 in 2011, that 10,000 persons would turn 65 every day—and continue to do so for the next 20 years. By 2030, almost one out of every five Americans—some 72 million— will be 65 years or older." To health care providers these statements indicate that we had better prepare for a healthy aging society. Prevention of disease and promotion of healthy aging must be a priority in our medical nursing and professional health care programs.

This text is an outgrowth of years dedicated to teaching advanced practice nurses, residents, interns, and physician assistants and attests to a dedication to care and treatment of older adults for many years. For me it has been 34 years since I graduated as a Geriatric Nurse Practitioner. The three of us, Dr. Knight, and Dr. Kim, share a common element: We are passionate about practice in care and treatment of older adults. Twenty-nine chapters, divided into chronic illness both physical and emotional, cover only the most common illnesses of older adults. The chapters are consistent in their framework and are embedded with current treatment modalities. One cannot undertake all that is needed to educate providers in one text. Many use multiple texts in their courses. This text is our beginning into what we perceive as needed to assess and treat the multiple challenges that face our older adults.

Providers, in many disciplines, are challenged, together with their colleagues, by the complexities of care, regulation, and standards that govern practice. They practice both independently and in partnership and must emphasize evidence-based knowledge and interventions to protect the health of older adults wherever they reside: in the community, a facility, institution, and/or at home. The recent Affordable Care Act (ACA) demands that we pay more attention to the older adult in the community, keeping them on target with screenings and promoting their health. The present older adults have fond memories of the doctor showing up at their homes with his "black bag." I am one of those persons who recall that scene. I know we will soon return to that effort. Some providers are already seeing patients in their homes.

This text incorporates the holistic framework that comprises geriatric care in partnership with physicians, gerontologists, and nurses. The uniqueness of this text lies not only in these identified partnerships but also in addressing the Healthy People 2020 objectives that all practitioners must incorporate into their practice. Additionally, the editors tried to explain the varied roles, education requirements, and certifications of the varied geriatric practitioners and how we all act in tandem for the care of the older adult. Each chapter lists electronic resources specific to the content of the chapter. The electronic resources include video, text, and websites to complement and support the textbook content. In addition, there is a list of general geriatric electronic resources that cross multiple chapters and support the textbook as a whole. In the ever-changing world of technology, these added resources provide up-to-date content for both the faculty and students who use the textbook.

Virginia Burggraf, RN, DNS, FAAN
Kye Y. Kim, MD
Aubrey L. Knight, MD

Acknowledgments

One cannot begin an enormous undertaking without support from many. We would collectively like to thank Ms. Kathy Kleppin. From the inception of this idea to its ending, she was a shining star developing all the IT resources, tracking permissions, formatting, and making certain we were all on the same page. All the contributors knew who she was, although they had not personally met. Thank you, Kathy. To our multiple contributors who were professionally attacked by us to revise and submit and rewrite often: you were wonderful. To our reviewers: many thanks for your comments that perfected our work. Ashley Fischer, our Lippincott Williams & Wilkins Wolters Kluwer Health Product Manager, was a true colleague and persevered with our multiple questions. This was a true effort from the publishing perspective and would not have been realized without Ashley's untiring efforts. Thank you. Shannon Magee, the Senior Acquisitions Editor and our first contact at Wolters Kluwer, could not have been more receptive to the text, our multiple suggestions, and constant questions. Thank you for believing in us and our efforts to promote healthy aging.

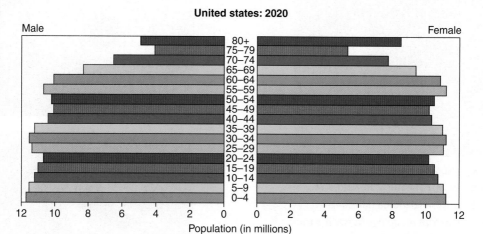

FIGURE 1.1. Population demographics. From U.S. Census Bureau, International database.

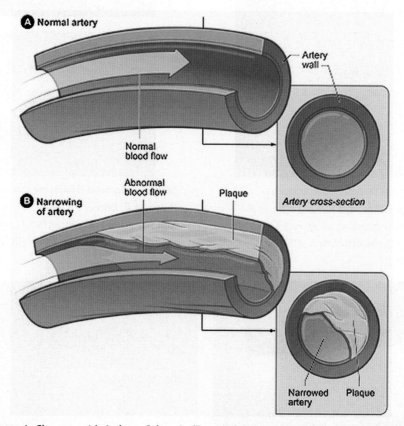

FIGURE 4.1. Anatomic Changes with Arthero-Sclerosis. (From U.S. Department of Health & Human Services. [2011, June 1]. What is atherosclerosis? Retrieved from http://www.nhlbi.nih.gov/health/health-topics/topics/atherosclerosis/)

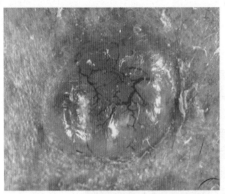

FIGURE 5.1. Nodular basal cell carcinoma. (From Nolen, M. E., Beebe, V. R., King, J. M., et al. [2011]. Nonmelanoma skin cancer: Part 1. *Journal of Dermatology Nurses Association, 3* [5], 260–281, with permission.)

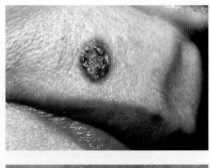

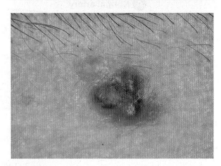

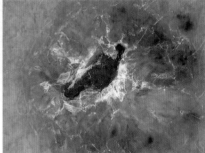

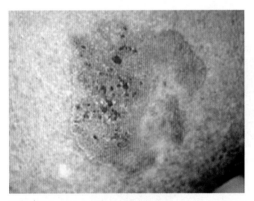

FIGURE 5.2. Superficial basal cell carcinoma. (From Nolen, M. E., Beebe, V. R., King, J. M., et al. [2011]. Nonmelanoma skin cancer: Part 1. *Journal of Dermatology Nurses Association, 3* [5], 260–281, with permission.)

FIGURE 5.3. Pigmented basal cell carcinoma. (From Nolen, M. E., Beebe, V. R., King, J. M., et al. [2011]. Nonmelanoma skin cancer: Part 1. *Journal of Dermatology Nurses Association, 3*[5], 260–281, with permission.)

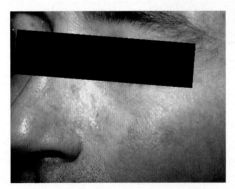

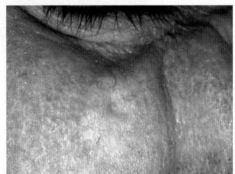

FIGURE 5.4. Morpheaform basal cell carcinoma. (From Nolen, M. E., Beebe, V. R., King, J. M., et al. [2011]. Nonmelanoma skin cancer: Part 1. *Journal of Dermatology Nurses Association, 3* [5], 260–281, with permission.)

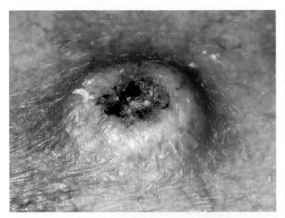
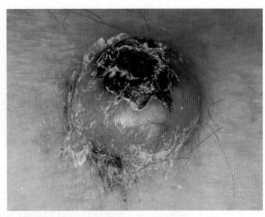

FIGURE 5.5. Keratoacanthoma. (From Nolen, M. E., Beebe, V. R., King, J. M., et al. [2011]. Nonmelanoma skin cancer: Part 1. *Journal of Dermatology Nurses Association, 3* [5], 260–281, with permission.)

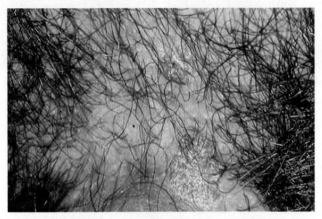

FIGURE 5.6. Bowenoid papulosis. (From Nolen, M. E., Beebe, V. R., King, J. M., et al. [2011]. Nonmelanoma skin cancer: Part 1. *Journal of Dermatology Nurses Association, 3* [5], 260–281, with permission.)

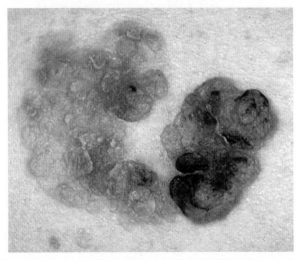

FIGURE 5.7. Squamous cell carcinoma, in situ. (From Nolen, M. E., Beebe, V. R., King, J. M., et al. [2011]. Nonmelanoma skin cancer: Part 1. *Journal of Dermatology Nurses Association, 3* [5], 260–281, with permission.)

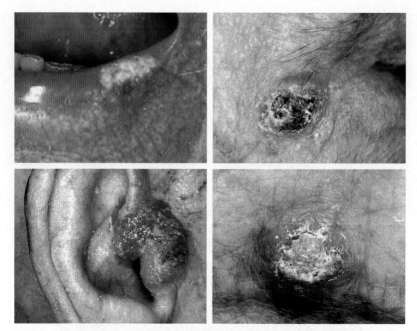

FIGURE 5.8. Squamous cell carcinoma, invasive. (From Nolen, M. E., Beebe, V. R., King, J. M., et al. Nonmelanoma skin cancer: Part 1. [2011]. *Journal of Dermatology Nurses Association, 3* [5], 260–281, with permission.)

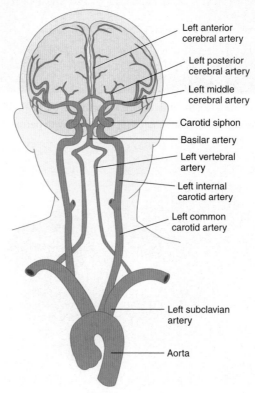

Left anterior cerebral artery

Left posterior cerebral artery

Left middle cerebral artery

Carotid siphon

Basilar artery

Left vertebral artery

Left internal carotid artery

Left common carotid artery

Left subclavian artery

Aorta

FIGURE 7.5. Circle of Willis. (From Waxman, S. G. [2009]. *Clinical neuroanatomy* [26th ed.]. New York, NY: McGraw-Hill, with permission.)

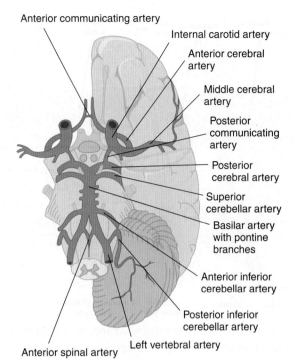

Anterior communicating artery

Internal carotid artery

Anterior cerebral artery

Middle cerebral artery

Posterior communicating artery

Posterior cerebral artery

Superior cerebellar artery

Basilar artery with pontine branches

Anterior inferior cerebellar artery

Posterior inferior cerebellar artery

Left vertebral artery

Anterior spinal artery

FIGURE 7.6. Vascular distribution of the brain. (From Waxman, S. G. [2009]. *Clinical neuroanatomy* [26th ed.]. New York, NY: McGraw-Hill, with permission.)

MyPlate for Older Adults

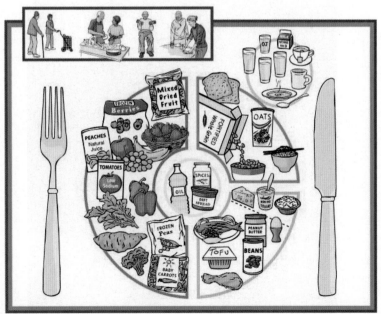

FIGURE 10.1. MyPlate for older adults. (From Tufts Now. [2011]. Tufts University nutrition scientists unveil MyPlate for older adults. Retrieved from http://now.tufts.edu/news-releases/tufts-university-nutrition-scientists-unveil-, with permission.)

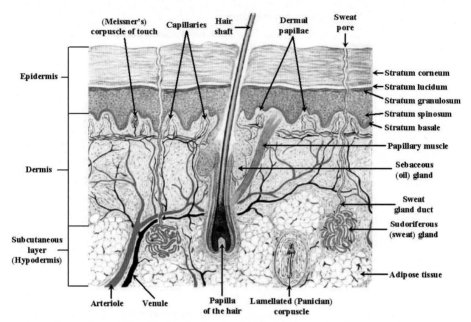

FIGURE 17.1. Basic skin anatomy of healthy intact skin. (From Lazaroff, M and Rollinson, D. The Anatomy of Hair. In: Forensics: An Online Textbook [online]. Retrieved from: http://shs2.westport.k12.ct.us/forensics/09-trace_evidence/splitting_hairs.htm#parts)

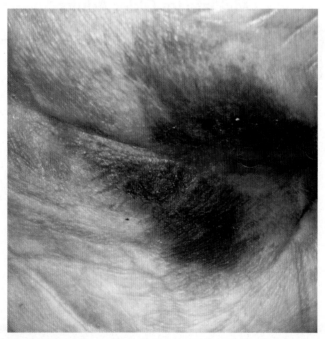

FIGURE 17.2. 85-Year-old female with prolonged immobility to sacral region. Note dark purple irregular wound indicative of deep tissue injury (bruise). (Photograph courtesy of David Mercer.)

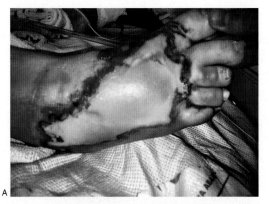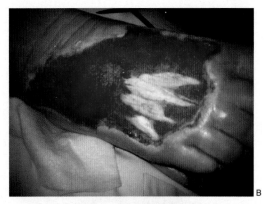

FIGURE 17.3. The debridement process. Note nonviable tissue in **(A)** prior to debridement strategy (a combination maggot biodebridement, conservative, sharp, enzymatic, and autolytic debridement used). A wound will only progress to **(B)** if and when devitalized tissue is removed. **A.** PU caused from foot pump pad in vulnerable patient. **B.** Same foot after debridement and wound healing therapies aimed at moist, clean, wound bed preparation. Healthy, robust granulation tissue with exposed tendons of foot (1 month allotted time). (Photographs courtesy of David Mercer.)

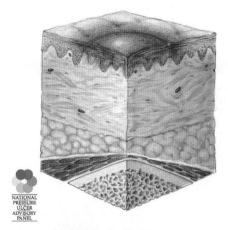

NATIONAL
PRESSURE
ULCER
ADVISORY
PANEL

TABLE 17.1. Stage I Image

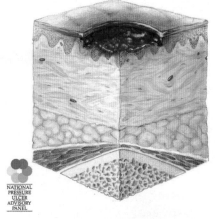

NATIONAL
PRESSURE
ULCER
ADVISORY
PANEL

TABLE 17.1. Stage II Image

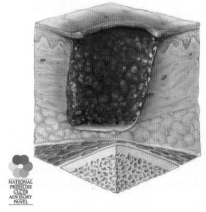

NATIONAL
PRESSURE
ULCER
ADVISORY
PANEL

TABLE 17.1. Stage III Image

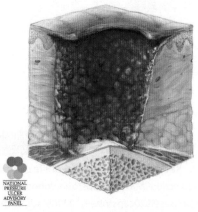

NATIONAL
PRESSURE
ULCER
ADVISORY
PANEL

TABLE 17.1. Stage IV Image

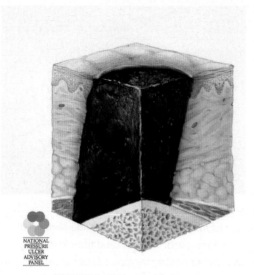

TABLE 17.1. Unstageable Image

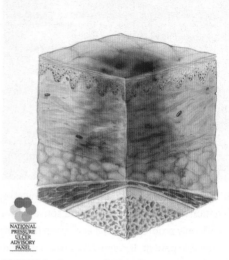

TABLE 17.1. Suspected Deep Tissue Injury Image

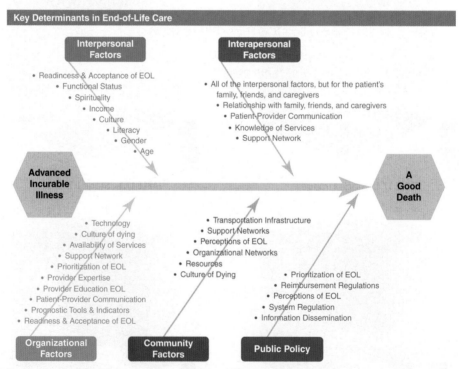

FIGURE 29.2. Key determinants in end-of-life care. (From Hess, S. G. [2009]. *Improving end-of-life care: A public health call to action* [Masters Capstone, Johns Hopkins University]. Retrieved from http://www.jhsph.edu/bin/q/n/Sally%20Hess%20capstone%202009.pdf, with permission.)

Contents

WHAT DO YOU SEE?*

What do you see, what do you see?
What are you thinking when you're looking at me?
A crabby old woman, not very wise,
Uncertain of habit, with faraway eyes.

Who dribbles her food and makes no reply
When you say in a loud voice, "I do wish you'd try?"
Who seems not to notice the things that you do,
And forever is losing a stocking or shoe.

Who, resisting or not, lets you do as you will.
With bathing and feeding, the long day to fill,
Is that what you're thinking? Is that what you see?
Then open your eyes, you're not looking at me.

I'll tell you who I am as I sit here so still,
As I use at your bidding, as I eat at your will.
I'm a small child of ten with a father and mother,
Brothers and sisters, who love one another.

A young person of sixteen, with wings on my feet,
Dreaming that soon now a lover I'll meet.
A bride/groom soon at twenty, my heart gives a leap,
Remembering the vows that I promised to keep.

At twenty-five now, I have young of my own,
Who need me to guide, and a secure happy home.
A woman/man of thirty, my young now grown fast,
Bound to each other with ties that should last.

At forty my young sons have grown and are gone,
But my spouse is beside me to see I don't mourn.
At fifty once more babies play around my knee,
Again we know children, my loved one and me.

Dark days are upon me, my spouse is now dead,
I look at the future, I shudder with dread.
For my young are all rearing young of their own,
And I think of the years and the love that I've known.

I'm now old and nature is cruel,
'Tis just to make old age look like a fool.
The body, it crumbles, grace and vigor depart,
There is now a stone where I once had a heart.

But inside this old carcass a young person still dwells,
And now and again my battered heart swells.
I remember the joys, I remember the pain,
And I'm loving and living life over again.

I think of the years, all too few, gone too fast,
And accept the stark fact that nothing can last.
So open your eyes, open and see,
Not a crabby old person, look closer—see ME!!

This was originally written for nurses and is listed as anonymous. The poem speaks to all individuals caring for older adults as well as the families we treat.

CHRONIC ILLNESS

Advanced Practice for Geriatric Clinicians

Virginia Burggraf, RN, DNS, FAAN

INTRODUCTION

The demographic realities of an aging population have been discussed for over 40 years. We hear the words "silver tsunami" and "age wave" when discussing the growing older population. The Alliance for Aging Research (2006) discusses the fact that 10,000 persons turn 65 years old every day—and will continue to do so for the next 20 years. By 2030, almost 1 out of every 5 Americans—some 72 million persons—will be 65 years or older. By 2050, the number of persons over 65 years is projected to be between 80 and 90 million, and those 85 years and older close to 21 million. A significant proportion of these individuals will suffer from chronic conditions such as heart disease, cancer, and cognitive impairment; these conditions challenge caregivers and impact their quality of life as well as impose an economic burden. Over 80% of health-care spending is for those with people with chronic health conditions; predictions are that health expenditures will skyrocket, with the expectation to reach $16 trillion by 2030 (Alliance for Aging Research, 2006) (Fig. 1.1).

A critical shortage exists in geriatrics-prepared professionals. Health Affairs (2002) discussed this shortage over a decade ago. At that time, there were 35 million persons over 65 years of age, and 23% of them were in poor or fair health, and 23% of them used authority care units, 48% of hospital days, and represented 83% of the residents in a long-term care facility. Nursing and medical schools had few facilities prepared or certified to teach in this specialty. It was agreed in this article that nurses in need for education, training, and givingback to the community are a necessity. In the year 2015, 13% of the population (46 million) will be over 65 years of age.

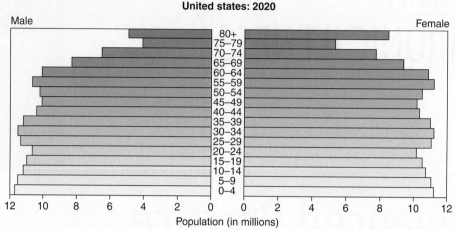

FIGURE 1.1. Population demographics. From U.S. Census Bureau, International database.

This chapter will discuss the varied clinicians who provide primary health care to older adults. It is meant to be an overview of the geriatrician, family practitioner, the physician assistant, and the advanced practice nurse. Who are these professionals, and what are their roles, educational preparation, and credentials? Accreditation of these clinicians as well as the schools they attend is a gold standard and benefits society with a reasonable assurance of quality and educational preparation for profession licensure and practice (Accreditation Review Commission on Education for the Physician Assistant [ARC-PA], 2013).

GERIATRICS

It is an exciting time to pursue a career in geriatric medicine: The Medical College of Wisconsin (n.d., http://www.mcw.edu/geriatrics/medgerresidency.htm) states the following:

- Baby boomers are here!
- Explosion of research in all subspecialties with respect to the geriatrics population;
- Anticipate public policy changes and growing public emphasis on geriatrics education;
- New government-sponsored loan repayment grants/scholarships for geriatrics practice;
- Geriatrics provides a unique niche for opportunities in medical education, research, and leadership at medical student, resident, and faculty levels.

There is a growth in geriatric education programs, but not sufficient to meet the growing need. In 2009, Weiss and Fain reported that as recently as 2006 there was only one geriatrician for every 5,000 Americans. They estimated that by 2030, as many as 36,000 geriatricians will be needed to care for the aging population.

The Accreditation Council for Graduate Medical Education (ACGME) is a private professional organization responsible for the accreditation of medical residency programs. It is the largest accrediting body in the country, if not in the world.

Geriatric Research and Education Centers (GREC) were established in 1975 by the Veterans Health Administration (VHA) to meet the needs of the aging veterans. The goals of the GRECC program are to advance scientific knowledge regarding medical, psychological, and social needs of the veterans; to develop improved and live models to provide clinical services; and to advance the quality of education in geriatrics and gerontology therapy the VHA health problem. GRECC are often affiliated with medical schools (The Association of Directors of Geriatric Programs, 2002).

A geriatrician is a physician who has completed a residency in either internal medicine or family medicine with an additional 1- or 2-year fellowship training in the medical, social, and psychological issues that concern older adults. They are Board-certified and carry a Certificate of Added Qualifications through the American Board of Medical Specialties (ABMS).

The American Geriatrics Society (AGS) is a not-for-profit organization. Practitioners and clinicians share their mission to improve the health, independence, and the quality of geriatric life of older people; and their mission—every older American will receive quality patient-centered care (American Geriatrics Society [AGS], 2013, http://www.americangeriatrics.org/about_us/life_we_are).

Geriatric Psychiatry

In 1991, the American Board of Psychiatry and Neurology (ABPN) began certifying geriatric psychiatrists, and required one year of fellowship training for certification. The purpose of the ABPN's initial certification examination is to test the qualifications of candidates in geriatric psychiatry. Geriatric psychiatry entails expertise in prevention, evaluation, diagnosis, and treatment of mental and emotional disorders in the older adults, and improvement of psychiatric care for healthy and ill older patients.

New Certification Information

- Effective January 1, 2012, ABPN will require a physician to become Board-certified within 7 years following successful completion of ACGME-accredited or ABPN-approved residency training in their primary specialty or ACGME-accredited subspecialty.
- Graduates can take the ABPN Certification Examination as many times as allowed during the 7-year period.
- Individuals who have completed an accredited residency program prior to January 1, 2012 will have until January 1, 2019 to become Board-certified.
- Individuals who do not become certified during the 7-year period (or before January 1, 2019 for those who completed residency training before January 1, 2012) will be required to (1) repeat the required clinical skills evaluations and (2) complete one stage of MOC (90 CME credits, 24 self-assessment CME credits, and 1 PIP Unit that includes a clinical and feedback module) in order to be credited to take the ABPN Certification Examination.

Specific Training Requirements

Applicants for certification in geriatric psychiatry must be certified by the Board in General Psychiatry by December 31 of the year prior to the examination. All applicants other than those initially admitted during the "grandfathering period" are required to submit documentation of successful completion of one year of ACGME-accredited fellowship training in psychiatry, including time spent in combined training programs. The exposure to geriatric psychiatry given to psychiatry residents as part of their basic psychiatry curriculum does not count toward the one year of training. All licensing and training requirements must be met by June 30 of the year of the examination.

The required one year of specialized training in geriatric psychiatry may be completed on a part-time basis as long as it is not less than 6 months; credit is not given for periods of training lasting less than one year except under special circumstances that must be approved by the ABPN Credentials Committee. In such cases, it is the responsibility of the applicant to provide detailed documentation from the respective training directors, including the exact dates (month/day/year) and outlining training content, duties, and responsibilities. Each case is considered on an individual basis (American Board of Psychiatry and Neurology [ABPN], 2013, http://www.abpn.com/cert_qp_html).

Family Practice Physician

In 2012, the Association of Directors of Geriatric Medicine reported that 21% of family physician practices consisted of ambulatory visits from adults who were 65 years and older. It projected that by 2020 at least 30% of family physicians will be in outpatient practices, 60% in hospitals, and 95% in home and home-care practices. The statistics were similar for those in internal medicine.

Family practice physicians encounter older patients with a variety of medical concerns. Geriatric programs in family medicine focus on the needs of older adults and include polypharmacy, cognitive issues, long-term care insurance, and psychosocial aspects of aging, including mistreatment. Each resident is assigned to nursing home care. The American Board of Family Medicine (ABFM) offers a Certificate of Added Qualifications (CAQ) in Geriatric Medicine. This CAQ recognizes a practice that emphasizes care of the older adult.

Certification Requirements

- Family physicians must be certified by the ABFM and must be Diplomates in good standing in order to apply and take the examination; they must maintain their primary certification with the ABFM to maintain a certification in a CAQ.
- Diplomates must hold a currently valid, full, and unrestricted license to practice medicine in the United States or Canada and be in continuous compliance with the ABFM Guidelines for Professionalism, Licensure, and Personal Conduct.
- Diplomates must satisfactorily complete an ACGME-accredited fellowship training program in Geriatric Medicine.
- Diplomates must submit an online application with appropriate application fee.
- Diplomates must achieve a satisfactory score on the one-day computer-based Geriatric Medicine Examination.

Recertification Requirements

The recertification process for Geriatric Medicine certificate may be completed in the 9th or 10th year of the certificate and includes the following requirements:

- Family physicians must be certified by the ABFM and must be Diplomates in good standing by the time of the examination.
- Diplomates must hold a currently valid, full, and unrestricted license to practice medicine in the United States or Canada and be in continuous compliance with the ABFM Guidelines for Professionalism, Licensure, and Personal Conduct.

- Diplomates must submit an online application with appropriate application fee.
- Diplomates must achieve a satisfactory score on the one-day computer-based Geriatric Medicine Examination.

Physician Assistant

A physician assistant (PA) is a person who works either at a clinic, hospital, or mental-care facility. They function under the direct supervision of a physician. In 2011, there were 151 accredited PA programs in the United States (Physician Assistant http://www.mypatraining.com Retrieved October 1, 2013). Prospective PAs must obtain formal training through an educational program approved by the ARC-PA. These programs often require applicants to have a bachelor's degree and some amount of experience in the health-care profession to gain admission. Most PAs serve as emergency medical technicians, nurses, or paramedics before pursuing admission to PA programs.

PA programs generally take 26 months' full-time study to complete. During the first year, students focus on classroom instruction in medical science and clinical preparation. Courses may include pathology, pediatrics, diagnosis, surgical technique, emergency medicine, pharmacology, and research methods. Afterward, the curriculum shifts to focus mainly on clinical rotations in various disciplines, such as general surgery, gynecology, and behavioral medicine. During these rotations, students gain first-hand experience in patient care under the supervision of licensed physicians.

PAs are required to be licensed by the state in which they practice. Along with completion of an accredited training program, the licensing process entails the passage of the Physician Assistant National Certifying Examination (PANCE, 2013). PANCE, administered by the National Commission of Certification of Physician Assistants (NCCPA), evaluates fundamental medical and surgical comprehension. Candidates who pass the PANCE may use the Physician Assistant-Certified (PA-C) designation.

PAs must maintain the PA-C designation by earning 100 continuing education credits every 2 years. They are also required to pass the Physician Assistant National Recertifying Exam every 6 years. PA-Cs are subject to recertification and testing fees.

PAs may choose to specialize in a particular field of medicine, such as internal medicine, surgery, or pediatrics. Becoming a specialist entails completion of an additional postgraduate training program and certification from the NCCPA. Candidates for specialty certification must hold a PA-C certification, have 2 years of experience, and complete a specialty certification program. They may then become certified by passing a specialty exam. Specialty certification must be renewed every 6 years.

The Advanced Practice Nurse

In July 2008, nursing's leading professional organizations, after meeting for over 4 years, reached a consensus on a model for advanced practice registered nurse (APRN) regulation. This landmark document, the collaborative work of the APRN Consensus Work Group and the National Council of State Boards of Nursing (NCSBN) APRN Committee, establishes clear expectations for licensure, accreditation, certification, and education for all APRNs. Since its completion in July 2008, 45 national nursing organizations have endorsed the Model, which can be accessed at http://www.aacn.nche.edu/education/pdf/APRNReport.pdf.

Broadly defined, regulation encompasses licensure, accreditation, certification, and education, now known as LACE. The difficult work to fully implement the Model by the targeted date of 2015 has begun, including the creation of a LACE electronic network or platform to support this work and to ensure transparent and ongoing communication among all stakeholder groups. For implementation to occur, it is imperative that each entity within LACE move forward in a timely and sequential manner. Certification organizations, state boards of nursing, and accrediting bodies have all begun to analyze what needs to be done and have begun to move forward to make these changes.

Education and certification are two of the critical components that must be addressed early in this process. The changes and impacts specifically pertaining to the redesign or expansion of APRN adult-gerontology program curricula and the APRN adult-gerontology certification examinations are outlined below. This list may not be all inclusive and may change over time as implementation moves forward.

- For graduates to meet licensure criteria by 2015, the target date for full implementation of the Consensus Model, changes in education programs and curricula must occur by 2012 to 2013.
- Changes in the certification exams will also occur by 2012 or 2013 so that graduates will be prepared to meet the eligibility criteria to sit for the new or revised certification exams by that date.
- APRN education must be formal education in a graduate degree or postgraduate certificate program.
- All new APRN programs/tracks must be preaccredited prior to admitting students. CCNE and NLNAC will be establishing or reviewing current practices to ensure that a process for preaccreditation of NP and CNS programs is in place. Nurse anesthesia and nurse-midwifery programs will continue to be preapproved or preaccredited by their respective accrediting bodies.
- All postgraduate certificate APRN programs will be accredited.
- All APRN programs must include, at a minimum, three separate comprehensive graduate-level courses (known as the APRN Core: competencies are delineated in the AACN *Essentials of Doctoral Education for Advanced Nursing Practice* or the AACN *Essentials of Master's Education for Advanced Practice Nursing*).

The three courses should be named on the transcript and are as follows:

1. Advanced physiology/pathophysiology, including general principles that *apply across the life span*;
2. Advanced health assessment, which includes assessment of all human systems, advanced assessment techniques, concepts, and approaches; and
3. Advanced pharmacology, which includes pharmacodynamics, pharmacokinetics, and pharmacotherapeutics of *all broad categories of agents*.

- All APRN education programs, in addition to the APRN Core, must prepare graduates with the nationally recognized core competencies for one of the four APRN roles and across at least one of the six population foci: across the life span, neonatal, gender-specific, pediatrics, adult-gerontology, and psychiatric/mental health (see Fig. 1.2).
- All current NP or CNS programs preparing individuals to provide care to the adult or gerontology populations, for example Adult Health CNS, Acute and Critical Care CNS-Adult, Gerontology CNS, Adult NP, Gerontology NP, and Adult Acute Care NP, must merge the programs so that graduates are prepared with the full complement of competencies necessary to provide comprehensive care to the entire adult population, which includes the young adult through the frail older adult. (See update below on JAHF-funded AACN initiative to develop separate sets of consensus-based competencies for the Adult-Gerontology NP and CNS.)
- Preparation in a specialty area of practice, for example oncology or gero-psych, is optional but if included cannot expand the individual's scope of practice and must build on and be in addition

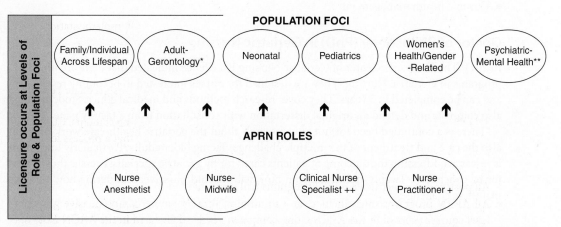

FIGURE 1.2. Consensus model for APRN regulation. (From APRN Joint Dialogue Group. [2008]. *Based on the work of the APRN Consensus Work Group and the NCSB APRN Advisory Committee*. Retrieved from http://www.aacn.nche.edu/education/pdf/APRNReport.pdf, with permission.)

to the APRN role/population-focused competencies. Clinical and didactic coursework must be comprehensive and sufficient to prepare the graduate to obtain certification for licensure in an APRN role with a specific population focus.

Presently, AACN, in collaboration with the Hartford Institute for Geriatric Nursing at New York University, developed national consensus-based competencies for the Adult-Gerontology NP and the Adult-Gerontology CNS. A validation panel of many organizations provided significant input. These competencies were distributed and can be obtained at (https://www.ncsbn.org/7_23_08_Consensue_APRN_Final.pdf).

Master of Science in Geriatric Nursing

These programs take 2 to 3 years to complete and may also be known as adult health nursing programs. Graduates may pursue advanced credentials, such as nurse practitioner certification from the American Nurse's Credentialing Center (ANCC). Common courses include the following:

- Pathophysiology
- Pharmacology
- Nursing research
- Nursing problems of older adults

Graduate Certificate in Geriatric Nursing

This program is for those who hold a master's degree in nursing and wish to become clinical nurse specialists or nurse practitioners who specialize in gerontology. Depending on the institution, its length ranges from 12 to 27 credits. Some classes may be available online. Topics include the following:

- Promoting health
- Issues in nursing the aged
- Nursing theories
- Chronic health management

Doctor of Philosophy (PhD) in Geriatric Nursing

In 2011, The Hartford's Center of Geriatric Nursing Excellence indicated that there are nine PhD programs in Geriatric Nursing. They are designed for nurses interested in becoming researchers and can be completed in 3 years. They cover research methods and medical ethics. Students must also complete and defend an original dissertation with consultation from a faculty panel.

There is a continued need for not only research about the geriatric health-care workforce but also the care and treatment of the multiple challenges facing older adults. Particularly important is research addressing the outcome of patients cared for by geriatric specialists versus those cared for by generalists. Twenty-five years from now, will we find ourselves wondering how we have met these challenges?

REFERENCES

Accreditation Council for Graduate Medical Education. (2006). Program requirements for fellowship education in internal medicine-geriatric medicine. Retrieved from http://www.acgme.org Accred . Council of Grad Med. Educ

Accreditation Review Commission on Education for the Physician Assistant, Inc. (2013). Retrieved from http://www.arc-pa.org

Alliance for Aging Research. (2006). Preparing for a silver tsunami. Retrieved from http://www.agingresearch.org/content/article/detail/826

American Association of Colleges of Nursing. (n.d.). Consensus Model. Retrieved from http://www.aacn.nche.edu/education-resources/aprn-consensus-process

American Board of Psychiatry and Neurology, Inc. (2013). Retrieved from http://www.abpn.com/

American Board of Physician Specialists. (2013). Retrieved from http://www.abpsus.org/

American Geriatrics Society. (2013). Retrieved from http://www.americangeriatrics.org

The Association of Directors of Geriatric Programs. (2002). *Geriatric medicine training and practice in the United States at the beginning of the 21st century*. Retrieved from http://www.americangeriatrics.org/files/documents/gwps/ADGAP%20Full%20Report.pdf

Hartford's Center of Geriatric Nursing Excellence. (n.d.). Retrieved from http://www.nursing.upenn.edu/cisa/Pages/HartfordCenterofGeriatricNursingExcellence.aspx

Kovner, C. T., Mezey, M., & Harrington, C. (2002). *Who cares for older adults? Workforce implications of an aging society*. Retrieved from http://content.healthaffairs.org/content/21/5/78.full

Medical College of Wisconsin. (n.d.). *Medicine-Geriatric Combined Residency Program*. Retrieved from http://www.mcw.edu/geriatrics/medgerresidency.htm

Physician Assistant: Educational requirements. (2012). Retrieved from http://education-portal.com/articles/physicians_Assistant_education_requirements.html

Physician Assistant National Certifying Examination. (2013). Retrieved from http://www.nccpa.net

Weiss, B. D., & Fain, M. (2009). Geriatric education for the physicians of tomorrow. *Archives of Gerontology and Geriatrics*, *49*(Suppl. 2), S17–S20.

Healthy People 2020: Implications for Practice

Virginia Burggraf, RN, DNS, FAAN

INTRODUCTION

Currently, the messages heard about prevention of illness and promotion of health are not new. Ben Franklin, I believe, is credited with the words that "an ounce of prevention is worth a pound of cure" (http://www.ushistory.org/franklin/quotable/singlehtml.htm). "Healthy People: The Surgeon General's Report on Health Promotion and Disease Prevention" was launched in 1979. Every decade since, the federal government has released its Healthy People program. Healthy People 2020 (HP2020) provides a comprehensive set of national goals and objectives that are designed to improve the health of all Americans. HP2020 contains 42 topic areas with nearly 600 objectives (and others still evolving) which encompasses 1,200 measures.

The goals of HP2020 are

- Attaining high-quality, longer lives, free of preventable disease, disability, injury, and premature death
- Achieving health equality, eliminating disparities, and improving health of all groups
- Creating social and physical environments that promote good health for all
- Promoting quality of life, healthy development, and healthy behaviors across the life span

HP2020 emphasizes the concept of social determinants of health—that is, the notion that health is impacted by many social, economic, and environmental factors that extend far beyond individual biology of disease. Improving health requires a broad approach to prevent disease and promote health. You can link to the updates at www.healthypeople.gov. The following information provided is from this link and in the public domain. ·

HEALTHY PEOPLE AND OLDER ADULTS

Why is HP2020 important for providers and clinicians of older adults? These words are directly from the Web site and its overview of HP and Older Adults (http://www.healthypeople.gov/2010/topoicsobjectssivesw0w0/overview.aspx?topicd=31).

Older adults are among the fastest-growing age group and the first baby boomers (adults born between 1946 and 1964) who turned 65 in 2011. More than 37 million people in this group (60%) will manage more than one chronic condition by 2030. We know that they are at high risk for chronic illnesses, including diabetes mellitus, arthritis, congestive heart failure, and dementia to name a few. Many experience hospitalizations, nursing home admissions, and low quality of care. They also lose the ability to live independently in their homes, and the strain on caregivers increases. One may ask why the health of older adults is important.

Preventative health services are valuable for maintaining the quality of life and wellness of older adults. The Patient Protection and Affordability Care Act (2010) includes many provisions related to relevant Medicare services. However, preventative services are underused, especially among certain racial and ethnic groups. Ensuring quality health care for older adults is difficult, but the Centers for Medicare and Medicaid Services (CMS) has programs designed to improve physician, hospital, and nursing home care as well as rehabilitation services and home care. Older adults use many health-care services, have complex conditions, and require professional expertise that meets their needs. Most providers receive some type of training on aging, but the percentage of those who actually specialize in this area is small. More certified specialists are needed to meet the needs of this group.

Quality of Life

The ability to complete basic daily activities may increase if illness, chronic disease, or injuries causing a decline in physical or mental abilities of older adults were prevented. These limitations make it hard for older adults to remain at home. Early prevention and physical activity can help prevent such declines. Unfortunately, less than 20% of older adults engage in physical activity, and fewer in strength training. Minority populations often have lower rates of physical activity. Most older adults wish to remain in their communities as long as possible. Unfortunately, when they acquire disabilities, there is often not enough support available to help them. States that invest in such services show lower rates of growth in long-term care expenditures. Caregivers, those informal unpaid caregivers at home, are often challenged by the constant care of their loved ones. Caregiver stress is well documented and must be considered by the clinician/provider.

Below, you will find objectives pertaining to older adults and the disease entities most commonly prevalent that this text is addressing (Table 2.1).

Older adults use many health-care services, have complex medical conditions, and require professional expertise that meets their needs. This expertise requires specialization. More certified specialists are needed. Preventive health services are valuable for maintaining the independence and quality of life of older adults. Clinical preventive services, such as routine disease screening and scheduled immunizations, are key to reducing death and disability and improving the nation's health. Yet despite the fact that these services are covered by Medicare, and many private insurers, many go without accessing clinical preventive services that can protect them

TABLE 2.1 · Healthy People 2020 Objectives—Older Adults

OA-1: Increase the proportion of older adults who use the Welcome to Medicare Benefit.

OA-2: Increase the proportion of older adults who are up to date on a core set of clinical preventive services.

OA-3: (Developmental) Increase the proportion of older adults with one or more chronic health conditions who report confidence in managing their conditions.

OA-7: Increase the proportion of the health care workforce with geriatric certification.

OA-9: (Developmental) Reduce the proportion of unpaid caregivers of older adults who report an unmet need for caregiver support services.

DH-7: (Developmental) Reduce the proportion of older adults with disabilities who use inappropriate medications.

from developing a number of serious diseases or help them treat certain health conditions before they worsen.

The HP2020 objectives are designed to promote healthy outcomes for this population. Many factors, the document discusses, affect the health, function, and quality of life of the older adult. These are individual behavioral determinants of health, the social environment of the person, and health services that are accessed. All these require a coordinated approach to care so that the older adult can manage their care, the establishment of quality measures in your practice, education of staff, and an evidence-based approach to care and treatment.

The goal is to decrease the economic burden of diabetes mellitus (DM) and improve the quality of life for all persons who have, or are at risk for, DM. Diabetes (DM) has three types: type 1, when the body cannot produce insulin; type 2, which results from a combination of resistance to the action of insulin and insufficient insulin production; and gestational diabetes, affecting pregnant women. This disease affects an estimated 27 million people in the United States and is the seventh leading cause of death. It decreases life expectancy, increases the risk of heart disease, and is the leading cause of kidney failure, lower limb amputations, and adult-onset blindness.

Many recent discoveries on the individual and societal benefits from improved diabetes management clearly indicate that prevention and treatment are to be employed. The Healthy People document emphasizes four transition points: primary prevention, testing and early diagnosis, access to care, and improved quality of care.

Evidence is emerging that diabetes is associated with additional comorbidities, including cognitive impairment, incontinence, fracture risk, and cancer risk. It is important that new public health initiatives emerge and that lifestyle changes are employed to lower the risk (Table 2.2).

The goal is to improve the health, function, and quality of life of older adults. Aging is a well-known risk factor for Alzheimer disease and other types of dementias. Among adults 65 years and older, the prevalence of this disease doubles every 5 years. Persons with a family history of Alzheimer disease are generally at risk for developing the disease. Three genes have been identified and linked to early-onset Alzheimer disease. Many individuals go undiagnosed. Early diagnosis can assist the individual and family in managing the challenges that this disease presents. The evidence has indicated appropriate medications to manage symptoms. It is also important to understand the influence of lifestyle factors on a person's risk of cognitive decline and dementia (Table 2.3).

The goal is to improve mental health through prevention and ensure access to appropriate, quality mental health services. Mental health is essential for personal well-being, family and

TABLE 2.2 · Healthy People 2020 Objectives—Diabetes

OA-4: Increase the proportion of older adults who receive Diabetes Self-Management Benefits.
D-1: Reduce the annual number of new cases of diagnosed diabetes in the population.
D-3: Reduce the diabetes death rate.
D-5: Improve glycemic control among the population with diagnosed diabetes.
D-7: Increase the proportion of the population with diagnosed diabetes whose blood pressure is under control.
D-8: Increase the proportion of persons with diagnosed diabetes who have at least an annual dental examination.
D-9: Increase the proportion of adults with diabetes who have at least an annual foot examination.
D-10: Increase the proportion of adults with diabetes who have annual dilated eye examination.
D-11: Increase the proportion of adults with diabetes who have glycosylated hemoglobin measurement at least twice a year.
D-12: Increase the proportion of persons with diagnosed diabetes who obtain an annual urinary microalbumin measurement.
D-13: Increase the proportion of adults with diabetes who perform self–blood glucose monitoring at least once daily.
D-14: Increase the proportion of persons with diagnosed diabetes who receive formal diabetes education.
D-15: Increase the proportion of persons with diabetes whose condition has been diagnosed.
D-16: Increase prevention behaviors in persons at high risk for diabetes with prediabetes.

interpersonal relationships, and the ability to contribute to community and society. Several factors have been linked to mental health, including race, ethnicity, gender, age, income level, education, sexual orientation, and geographic location. Mental health disorders are the most common causes of disability, with suicide the 11th leading cause of death in the United States. Mental health is closely allied with physical health, and plays a role in a person's ability to maintain good physical health. Mental disorders, such as depression and anxiety, affect people's ability to participate in health-promoting behaviors. In turn, problems with physical health, such as chronic diseases, can have a serious impact on mental health and decrease a person's ability to participate in treatment and recovery (Table 2.4).

One may also refer to the following two resources:

Preventing mental, emotional, and behavioral disorders among young people: progress and possibilities, by the Committee on Prevention of Mental Disorders and Substance Abuse among Children, Youth and Young Adults, National Research Council and Institute of Medicine. This book, which can be read online for free (http://www.whyy.org/news/sci20090302Mentalprepub.pdf), provides the most current evidence on preventing mental, emotional, and behavioral disorders among young people.

TABLE 2.3 · Healthy People 2020 Objectives—Dementias

DIA-1: (Developmental) Increase the proportion of persons with diagnosed Alzheimer's disease and other dementias, or their caregivers, who are aware of the diagnosis.
DIA-2: (Developmental) Reduce the proportion of preventable hospitalizations in persons with diagnosed Alzheimer disease and other dementias.

TABLE 2.4 · Healthy People 2020 Objectives—Mental Health

MHMD-1: Reduce the suicide rate.

MHMD-4: Reduce the proportion of persons who experience major depressive episodes (MDEs).

MHMD-9: Increase the proportion of adults with mental health disorders who receive treatment.

MHMD-10: Increase the proportion of persons with co-occurring substance abuse and mental disorders who receive treatment for both disorders.

MHMD-11: Increase depression screening by primary care providers.

Effective programs to treat depression in older adults: implementation strategies for community agencies (http//www.prc-han.org/docs/2008-conference-program-brochure.pdf)

The goal is to increase immunization rates and reduce preventable infectious diseases. Vaccines are among the most cost-effective prevention services. Despite the progress made, over 40,000 adults reportedly do not avail themselves of needed vaccines. Acute respiratory infections, including pneumonia and influenza, are the eighth leading cause of death in the United States. In the coming decade it is anticipated that the public health infrastructure will change. Due to the increasing immigrant demographics and threats of bioterrorism, not only providing culturally appropriate preventive measures but also anticipating environment changes need to be a priority (Table 2.5).

The goal is to reduce new cases of chronic kidney disease (CKD) and its complications, disability, death disability, and economic burden. CKD and end-stage renal disease (ESRD) are significant public health problems in the United States and major causes of suffering and poor quality of life for those afflicted. They are responsible for premature death and exact high economic prices from both the private and public sectors (Table 2.6).

The goal is to promote respiratory health through better prevention, detection, treatment, and education efforts. Asthma and chronic obstructive pulmonary disease (COPD) are significant public health burdens. Asthma has affected over 23 million people and COPD has affected 14 million according to the Centers for Disease Control and Prevention. COPD is the fourth leading cause of death in the United States, and tobacco cessation is key to preventing this disease in the future. Specific methods of detection and treatment exist that may reduce this burden and promote health in patients with these respiratory challenges. Asthma, a chronic inflammatory disease that can be episodic in nature, can be controlled by preventive treatment. Genetic factors also play a role in asthma.

TABLE 2.5 · Healthy People 2020 Objectives—Immunizations and Infectious Disease

IID-1: Reduce, eliminate, or maintain elimination of vaccine-preventable disease.

IID-3: Increase the percentage of adults who are vaccinated against pneumococcal disease.

IID-4: Reduce invasive pneumococcal infections.

IID-12: Increase the proportion of children and adults who are vaccinated annually against seasonal influenza.

IID-14: Increase the percentage of adults who are vaccinated against zoster (shingles).

TABLE 2.6 • Healthy People 2020 Objectives—Chronic Kidney Disease (CKD)

CKD-1: Reduce the proportion of the U.S. population with CKD.

CKD-2: Increase the proportion of persons with CKD who know they have impaired renal function.

CKD-4: Increase the proportion of persons with diabetes and CKD who receive recommended medical evaluation.

CKD-6: Improve cardiovascular care in persons with CKD.

CKD-9: Reduce kidney failure due to diabetes.

Many issues are emerging that affect the pulmonary system, particularly as we become more conscious of global warming, the environment, and pollutants (Table 2.7).

The goals are to improve the visual health of the nation, prevention, early detection, timely treatment, and rehabilitation and to reduce the prevalence and severity of disorders of hearing and balance, smell and taste, and voice speech and language.

Vision is an essential part of everyday life, influencing how Americans of all ages learn. The vision objectives focus on preserving sight and preventing blindness. Referral to an ophthalmologist is imperative for older adults to avoid diabetic retinopathy, glaucoma, cataract, and age-related macular degeneration. The number of older adults with eye disease is increasing and medical care is imperative. By 2020 it is predicted that the number of those blind or having low vision will be over 5 million.

Hearing/communication and other sensory processes contribute to our overall health and well-being. Protecting these processes is critically important, particularly for those whose age, race, ethnicity, gender, occupation, genetic background, and health status place them at increased risk. Combat situations will place our veterans as well as the adolescent population at risk, in the future, with noise-induced injury to the inner ear (Table 2.8).

The goal is to prevent illness and disability related to arthritis and other rheumatic conditions, osteoporosis, and chronic back conditions. There are over 100 types of arthritis, and the disease commonly occurs with other chronic conditions, such as diabetes, heart disease, and obesity. Interventions to treat pain and reduce functional limitations are important. It affects 1 in 5 adults and is a cause of functional disability.

TABLE 2.7 • Healthy People 2020 Objectives—Respiratory Diseases

IID-4: Reduce invasive pneumococcal infections.

RD-4: Reduce activity limitations among persons with current asthma.

RD-6: Increase the proportion of persons with current asthma who receive formal patient education.

RD-7: Increase the proportion of persons with current asthma who receive appropriate asthma care according to the National Asthma Education and Prevention Program (NAEPP) guidelines.

RD-9: Reduce activity limitations among adults with chronic obtrusive pulmonary disease (COPD).

RD-11: Reduce hospitalizations for COPD.

RD-13: (Developmental) Increase the proportion of adults with abnormal lung function whose underlying obstructive disease has been diagnosed.

TABLE 2.8 • Healthy People 2020 Objectives—Sensory: Vision and Hearing

V-4: Increase the proportion of adults who have a comprehensive eye examination, including dilation, within the past 2 years.
V-5: Reduce visual impairment.
V-7: Increase vision rehabilitation.
ENT-VSL-3: Increase the proportion of persons with hearing impairments who have ever used a hearing aid or assistive listening device or who have cochlear implants.
ENT-VSL-4: Increase the proportion of adults who had a hearing evaluation on schedule.
ENT-VSL-9: Increase the proportion of adults bothered by tinnitus who have seen a doctor or other health care professionals.
ENT-VSL-15.2: Reduce the proportion of adults with balance and dizziness problems who have been injured as a result of a fall for any reason in the past 12 months.

Osteoporosis is a disease marked by reduced bone strength, leading to an increased risk of fractures. It mostly affects women. The osteoporosis objectives **identify** bone mineral density as a measure of the major risk factor for fractures. Hip fracture is the most serious of osteoporosis-related fracture. Chronic back pain (CBP) is often progressive, and its cause(s) can be difficult to determine. There are many emerging issues related to these conditions: fatigue, loss of independence, anxiety and depression, and a decreased quality of life to mention only a few (Table 2.9).

The goal is to promote health and reduce chronic disease risk through the consumption of healthful diets and achievement and maintenance of healthy body weight. Good nutrition, physical activity, and a healthy body weight are essential parts of a person's overall health and well-being. Together, these can help decrease a person's risk of developing serious health conditions.

TABLE 2.9 • Healthy People 2020 Objectives—Bone and Joint

AOCBC-1: Reduce the mean level of joint pain among adults with doctor-diagnosed arthritis.
AOCBC-2: Reduce the proportion of adults with doctor-diagnosed arthritis who experience a limitation in activity due to arthritis or joint symptoms.
AOCBC-3: Reduce the proportion of adults with doctor-diagnosed arthritis who find it difficult to perform joint-related activities.
AOCBC- 4: Reduce the proportion of adults with doctor-diagnosed arthritis who have difficulty in performing two or more personal care activities, thereby preserving independence.
AOCBC-7: Increase the proportion of adults with doctor-diagnosed arthritis who receive health care provider counseling.
AOCBC-8: Increase the proportion of adults with doctor-diagnosed arthritis who have had effective, evidence-based arthritis education as an integral part of the management of their condition.
AOCBC-9: Increase the proportion of adults with chronic joint symptoms who have seen a health care provider for their symptoms.
ABOCB-10: Reduce the proportion of adults with osteoporosis.
ABOCB-11: Reduce hip fractures among older adults.

TABLE 2.10 · Healthy People 2020 Objectives—Nutrition

NWS-5: Increase the proportion of primary care physicians who regularly assess body mass index (BMI) in their adult patients.

NWS-6: Increase the proportion of physician office visits that include counseling or education related to nutrition or weight.

Most Americans, however, do not eat a healthy diet and are not physically active at levels needed to maintain proper health. As a result, there is a marked increase in obesity.

Together, a healthful diet and regular physical activity can help people achieve and maintain their appropriate weight, reduce the risk of heart disease and stroke, reduce the risk of certain forms of cancer, strengthen muscles, bones, and joints, and improve mood and energy level (Table 2.10).

The goal is to improve health, fitness, and the quality of life through daily physical activity. More than 80% of adults do not meet the guidelines for both aerobic and muscle-strengthening activities. Regular physical activity can improve the health and quality of life of Americans of all ages, regardless of the presence of chronic diseases. Physical activity for older adults can lower the risk of early death, coronary heart disease, stroke, high blood pressure, type 2 diabetes, breast and colon cancer, falls, and depression. Older adults may have additional factors that keep them from being physically active, including lack of social support, lack of transportation to facilities, fear of injury, and cost of programs (Table 2.11).

The goal is to improve cardiovascular health and quality of life through prevention, detection, and treatment of risk factors for heart attack and stroke; early identification and treatment of heart attacks and strokes; and prevention of repeat cardiovascular events.

Heart disease is the leading cause of death in the United States and stroke is the third. Together, they are the most widespread and costly health problems facing the nation. They are preventable.

The leading modifiable (controllable) risk factors for heart disease and stroke are high blood pressure, high cholesterol, cigarette smoking, diabetes, poor diet and physical activity, and overweight and obesity. The burden of these diseases is disproportionately distributed across the population and is based on age, race, gender, geographic area, and socioeconomic status (Table 2.12).

The goal is to reduce the number of new cancer cases, as well as the illness, disability, and death caused by cancer. Although significant strides have been made in the detection and treatment of all cancers, it remains the number 2 killer, second only to heart disease. The HP2020 objectives support the continued monitoring of cancer incidence, mortality, and survival to better assess the progress made toward decreasing the burden of cancer in the United States. The objectives stress

TABLE 2.11 · Healthy People 2020 Objectives—Physical Activity

OA-5: Reduce the proportion of older adults who have moderate to severe functional limitations.

OA-6: Increase the proportion of older adults with reduced physical or cognitive function who engage in light, moderate, or vigorous leisure-time physical activities.

PA-11: Increase the proportion of physician office visits that include counseling or education related to physical activity.

TABLE 2.12 • Healthy People 2020 Objectives—Cardiovascular Disease and Stroke

HDS-1: (Developmental) Increase overall cardiovascular health in the U.S. population.

HDS-2: Reduce coronary heart disease deaths.

HDS-3: Reduce stroke deaths.

HDS-5: Reduce the proportion of persons with hypertension in the population.

HDS-6: Increase the proportion of adults who have had their blood cholesterol checked within the preceding 5 years.

HDS-7: Reduce the proportion of adults with high blood cholesterol levels among adults.

HDS-10: (Developmental) Increase the proportion of adults with hypertension who meet the recommended guidelines.

HDS-11: Increase the proportion of adults with hypertension who are taking the prescribed medications to lower their blood pressure.

HDS-12: Increase the proportion of adults with hypertension whose blood pressure is under control.

HDS-13: (Developmental) Increase the proportion of adults with elevated LDL cholesterol who have been advised by a health care provider regarding cholesterol-lowering management, including lifestyle changes and, if indicated, medication.

HDS-14: (Developmental) Increase the proportion of adults with elevated LDL cholesterol who adhere to the prescribed LDL cholesterol lowering management lifestyle changes and, if indicated, medication.

HDS-15: (Developmental) Increase aspirin use as recommended among adults with no history of cardiovascular disease.

HDS-19: Increase the proportion of eligible heart attack/stroke patients who receive timely artery-opening therapy as specified by current guidelines.

HDS-22: (Developmental) Increase the proportion of adult heart attack survivors who are referred to a cardiac rehabilitation program following discharge.

HDS-23: (Developmental) Increase the proportion of adult stroke survivors who are referred to a stroke rehabilitation program at discharge.

the importance of evidence-based screening for cervical, colorectal, and breast cancer by measuring the use of screening tests identified in the U.S. Preventive Services Task Force (USPSTF) recommendations.

Many cancers are preventable by reducing risk factors such as use of tobacco products, physical inactivity and poor nutrition, obesity, ultraviolet light exposure. Screening is very effective in detecting many cancers (Table 2.13).

TABLE 2.13 • Healthy People 2020 Objectives—Cancer

C-1: Reduce the overall cancer death rate.

C-3: Reduce the female breast cancer death rate.

C-4: Reduce the death rate from cancer of the uterine cervix.

C-7: Reduce the prostate cancer death rate.

C-8: Reduce the melanoma cancer death rate.

(Continued)

TABLE 2.13 • Healthy People 2020 Objectives—Cancer *(Continued)*

C-9: Reduce invasive colorectal cancer.

C-13: Increase the proportion of cancer survivors who are living 5 years or longer after diagnosis.

C-14: (Developmental) Increase the *mental and physical health-related* quality of life of cancer survivors.

C-15: Increase the proportion of women who receive a cervical cancer screening based on the most recent guidelines.

C-16: Increase the proportion of adults who receive a colorectal cancer screening based on the most recent guidelines.

C-17: Increase the proportion of women who receive breast cancer screening based on the most recent guidelines.

C-19: (Developmental) Increase the proportion of men who have discussed with their health care provider whether or not to have a prostate-specific antigen (PSA) test to screen for prostate cancer.

C-20: Increase the proportion of persons who participate in behaviors that reduce their exposure to harmful ultraviolet (UV) irradiation and avoid sunburn.

TU-4: Increase smoking cessation attempts by adult smokers.

TU-5: Increase recent smoking cessation success by adult smokers.

TU-9: Increase tobacco screening in health care settings.

TU-10: Increase tobacco cessation counseling in health care settings.

The goal is to reduce substance abuse to protect the health, safety, and quality of life for all. Many Americans struggle with alcohol and/or substance abuse. Substance abuse refers to a set of related conditions associated with the consumption of mind- and behavior-altering substances that have negative behavioral and health outcomes. Societal attitudes and political and legal responses to the consumption of alcohol and illicit drugs make substance abuse one of the most complex public health problems.

Advances in research have led to the development of evidence-based strategies to effectively address substance abuse. The HP2020 overview of substance abuse discusses that in 2005 22 million Americans struggled with this problem and that 95% of them were unaware that a problem existed. And, many unsuccessful attempts at treatment have also been made on those who recognized their problems. Substance abuse has a major impact not only on the individual but also on the family and community (Table 2.14).

TABLE 2.14 • Healthy People 2020 Objectives—Substance Abuse

S-15: Reduce the proportion of adults who drank excessively in the previous 30 days.

S-16: Reduce average annual alcohol consumption.

S-19: Reduce the past-year nonmedical use of prescription drugs.

S-20: Decrease the number of deaths attributable to alcohol.

SUGGESTED READING

Healthy People 2020 Objectives—Older Adults References

Administration on Aging. (2009). *A profile of older Americans.* Washington, DC: U.S. Department of Health and Human Services. Retrieved from http://www.aoa.gov/aoaroot/aging_statistics/profile/2009/docs/2009profile_508.pdf

American Hospital Association; First Consulting Group. (2007). *When I'm 64: How boomers will change health care* (p. 23). Chicago, IL: American Hospital Association. Retrieved from http://www.aha.org/content/00-10/070508-boomerreport.pdf

Centers for Disease Control and Prevention. (2003). Public health and aging: Trends in aging—United States and Worldwide. *Morbidity and Mortality Weekly Report, 52*(06), 101–106. Retrieved from http://www.cdc.gov/mmwr/preview/mmwrhtml/mm5206a2.htm

Centers for Disease Control and Prevention. (2009). *Health, United States, 2009.* Hyattsville, MD: National Center for Health Statistics. Retrieved from http://www.cdc.gov/nchs/data/hus/hus09.pdf

Federal Interagency Forum on Aging-Related Statistics. (2010). *Older Americans 2010: Key indicators of well-being.* Washington, DC: U.S. Government Printing Office. Retrieved from http://www.agingstats.gov/Main_Site/Data/2010_Documents/docs/Introduction.pdf

Institute of Medicine, Committee on the Future Health Care Workforce for Older Americans. (2008). *Retooling for an aging America: Building the healthcare workforce.* Washington, DC: National Academies Press. Retrieved from http://www.iom.edu/Activities/Workforce/agingamerica.aspx

Kramarow, E., Lubitz, J., Lentzner, H., & Gorina, Y. (2007). Trends in the health of older Americans, 1970–2005. *Health Affairs, 26*(5), 1417–1425. Retrieved from http://www.content.healthaffairs.org/content/26/5/1417.full

U. S. Department of Health and Human Services, Centers for Medicare & Medicaid Services. (n.d.). *Medicare claims data.* Baltimore, MD: Author. Retrieved from http://www.hhs.gov/open/contacts/cms.html

Healthy People 2020 Objectives—Diabetes References

Centers for Disease Control and Prevention. (2011). *National diabetes fact sheet: National estimates and general information on diabetes and prediabetes in the United States.* Atlanta, GA: Author. Retrieved from http://www.cdc.gov/diabetes/pubs/factsheet11.htm

Knowler, W. C., Fowler, S. E., Hamman, R. F., Christophi, C. A., Hoffman, H. J., Brenneman, A. T., & Nathan, D. M. (2009). Ten-year follow-up of diabetes incidence and weight loss in the diabetes prevention program outcomes study. *Lancet, 374*(9702), 1677–1686. Retrieved from www.thelancet.com/journals/lancet/article/PIIS0140-6736(09)61457-4/abstract

Healthy People 2020 Objectives—Dementias References

Centers for Disease Control and Prevention. (n.d.). Surveillance: Impact of cognitive impairment module—Behavioral Risk Factor Surveillance System (BRFSS). Retrieved from http://www.cdc.gov/aging/healthybrain/surveillance.htm

Healthy People 2020 Objectives—Mental Health References

Lando, J., Williams, S. M., Sturgis, S., & Williams, B. (2006). A logic model for the integration of mental health into chronic disease prevention and health promotion. *Preventing Chronic Disease, 3*(2), A61. Retrieved from http://www.ncbi.nlm.nih.gov/pmc/articles/PMC1563949/

National Institutes of Health, National Institute of Mental Health (2008). *National Institute of Mental Health Strategic Plan.* Bethesda, MD: Author. Retrieved from http://www.nimh.nih.gov/about/strategic-planning-reports/index.shtml

Healthy People 2020 Objectives—Immunizations and Infectious Disease References

Centers for Disease Control and Prevention. (1999). Achievements in public health, 1900–1999: Control of infectious diseases. *Morbidity and Mortality Weekly Report, 48*(29), 621–629. Retrieved from www.cdc.gov/mmwr/preview/mmwrhtml/mm4829a1.htm

Healthcare IT News. (2013, January 9). *NQF OKs 14 infectious disease measures.* Retrieved from http://www.healthcareitnews.com/news/nqf-oks-14-infectious-disease-measures

Healthy People 2020 Objectives—Chronic Kidney Disease (CKD) References

Barnett, A. (2006). Prevention of loss of renal function over time in patients with diabetic nephropathy. Review. *The American Journal of Medicine, 119*(5A), S40–S47. Retrieved from http://w3.csmu.edu.tw/~chr/PDF/int2006%20prevention%20of%20loss%20of%20renal%20function%20in%20DM%20Nephropathy_AJM.pdf

Peralta, C. A., Kurella, M., Lo, J. C., & Chertow, G. M. (2006). The metabolic syndrome and chronic kidney disease. *Current Opinion in Nephrology and Hypertension, 15*(4), 361–365. Retrieved from http://www.ncbi.nlm.nih.gov/pubmed/16775449

Ravera, M., Re, M., Deferrari, L., Vettoretti, S., & Deferrari, G. (2006). Importance of blood pressure control in chronic kidney disease. *Journal of the American Society of Nephrology,* 17(4 Suppl. 2), S98–S103. Retrieved from http://jasn.asnjournals.org/content/17/4_suppl_2/S98.full.pdf+html

U.S. Renal Data System. (2012). *2012 USRDS Annual Data Report: Atlas of end-stage renal disease in the United States.* Bethesda, MD: National Institutes of Health, National Institute of Diabetes, and Digestive and Kidney Diseases. Retrieved from http://www.usrds.org/atlas.aspx

Healthy People 2020 Objectives—Respiratory Diseases References

National Institutes of Health, National Heart, Lung, and Blood Institute. (n.d.). *National Asthma Education and Prevention Program.* Retrieved from http://www.nhlbi.nih.gov/about/naepp/

National Institutes of Health, National Heart, Lung, and Blood Institute. (2007). *Guidelines for the diagnosis and management of Asthma (EPR-3).* Bethesda, MD: Author. Retrieved from http://www.nhlbi.nih.gov/guidelines/asthma/

Healthy People 2020 Objectives—Sensory: Vision and Hearing References

National Institutes of Health, National Institute on Deafness and Other Communication Disorders. (n.d.). *Statistics on voice, speech, and language* [Fact sheet]. Bethesda, MD: Author. Retrieved from http://www.nidcd.nih.gov/health/statistics/pages/vsl.aspx

Alliance for Aging Research. (n.d.). *The silver book: Vision loss.* Washington, DC: Author. Retrieved from http://www.silverbook.org/visionloss

Healthy People 2020 Objectives—Bone and Joint References

Arthritis Foundation, Association of State and Territorial Health Officials, & Centers for Disease Control and Prevention. (1999). *National arthritis action plan: A public health strategy.* Atlanta, GA: Arthritis Foundation. Retrieved from http://www.arthritis.org/files/images/Delia/NAAP_full_plan.pdf

Hootman, J. M., & Helmick, C. G. (2006). Projections of U.S. prevalence of arthritis and associated activity limitations. *Arthritis and Rheumatism, 54*(1), 226–229. Retrieved from http://www.ncbi.nlm.nih.gov/pubmed/16385518

Martin, B. I., Turner, J. A., Mirza, S. K., Lee, M. J., Comstock, B. A., & Deyo, R. A. (2009). Trends in health care expenditures, utilization, and health status among us adults with spine problems, 1997–2006. *Spine, 34*(19), 2077–2084. Retrieved from http://www.ncbi.nlm.nih.gov/pubmed/19675510

U.S. Department of Health and Human Services, Public Health Service, Office of the Surgeon General. (2004). *Bone health and osteoporosis: A report of the surgeon general.* Rockville, MD: U.S. Government Printing Office. Retrieved from http://www.surgeongeneral.gov/library/reports/bonehealth/

Healthy People 2020 Objectives—Nutrition References

Institute of Medicine. (2004). *Dietary reference intakes for water, potassium, sodium, chloride, and sulfate* (1st ed.). Washington, DC: National Academies Press. Retrieved from http://www.iom.edu/Reports/2004/Dietary-Reference-Intakes-Water-Potassium-Sodium-Chloride-and-Sulfate.aspx

Healthy People. (n.d.). Nutrition and weight status. Retrieved from http://www.healthypeople.gov/2020/topicsobjectives2020/overview.aspx?topicid=29

Healthy People. (n.d.). Nutrition, physical activity, and obesity. Retrieved from http://www.healthypeople.gov/2020/LHI/nutrition.aspx and http://www.cdc.gov/healthyyouth/npao/index.htm

Healthy People 2020 Objectives—Physical Activity References

Belza, B., Walwich, J., Shiu-Thornton, S., Schwartz, S., Taylor, M., & LoGerfo, J. (2004). Older adult perspectives on physical activity and exercise: Voice from multiple cultures. *Preventing Chronic Disease, 1*(4), A09. Retrieved from http://www.cdc.gov/pcd/issues/2004/oct/04_0028.htm

Centers for Disease Control and Prevention. (2004). Strength training among adults age > 65 years—United States, 2001. *Morbidity and Mortality Weekly Report, 53*(2), 25–28. Retrieved from http://www.cdc.gov/mmwr/preview/mmwrhtml/mm5302a1.htm

Hornbrook, M. C., Stevens, V. J., Wingfield, D. J., Hollins, J. F., Greenlick, M. R., & Ory, M. G. (1994). Preventing falls among community-dwelling older persons: Results from a randomized trial. *Gerontologist, 34*(1), 16–23. Retrieved from http://www.ncbi.nlm.nih.gov/pubmed/8150304

Healthy People. (n.d.). Physical activity. Retrieved from http://healthypeople.gov/2020/topicsobjectives2020/overview.aspx?topicid=33

U.S. Department of Health and Human Services, Office of Disease Prevention and Health Promotion. (2008). *2008 Physical activity guidelines for Americans.* Washington, DC: Author. Retrieved from http://www.health.gov/paguidelines/

Healthy People 2020 Objectives—Cardiovascular Disease and Stroke References

Agency for Healthcare Research and Quality, U.S. Preventive Services Task Force. (2009). *Aspirin for the prevention of cardiovascular disease.* Retrieved from http://www.uspreventiveservicestaskforce.org/uspstf/uspsasmi.htm

Lloyd-Jones, D., Adams, R. J., Brown, T. M., Carnethon, M., Dai, S., De Simone, G., ... Wylie-Rosett, J. (2010). Heart disease and stroke statistics—2010 update: A report from the American Heart Association Statistics. *Circulation, 121*(7), e46–e215. Retrieved from http://www.ncbi.nlm.nih.gov/pubmed/20019324

Healthy People 2020 Objectives—Cancer References

Danaei, G., Ding, E., Mozaffarian, D., Taylor, B., Rehm, J., Murray, C. J., & Ezzati, M. (2009). The preventable causes of death in the United States: Comparative risk assessment of dietary, lifestyle, and metabolic risk factors. *PLoS Medicine, 6*(4), e1000058. Retrieved from http://www.plosmedicine.org/article/info:doi/10.1371/journal.pmed.1000058

Edwards, B. K., Ward, E., Kohler, B. A., Eheman, C., Zauber, A. G., Anderson, R. N., ... Ries, L. A. (2010). Annual report to the nation on the status of cancer 1975–2006 featuring colorectal cancer trends and impact of interventions to reduce future rates. *Cancer, 116*(3), 544–573. Retrieved from http://www.ncbi.nlm.nih.gov/pubmed/19998273

Innovations Exchange Team. (2013). *Trends in cancer screening: A conversation with two cancer researchers.* Rockville, MD: Agency for Healthcare Research and Quality. Retrieved from http://innovations.ahrq.gov/content.aspx?id=3816

Schueler, K. M., Chu, P. W., & Smith-Bindman, R. (2008). Factors associated with mammography utilization: A systematic quantitative review of the literature. *Journal of Women's Health, 17*(9), 1477–1498. Retrieved from http://www.ncbi.nlm.nih.gov/pubmed/18954237

Danaei, G., Ding, E., Mozaffarian, D., Taylor, B., Rehm, J., Murray, C. J., & Ezzati, M. (2009). The preventable causes of death in the United States: *Comparative risk assessment of dietary lifestyle, and metabolic risk factors.* Retrieved from http://www.ncbi.nlm.nih.gov/pubmed/19399161

Healthy People 2020 Objectives—Substance Abuse References

National Institutes of Health, National Institute on Drug Abuse. (2008). *Prescription drug abuse.* Bethesda, MD: Author. Retrieved from http://www.drugabuse.gov/publications/topics-in-brief/prescription-drug-abuse

U.S. Department of Health and Human Services, Office of Disease Prevention and Health Promotion. (2006). *Healthy People 2010 Midcourse Review: Focus Area 26, substance abuse.* Washington, DC: Author. Retrieved from http://www.healthypeople.gov/2020/topicsobjectives2020/overview.aspx?topicid=40

Comprehensive Geriatric Assessment

Lisa Campo, DNP, ANP-BC

INTRODUCTION

When you think of an older person, it brings to mind a window, a systemic window. Burggraf (1993) wrote these words, in an article of the same title, two decades ago, and they are worth repeating as we begin this chapter on comprehensive assessment. "A window is an opening in the wall of a building that can admit light: it also can be and sometimes admits air. A window allows one to see in as well as out" (Burggraf, 1993). More recently, American astronauts have referred to a "window" when entering space, giving one the impression that a window can be a "transparent patch." When we observe an older person, what type of window do we find? Are we observing objectively? After many years of life, there may be some cloudiness and cracks—which are in the form of multiple chronic illnesses and a fragility of body, mind, and spirit. Does one value an antique glass or discard it? Do we raise this question when considering the older adult? The concept of aging being a systemic window begins for providers when they initially encounter the older patient. On the initial inspection, the lines on the face and body provide a window that gives multiple answers to questions frequently not asked. Rough-looking skin and knobby joints tell us about the years of environmental hazards and possible pain. Varicosities may reveal to us information about former occupations, pregnancies, and lifestyle. The coarse skin of a lifelong smoker, the sun exposure of a farmer, or the calloused hands of a laborer all reveal years of hard work and survival. These are simple details to investigate; however, they are often the questions that are never asked. Breathing patterns, pursed lips, skin blushing, cyanosis, or pallor may indicate the values that will show up when taking vital signs, drawing blood for a hematocrit or hemoglobin, or listening for heart sounds. Dilated veins; whiskey nose; the inspection of gait alone, with walker, cane, or wheelchair; dress; and communication patterns further open the window to reveal patterns of coping. Diminished senses, tone of voice, weak handshake, and the patient's affect speak to us about the functional capacity of this older person to accept the future. This window appears within the first 5 minutes of contact with the provider. We immediately assess and make a judgment that will determine whether the window will remain transparent or become cloudier with inappropriate treatment, medications, lack of social support, education, and follow-up. Integrating these signs is the key to assessment of the older person. The following are factors to think about when assessing older persons: What does he or she look like? Appearance and grooming provide information about their self-image and life satisfaction. Is the older person accompanied by others and/or frequent visitors who are helpful, concerned, and/or stressed by a caregiving situation? This information is important to discern when preparing a discharge or follow-up plan of care. Does the older person have a positive or negative attitude toward the future? Unresolved problems are frequently manifested by anger and hostility. The grief of loss is frequently reflected in a depressed face or a desire to be left alone. Be alert to the need for consultation with professionals from other disciplines to clear the window. Does the older person make his or her own decisions regarding treatment? Loss of control over decision making is something we all fear. The desire to survive may mean undergoing an amputation or bypass; this decision requires time to reorder thinking and consider their future body image. Control and power over one's future and how one will lead it must be an informed decision. Control may be as simple as deciding the menu of the day or when to take medications. Decision making is important in maintaining some individual control, self-image, and self-worth. Is medication administration assessed in a thorough manner, whether the older person is in an acute care, outpatient, or institutional setting? Polypharmacy clouds the window to a point of fragility, incoherence, and diminished stamina and threatens survival. The window may be further clouded if the person believes that he or she is capable of self-medication yet seems to need additional guidance. This may impact adherence to medication regimen. Are the lines of communication kept open? Listen carefully when making decisions with patients and their families. Take these concepts into consideration as you begin your assessment.

Assessment of patients over the age of 65 differs significantly from a standard annual medical evaluation of a younger patient (Rosen & Reuben, 2011). It is currently estimated that approximately 50% of Americans over 65 live with two or more chronic diseases, and 80% with one or more (Centers for Disease Control and Prevention & The Merck Company Foundation, 2007). The goals of the assessment of a patient over the age of 65 emphasize the functional status and quality of life, as well as concentrating on the prognosis and outcome of illnesses. Often, your assessment uncovers multiple chronic complaints that decrease the quality of life and functional status (Centers for Disease Control and Prevention & The Merck Company Foundation, 2007). Identifying these issues early and intervening may allow for patients to have a longer quality of life even if the illness cannot be cured. Assessment of risk for illness and disease should also be considered to promote health and the quality of life of the individual. By the year 2049, it is expected that the number of Americans whose functional ability has been affected by chronic disease will rise by 300% (Kass-Bartelmes, 2002). These chronic medical conditions along with potential functional, cognitive, and/or sensory impairments create unique needs and health issues for the geriatric patient.

When working with a geriatric patient, care must be taken to recognize that many older patients with a common illness will present in atypical fashion (Fig. 3.1). Advanced practice

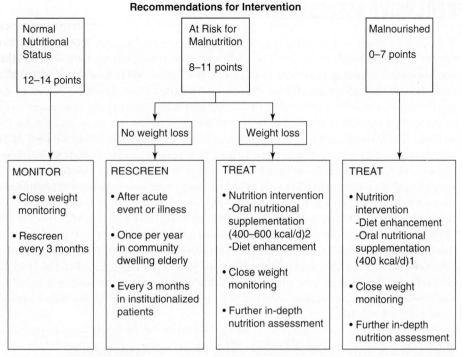

Recommendations for Intervention

| Normal Nutritional Status 12–14 points | At Risk for Malnutrition 8–11 points | Malnourished 0–7 points |

No weight loss   Weight loss

MONITOR

- Close weight monitoring
- Rescreen every 3 months

RESCREEN

- After acute event or illness
- Once per year in community dwelling elderly
- Every 3 months in institutionalized patients

TREAT

- Nutrition intervention
  -Oral nutritional supplementation (400–600 kcal/d)2
  -Diet enhancement
- Close weight monitoring
- Further in-depth nutrition assessment

TREAT

- Nutrition intervention
  -Diet enhancement
  -Oral nutritional supplementation (400 kcal/d)1
- Close weight monitoring
- Further in-depth nutrition assessment

(Gabriballa & Powers, 2006)

FIGURE 3.1. Recommendations for intervention. (From Gariballa, F., & Powers, W. (2006). The benefits of nutritional supplements in hospitalized older adults. *American Journal of Medicine*, 693–699.)

nurses must be aware of these atypical symptoms and be ready to evaluate patients presenting in this unusual way; for example, a patient with pneumonia who presents without fever and cough, but instead with confusion, anorexia, and malaise (Besdine, 2009) (Table 3.1).

TABLE 3.1 · Examples of Atypical Illness Presentation in Elderly Patients

Illness	Presentation in the Elderly
Pneumonia	Malaise, anorexia, confusion, may have tachycardia and tachypnea, fever usually absent, coughing mild without much sputum
MI	Diaphoresis, dyspnea, epigastric distress, syncope, weakness, vomiting or confusion instead of chest pain
UTIs	Dizziness, confusion, anorexia, falls, fatigue, weakness
Bacteremia	Low-grade temperature, general malaise, anorexia, unexplained mental status change
Acute abdomen	Acute confusion, usually abdominal pain absent

From Besdine, R. (2009). *Merck manual of geriatrics*. Retrieved from Merck Manual Web site: http://www.merckmanuals.com/professional/geriatrics/approach_to_the_geriatric_patient/unusual_presentations_of_illness_in_the_elderly.html

COMPREHENSIVE ASSESSMENT

A multidisciplinary comprehensive geriatric assessment utilizes many tools to assess not only a patient's physical health issues but also their cognitive, functional, spiritual and mental health, and socioenvironmental circumstances (Elsawy & Higgins, 2011; Rosen & Reuben, 2011). The tools that are utilized specifically for each part of the assessment should be chosen by considering the knowledge level and comfort of the provider administering the assessment tool, as well as the appropriateness of the tool according to the clinical site, resources, and patient (Rosen & Reuben, 2011). Many tools may be reprinted and used without permission and fees, while others may be expensive for a practice or clinic to purchase. Ease of use for patients who are cognitively impaired as well as concerns for time in a busy office or clinic must also be considered. Allowing enough time for a comprehensive visit to be completed over more than one appointment may be necessary. A specific area may be targeted for assessment at different visits. For example, functional assessment could be completed at one visit and cognitive assessment at another (Elsawy & Higgins, 2011). Including members of a multidisciplinary team such as Physicians, Specialists, Advanced Practice Nurses, Physician Assistants, Registered Nurses, Physical Therapists, Occupational Therapists, Pharmacists, Social Workers, Registered Dieticians, Psychologists, Spiritual Leaders, and family members can provide valuable information as well as a more complete assessment for the older patient with the potential of more comorbidities and chronic diseases (Rosen & Reuben, 2011).

Taking a Comprehensive History and Physical Assessment

Health History

A detailed medical and surgical history should be completed to identify inactive and active medical problems as well as risks for potential medical issues. Family history, allergies, and vaccination history should be included as well as a detailed social history that includes occupation information, marital status, alcohol intake, smoking, and current living arrangements. Establishing whether the older patient is currently sexually active, number of sexual partners, sex of partners, and safe sex practices should be sensitively evaluated in order to assess the need for information regarding safe sex education and additional screening exams (Besdine, 2009). Evaluation of current medications should include an inventory of all over-the-counter and prescription medications brought to each visit by the patient in a bag. Identification of the purpose of each drug with the patient may help to reduce unnecessary medications and assist with reducing potential negative effects of polypharmacy (Hajjar et al., 2007). "The 2012 Beers criteria for potentially inappropriate medication use in older adults" (American Geriatric Society, 2012) should be consulted for medications that may cause adverse side effects. Patients may be asked to complete health history forms as well as some screening forms prior to their visit, or while they are waiting for the provider in the office. Review of systems should include special attention to geriatric concerns such as falls, sensory or motor changes, depression, incontinence, and nutrition. Many patients consider falls, change in hearing, and incontinence a normal part of aging and fail to mention them to their health-care provider (Rosen & Reuben, 2011). It is best to allow the patient to give their own history privately with the provider. This can help to develop a rapport with the patient and allow for the clinician to evaluate many verbal and nonverbal clues for mental status and depression. The provider should ask for the patient's permission prior to asking a caregiver or relative to join the interview (Besdine, 2009).

The Physical Exam

As a part of the assessment, a patient's height and weight must be recorded along with vital signs. Geriatric patients are more prone to orthostatic hypotension and may require orthostatic hypotension blood pressure checks. Observation of the patient's hygiene, general appearance, eye contact, and gait as they enter the exam room will give the examiner valuable information (Besdine, 2009).

When completing a physical assessment, the clinician must use caution to evaluate for normal aging changes as well as abnormal findings that are not attributed to the aging process. Other concerns are issues of disuse or lack of use, which may be able to be improved with therapy and exercise versus active disease. Many times these can be difficult to distinguish, and tools that will be discussed later in the chapter can help with this evaluation. Table 3.2 identifies red flags or abnormal findings on physical exam that require immediate evaluation, which should be identified immediately so as not to delay treatment.

TABLE 3.2 · Identification of Normal versus Abnormal Assessment

Body System	Normal Changes with Aging	Abnormal Findings on Exam	Red Flags on Exam
Skin	Ecchymosis occur more easily as dermis thins, nails become more brittle and dry, skin may be more dry	Tissue ischemia, pressure ulcers, unexplained bruises	Malignant or premalignant lesions
Eyes	Entropion, ectropion, arcus senilis, loss of orbital fat causing gradual sinking of eye back into orbit, presbyopia develops with age	Cataracts, narrowing field of vision, visual changes; although presbyopia occurs with age, it warrants a further evaluation for treatment	Sudden visual changes, loss of vision, or severe pain in the eye
Ears	Presbycusis—gradual bilateral symmetrical predominately high-frequency hearing loss	Sudden severe hearing loss, ringing in the ears, pain in the ears; note that ears need to be assessed for cerumen impaction	
Mouth	Teeth may become stained, mouth becomes more dry	Bad breath usually indicates underlying disorder from dental caries to periodontitis. Bleeding gums, oral thrush, pain in the mouth	
Neck	May be less flexible	Carotid bruit, palpable thyroid, lymphadenopathy	
Pulmonary	Bibasilar rales may be heard in absence of disease but should clear with a few deep breaths	Rales that do not clear, wheezing, absence of breath sounds, decreased breath sounds, shortness of breath, tachypnea	Absence of breath sounds in a lobe
Cardiac	Fourth heart sound is common	Diastolic murmurs and new systolic murmurs that have not yet been evaluated, arrhythmias, irregular heartbeats, hypertension, hypotension	Chest pain, new-onset arrhythmia

(Continued)

TABLE 3.2 · Identification of Normal versus Abnormal Assessment *(Continued)*

Body System	Normal Changes with Aging	Abnormal Findings on Exam	Red Flags on Exam
GI	Normal aorta may be palpable, weak abdominal muscles	Pain, palpable masses, enlargement of organs, positive fecal occult blood testing	Pulsatile mass on exam may indicate abdominal aortic aneurysm
Male reproductive system		Nodules tenderness and enlargement of prostate, urinary incontinence	
Female reproductive system	Atrophy of vaginal mucosa	Palpable ovaries, prolapse of uterus, vagina, urinary incontinence	
Musculoskeletal system	Decreased range of motion, gait may be slightly slower; typically aging should have little effect on walking unless disorder present	Joint deformities, pain, crepitus—warmth, redness, swelling	
Neurologic	Results should be similar to any other adult[a] Information processing may be slightly slower but should be unchanged	Pathologic reflexes, numbness in extremities or decreased sensation, change in mental status	

[a]Must consider other issues, for example, hearing deficits or visual loss, which may affect findings.

From Besdine, R. (2009). *Merck manual of geriatrics*. Retrieved from Merck Manual: http://www.merckmanuals.com/professional/geriatrics/approach_to_the_geriatric_patient/evaluation_of_the_elderly_patient.html

SCREENING AND PREVENTIVE CARE RECOMMENDATIONS FOR THE GERIATRIC PATIENT

When considering screening recommendations for the geriatric patient, the patient's life expectancy, comorbid conditions, as well as functional status must be considered (Spalding & Sebasta, 2008). According to the 2010 Centers for Disease Control (CDC) National Vital Statistic System, the leading cause of death for people aged 65 and over in the United States is heart disease, and the second is malignant neoplasms (Centers for Disease Control and Prevention, National Vital Statistics System, 2010). These statistics must be considered when prioritizing screening exams for older adults. A patient may not receive the complete benefit from a cancer screening unless they will live for 5 years after the screening (Spalding & Sebasta, 2008).

The goal of preventive care screening exams is not only to prevent disease but also to promote successful healthful aging. However, many evidence-based prevention guidelines are limited for older adults since the older adult is not included in many clinical trials (Bluestein, 2005). With this in mind, The U.S. Preventive Services Task Force (USPSTF, 2010–2011) recommends smoking cessation counseling for patients at any age. Quitting smoking at the age of 65 can add 2 years to a man's and 3.7 years to a woman's life expectancy (Taylor et al., 2002). The USPSTF

(2010–2012) also recommends that all females 65 years and older be screened for osteoporosis using bone density testing. All men who have ever smoked should be screened for an abdominal aortic aneurysm by ultrasound between the age of 65 and 75 (Spalding & Sebasta, 2008). The CDC recommends that patients over the age of 65 should be given an influenza vaccine annually, a pneumococcal vaccine once after age 65, zoster vaccine once after age 60 (regardless of previous herpes zoster or chickenpox infection history), and Tetanus diphtheria (Td) every 10 years with one dose of Tetanus, diphtheria, and pertussis (Tdap) for any adult who has not had at least one dose of pertussis (Centers for Disease Control and Prevention, 2011).

Both visual and hearing impairment can have a major impact on the quality of life of an older individual. The accuracy of the Snellen exam and a fundoscopic exam, which are both commonly used in primary care to diagnose visual impairment in older adults, have been questioned (Chou et al., 2009). The USPSTF (2010–2011) recommends periodic complete visual eye examinations for asymptomatic patients over the age of 65 with an eye specialist (Bluestein, 2005). Patients who report hearing loss should be referred to an audiologist for hearing evaluation. Hearing should be assessed during each periodic health exam beginning at age 60. The patient's medications should be reviewed for the presence of any ototoxic medications. Many older adults consider hearing loss a normal part of aging or may not recognize a gradual change in their hearing. Patients should be asked if they have any difficulty hearing and then screened using the Whisper Test. The Whisper Test is performed by whispering a series of at least two different combinations of numbers or letters from 2 ft behind the patient while they are occluding one ear. The test is then repeated on the other side. If the patient is able to repeat three of the six items, they pass the test. Prior to referring a patient on for further evaluation to a specialist, the clinician should examine the ear canal and tympanic membrane carefully for abnormality or obstruction such as cerumen (Walling & Dickson, 2012).

Cancer screening recommendations for patients over the age of 65 vary according to different agencies. Mammography is recommended by the American Geriatrics Society annually or biannually until age 75 and then every 2 years in women with a life expectancy of four or more years. (Bluestein, 2005). The American Cancer Society recommends beginning annual mammography at age 40 and continuing for as long as the patient is in good health (Smith et al., 2012), while the USPSTF (2010–2011) recommends biennial mammography from age 50 to 74. Recommendations regarding prostate, cervical, and colon cancers also differ by agency. Table 3.3 summarizes these recommendations.

Cognitive Screening

The demographic realities of an increasing aging population demands that clinicians screen patients for cognitive impairment in all settings. The rapid growth of the population brings an increase in the incidence of Alzheimer disease and dementia. Unfortunately, many older adults with cognitive impairment are not identified by their primary care provider. The early presentation of mild cognitive impairment may be missed during their brief encounter with their healthcare providers, as the patient may present in a pleasant cooperative manner and is able to follow instructions (Finkel, 2003). While numerous methods and tools to screen for dementia are currently available, the differences between the tools are the length of time they take to administer, cost, need for special equipment or props, ease of scoring, and their sensitivity and specificity for cognitive impairment identification (Harvan & Cotter, 2006; Holsinger et al., 2012). Although current recommendations from the USPSTF (2010–2011) do not recommend screening all older

TABLE 3.3 · Cancer Screening Recommendations

	American Society of Geriatrics	USPSTF	American Cancer Society
Breast cancer	Mammography every 1–2 years until age 75 then every 2 years until life expectancy is <4 years	Biennial mammography for women aged 50–74	Annual mammography every 1 year starting at age 40 and continuing while the woman is in good health
Cervical cancer	Follow USPSTF guidelines/ American Cancer Society Guideline after considering the patient's life expectancy and comorbid conditions	Pap smear recommended until age 65	Women over age 70 who have had three or more normal pap smear or no abnormal pap smear in the last 10 years or who have had a hysterectomy may stop screening
Colon cancer	Colon cancer screening should continue for patients with a life expectancy of 10 years	Adults aged 50–75 using fecal occult blood testing, sigmoidoscopy or colonoscopy	Fecal occult blood testing annually starting at age 50, sigmoidoscopy every 5 years at age 50, or colonoscopy every 10 years starting at age 50
Prostate cancer	Recommend following the USPSTF or American Cancer Society recommendations after a careful history physical and discussion regarding benefits versus risks with patient	No recommendation for or against digital rectal examination or PSA, patients should consult with their health-care provider	Digital rectal exam and PSA in men over age 50 who have at least a 10-year life expectancy, after consultation with their health-care provider

patients for dementia, early identification and treatment of dementia has been shown to have many significant benefits (Harvan & Cotter, 2006).

The Mini-Cog Exam is a brief screening tool for dementia, which can be administered in approximately 3 minutes, is easily scored, does not require any special props or equipment, and works well in all types of health-care settings (Harvan & Cotter, 2006; Holsinger et al., 2012). This tool, which has a sensitivity of 76% to 99% and a specificity of 89% to 96% (Borson et al., 2000), tests the patient's memory with a three-item recall and their executive function through a clock-drawing test. The examiner begins by giving the patient three unrelated words to remember and then asks the patient to repeat those words. Then the examiner asks the patient to draw a clock face on a sheet of paper and put the numbers on the clock face. After they have completed the clock face, the examiner then asks the patient to draw the hands of the clock to read a specific time. After completing the clock-drawing test, the patient is asked to recall the previously stated three words. The patient receives 1 point for each of the correctly remembered words. They are classified as demented if they score 0 and not demented if they score a 3, remembering all of the words. If the patient scores a 1 or 2 on the word recall, then they are classified on the basis of their clock-drawing test score. If the clock drawing was normal, they are nondemented. If it was abnormal, they are classified as demented (Borson et al., 2000). If a patient's results show they are demented, then a more detailed exam should be considered.

Another useful tool for assessing cognition is the Confusion Assessment Method (CAM), which is used to detect delirium. Delirium is one of the most common acute neuropsychiatric illnesses that affects one third of hospitalized older adults (Inouye, 2006; Scheffer et al., 2010). The characteristics of delirium are a sudden onset of four features: mental status altered from baseline, inattention, disorganized thinking, and altered level of consciousness, all which can be transient in nature. Identifying delirium, which is considered an acute emergency, quickly is important as early identification and treatment of the underlying causes has been shown to reduce the negative outcomes associated with delirium (Inouye, 2006). There is both a nine-item and a four-item version of the CAM. Both have been tested for reliability and validity. The four-item version can be completed in less than 5 minutes and is frequently used in acute care and long-term-care settings.

1. Assessing Change in Mental Status from Baseline:
   - May be assessed through observation and with input from family members or close friends, primary care providers, or medical records that describe the patient's earlier mental status.
2. Assessing Patient for Signs of Inattention:
   - Inability to focus on tasks may be determined by asking the patient to spell the word "world" backward or recite days of the week backward. Patients without delirium and mild dementia can perform simple attention tasks such as counting backward from 20 to 1.
3. Assessing Disorganized Thinking:
   - Using standard orientation questions such as "What year is it? What season is it? What month is it?" Patients with dementia will have difficulty with these questions also.
4. Assessing Level of Consciousness:
   - The result for this item is considered positive if they are anything but alert and oriented.

Scoring for the CAM: There is evidence of delirium in the patient if the patient has 1 and 2 along with either 3 or 4 (or both 3 and 4) (Inouye, 2006; Scheffer et al., 2010; Waszynski & Petrovic, 2008).

Nutritional Screening

Although a separate chapter is dedicated to this topic, it is an important part of the initial assessment of an older adult. The USPTSF (2010–2011) recommends nutritional counseling for all older adults with a history of illnesses such as diabetes, hypertension, or coronary heart disease. The patient's height and weight should be evaluated and body mass index (BMI) obtained. It should be noted that BMI has limitations in older adults, for instance height loss due to osteoporosis. Both unintentional weight loss and elevated BMI should be assessed. Although the risks associated with an elevated BMI are not the same in an older person as in a younger person, they are associated with an increased risk of mortality from diabetes, hypertension, and cardiovascular disease. A 24-hour or 7-day diet recall can be a helpful tool for evaluating both inadequate nutrition and overeating (Spalding & Sebasta, 2008).

Physiologic changes with aging such as decreased sense of taste and smell, feeling a sense of fullness with a smaller meal than when they were younger, and feeling hungry less are believed to contribute to weight loss in the older adult. Many healthy older adults eat smaller less frequent meals and are hungry less often than when younger. This decreased appetite can lead to nutritional deficiencies. Oral problems such as loose, poorly fitting dentures and poor dentition should be carefully screened for during a physical exam. Poor nutrition in the older adult can lead to increased risk of morbidity and mortality (Ahmed & Haboubi, 2010).

One well-validated tool for screening for malnutrition is the full Mini Nutritional Assessment. This assessment tool, which takes approximately 15 minutes to complete and contains 18 items, was developed specifically for use in the older adult population (Ahmed & Haboubi, 2010). The Mini Nutritional Assessment–Short Form has also been validated as a reliable method of identifying older patients who are either at risk for malnutrition or are already malnourished. The short form only takes 5 minutes to complete and is simple and easy for providers to use (see Fig. 3.2).

Mini Nutritional Assessment
MNA®

Last name:		First name:		
Sex:	Age:	Weight, kg:	Height, cm:	Date:

Complete the screen by filling in the boxes with the appropriate numbers. Total the numbers for the final screening score.

Screening

A Has food intake declined over the past 3 months due to loss of appetite, digestive problems, chewing or swallowing difficulties?

0 = severe decrease in food intake
1 = moderate decrease in food intake
2 = no decrease in food intake ☐

B Weight loss during the last 3 months

0 = weight loss greater than 3 kg (6.6 lbs)
1 = does not know
2 = weight loss between 1 and 3 kg (2.2 and 6.6 lbs)
3 = no weight loss ☐

C Mobility

0 = bed or chair bound
1 = able to get out of bed / chair but does not go out
2 = goes out ☐

D Has suffered psychological stress or acute disease in the past 3 months?

0 = yes   2 = no ☐

E Neuropsychological problems

0 = severe dementia or depression
1 = mild dementia
2 = no psychological problems ☐

F1 Body Mass Index (BMI) (weight in kg) / (height in m²)

0 = BMI less than 19
1 = BMI 19 to less than 21
2 = BMI 21 to less than 23
3 = BMI 23 or greater ☐

IF BMI IS NOT AVAILABLE, REPLACE QUESTION F1 WITH QUESTION F2.
DO NOT ANSWER QUESTION F2 IF QUESTION F1 IS ALREADY COMPLETED.

F2 Calf circumference (CC) in cm

0 = CC less than 31
3 = CC 31 or greater ☐

Screening score (max. 14 points)

12 - 14 points: Normal nutritional status
8 - 11 points: At risk of malnutrition
0 - 7 points: Malnourished ☐☐

References
1. Vellas B, Villars H, Abellan G, *et al.* Overview of the MNA® - Its History and Challenges. *J Nutr Health Aging.* 2006;**10**:456-465.
2. Rubenstein LZ, Harker JO, Salva A, Guigoz Y, Vellas B. Screening for Undernutrition in Geriatric Practice: Developing the Short-Form Mini Nutritional Assessment (MNA-SF). *J. Geront.* 2001; **56A**: M366-377
3. Guigoz Y. The Mini-Nutritional Assessment (MNA®) Review of the Literature - What does it tell us? *J Nutr Health Aging.* 2006; **10**:466-487.
4. Kaiser MJ, Bauer JM, Ramsch C, et al. Validation of the Mini Nutritional Assessment Short-Form (MNA®-SF): A practical tool for identification of nutritional status. *J Nutr Health Aging.* 2009; **13**:782-788.
® Société des Produits Nestlé, S.A., Vevey, Switzerland, Trademark Owners © Nestlé, 1994, Revision 2009. N67200 12/99 10M
For more information: www.mna-elderly.com

FIGURE 3.2. Mini nutritional assessment. (From Société des Produits Nestlé, S.A., Vevey, Switzerland, Trademark Owners © Nestlé, 1994, Revision 2009. N67200 12/99 10M, with permission.) For more information: www.mna-elderly.com.

PAIN ASSESSMENT

Although pain was labeled the fifth vital sign by the Joint Commission on Accreditation of Healthcare Organizations over 10 years ago, older adults continue to be underassessed and undertreated for pain. According to the CDC, adults older than 65 are the least likely to report feeling pain, even though three fifths of adults in this age group were found to have pain that had lasted for a year or more (Flaherty, 2008). Pain assessment in the older adult may appear similar to any-age adult, but may be complicated by the reluctance of the older adult to report pain, which may be due to fears of expensive testing or thoughts that pain is a normal part of the aging process. The assessment of the older adult in pain may be further complicated by comorbidities, which affect how the patient's pain presents, such as cognitive or sensory impairments, for example dementia. A complete pain assessment should include a detailed history of the pain complaint including onset, duration, frequency, intensity, and relieving and contributing factors. All past medical and surgical history, sensory deficits, and current medications, including over-the-counter medications, should be noted (Bruckenthal, 2008).

Whenever possible, the self-report of pain is considered the gold standard for pain assessment. There are many simple pain assessment scales that have been widely used and tested for validity with patients of all ages. Examples of three of these scales are given below:

1. Number Rating Scale: Patients are asked to rate their pain on a scale of 0 to 10, 0 being no pain and 10 being the worst pain that they can imagine.
2. Verbal Descriptor Scale: Patients are asked to describe their pain using no pain, mild pain, moderate pain, or pain as bad as it could be.
3. Faces Pain Scale–Revised (FPS-R): Patients are shown a visual scale with pictures of a facial expression and asked to pick the one that corresponds with their pain level. A smiling face would be no pain and a harsh grimace would be severe pain (Flaherty, 2008).

When choosing a pain scale, the patient's special needs such as mild dementia, hearing loss, visual impairment, verbal communication impairment, or a patient who does not speak the same language as the examiner must be taken into account. Research has shown that these three simple methods work well with older adults when chosen with the patient's individual needs in mind (Flaherty, 2008).

The Pain Assessment in Advanced Dementia Scale (PAINAD) is a pain assessment tool that relies on behavior observation. This tool does require some basic training for staff before they administer it the first time and can then be completed in about 5 minutes' time (Horgas & Miller, 2008). Studies have found the PAINAD a reliable and valid tool to use for assessing pain in cognitively impaired patients (Liu et al., 2010). The PAINAD asks the examiner to rate the patient in five areas: breathing, vocalization, facial expression, body language, and consolability. Each area is given a score of 0, 1, or 2, and then all five areas are totaled. A score of 0 is no pain and a score of 10 is severe pain (Warden et al., 2003) (see Fig. 3.3).

SLEEP ASSESSMENT

It is important to assess older adults for sleep problems, since poor sleep has the potential of placing an older adult at risk for fatigue and greater risk for falls and mortality. The first indication of sleep disturbances may be interference with daytime functioning. If the patient, the patient's significant other, or caregiver begins to complain of or report that the patient has excessive daytime sleepiness, a complete sleep assessment should be undertaken.

Pain Assessment in Advanced Dementia Scale (PAINAD)

Instructions: Observe the patient for five minutes before scoring his or her behaviors. Score the behaviors according to the following chart. Definitions of each item are provided on the following page. The patient can be observed under different conditions (e.g., at rest, during a pleasant activity, during caregiving, after the administration of pain medication).

Behavior	0	1	2	Score
Breathing Independent of vocalization	■ Normal	■ Occasional labored breathing ■ Short period of hyperventilation	■ Noisy labored breathing ■ Long period of hyperventilation ■ Cheyne-Stokes respirations	
Negative vocalization	■ None	■ Occasional moan or groan ■ Low-level speech with a negative or disapproving quality	■ Repeated troubled calling out ■ Loud moaning or groaning ■ Crying	
Facial expression	■ Smiling or inexpressive	■ Sad ■ Frightened ■ Frown	■ Facial grimacing	
Body language	■ Relaxed	■ Tense ■ Distressed pacing ■ Fidgeting	■ Rigid ■ Fists clenched ■ Knees pulled up ■ Pulling or pushing away ■ Striking out	
Consolability	■ No need to console	■ Distracted or reassured by voice or touch	■ Unable to console, distract, or reassure	
TOTAL SCORE				

(Warden et al., 2003)

Scoring:

The total score ranges from 0-10 points. A possible interpretation of the scores is: 1-3=mild pain; 4-6=moderate pain; 7-10=severe pain. These ranges are based on a standard 0-10 scale of pain, but have not been substantiated in the literature for this tool.

Source:

Warden V, Hurley AC, Volicer L. Development and psychometric evaluation of the Pain Assessment in Advanced Dementia (PAINAD) scale. J Am Med Dir Assoc. 2003;4(1):9-15.

PAINAD Item Definitions

(Warden et al., 2003)

Breathing

1. *Normal breathing* is characterized by effortless, quiet, rhythmic (smooth) respirations.
2. *Occasional labored breathing* is characterized by episodic bursts of harsh, difficult, or wearing respirations.

3. *Short period of hyperventilation* is characterized by intervals of rapid, deep breaths lasting a short period of time.
4. *Noisy labored breathing* is characterized by negative-sounding respirations on inspiration or expiration. They may be loud, gurgling, wheezing. They appear strenuous or wearing.
5. *Long period of hyperventilation* is characterized by an excessive rate and depth of respirations lasting a considerable time.
6. *Cheyne-Stokes respirations* are characterized by rhythmic waxing and waning of breathing from very deep to shallow respirations with periods of apnea (cessation of breathing).

Negative Vocalization
1. *None* is characterized by speech or vocalization that has a neutral or pleasant quality.
2. *Occasional moan or groan* is characterized by mournful or murmuring sounds, wails, or laments. Groaning is characterized by louder than usual inarticulate involuntary sounds, often abruptly beginning and ending.
3. *Low level speech with a negative or disapproving quality* is characterized by muttering, mumbling, whining, grumbling, or swearing in a low volume with a complaining, sarcastic, or caustic tone.
4. *Repeated troubled calling out* is characterized by phrases or words being used over and over in a tone that suggests anxiety, uneasiness, or distress.
5. *Loud moaning or groaning* is characterized by mournful or murmuring sounds, wails, or laments in much louder than usual volume. Loud groaning is characterized by louder than usual inarticulate involuntary sounds, often abruptly beginning and ending.
6. *Crying* is characterized by an utterance of emotion accompanied by tears. There may be sobbing or quiet weeping.

Facial Expression
1. *Smiling or inexpressive.* Smiling is characterized by upturned corners of the mouth, brightening of the eyes, and a look of pleasure or contentment. Inexpressive refers to a neutral, at ease, relaxed, or blank look.
2. *Sad* is characterized by an unhappy, lonesome, sorrowful, or dejected look. There may be tears in the eyes.
3. *Frightened* is characterized by a look of fear, alarm, or heightened anxiety. Eyes appear wide open.
4. *Frown* is characterized by a downward turn of the corners of the mouth. Increased facial wrinkling in the forehead and around the mouth may appear.
5. *Facial grimacing* is characterized by a distorted, distressed look. The brow is more wrinkled, as is the area around the mouth. Eyes may be squeezed shut.

Body Language
1. *Relaxed* is characterized by a calm, restful, mellow appearance. The person seems to be taking it easy.
2. *Tense* is characterized by a strained, apprehensive, or worried appearance. The jaw may be clenched. (Exclude any contractures.)
3. *Distressed pacing* is characterized by activity that seems unsettled. There may be a fearful, worried, or disturbed element present. The rate may be faster or slower.
4. *Fidgeting* is characterized by restless movement. Squirming about or wiggling in the chair may occur. The person might be hitching a chair across the room. Repetitive touching, tugging, or rubbing body parts can also be observed.

(Continued)

Pain Assessment in Advanced Dementia Scale (PAINAD) *(Continued)*

5. *Rigid* is characterized by stiffening of the body. The arms and/or legs are tight and inflexible. The trunk may appear straight and unyielding. (Exclude any contractures.)

6. *Fists clenched* is characterized by tightly closed hands. They may be opened and closed repeatedly or held tightly shut.

7. *Knees pulled up* is characterized by flexing the legs and drawing the knees up toward the chest. An overall troubled appearance. (Exclude any contractures.)

8. *Pulling or pushing away* is characterized by resistiveness upon approach or to care. The person is trying to escape by yanking or wrenching him- or herself free or shoving you away.

9. *Striking out* is characterized by hitting, kicking, grabbing, punching, biting, or other form of personal assault.

Consolability

1. *No need to console* is characterized by a sense of well-being. The person appears content.

2. *Distracted or reassured by voice or touch* is characterized by a disruption in the behavior when the person is spoken to or touched. The behavior stops during the period of interaction, with no indication that the person is at all distressed.

3. *Unable to console, distract, or reassure* is characterized by the inability to soothe the person or stop a behavior with words or actions. No amount of comforting, verbal or physical, will alleviate the behavior.

FIGURE 3.3. The PAINAD Tool. (From Warden, V., Hurley, A. C., & Volicer, L. (2003). Development and psychometric evaluation of the Pain Assessment in Advanced Dementia (PAINAD) scale. *Journal of the American Medical Directors Association, 4*(1), 9–15, with permission).

Sleep disturbances in the older adult may be associated with undertreated pain in them. Research has shown that behaviors associated with pain such as certain medications, daytime napping, decreased activity, and exercise may also be associated with developing insomnia, while sleep deprivation can cause a reduction in pain tolerance (Dzierzewski et al., 2010). While many believe that poor sleep is a problem that occurs with normal aging, healthy older adults without comorbidities have been found to rarely suffer from sleep disturbances. Normal aging does not change the need for sleep. However, comorbidity and other medical, psychiatric, and environmental issues may affect the person's ability to get the sleep that they need. A person who has suffered the loss of a spouse and is now living in a long-term-care facility being treated for depression may be experiencing many changes that affect his or her ability to sleep (Neikrug & Ancoli-Israel, 2009).

The three sleep disorders that are most often found in older adults are restless leg syndrome, sleep-disordered breathing, and rapid eye movement (REM) sleep behavior disorder. Restless leg syndrome may happen when the patient is in a relaxed state or while asleep. Some patients refer to this as feeling an uncomfortable creepy crawly sensation, pin and needle sensation, crazy leg, or electric current, which is relieved temporarily by moving the leg. Screening for this type of disorder includes asking the patient a question such as "Do you ever feel unpleasant restless feelings in your legs when you are relaxing that can be relieved by moving?" These patients may also have repeated jerky leg movements in their sleep periodically, which may affect their REM sleep. They may not remember these movements, but interviewing their significant other or caretaker who has observed them sleep may reveal these types of sleep disturbances.

Sleep-disordered breathing can be classified in a wide range of respiratory events from mild snoring to patients who have complete apnea while sleeping. Older adults with a history of snoring and excessive daytime sleepiness should be screened for sleep-disordered breathing. After a complete history has been taken and the patient has been evaluated for risk factors such as obesity, age, gender, alcohol consumption, smoking, upper airway congestion, use of sedating medications, and family history, the patient should be sent for a sleep study. Sleep-disordered breathing in the older adult is associated with functional impairment, increased cognitive impairment, and greater risk of nocturia, hypertension, and cardiovascular disease. Treatment with continuous positive airway pressure (CPAP) has been found to be a reliable treatment for this sleep disorder (Neikrug & Ancoli-Israel, 2009).

REM sleep behavior disorder occurs when the patient displays uncontrolled possibly violent movements during their REM sleep cycle. This disorder is thought to possibly be related to an underlying neurologic disorder and may require a detailed sleep study as well as a referral to a neurologist (Neikrug & Ancoli-Israel, 2009).

Although many patients feel that poor sleep is a normal part of aging, healthy older adults should have a healthy sleep pattern. Comorbidities as well as complex environmental and psychosocial changes may make sleep more difficult for older adults. A careful and detailed sleep and medical history as well as information from any bed partner or caregiver is very important in order to prevent the potential negative complications from not getting enough sleep.

FUNCTIONAL ASSESSMENT

According to the CDC, 2.4 million nonfatal fall injuries among older adults were treated in United States emergency rooms (Centers fo Disease Control and Prevention, 2012). About 30% to 40% of older adults over the age of 65 who are living in the community report falling at least once per year, making falls the leading cause of injury in this age group of adults (Moyer, 2012). All patients over the age of 65 should be assessed for their risk of falls at their annual primary care visit. The patient should be asked if they have fallen in the past year. The American Geriatric Society algorithm for evaluating falls in older adults recommends evaluating the patient for gait and balance disturbances if they report one fall in the past year. If the patient reports two or more falls in the past year, the patient is then given a full multifactorial evaluation to determine their fall risk and potential preventive measures (Falls, 2011).

The Timed Get Up and Go test is a simple-to-use evaluation tool that was developed to further evaluate a patient's risk for fall that requires no special equipment or training to perform. This test is performed by asking the patient to rise from a sitting position, walk 10 ft, turn around, return to chair, and sit down. If the patient takes less than 20 seconds to perform the tasks, they are screened as able to perform independent transfers and mobility. If they take longer than 30 seconds to perform the task, then their results suggest a high risk for falls. Results between 20 and 30 seconds indicate a possible risk for fall.

Another test for gait and balance is the Functional Gait Test, which asks the patient to perform 10 items such as walking at normal, fast, and slow speeds with their head at different angles and also when their eyes are closed. The results are then scored depending on the patient's ability to perform these tests. The Berg Balance Scale is a 14-item clinical balance test that evaluates the patient's ability to perform sitting and standing activities such as standing from a chair, reaching forward while standing with feet together. The results are scored on a 1-to-4-point Likert Scale; the lower the score, the more likely the patient is to fall. Both the Berg Balance and Functional

Gait Test require instruction for providers performing the evaluation. Whichever screening tool is used to test a patient's gait and balance as well as risk for falls, it is important to use these results as one part of a comprehensive fall risk assessment (Wrisley & Kumar, 2010).

Older adults must also be assessed for the ability to complete their activities of daily living as well as their instrumental activities of daily living. The Katz Index of Independence in Activities of Daily Living is a well-validated and reliable tool used to evaluate a patient's ability to perform basic activities of daily living such as bathing, dressing, toileting, transferring, continence, and feeding. The patient is given a yes or no for being able to perform each of the six activities independently. A yes answer is scored as a 1. The total score of 6 reveals complete function without impairment, a score of 4 or below reveals moderate impairment of function, and a score of 2 or below reveals a severe impairment of function (Wallace & Shelkey, 2008). The Lawton Instrumental Activities of Daily Living Scale assesses a patient's ability to perform higher-level activities such as dialing a phone, shopping, meal preparation, housekeeping, laundry, transportation, responsibility for medications, and ability to handle finances. There are multiple choices under each category with corresponding scores. The total score reveals a range of a patient being low-function and high-dependent to a patient who is high-function and independent. These screens should be used to determine an individual patient's needs and may trigger need for further evaluation (Graf, 2008).

Many older adults are faced with loss of function after an acute illness or as they age or deal with a chronic illness. Modifications of their home environment may allow patients to remain in their own home instead of moving into a long-term-care facility. A home safety assessment may be necessary to ensure that the home environment does not contain hazards that could pose a fall risk for older adults. Home Screening Checklists for patients to use at home to evaluate and remediate any potential fall risk areas are available on the CDC Web site as well as through many local areas' National Association of Area Agencies on Aging. These checklists usually concentrate on issues such as lighting, scatter rugs, steps, color contrast, grab bars in showers and tubs, and items within easy reach without a step ladder. Patients with dementia or certain medical illnesses may be eligible for home occupational therapy assessment depending on their coverage and insurance plan (Unwin et al., 2009).

The Hendrich II Fall Risk Model was designed by nurses as a quick reliable method to identify a hospitalized older adult who is at increased risk for falls. The model screens patients for confusion, depression, altered elimination, dizziness, male gender, any administered antiepileptics or benzodiazepines, as well as a get-up-and-go test. A total score of 5 or more indicates a patient who is at high risk for fall. As with any of the risk-for-fall screening evaluations, the next step would be to implement further steps to prevent the patient from falling (Hendrich, 2007).

Mental Health Assessment Screening Tools

While the majority of older adults are not depressed, older adults with chronic illnesses are at increased risk for depression. Symptoms of depression in older adults may be mistaken for normal aging changes and are often underrecognized and undertreated. Studies have shown that up to 75% of older adults who commit suicide had visited their primary care provider within the month prior to their death. Careful screening for signs and symptoms of depression in older adults can reduce the risks associated with depression (Centers for Disease Control and Prevention, 2005).

The Geriatric Depression Scale (GDS) is a 30-item questionnaire, which is specifically designed to screen for depression in older adults (Roman & Callen, 2008). Another version was later developed, which only contains 15 questions and is called the Geriatric Depression Scale–Short Form (GDS-15). The GDS-15 has been shown to be both sensitive and specific for screening for depression in the older adult (Sheikh & Yesavage, 1986). This questionnaire provides a simple form that patients may complete for themselves or may be completed by a provider asking them the questions if they are unable to fill out the form. This screening tool has been widely used in multiple clinical settings such as long-term care, acute care, and primary care (see Fig. 3.4).

Addressing spiritual needs in the older adult, especially in palliative care or end-of-life settings, is an important aspect of improving the patient's satisfaction with their care. The Faith, Importance and Influence, Community and Address (FICA) Spiritual History Tool was developed by Dr. Puchalski and a group of primary care physicians and has been validated with oncology patients (Lunder et al., 2011). This tool provides an easy way for clinicians to conduct a spiritual history of older adults and open a dialog with the patient regarding their spiritual needs. The FICA tool is a short questionnaire that can be self-administered or administered with help from a provider if necessary. The FICA assessment is not only a reliable way for patients' spiritual needs to be identified, but also for a patient to let their provider know that their spiritual needs are already being met. Spiritual histories should be included as part of the patient's regular annual exam or new patient visit and then updated as needed. As with any screening tool, the FICA spiritual history tool should be used as a guide for the patient and clinician to begin to talk about the patient's spiritual concerns and needs (Bourneman et al., 2010; Puchalski, 2006; Puchalski & Romer, 2000) (see Fig. 3.5).

While 50% of adults over the age of 65 have been found to drink alcohol, 1% to 3% of older adults are affected by alcohol use disorder. Alcohol use disorder is defined as alcohol dependence, alcohol abuse, or harmful drinking. Alcohol use disorders are thought to be underidentified in the older adult, yet believed to cause an increased risk of physical and psychological morbidity. There are two tools that are used frequently to assess for the presence of the misuse of alcohol in an older adult—the four-item CAGE questionnaire and the short-version Michigan Alcoholism Screening Test. Many researchers encourage the use of both tools to enhance the specificity and sensitivity of identifying alcohol abuse issues in the older adult (Caputo et al., 2012).

To perform the CAGE test, the examiner asks the patient four questions that deal with C, cut off; A, annoyed; G, guilty; and E, eye opener. If the patient answers yes to two or more of the following questions, the results suggest that the patient has an alcohol-related problem.

C: Have you ever felt that you should cut down on your drinking?
A: Have people annoyed you by criticizing your drinking?
G: Have you ever had guilty feelings about drinking?
E: Have you ever had a drink first thing in the morning to steady your nerves or get rid of a hangover? (Ewing, 2008)

The short-form Michigan Alcohol Screening Test–Geriatric Version, which was developed to identify hazardous drinking in the older adult patient, is composed of 10 "yes or no" questions. This assessment may be either self-administered or completed by a health-care provider during an interview. Two or more "yes" responses to the questions would indicate that the patient has a problem with alcohol. Further evaluation and medical workup would be warranted, including possible referral for treatment (Johnson-Greene et al., 2009).

Although elder abuse has been the topic of many studies of the last decade, it is believed that the incidence of elder abuse remains higher than what is reported. Elder abuse can be defined as any act, one time or repeated, or lack of action, that causes harm or stress to an older adult. This abuse occurs when there is a trusted relationship between the older adult and the abuser. This abuse can be in the form of physical, psychological, neglect, sexual, or financial abuse. Many cases may go unreported because the older adult is ashamed to report the abuse, frightened to report the abuse, or the patient's health-care providers fail to identify and report it. Older adults

Geriatric Depression Scale (short form)

Instructions: Circle the answer that best describes how you felt over the <u>past week</u>.

1.	Are you basically satisfied with your life?	yes	no
2.	Have you dropped many of your activities and interests?	yes	no
3.	Do you feel that your life is empty?	yes	no
4.	Do you often get bored?	yes	no
5.	Are you in good spirits most of the time?	yes	no
6.	Are you afraid that something bad is going to happen to you?	yes	no
7.	Do you feel happy most of the time?	yes	no
8.	Do you often feel helpless?	yes	no
9.	Do you prefer to stay at home, rather than going out and doing things?	yes	no
10.	Do you feel that you have more problems with memory than most?	yes	no
11.	Do you think it is wonderful to be alive now?	yes	no
12.	Do you feel worthless the way you are now?	yes	no
13.	Do you feel full of energy?	yes	no
14.	Do you feel that your situation is hopeless?	yes	no
15.	Do you think that most people are better off than you are?	yes	no

Total Score _____

Geriatric Depression Scale (GDS) Scoring Instructions

Instructions: Score 1 point for each bolded answer. A score of 5 or more suggests depression.

1.	Are you basically satisfied with your life?	yes	**no**
2.	Have you dropped many of your activities and interests?	**yes**	no
3.	Do you feel that your life is empty?	**yes**	no
4.	Do you often get bored?	**yes**	no
5.	Are you in good spirits most of the time?	yes	**no**
6.	Are you afraid that something bad is going to happen to you?	**yes**	no
7.	Do you feel happy most of the time?	yes	**no**
8.	Do you often feel helpless?	**yes**	no
9.	Do you prefer to stay at home, rather than going out and doing things?	**yes**	no
10.	Do you feel that you have more problems with memory than most?	**yes**	no
11.	Do you think it is wonderful to be alive now?	yes	**no**
12.	Do you feel worthless the way you are now?	**yes**	no
13.	Do you feel full of energy?	yes	**no**
14.	Do you feel that your situation is hopeless?	**yes**	no
15.	Do you think that most people are better off than you are?	**yes**	no

A score of ≥ 5 suggests depression   *Total Score* _____

Ref. Yes average: The use of Rating Depression Series in the Elderly, in Poon (ed.): Clinical Memory Assessment of Older Adults, American Psychological Association, 1986

FIGURE 3.4. Geriatric Depression Scale—Short Form. (From The use of Rating Depression Series in the elderly. (1986). In Poon (Ed.), *Clinical memory assessment of older adults.* American Psychological Association, may be copied without permission). Retrieved from http://www.chcr.brown.edu/GDS_SHORT_FORM.PDF

Spiritual Assessment Tool

An Acronym *that can be used to remember what is asked in a spiritual history is:*

F : Faith or Beliefs

I : Importance and influence

C: Community

A: Address

Some specific questions you can use to discuss these issues are:

F: What is your faith or belief?

 Do you consider yourself spiritual or religious?

 What things do you believe in that give meaning to your life?

I: Is it important in your life?

 What influence does it have on how take care of yourself?

 How have your beliefs influenced your behavior during this illness?

 What role do your beliefd play in regaining your health?

C: Are you part of a spiritual or religious community?

 Is this of support to you and how?

 Is there a person or group of people you really love or who are really important to you?

A: How would you like me, your healthcare provider, to address these issues in your healthcare?

General recommendations when taking a spiritual histry:

1. Consider spirituality as a potentially important component of every patient's physical well being and mental health.

2. Address spirituality at each complete physical examination and continue addressing it at follow-up visits if appropriate. In patient care, spirituality is an ongoing issue.

3. Respect a patient's privacy regarding spiritual beliefs; don't impose your beliefs on others.

4. Make referrals to chaplains, spiritual directors, or community resources as appropriate.

5. Be aware that your own spiritual beliefs will help you personally and will overflow in your encounters with those for whom you care to make the doctor-patient encounter a more humanistic one.

© 1999 Christina Puchalski, M.D. Reprinted with permission from Christina Puchalski, M.D.

FIGURE 3.5. FICA Spiritual History Tool. (From Christina Puchalski, MD, ©1999, reprinted with permission.)

may have medical conditions that may complicate the identification of abuse, for instance, medication side effects such as malnutrition or easy bruising (Cohen, 2011).

The Elder Abuse Instrument has been used in all types of clinical setting to screen for signs and symptoms and subjective complaints associated with elder abuse (Stark, 2012). This 41-item assessment tool was developed to be administered by a provider to screen for possible abuse. The results are not given in a total score. Instead, after completing the tool if the provider finds any evidence of mistreatment that cannot be explained, a subjective complaint of elder mistreatment, or high risk of elder abuse, neglect, abandonment, or exploitation, the patient should be referred to social services for a further evaluation of potential maltreatment. The goal of this assessment is to provide a brief screening that would then allow for potential mistreatment to be identified and for a more in-depth screening by Adult Protective Services to be initiated (Fulmer, 2008).

SUMMARY

There are multiple screening tools available for use in assessing the older adult. Choosing the appropriate tool requires careful evaluation by the advance practice nurse of the setting, needs of the patient, and benefits of the tool. The unique health-care needs of the older patient require critical thinking, excellent communication skills to involve all members of the multidisciplinary health-care team, the patient, the family of the patient, and caretakers in order to increase the patient's functional status and quality of life.

REFERENCES

Ahmed, T., & Haboubi, N. (2010). Assessment and management of nutrition in older people and its importance to health. *Clinical Interventions in Aging, 5,* 207–216.

American Geriatric Society. (2012). *The American Geriatrics Society 2012 Beers Criteria Update Expert Panel.* New York, NY: Author.

Besdine, R. (2009, June). *Merck manual of geriatrics.* Retrieved from http://www.merckmanuals.com/professional/geriatrics/approach_to_the_geriatric_patient/evaluation_of_the_elderly_patient.html

Bluestein, D. (2005). Preventive services: Screening. Health maintenance examinations include screening for diabetes, heart disease, cancer, osteoporosis, hearing and vision loss. *Geriatrics, 60*(2), 34–39.

Borson, S., Scanlan, J., Brush, M., Vitaliano, P., & Dokmak, A. (2000). The mini-cog: A cognitive "vital signs" measure for dementia screening in multi-lingual elderly. *International Journal of Geriatric Psychiatry, 15*(11), 1021–1027.

Bourneman, T., Ferrell, B., & Puchalski, C. (2010). Evaluation of the FICA tool for spiritual assessment. *Journal of Pain and Symptoms Management, 40*(2), 163–173.

Brink, T.L., Yesavage, J.A., Lum, O., Heersema, P., Adey, M.B., Rose, T.L. (1982). Screening tests for geriatric depression. *Clinical Gerontologist 1,* 37–44.

Bruckenthal, P. (2008). Assessment of pain in the eldery adult. *Clinical Geriatrics Medicine, 24*(2), 213–236.

Burggraf, V. (1993). A systemic window: Revelations of aging. *Journal of Gerontologic Nursing, 19*(12), 5–6.

Caputo, F., Leggio, L., Addolorato, G., Zoli, G., & Bernardi, M. (2012). Alcohol use disorders in the elderly: A brief overview from epidemiology to treatment options. *Experimental Gerontology, 47*(6), 411–416.

Centers for Disease Control and Prevention. (2005). National Center for Injury Prevention and Control. Retrieved from www.cdc.gov/ncipc/wisqar

Centers for Disease Control and Prevention, National Vital Statistics System. (2010). Ten leading causes of death by age group, U.S.–2010. Retrieved fromwww.cdc.gov/injury/wisqars/Leadingcauses.html

Centers for Disease Control and Prevention. (2011). Summary of recommendations for adult immunization. Retrieved from www.immunize.org/catg.d/p2011.pdf

Centers fo Disease Control and Prevention. (2012, September 20). Costs of falls among older adults. Retrieved from http://www.cdc.gov/HomeandRecreationalSafety/Falls/fallcost.html

Centers for Disease Control and Prevention & The Merck Company Foundation. (2007). *The state of aging and health in America 2007.* Whitehouse Station, NJ: Author.

Chou, R., Dana, T., & Bougatsos, C. (2009). Screening older adults for impaired visual acuity: A review of the evidence for the U.S. Preventive Services Task Force. *Annals of Internal Medicine, 151*(1), 44–58.

Cohen, M. (2011). Screening tools for the identification of elder abuse. *Journal of Clinical Outcomes Management, 18*(6), 261–270.

Dzierzewski, J., Williams, J., Roditi, D., Marsiske, M., McCoy, K., McNamara, J., … McCrae, C. (2010). Daily variations in objective nighttime sleep and subjective morning pain in older adults with insomnia: Evidence of covariation over time. *Journal of the American Geriatric Society, 58*(5), 925–930.

Elsawy, B., & Higgins, K. E. (2011). The geriatric assessment. *American Family Physician, 83*(1), 48–56.

Ewing, J. (2008). The CAGE Questionnaire for detection of alcoholism. *Journal of American Medical Association, 300*(17), 2054–2056.

Falls, P. O. (2011). Summary of the updated American Geriatrics Society/British Geriatrics Society clinical practice guidelines for prevention of falls in older persons. *Journal of the American Geriatrics Society, 59*(1), 148–157.

Finkel, S. (2003). Cognitive screening in the primary care setting. The role of physicians at the point of entry. *Geriatrics, 58*(6), 43–44.

Flaherty, E. (2008). Using pain-rating scales with older adults. *American Journal of Nursing, 108*(6), 40–47.

Fulmer, T. (2008). Screening for mistreatment of older adults. *American Journal of Nursing, 108*(12), 52–59.

Gariballa, S., Forster, S., Walters, S., & Powers, H. (2006). A randomized, double-blind, placebo-controlled trial of nutritional supplementation during acute illness. *American Journal of Medicine, 119,* 693–699.

Graf, C. (2008). The Lawton instrumental activities of daily living scale. *American Journal of Nursing, 108*(4), 52–62.

Hajjar, E. R., Cafiero, A. C., & Hanlon, J. T. (2007). Polypharmacy in elderly patients. *American Journal of Geriatric Pharmacotherapy, 5*(4), 345–351.

Harvan, J., & Cotter, V. (2006). An evaluation of dementia screening in the primary care setting. *Journal of the American Academy of Nurse Practitioners, 18*(8), 351–360.

Hendrich, A. (2007). How to try this: Predicting patient falls. Using the Hendrich II Fall Risk Model in clinical practice. *American Journal of Nursing, 107*(11), 50–58.

Holsinger, T., Plassman, B., Stechuchak, K., Burke, J., Coffman, C., & Williams, J. (2012). Screening for cognitive impairment: Comparing the performance of four instruments in primary care. *Journal of the American Geriatric Society, 60*(6), 1027–1036.

Horgas, A., & Miller, L. (2008). Pain assessment in people with dementia. *American Journal of Nursing, 108*(7), 62–70.

Inouye, S. (2006). Current concepts: Delirium in older persons. *New England Journal of Medicine, 354,* 1157–1165.

Johnson-Greene, D., McCaul, M., & Roger, P. (2009). Screening for hazardous drinking using the Michigan Alcohol Screening Test-Geriatric Version (MAST-G) in elderly persons with acute cerebrovascular accidents. *Alcoholism Clinical and Experimental Research, 33*(9), 1555–1561.

Kass-Bartelmes, B. L. (2002, April). *Preventing disability in the elderly with chronic disease.* Retrieved from Agency for Healthcare Research and Quality Web site: http://www.ahrq.gov/research/elderdis.htm

Liu, J., Briggs, M., & Closs, J. (2010). The psychometric qualities of four observation pain tools for the assessment of pain in elderly people with osteoarthritic pain. *Journal of Pain and Symptoms Management, 40*(4), 582–589.

Lunder, U., Furlan, M., & Simonic, A. (2011). Spiritual needs assessment and measures. *Current Opinions in Supportive and Palliative Care, 5*(3), 273–278.

Moyer, V. (2012). Prevention of falls in community-dwelling older adults: U.S. Preventive Services Task Force recommendation statement. *Annals of Internal Medicine, 157*(3), 197–204.

Neikrug, A., & Ancoli-Israel, S. (2009). Sleep disorders in the older adult—A mini review. *Gerontology, 56*(2), 181–189.

Puchalski, C. (2006). Spiritual assessment in clinical practice. *Psychiatric Annals, 36*(3), 150–155.

Puchalski, C., & Romer, A. L. (2000). Taking a spirtiual history allow clinicians to understand patients more fully. *Journal of Palliative Medicine, 3*(1), 129–137.

Roman, M., & Callen, B. (2008). Screening instruments for older adult depression disorders: Updating the evidence-based toolbox. *Issues In Mental Health Nursing, 29*(9), 924–941.

Rosen, S. L., & Reuben, D. B. (2011). Geriatric Assessment Tools. *Mount Sinai Journal of Medcine, 78*(4), 489–497.

Scheffer, A., van Munster, B., Schuurmans, M., & de Rooij, S. (2010). Assessing severity of delirium by the Delirium Observation Screening Scale. *International Journal of Geriatric Psychiatry, 26*(3), 284–291.

Sheikh, J. I., & Yesavage, J. A. (1986). Geriatric Depression Scale (GDS). *Clinical Gerontology, 5,* 165–173.

Smith, R. A., Cokkinides, V., & Brawley, O. W. (2012). Cancer screening in the United States, 2012: A review of current American Society guidelines and current issues in cancer screening. *A Cancer Journal for Clinicians, 62*(2), 129–142.

Spalding, M., & Sebasta, S. (2008). Geriatric screening and preventive care. *American Family Physicians, 78*(2), 206–215.

Stark, S. (2012). Elder abuse: Screening, intervention and prevention. *Nursing, 42*(10), 24–29.

Taylor, D., Hasselblad, V., Henley, J., Thun, M., & Sloan, F. (2002). Benefits of smoking cessation for longevity. *American Journal of Public Health, 92*(6), 990–996.

Unwin, B., Andrews, C., Andrews, P., & Hanson, J. (2009). Therapeutic home adaptions for older adults with disabilites. *American Family Physicians, 80*(9), 963–970.

U.S. Preventive Services Task Force. (2010–2011). Guide to clinical preventive services, 2010–2011. Recommendations of the U.S. Preventive Services Task. Retrieved from http://www.uspreventiveservicestaskforce.org/tfolderfocus.htm#current

Wallace, M., & Shelkey, M. (2008). Monitoring functional status in hospitalized older adults. *American Journal of Nursing, 108*(4), 64–71.

Walling, A., & Dickson, G. (2012). Hearing loss in older adults. *American Academy of Family Physicians, 85*(12), 1150–1156.

Warden, V., Hurley, A., & Volicer, L. (2003). Development and psychometric evaluation of the Pain Assessment in Advanced Dementia (PAINAD) scale. *Journal of American Medical Directors Association, 4*(1), 9–15.

Waszynski, C., & Petrovic, K. (2008). Nurses' evaluation of the confusion assessment method: A pilot study. *Journal of Gerontological Nursing, 34*(4), 49–56.

Wrisley, D., & Kumar, N. (2010). Functional gait assessment: Concurrent, discriminative, and predictive validity in community-dwelling older adults. *Physical Therapy, 90*(5), 761–773.

CHAPTER 3: IT RESOURCES

Websites

Hartford Institute for Geriatric Nursing—General Assessment Series
http://www.hartfordign.org/practice/try_this/

American Family Physician—The Geriatric Assessment
http://www.aafp.org/afp/2011/0101/p48.html

Geriatric Examination Tool Kit
http://web.missouri.edu/~proste/tool/

The University of Iowa—Geriatric Assessment Tools
http://www.healthcare.uiowa.edu/igec/tools/

MNA as part of the Comprehensive Geriatric Assessment (CGA)
http://www.mna-elderly.com/geriatric_assessment.html

Geriatric Assessment Methods for Clinical Decision Making
http://consensus.nih.gov/1987/1987geriatricassessment065html.htm

Inpatient Geriatric Assessment
http://www.amh.org/services/senior-health/geriatric-assessments/
geriatric-assessments-inpatient/

Outpatient Geriatric Assessment
http://www.amh.org/services/senior-health/geriatric-assessments/
geriatric-assessments-outpatient/

Geriatric Assessment: Essential Skills for Nurses
http://www.americannursetoday.com/article.aspx?id=8038&fid=7986

Individualizing Cancer Screening in Older Adults
http://www.uspreventiveservicestaskforce.org/uspstf12/cancerolder.htm

Recommendations for Adults
http://www.uspreventiveservicestaskforce.org/adultrec.htm

Clinical Preventive Services in Older Adults
http://www.cdc.gov/features/preventiveservices/

Fact Sheet: Screening for Older Adults
http://www.medscape.com/viewarticle/501880

Screening for Cognitive Impairment
http://www.medscape.com/viewarticle/765925

Retooling Pain Assessment for Older Adults
http://www.medscape.com/viewarticle/804127

Pain Assessment in Advanced Dementia—PAINAD Instructions
http://www.geriatricpain.org/Content/Assessment/Impaired/Pages/PAINAD
ToolInstructions.aspx

US Department of Health & Human Services HealthBeat—An Eye on Independence
http://www.hhs.gov/news/healthbeat/2013/01/20130123a.html

PDF Documents

Geriatric Assessment Tool Kit
http://www.chcr.brown.edu/geriatric_assessment_tool_kit.pdf

Comprehensive Geriatric Assessment
  http://ocw.tufts.edu/data/42/499797.pdf
Summary of Recommendations for Adult Immunizations
  http://www.amc.edu/Patient/Immunization/documents/Adult_2011.pdf
History and Physical Examination of the Older Adult
  http://www.galter.northwestern.edu/geriatrics/chapters/history_physical_exam.pdf
Assessment of the Older Adult
  http://www.ouhsc.edu/geriatricmedicine/documents/GRS5-Geriatric_Assessment.pdf
General Screening Recommendations for Chronic Disease and Risk Factors in Older Adults
  http://consultgerirn.org/uploads/File/trythis/try_this_27.pdf
Cognitive Screening of Older Adults
  http://med.brown.edu/neurology/articles/jg805.pdf
Confusion Assessment Method (CAM)
  http://consultgerirn.org/uploads/File/Confusion%20Assessment%20Method%20
  (CAM).pdf
Nutritional Checklist—Determine your Nutritional Health
  http://www.cdaaa.org/images/Nutritional_Checklist.pdf
Mini Nutritional Assessment Tool
  http://www.cdaaa.org/images/Nutritional_Checklist.pdf
Pain Assessment for Older Adults
  http://consultgerirn.org/uploads/File/trythis/try_this_7.pdf
What Is Pain Assessment in Older Adults?
  http://www.ebscohost.com/uploads/poc/pdf/NRC_skillPaper.pdf
Using Pain-Rating Scales with Older Adults
  http://tufts-health.org/providers/pdf/pain_assessment.pdf
Pain Assessment in Advanced Dementia (PAINAD) Scale
  http://web.missouri.edu/~proste/tool/cog/painad.pdf
Pain Assessment in People with Dementia
  http://www.nursingcenter.com/pdf.asp?AID=800535

Videos

Physical Examination of the Older Adult (2012)
  A geriatric practitioner will demonstrate the routine physical examination he performs during the course of a comprehensive geriatric assessment. The challenge is to package all the high-yield maneuvers into an exam that can be done in 10 minutes
  http://youtube/OeXVV3elJx8 (26 minutes)
2013 Adult Immunization Schedule: A Quick Overview
  Dr. Sandra Fryhofer discusses the key points of the new adult immunization schedule from Advisory Committee on Immunization Practices.
  http://links.email.empr.com/servlet/MailView?ms=NTgzMDUwOAS2&r=MzEwODAwMTU
  zNjcS1&j=NjkyOTAxNjYS1&mt=1&rt=0 (3:07 minutes)
Pain Assessment in Older Adults (1 hour)
  http://www.geriatricpain.org/Content/Assessment/Impaired/Pages/Howtovideo.aspx
Pain Assessment in Older Adults (1 hour)
  http://vimeo.com/4669429

Pain-Behavioral Assessment Tools in the Nursing Home (2011)

To help healthcare providers identify clinically useful pain-behavioral assessment tools for use in the nursing home, the MayDay Fund provided support for an expert panel to evaluate the currently available tools. Fourteen tools were rated using newly developed criteria, which included reliability, validity, and utility in the nursing home setting. As a result, the Pain Assessment in Advanced Dementia scale and the Pain Assessment Checklist for Seniors with Limited Ability to Communicate were selected as the most clinically relevant and applicable tools for everyday practice. Kella Herr, PhD, RN, FAAN, AGSF

http://youtube/D4LVpgEjZCs (1:43 minutes)

Persistent pain in older people—Tricia Moylan (2013)

Dr. Moylan is a Consultant in Care of the Elderly; she outlines difference in pain assessment and adjustments to analgesic treatments in this patient demographic.

http://youtube/AoDym73Lwn8 (44 minutes)

Assessment and Diagnosis of Older Adults (2011)

Capacity to Care: Building Competency in Geriatric Mental Health Care—Eve H. Byrd, MSN, MPH, APRN-BC

http://youtube/NadEQBnVTZ4 (1:28 minutes)

Basic Head-to-Toe Assessment with Geriatric Focus (2007)

A thorough physical assessment is necessary for all clients whether in long-term care, acute care, or home health. Our focus is to take the professional through a comprehensive physical assessment, divided into upper body and lower body and put it all together. Includes proper documentation guidelines.

http://youtube/vnMbuVddRok (1:59 minutes)

Mini Nutritional Assessment (2009)

MNA Video demonstrates step-by-step directions for using the MNA in clinical practice to identify malnutrition in the elderly.

http://youtube/9oT7pF_Gck8 (10:59 minutes)

Images

Google images for Geriatric Assessment

http://www.google.com/search?q=geriatric+assessment&source=lnms&tbm=isch&sa=X&ei=vI6jUdbWDNbh4AOtv4DAAg&ved=0CAcQ_AUoAQ&biw=1011&bih=220

Google images for Mini Nutritional Assessment

http://www.google.com/search?q=mini+nutritional+assessment&tbm=isch&tbo=u&source=univ&sa=X&ei=UpSjUeSYHOfi0gGO94HYCw&sqi=2&ved=0CDwQsAQ&biw=1011&bih=220

Google images for Pain Assessment in Advanced Dementia Scale

http://www.google.com/search?q=Pain+Assessment+in+Advanced+Dementia+Scale&tbm=isch&tbo=u&source=univ&sa=X&ei=75WjUY_XB-v00QH8yYHgDg&ved=0CDsQsAQ&biw=1011&bih=220

Cardiovascular Disease

DeEtta Compton, DNP, FNP-BC

INTRODUCTION

This chapter discusses the following cardiovascular diseases (CVDs): coronary artery disease (CAD), heart failure (HF), atrial fibrillation (AF), and aortic stenosis (AS), dyslipidemia. The disease processes are some of the most common in the aging population, and this chapter will discuss the incidence of these disease processes, basic pathophysiology, management guidelines, and special considerations in the older adult.

CVD is an insidious process that affects many in the aging population. Chapman and Perry (2008) acknowledge that, as the population ages, older adults will account for most of the US population. CVD is the leading cause of mortality in both men and women over the age of 65 (Bonow et al., 2012). Owing to the high incidence of mortality and morbidity due to CVD in the older adult, it is important to be aggressive with prevention and treatment. Convincing data exist that demonstrate a decreased morbidity and mortality when CVD is aggressively treated in patients up to age 74. However, limited data exist regarding patients 75 years and older (Bonow et al., 2012). Multiple age-related changes that occur in the cardiovascular system are outlined in Table 4.1.

The literature suggests an increase in CVD deaths in women, which is partly due to the higher percentage of women compared with men greater than 55 years old. CVD is commonly thought to be a man's disease; this is a widespread misconception (Ridker et al., 2005). The Centers for Disease Control and Prevention (CDC, 2010) reported that CVD is the leading cause of death in women in the United States. In 2010, CDC reported that about 600,000 people die of heart disease in the United States every year—that is 1 in every 4 deaths. More than half of the deaths due to heart disease in 2009 were in men (CDC, 2010). The CDC reported results of a 2005 survey showing 36% of women did not recognize they were at risk for CVD (2010). Risk factors for

TABLE 4.1 · Age-Related Cardiovascular Changes

- Increased intimal thickness
- Arterial stiffening
- Decreased vessel elasticity
- Increased pulse pressure
- Increased pulse wave pressure
- Early central wave reflections
- Decreased endothelium-mediated vasodilatation
- Increased left atrial size
- Premature atrial complexes
- Maximal heart rate decreased
- Heart rate variability decreased
- Conduction time increased
- Calcification
- Sclerosis
- Pigmentation of lipofuscin granules
- Increased left ventricular wall tension
- Prolonged contraction of the myocardium
- Early diastolic filling time prolonged
- Decreased maximal cardiac output
- Right bundle branch block
- Premature ventricular complexes

Adapted from Bonow, R. O., Mann, D. L., Zipes, D. P., & Libby, P. (2012). *Braunwald's heart disease* (9th ed.). Philadelphia, PA: Elsevier Inc., with permission.

CVD in women include diabetes, hypertension (HTN), hyperlipidemia, metabolic syndrome, obesity, depression, postmenopausal syndrome, rheumatologic disease, and sedentary lifestyle (Ridker et al., 2005).

CORONARY ARTERY DISEASE

CAD is the most common type of CVD and is the leading cause of death in the United States. The severity and prevalence increases with age in both men and women, and by the age of 80, symptomatic CAD is present in 20% to 30% of people (Bonow et al., 2012).

The threat of CAD is that it can lead to myocardial ischemia and myocardial infarction (MI). Plaque buildup (atherosclerosis) becomes hard and narrows the artery, causing decreased blood supply and oxygen to the heart. Figure 4.1A shows a normal coronary artery with normal blood flow. Figure 4.1B shows a coronary artery with plaque buildup (atherosclerosis).

The risk factors for CAD include age, family history, tobacco abuse, HTN, dyslipidemia, diabetes, obesity, physical inactivity, male gender, and high stress (U.S. Department of Health & Human Services [HHS], 2011a). Although, not incorporated into risk models, chronic kidney disease is also considered a risk factor for CAD (Bonow et al., 2012). Older patients have many of these risk factors that increase their risk of CAD. In the United States, the typical cardiology patient is older with multiple comorbidities that are associated with increased age (Forman et al., 2011). The Framingham risk assessment score is a model that is used to predict a person at risk for coronary heart disease over the 10 years (Sheridan et al., 2003).

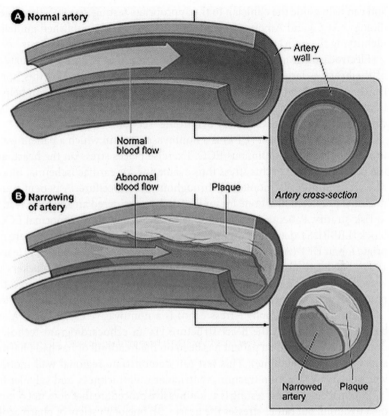

A Normal artery

Artery wall

Normal blood flow

Abnormal blood flow

Plaque

Artery cross-section

B Narrowing of artery

Narrowed artery   Plaque

FIGURE 4.1. Anatomic Changes with Arthero-Sclerosis. (From U.S. Department of Health & Human Services. [2011, June 1]. What is atherosclerosis? Retrieved from http://www.nhlbi.nih.gov/ health/health-topics/topics/atherosclerosis/)

Signs and Symptoms

The typical presentation of symptoms of CAD is angina. Angina is described as stable or unstable. Stable angina is described as poorly localized chest discomfort that is brought on by exertion or emotional stress. The symptoms are relieved within 5 to 10 minutes with rest or nitroglycerine taken sublingually. Unstable angina presents with at least one of the following: chest discomfort with minimal exertion or at rest and lasts 20 minutes or more unless given nitroglycerine or pain medications, patients describe chest pain that may be severe, and may have a crescendo pattern (HHS, 2011b). They may present with atypical symptoms that may include dyspnea, back or shoulder pain, fatigue, weakness, or epigastric discomfort. Some older patients may have no symptoms or are not able to identify symptoms owing to cognitive impairment (Bonow et al., 2012).

Cardiac Testing

Cardiac testing is used to help identify patients with CAD or identify those at risk for CAD. Testing includes invasive and noninvasive procedures. Patient history and physical exam is important and can help guide the clinician to the appropriate testing. In 2002, the American College of Cardiology (ACC) and American Heart Association (AHA) published guidelines for stress testing, identifying the indications as well as contraindications for specific tests.

Electrocardiogram (ECG) is a noninvasive test that is used to evaluate the electrical activity of the heart. A large amount of information can be obtained by this noninvasive test such as heart rate and rhythm, evidence of hypertrophy, pericarditis, and can help identify an ST elevation myocardial infarction (STEMI) or non-ST elevation myocardial infarction (NSTEMI) as discussed in the "Acute Coronary Syndrome" section.

Exercise tolerance test (ETT) is a noninvasive test in which a patient walks on a treadmill being monitored by a continuous ECG. Exercise places stress on the heart, and this test monitors the heart's response to this stress thus evaluating for cardiac ischemia. Blood pressure and heart rate are continuously monitored throughout the procedure. A patient must reach 85% of their maximal predicted heart rate for an ETT to be considered an adequate test. This test can be used to risk-stratify. Patients such as those with unstable angina, abnormal ECG (left bundle branch block [LBBB], ST depression at rest, or a paced rhythm), and severe AS are not considered appropriate for an ETT (American College of Cardiology [ACC], American Heart Association [AHA], 1997). Medications such as beta-blockers and calcium-channel blockers (CCB) may interfere with the interpretation of the test. Many older patients cannot undergo this testing because it requires a patient to walk on a treadmill and many are not physically able to do so.

Stress echocardiography (stress echo) is a noninvasive cardiac test. A stress echo includes a baseline evaluation of the heart structure via an echocardiogram (echo), and then another is done immediately after a patient has been on the treadmill or has had pharmacologically induced stress (usually dobutaime). This test can demonstrate regional wall motion abnormalities, left ventricular (LV) ejection fraction, ventricular wall thickness, and valvular function.

Pharmacologic stress testing is a noninvasive procedure that does not require the patient to walk on a treadmill but rather stresses the heart with one of a variety of pharmacologic agents. Myocardial perfusion imaging (MPI) is often done in conjunction with this testing (Henzlova et al., 2009).

MPI allows more accurate diagnosis of obstructive CAD than the ETT or stress testing alone. MPI is noninvasive but does require insertion of a radioactive tracer via an intravenous (IV) route. This allows visualization of coronary blood flow while the patient is at rest or after stress (treadmill or chemically induced). Images are taken by a nuclear medicine gamma camera. A positive test is one that shows reversible ischemia, which means a potential coronary blockage is present. This test can also determine LV ejection fraction, and can detect a scar from a previous MI. Unlike an ETT, the nuclear stress test can be used in patients with ECG abnormalities such as LBBB or who have a paced rhythm and is used in patients on beta-blockers, CCB, and digoxin. This test is particularly useful in older patients since there is no requirement to walk on the treadmill. Inadequate imaging can occur in patients with morbid obesity and in women with large breast tissue (Henzlova et al., 2009).

Cardiac magnetic resonance imaging (MRI) and cardiac computed tomography (CT) are newer advanced noninvasive procedures. Cardiac MRI is used to examine the heart's structure and function. Images are taken while the heart is beating and can be used in the diagnosis of conditions such as CAD, HF, valvular abnormalities, congenital heart defects, and cardiac tumors. Cardiac CT is used for evaluating coronary calcium, which can be an early sign of CAD (Henzlova et al., 2009).

Cardiac catheterization is an invasive procedure where dye is inserted into the coronary arteries while under fluoroscopy to assess for the presence of CAD as well as for overall cardiac function.

Acute Coronary Syndrome

Acute coronary syndrome (ACS) is often called "heart attack" and happens when there is an interruption of blood flow and, thus, oxygen to the coronary arteries. This can be complete blockage from plaque rupture or buildup.

Two percent of patients with ACS are misdiagnosed. This misdiagnosis leads to a twofold increase in mortality as compared with those patients who are admitted to the hospital. Many misdiagnosed patients are given noncardiac diagnosis such as abdominal viscera problems, musculoskeletal conditions, and psychological diagnosis. Chest pain may be an unreliable guide to diagnosis. As many as 33% of patients who have MI may not have chest pain (Panteghini, 2002). Misdiagnosis is particularly common in older persons.

ACS is broken into three types: STEMI, NSTEMI, and unstable angina (UA). Reeder and Kennedy (2011) discuss the diagnostic criteria for acute MI in the presence of rise and fall of cardiac biomarkers (CK-MB and troponin), which include the following:

- Ischemic symptoms
- ECG changes (ST elevation, depression, or new LBBB)
- Pathologic Q wave development on ECG
- Loss of viable myocardium or new wall motion abnormality as evidenced by imaging (Fig. 4.2)

Management of STEMI and NSTEMI

The ACC and AHA Guidelines for acute management of a STEMI that is diagnosed by ECG criteria (ST elevation, new left bundle branch, or true posterior MI wall pattern) is percutaneous coronary intervention (PCI). The recommended time for PCI is within 90 minutes of presentation, often referred to as "door to balloon time." PCI is a procedure that involves inflation of a balloon into a coronary artery to crush plaque that is built up inside the coronary artery and often involves stent placement, brachytherapy, and possibly athrectomy (Campbell-Scherer & Green, 2009). Rural hospitals may not have access to PCI nor be able to transfer patients quickly enough to a facility equipped to perform PCI; in those cases, fibrinolytics may be used for management.

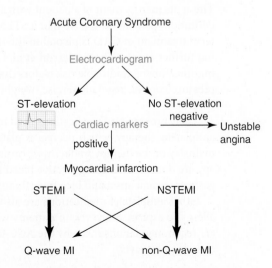

FIGURE 4.2. Algorithm for defining myocardial infarction. (From Alpert, J. S., Thygesen, K., Antman, E., & Bassand, J. P. [2000]. Myocardial infarction—A consensus document of the Joint European Society of Cardiology/American College of Cardiology committee for the redefinition of myocardial infarction. *Journal of the American College of Cardiology, 36*[3], 959–969, with permission.)

Fibrinolytics are also used in the acute management of a STEMI if PCI cannot be done within 90 minutes of presentation. Fibrinolytics cause clot dissolution and restore blood flow to the coronary artery. There are absolute contraindications to fibrinolytic therapy and some of those include history of intracranial hemorrhage, known structural cerebral lesions, malignant intracranial neoplasms, or active bleeding. Some relative contraindications also exist (ACC/AHA, 2009).

General treatment measures of STEMI include the following:

- Control of pain
  - Nitroglycerine
  - Analgesics (typically morphine)
  - Oxygen
  - Beta-adrenergic agents (beta-blockers)
- Antiplatelet therapy
- Anticoagulant therapy
- Statin therapy

NSTEMI and UA have the same general treatments of a STEMI that include control of pain via nitroglycerine, analgesics, oxygen, and beta-blockers and antiplatelet, anticoagulant, and statin therapies (Bonow et al., 2012). Finally, coronary artery bypass surgery (CABG) may be indicated in the treatment of CAD.

Older patients may present with nondiagnostic ECG changes. An estimated majority of STEMI (60% to 65%) occurs in patients aged 65 or older, and 80% of all deaths related to MI occur in patients aged 65 and older (Alexander et al., 2007). Morbidity and mortality from CAD increases with age, especially in patients aged 75 and older. Decisions regarding medical therapy versus PCI or CABG in the older person should be done on an individual basis. Consideration should include such considerations as the degree to which the CAD is affecting their overall health and function of the individual, the comorbidities and life expectancy of the individual, and the patient's preference regarding management (Bonow et al., 2012).

Coronary Artery Disease Management

The acute management of a patient with a STEMI, NSTEMI, or UA was discussed previously. By definition, patients who have had a STEMI, NSTEMI, or UA have established CAD. The long-term treatment of CAD is pivotal in the management of these patients with the aim of preventing further events. The Anderson et al. (2007) recommendations for the management include modification of modifiable risk factors that include smoking cessation, cholesterol control, blood pressure control, regular exercise, weight control, stress control, and, if diabetic, tight glucose control.

There are standard medications used in the long-term management of patients with CAD: In antiplatelet therapy, which decreases platelet aggregation and thrombus formation, aspirin is a mainstay of the therapy to decrease thrombus formation. The contraindications to aspirin therapy are documented allergy, active bleeding, or a platelet disorder. Potential side effects include gastrointestinal upset and bleeding (Bonow et al., 2012).

Other antiplatelet medications are also available. They may be prescribed if patients have an allergy to aspirin. However, in patients with STEMI, NSTEMI, PCI, and coronary stents, there are recommendations made by the ACC for dual antiplatelet therapy (Kushner et al., 2009) with clopidogrel (Plavix).

Beta-blockers are used to relax the blood vessels and have antiarrhythmic, antiremodeling, anti-ischemic, and antiapoptotic properties. In addition, they decrease the heart rate, and cause a decrease in myocardial oxygen consumption. Potential side effects include severe bronchospasm, hypotension, bradycardia, fatigue, worsening depression, and potentially increased blood glucose (Hobbs & Boyle, 2010). Unless contraindicated, beta-blockers should be prescribed in patients with CAD.

CCB cause vasodilation of blood vessels and decreased workload on the heart. They are effective for vasospastic syndrome. CCB are divided into two groups: dihydropyridines and non-dihydropyridines. The dihydropyridines are considered to be more potent vasodilators than nondihydropyridines. Beta-blockers are preferred over CCB for stable angina; however, when beta-blockers are not effective or a patient has side effects, CCB may be used. Combination therapy of beta-blockers and CCB is sometimes used if patients do not have symptom relief with beta-blockers or for patients with coronary spasm (Fraker & Fihn, 2007). Some potential side effects of CCB include bradycardia, constipation, worsening HF, and pedal edema.

Angiotensin-converting enzymes (ACE) inhibitors are considered the cornerstone of HF therapy related to systolic dysfunction. This includes patients with HF following MI (Gring & Francis, 2004). ACE inhibitors have been shown to decrease mortality and encourage remodeling (Gring & Francis, 2004; Strippoli et al., 2004).

Angiotensin receptor blockers (ARBs) have somewhat different indications for use. At times they are prescribed in patients who are on an ACE inhibitor owing to the phenomenon of ACE-escape, which results in steady increase of the serum angiotensin II and aldosterone levels, even though ACE inhibitors are being used to cause renin-angiotensin aldosterone system (RAAS) inhibition. Other indications for the use of ARBs are for more specific angiotensin II blockade, preservation of unopposed angiotensin II agonism, and for patients who cannot take ACE inhibitor owing to allergy (Gring & Francis, 2004).

ACE inhibitors and ARBs have been proven to delay the progression of diabetic nephropathy (Strippoli et al., 2004). They have potential side effects that include hyperkalemia; this is a particular problem in patients aged 75 years and older because much of the increased incidence of renal dysfunction takes place in that population (Strippoli et al., 2004). Up to 25% of patients who take ACE inhibitors develop a dry cough (Simon et al., 1992). Two uncommon side effects but important to keep in mind with ACE inhibitors are angioedema and acute renal failure (usually caused by bilateral renal artery stenosis); both require discontinuation of the drug (Hobbs & Boyle, 2010).

Nitrates decrease myocardial oxygen demand by their vasodilatory effect. They are used in the acute treatment of STEMI, NSTEMI, UA, and chronic angina. The most common side effects of this medication are hypotension and headache (Fraker & Fihn, 2007).

Ranexa is used to treat angina. The exact mechanism of action is unknown, but it appears to improve blood flow. It should be reserved for patients who have not achieved symptom relief with other antianginal medications. Some common reactions to ranexa include constipation, nausea, and dizziness. QT prolongation also can occur, and it should not be given to patients who have a preexisting QT prolongation, with other medications that can cause QT prolongation, or to patients with liver impairment (Antonopoulos et al., 2007).

Statin therapy has shown to reduce first cardiovascular events and recurrent events. Statins are also used in the treatment of ACS (Murphy et al., 2009). The most common side effect of statins is myopathy (Sinzinger et al., 2002). In addition, 0.5% to 2.0% of patients on statin have elevated hepatic transaminases; this is a dose-dependent phenomenon (Cleeman et al., 2002). Patients who complain of myalgia or myopathy should have a total creatine kinase drawn and, if elevated, statin use may need to be reconsidered. Also, other medications that could interact with statin medications should be considered (Sinzinger et al., 2002).

Although medications are needed in the treatment of CAD, considerations in the older patients exist. Metabolism, absorption, and excretion may be altered in the patients owing to age-related changes. Many of these patients have multiple comorbidities and are on multiple medications, so drug-to-drug interactions should also be considered (Forman et al., 2011).

Summary

CVD is an insidious process that affects many people but has an increased burden when older. CVD is the leading cause of mortality in both men and women over the age of 65. Data have shown that treatment of CVD improves morbidity and mortality in older patients up to age 74; however, limited data exist regarding patients 75 years and older. Age-related changes impact the presence of CVD (Bonow et al., 2012).

CAD is the most common type of CVD and is the leading cause of death in the United States. The severity and prevalence increase with age in both men and women and by the age of 80, symptomatic CAD is present in 20% to 30% of people (Bonow et al., 2012). Plaque buildup becomes hard and narrows the artery, causing decreased blood supply and oxygen to the heart. This can lead to myocardial ischemia and MI. Typical presentation of symptoms of CAD present as angina. Angina is described as stable or unstable. Older patients may present with atypical symptoms, have no symptoms at all, or may not be able to identify symptoms owing to mental impairment (Bonow et al., 2012).

Risk factors that increase the risk for CAD were described, and it is imperative to remember that many older patients have many of these risk factors present. The typical cardiology patient in the United Stated is older with multiple comorbidities that are associated with increased age (Forman et al., 2011).

Specific criteria exist for the identification and management of ACS and CAD. Older patients may present with nondiagnostic ECG changes. Estimated majorities of STEMI (60% to 65%) occur in patients aged 65 or older, and 80% of all deaths related to MI occur in patients aged 65 and older (Alexander et al., 2007).

Cardiac testing involves both invasive and noninvasive procedure. A careful history should be taken from all patients, and providers should be aware of the different tests that can be done to evaluate for cardiac problems.

Older adult patients should have special consideration with regard to the management of CVD owing to age-related changes that may affect the metabolism, absorption, and excretion of medications. Drug-to-drug interactions should also be considered owing to multiple comorbidities that exist with older persons. These may also require medications for management (Forman et al., 2011).

HEART FAILURE

HF is a chronic health condition that affects nearly 5 million people in the United States, and approximately 550,000 new cases are diagnosed each year (White et al., 2010). HF is a terminal diagnosis and is not curable but the symptoms can be managed. HF is associated with poor quality of life, recurrent hospital readmissions, increased cost of care, disability, and early mortality (Kleinpell & Avitall, 2005).

In the United States, HF is the leading readmission diagnosis for patients over the age of 65 (Phillips et al., 2004). Complex care for HF patients includes medication management and extensive education about the importance of proper diet, regular exercise, symptom management, and fluid monitoring. This complex care of HF places financial burdens on our health-care system and consumes approximately 60% of the Medicare budget (Phillips et al., 2004). This chapter will discuss the different types, classes, signs and symptoms, diagnostic tests, and management of HF.

Types of Heart Failure

Many types of HF are described. Left-sided HF, which includes systolic and diastolic, is the most common form that results in LV dysfunction. LV dysfunction can be caused by many different conditions or exposures such as CAD, valvular disease, HTN, neurologic diseases, metabolic problems, heavy metals (iron), viruses (myocarditis), inherited diseases, connective tissue diseases (lupus), and drugs (cocaine) (Bullock, 1996).

Systolic HF is also known as heart failure with low ejection fraction (HFLEF). Systolic HF account for 60% of all HF and is present in patients with ejection fraction (EF) less than 50%. Systolic HF is primarily a problem with backward flow. The LV output is less than the total volume of blood received (Bullock, 1996). Systolic HF is common in patients with known CAD who have suffered an MI. The estimated annual mortality rate of patients with systolic HF is 10% to 15% (Dhar et al., 2008).

Diastolic HF is also known as heart failure with normal ejection fraction (HFNEF). Abnormal filling pressures and altered ventricular relaxation result in an elevated left ventricular end diastolic pressure (LVEDP), which is diagnostic of diastolic HF (Zile & Colucci, 2011). The incidence of diastolic HF increases with age, and the most commonly affected are women. The common medical conditions that are associated with diastolic HF include diabetes mellitus, renal dysfunction, HTN, myocardial ischemia, and left ventricular hypertrophy (LVH). The annual mortality rate associated with diastolic HF is 5% to 8% (Dhar et al., 2008). What is important to keep in mind is that diastolic HF may be a precursor of systolic HF (Paulus et al., 2007).

Diagnosis of Heart Failure

Systolic HF and its diagnosis have been validated in the literature and can be diagnosed by the following tests: cardiac catheterization, echocardiogram with tissue Doppler, brain natriuretic peptide (BNP), cardiac nuclear stress testing, and cardiac MRI. Systolic HF is diagnosed when systolic dysfunction is confirmed, and the EF is determined to be less than 50% (Kumar et al., 2006).

To confirm the presence of mildly decreased or normal systolic function or evidence of diastolic dysfunction, several different diagnosis procedures can be done: cardiac catheterization, echocardiogram with tissue Doppler, BNP, and cardiac MRI (Paulus et al., 2007). Although all the above tests can be used to determine diastolic HF, the gold standard and least invasive test is the echocardiogram with tissue Doppler.

According to Paulus and his colleagues (2007), diastolic HF has three essential stipulations that should be met for the diagnosis, which is given below:

- Signs and symptoms of HF must be present (crackles on exam, pulmonary edema, peripheral edema, dyspnea on exertion, and fatigue)
- Presence of normal or mildly decreased systolic function (EF 50% or less)
- Evidence of diastolic dysfunction

Classes of Heart Failure

Activity tolerance is an important indication of the HF class. Asking patients about their normal activity level is important. The New York Heart Association (NYHA) classification for HF was established and is important to understand (Hunt et al., 2009). This is a subjective system for the identification of patient HF class and can change on the basis of symptoms.

Class I: no symptoms with activity
Class II: symptoms with normal activity
Class III: shortness of breath with less than usual activity
Class IV: shortness of breath at rest or with little exertion

Stages of Heart Failure

The ACC and AHA developed a classification of HF based on stages (Table 4.2) in 2005.

Signs and Symptoms

The signs and symptoms of systolic HF include dyspnea (at rest or on exertion), fatigue, peripheral edema, orthopnea, paroxysmal nocturnal dyspnea (PND), nausea, crackles on lung exam, jugular venous distension, and S3 or S4 on auscultation (Trochelman et al., 2010). Muscle fatigue is common in systolic HF owing to decreased cardiac output, abnormalities of skeletal muscle metabolism, and deficient vasodilator capacity (Paulus et al., 2007).

Diastolic HF signs and symptoms are similar to those of systolic HF; however, they may come on slowly and thus may be somewhat harder to recognize. The chief presenting complaint of diastolic HF is dyspnea, but often with no other initial signs of clinical HF such as peripheral edema or pulmonary edema (Paulus et al., 2007).

Medication Management of Heart Failure

Many medications used for HF improve symptoms, but have not proven to have any effect on mortality. Diuretics have been shown to improve symptoms, but there is limited data on the long-term benefits and mortality (Faris et al., 2006; Hobbs & Boyle, 2010). According to CHF guidelines published by the Heart Failure Society of America, diuretics are first-line therapy in the treatment of CHF (Congestive Heart Failure) (Colucci, 2009). A meta-analysis by Faris et al. (2006) reviewed 14 clinical trials that revealed that participants who were treated with diuretics had reduced readmission rates (OR = 0.7, P = .01, in 2 clinical trials) and improvement of exercise capacity (OR = 0.72, $P < $ .001, in 4 trials); the participants in the control group were treated with placebo.

The accumulation of fluid/extra volume in HF patients causes shortness of breath; diuretics can relieve these symptoms more quickly than any other medication for HF. The most common type of diuretics used for decompensated HF are loop diuretics; however, thiazide diuretics may also be added for patients with resistant symptoms (Faris et al., 2006; Hobbs & Boyle, 2010; Sterns & Colucci, 2010). Decompensated HF patients may require hospitalization and IV diuretics owing to symptoms related to mucosal edema and decreased intestinal perfusion. Once the patient's HF is compensated, they may be changed to oral diuretics. The effective dose of diuretics in patients with HF is higher than in patients without HF (Brater, 2000).

Although diuretics are used daily for the treatment of HF and considered a mainstay of treatment, they are not without concerns. Orthostatic hypotension, hypokalemia, metabolic alkalosis, elevation of neurohormone levels, cardiorenal syndrome, resistance to therapy, and worsening renal

TABLE 4.2 · Classification of Heart Failure Stages

Stage	Incidence in the United States	Symptoms	Findings	Goal of Treatment
Stage A	60 million	Patients at risk for developing HF includes patients with diabetes mellitus, hypertension, cardiotoxin exposure, history of rheumatic fever, and hemochromatosis	No structural heart disease	The goal is to decrease the risk of progression
Stage B	32.6 million	Asymptomatic heart disease	Decreased LV ejection fraction, LVH, regional wall motion abnormality, or valve disorder	The goal is prevention of LV remodeling
Stage C	6.2 million	Symptomatic HF	Structural heart disease, dyspnea, fatigue, and impaired exercise tolerance	The goal is medication adjustment to help with symptoms. CRT also may be considered
Stage D	200,000	Severe refractory HF	End-of-life care or high-technology therapies such as cardiac transplantation or mechanical circulatory support, based on individual cases	The goal is symptom management

From the ACC/AHA classification of chronic heart failure, Hunt, S. A., Abraham, W. T., Chin, M. H., Feldman, A. M., Francis, G. S., Ganiats, T. G., ... Yancy, C. W. (2009). 2009 focused update incorporated into the American College of Cardiology/American Heart Association 2005 Guidelines for the diagnosis and management of heart failure in adults: A report of the American College of Cardiology Foundation/American Heart Association Task Force on Practice Guidelines: Developed in collaboration with the International Society for Heart and Lung Transplantation. *Circulation, 119*(14), e391–e479.

function can occur (Hobbs & Boyle, 2010; Sterns & Colucci, 2010). Owing to these potential side effects, the importance of regular monitoring of labs such as a basic metabolic panel is imperative.

Nitrates are another medication that can be used for symptom relief of HF. The most beneficial use of nitrates is when added to diuretics. Nitroglycerine is the most commonly used nitrate. Nitroglycerine causes venodilation and thus decreases LV filling pressure (Colucci, 2011). The most common side effects of this medication are hypotension and headache. Although the use of nitrate alone has not shown any reduction in mortality, the use of nitrates plus hydralazine provides symptomatic relief and reduces mortality benefit in selected patients with systolic HF.

The use of hydralazine plus oral nitrate therapy is recommended for patients with persistent NYHA class III to IV HF and LVEF less than 40% and/or those who exhibit contraindications to ACE inhibitors and ARBs owing to renal insufficiency (Colucci, 2009; Falvey & Blaxall, 2009). Nitrates should be avoided within 24 hours of a patient's use of the phosphodiesterase inhibitors. In addition, the clinician should consider holding nitrates if systolic blood pressure is less than 90 mm Hg to avoid syncope. Finally, it is important to note that nitrate tolerance can occur (Colucci, 2011).

Digoxin has been used for over 200 years in the treatment of HF. However, there is no literature to suggest that it improves survival. Digoxin can be beneficial in patients with systolic HF and has shown a decrease in the rate of admission for these patients. Digoxin is recommended for patients with EF less than 40% and who continue to have NYHA functional class II, III, and IV symptoms even with optimal therapy. Literature suggests that maintaining digoxin levels between 0.5 and 0.8 ng/ml in both men and women will decrease the likelihood of toxicity. Bradycardia, anorexia, nausea, and dizziness can be seen in patients who have digoxin toxicity (Colucci, 2009).

ACE inhibitors are considered the cornerstone of HF therapy related to systolic dysfunction and post-MI (Gring & Francis, 2004). ACE inhibitors have been shown to decrease mortality and promote remodeling (Gring & Francis, 2004; Strippol et al., 2004). A meta-analysis by Shekelle et al. (2003) of six different studies of ACE inhibitors found that patients with LV systolic dysfunction have a reduced rate of all-cause mortality when ACE inhibitors are used. Thus, ACE inhibitors are the most important antagonist of the RAAS and are prescribed routinely in patients with HF and reduced LV systolic function (Gring & Francis, 2004).

ARBs have different validations for use. Often they are prescribed in patients who are already on ACE inhibitors owing to the phenomenon of ACE-escape, which results in steady increase of the serum angiotensin II and aldosterone levels, even though ACE inhibitors are being used to cause RAAS inhibition. Other reasons for the use of ARBs are for more specific angiotensin II blockade, preservation of unopposed angiotensin II agonism, and for patients who cannot take ACE owing to allergy or intolerance (Gring & Francis, 2004).

ACE inhibitors and ARBs have been proven to delay the progression of diabetic nephropathy (Strippoli et al., 2004). They also have potential side effects that include hyperkalemia, especially in patients 75 years and older, usually as a result of renal dysfunction (Strippoli et al., 2004). As mentioned earlier, a dry cough may develop in up to 25% of patients who take ACE inhibitors (Simon et al., 1992). Two uncommon side effects but that need to to be kept in mind with ACE inhibitors are angioedema and acute renal failure (caused by bilateral renal artery stenosis); both require discontinuation of the drug (Hobbs & Boyle, 2010).

Statins have been shown to have benefits in patients with HF regardless of atherosclerosis or lipid levels. They have pleiotropic effects that include inhibition of inflammatory cytokines, improvement in endothelial function, repair of damaged autonomic function, potentiation of nitric oxide synthesis, and reversal of myocardial remodeling (Horwich et al., 2004). The most common side effect of statins is myopathy (Sinzinger et al., 2002). In addition, 0.5% to 2.0% of patients on statin have elevated hepatic transaminases. Both side adverse effects are dose-dependent (Cleeman et al., 2002). Baseline liver function test should be obtained before initiation of statin therapy and then again every 3 months to ensure there is no increase in hepatic transaminase levels (Murphy, 2011). For patients who complain of myalgias or myopathy, a total creatine kinase can be drawn, and if elevated, statin use may need to be reconsidered. Finally, the clinician should be on the lookout for drug-to-drug interactions when prescribing statins (Sinzinger et al., 2002).

Aldosterone agonists prevent sodium and water retention, endothelial dysfunction, and myocardial fibrosis. Spironolactone and eplerenone are two aldosterone agonists that are approved for HF. Spironolactone has a 30% decrease in hospitalization and mortality when added to standard therapy in patients with NYHA class III or IV and a serum creatine less than 2.5. Eplerenone has shown a 15% decrease in hospitalization and risk of death in patients with HF after an MI and EF less than 40%. A potential side effect of these medications is hyperkalemia, so these medications should be avoided in patients with creatinine greater than 2.5. Also, gynecomastia is reported in 8% of patients who take spironolactone, and hirsutism is a potential side effect (Hobbs & Boyle, 2010).

Beta-blockers improve survival in patients with HF, although the precise mechanism of action is unknown. It is suspected to be due to one or more of antiarrhythmic, antiremodeling, anti-ischemic, and antiapoptotic properties, a decrease in heart rate, and a decrease in myocardial oxygen consumption. Potential side effects include severe bronchospasm, hypotension, bradycardia, fatigue, worsening depression, and potentially increase blood glucose (Hobbs & Boyle, 2010).

Inotropes that are used in the treatment of acute decompensated HF are divided into two types: beta-adrenergic agonists and phosphodiesterase-III inhibitors. These are IV medications most often administered in the hospital setting. Each type works differently, but the overall goal is to temporarily improve heart function and cardiac output, thus temporarily improving the patient's symptoms from HF. Inotropes have a risk of irregular heart rhythm and increased demand for oxygen by the heart. These medications should only be used in severe cases of symptomatic HF with evident hypoperfusion (Peterson & Felker, 2008).

Vasopressin antagonists cause arterial and venous vasodilation, thus leading to an increase in cardiac output through afterload reduction. Vasopressin antagonists are IV medications, and the dose is calculated by weight and is used for patients with acute decompensated HF (Hobbs & Boyle, 2010). Natrecor was a popular drug in this class of medications for use in HF in 2004. However, in 2006, questions arose about its safety in renal patients and was found to have a high rate of mortality in these patients. Although natrecor is still in use, it has been recommended that more studies need to be conducted regarding the safety and efficacy of this medication (Kesselheim et al., 2006). There are other vasopressin antagonists that may be considered if a patient with acute decompensated HF cannot get symptom relief with IV loop diuretics.

Device Therapy for Heart Failure

Cardiac resynchronization therapy (CRT), implantable cardioverter defibrillator (ICD), and ventricular assist device (VAD) are devices that can be used in HF patients. CRT improves ventricular contraction, ventricular reverse-remodeling, and reduces mitral regurgitation. Approximately 70% of patients have symptomatic improvement with CRT therapy (Hobbs & Boyle, 2010). Current ACC criteria, discussed by Leclercq (2007), that should be met for CRT to be considered are given below:

- NYHA class III or IV HF symptoms
- Despite medications continues to be symptomatic
- EF less than or equal to 35%
- Wide QRS greater than 120 msec; intraventricular conduction delay; LBBB
- Evidence of dyssynchrony

An ICD is recommended for patients at risk for sudden death due to ventricular arrhythmias and has been shown to be superior to antiarrhythmic medications. Estimates suggest that 50% of HF patients die from sudden death. CRT can be combined with an ICD in one device if the patient meets the criteria for both therapies, as is often the case. ACC guidelines recommend a 40-day waiting period after an acute MI, coronary stenting, or bypass surgery prior to ICD implantation. Recommended guidelines for ICDs published by the ACC in 2008 (Diagnostic and Interventional Cardiology, 2008) are given below:

- LVEF less than 35% with ischemic cardiomyopathy
- LVEF less than 35% and symptomatic with dilated cardiomyopathy
- Survivor of cardiac arrest
- Sustained ventricular tachycardia
- Inducible ventricular tachycardia

VAD therapy is used for NYHA class III or IV HF to increase cardiac output and to thus reduce HF symptoms. This device is a mechanical pump that is implanted into the weak ventricle of the heart to help pump blood throughout the body. VAD can be used as a bridge to transplant or may be used long-term (Samala et al., 2011).

Surgical Therapy for Heart Failure

Surgical options that are available for HF patients include cardiac support device, LV reconstructive surgery, mitral valve replacement, aortic valve replacement, and cardiac transplantation. A cardiac support device uses mesh to create and support the heart and recreates the elliptical shape of the heart and is designed to resist or reverse cardiac remodeling. Indications are NYHA class III or IV patients and the improvements in cardiac size and shape last for several years (Dua et al., 2011; Stiles, 2007).

LV reconstruction surgery is done to remove scar tissue and/or an aneurysm. To restore the left ventricle to normal shape or as close as possible to the normal shape, scarred or dead tissue is removed from the LV, and healthy tissue is sewn back together. The goal of this surgical procedure is to decrease HF symptoms and improve the pumping ability of the heart (Dor et al., 2004).

Mitral valve replacement is performed when there is mitral valve stenosis to ensure adequate blood flow to the LV or for mitral valve regurgitation to prevent blood from flowing back into the left atrium and back up into the lungs. The replacement of the mitral valve helps with the symptoms of HF and general improvement of LV function (Gangemi & Hicks, 2009).

When there is aortic insufficiency, regurgitation, or AS, the aortic valve is often replaced (Gangemi & Hicks, 2009). This can be done via an open heart procedure or a less invasive catheter-based approach called percutaneous aortic valve replacement. This is a new procedure and is done at a few selected heart centers in the United States and Europe. Aortic valve replacement can lead to improved LV function and reduction or resolution of HF symptoms (Dua et al., 2011).

Cardiac transplantation is currently performed in approximately 1% of patients with HF. This procedure is considered for patients with NYHA class III and IV HF, EF less than 25%, all medical therapy has failed, all other surgical options have been excluded because of the heart's poor condition, and the patient has a prognosis of less than a year to live without transplant (Botta, 2011).

Consideration should be given on a case-by-case basis for frail older adults prior to invasive therapies. Survival benefit, comorbidities, functional status, and consideration for social support should be considered when evaluating for the appropriateness of invasive interventions (Samala et al., 2011).

Palliative Medicine

HF is considered a terminal disease, and identification of patients with advanced or end-stage HF (stages C and D) is an important role of clinicians. Some patients with HF may not be candidates for device or surgical intervention, have undergone device or surgical intervention and symptoms persist, or chose not to undergo device or surgical therapy. These patients have obvious symptoms of fatigue and dyspnea with minimal exertion. Collaboration between clinicians can provide the best comprehensive care. However, despite maximal medical therapy, HF symptoms will continue to advance and focus should be on symptom management and end-of-life care.

Advanced or end-stage HF symptom management can be challenging because clinicians often lack expertise. Palliative care physicians are experts in symptom management and are comfortable

TABLE 4.3 · Approach to Older Patients with Heart Failure

1. Signs and symptoms may be nonspecific such as fatigue, intolerance of exercise, or dyspnea.
2. Serum biomarkers such as BNP or echocardiogram are helpful in the diagnosis of HF.
3. Diastolic HF is often present in older women and patients with diabetes.
4. Improvement in HF outcomes may be received from aggressive treatment of hypertension and diabetes.
5. Improving quality of life and morbidity with the treatment of blood pressure control, treatment of ischemia, AF rate control, and encouraging physical activity.
6. Age adjustment for medications, disease-related changes in kinetics.
7. Educate patient, family, and caregivers in HF management (daily weight, medication, and dietary compliance).
8. Multidisciplinary team approach (cardiologist, nurse practitioner, dietician, cardiac rehabilitation, diabetic education, and palliative medicine).

Adapted from Bonow, R. O., Mann, D. L., Zipes, D. P., & Libby, P. (2012). *Braunwald's Heart Disease* (9th ed.). Philadelphia, PA: Elsevier, with permission.

with end-of-life care. Table 4.3 discusses common threads and approaches for the clinician assessing older adults with HF.

Summary

HF is a debilitating progressive disease whose incidence will continue to rise as the population continues to age (Phillips et al., 2004). Early diagnosis and treatment as well as appropriate management may improve quality of life, reduce hospital admissions, and slow the rate of mortality (Shamsham & Mitchell, 2000).

Treatment of HF starts with medications, some of which increase survival and others that help with symptom management. Device therapy may be used in addition to medications for the treatment and management of this debilitating disease. Surgical options are also available for HF treatment. Ultimately, HF is a terminal diagnosis, and focus on symptom control will be the goal of management.

ATRIAL FIBRILLATION

AF is a common rhythm disturbance whose prevalence increases with increasing age and affects approximately 2.2 million people in the United States. AF incidence doubles after each decade starting at the age of 60. It is estimated that 8% to 10% of patients between the ages of 80 and 89 will have AF (Bonow et al., 2012).

Pathophysiology of Atrial Fibrillation

In the normal heart, during each heart beat the atria contract, and this is followed by ventricular contraction. These contractions are regulated by the electrical conduction system of the heart. Normally in sinus rhythm, the electrical impulse through the heart is as follows:

Originates in the sinoatrial (SA) node (located in the right atrium) → atrioventricular (AV) node (located between the atrial and ventricles) → impulse is conducted to the bundle of His → branches to the right and left bundle branches → Purkinje fibers.

In patients with AF, the SA node is not directing the electrical rhythm. Instead, there are many different impulses that may be fast, disorganized, and firing all at once. Because of this chaos, the atria cannot contract effectively, resulting in inefficient transmission of blood into the ventricles. Subsequently, the ventricles contract irregularly, leading to an irregular heartbeat. AF can cause stasis of blood in the atria. This increases the risk of thrombus (clot) formation in the atria, which can be dislodged and cause stroke.

Classification of Atrial Fibrillation

AF is classified as paroxysmal, persistent, or permanent.

Paroxysmal: Two or more episodes of AF that spontaneously stop within 7 days of onset.
Persistent: AF events last more than 7 days. These events may necessitate pharmacologic or electrical intervention (electrical cardioversion).
Permanent: AF that is persistent for more than 1 year despite cardioversion (pharmacologic or electrical) or neither has been attempted.

Medical Conditions Associated with Atrial Fibrillation

Many common medical conditions in the older adult are associated with AF, which include CAD, hypertensive heart disease, valvular heart disease, HF, cardiomyopathy, endocrine disorders, and heart valve disease (Bonow et al., 2012).

AF increases a person's risk for ischemic stroke. Stroke is the third leading cause of death and the leading cause of disability in the United States (Virginia Department of Health [VDH], 2005). Approximately 15% of ischemic strokes are secondary to AF. Owing to the risk of stroke with AF and the incidence of other risk factors for stroke in the older patient, the focus is on the management of the common conditions associated with AF, rate control, and anticoagulation (Bonow et al., 2012). "The prevalence of AF is strongly associated with increasing age, rising to 5% in people older than 65 years and nearly 10% in those ages 80 years" (Font et al., 2011).

Signs and Symptoms of Atrial Fibrillation

Many patients with AF are asymptomatic. However, with patients who are symptomatic, the history should focus on date of onset, duration, frequency, and precipitating factors. Symptoms for AF can vary. Some patients are asymptomatic; those who have symptoms complain of palpitations, dizziness, tachycardia, and decreased exercise tolerance.

Diagnosis of Atrial Fibrillation

An ECG should be done to confirm the diagnosis of AF. The following ECG findings are representative of AF: substitution of P waves by fibrillating waves that may vary in shape, timing, amplitude, and irregular ventricular response (Fig. 4.3).

Further evaluation should be done for the patient with AF. An echocardiogram can provide the clinician with valuable information. The echocardiogram can identify the potential cause of the AF such as valvular disease (Fuster et al., 2011) and can also demonstrate the presence of or risk for atrial thrombosis. Evaluation for CAD being responsible for AF should also be considered and done via a stress test or potentially heart catheterization if indicated.

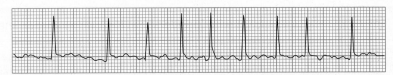

FIGURE 4.3. Rhythm strip of atrial fibrillation. (From Goodacre, S., & Irons, R. [2002]. ABC of clinical electrocardiography: Atrial arrhythmias. *British Medical Journal, 324* [7337], 594–597, with permission.)

Management of Atrial Fibrillation

In older patients, rate control instead of the maintenance of sinus rhythm may be a reasonable option; this, however, depends on symptoms (Fuster et al., 2011). The three main goals in the management of AF are return to sinus rhythm, rate control, and anticoagulation. Medications that can be used for the management of AF include antiarrhythmics to return or to maintain sinus rhythm, or rate control medications such as beta-blockers, non-dihydropyridine CCB, and digoxin. Anticoagulation is an important part of medical management of AF. When considering anticoagulation, the Cardiac Failure, Hypertension, Age (Doubled), Diabetes, Stroke (Doubled), Vascular disease, Age and Sex (CHA$_2$DS$_2$-VASc) classification system should be used (Table 4.4).

The CHA$_2$DS$_2$-VASc classification is a points system that estimates the patient's risk for stroke in patients with nonrheumatic AF. This points system can also be used to determine whether treatment is required with anticoagulation or antiplatelet therapy. Gage and colleagues (2004) addressed this therapy as outlined in Table 4.5.

Several anticoagulants exist today (warfarin, dabigatran, and rivaroxaban). Each patient with AF should be considered for anticoagulation unless there is a contraindication or risk outweighs the benefits. The main risk of all of the anticoagulants is bleeding. The warfarin dose can be monitored and appropriately adjusted by using the prothrombin time and international normalized ratio (PT/INR). As with many medications, this necessitates responsibility of the patient and

TABLE 4.4 · Vascular Disease Classification System

	Condition	Point Value
C	Congestive HF or LV dysfunction	1
H	Hypertension (this includes controlled hypertension on medication)	1
A$_2$	Age ≥75	2
D	Diabetes mellitus	1
S$_2$	Prior stroke or TIA or thromboembolism	2
V	Vascular disease	1
A	Age 65–74	1
Sc	Sex category (female gender confers higher risk)	1

From Fuster, V., Ryden, L. E., Cannom, D. S., Crijns, H. J., Curtis, A. B., Ellenbogen, K. A., … Wann, L. S. (2011). 2011 ACCF/AHA/HRS focused updates incorporated into the AC/AHA/ESC 2006 guidelines for the management of patients with atrial fibrillation: A report of the American College of Cardiology Foundation/American Heart Association Task Force on practice guidelines developed in partnership with the European Society of Cardiology and in collaboration with the European Heart Rhythm Association and the Heart Rhythm Society. *Journal of the American College of Cardiology, 57*(11), e101–e198, with permission.

TABLE 4.5 · Treatment Considerations for Anticoagulation Therapy with AF

Score	Stroke Risk	Anticoagulation Therapy	Considerations
0	Low	No antithrombotic therapy (or aspirin)	No antithrombotic therapy (or aspirin 75–325 mg daily)
1	Moderate	Oral anticoagulation or aspirin	Oral anticoagulation with anticoagulant
2 or greater	Moderate or high	Anticoagulation	Unless contraindications, use oral anticoagulants and if coumadin is used, then keep INR 2.0–3.0

From Gage, B. F., van Walraven, C., Pearce, L., Hart, R. G., Koudstall, P. J., Boode, B. S., & Petersen, P. (2004). Selecting patient with atrial fibrillation for anticoagulation: Stroke risk stratification in patients taking aspirin. *Circulation, 110*(16), 2287–2292.

provider. Patients who are not capable of compliance with medication (dementia, psychosis, etc.), with the frequent need for PT/INR, or do not have a caregiver who can be responsible would not be considered good candidates for coumadin. Although older patients are considered high risk for stroke due to AF, these patients may also have frequent falls that could result in serious bleeding if on an anticoagulant, so it is imperative that the benefits outweigh the risk of the medication.

When the restoration of sinus rhythm is warranted and cannot be obtained with medications, there are procedures that can be performed that can restore sinus rhythm, and these include the following:

Electrical cardioversion: An electrical shock to restore sinus rhythm.

Ablation: Done to destroy or scar the tissue in the heart that causes the AF.

Pacemaker: A small device implanted under the skin that may be used to set a pace and normalize the heart rhythm.

Surgery: This is done only on patients who have not responded to other treatments for AF and have severe symptoms. The "maze" procedure is usually done during bypass or valve repair or replacement. The surgeon makes multiple incisions into the atria and ultimately creates scar tissue that does not conduct electrical activity, resulting in a blockage of the abnormal electrical impulses that cause the AF. The scar created causes the electrical impulses to go through a structured pathway to the ventricles. This is called the "maze" because the incisions made into the atria are in a mazelike pattern.

Summary

AF is a common rhythm disturbance in the older patient. Treatment should be focused on rate control, return to sinus rhythm, and anticoagulation. Depending on symptoms, rate control may be a reasonable option (Fuster et al., 2011). Medications such as antiarrhythmics, beta-blockers, nondihydropyridine CCB, and digoxin can be prescribed for the maintenance of sinus rhythm or rate control. Anticoagulation should be considered for patients with AF and the CHA_2DS_2-VASc classification system can be used for patients with nonvalvular AF to assess patients' risk for stroke and whether treatment is required with anticoagulation or antiplatelet therapy (Gage et al., 2004). The older patients with AF are considered to be at high risk for stroke, so anticoagulation should be considered once the clinician determines that the risk outweighs the benefit. When the return of sinus rhythm is clinically indicated and has not been able to be obtained with medications, other options such as electrical cardioversion, ablation, pacemaker, or surgery may be considered.

AORTIC VALVE STENOSIS

AS is a valvular condition that leads to a narrowing that obstructs blood flow to the heart, aorta, and thus the rest of the body. AS causes the heart to work harder, and over time this leads to weakening of the heart. Approximately 50% of patients with severe AS have CAD (Bonow et al., 2012).

Aortic sclerosis is a condition where patients have mild aortic calcification and the aortic valve leaflets are stiff. Many of the same risk factors for CAD (diabetes, HTN, dyslipidemia, and advanced age) are associated with aortic valve sclerosis (Otto, 2004). Aortic valve sclerosis is present in approximately 30% of older patients, and the prevalence increases with age. Risk factors that increase the development from aortic sclerosis to AS to aortic sclerosis include bicuspid aortic valve, HTN, diabetes, dyslipidemia, smoking, and end-stage renal disease (Bonow et al., 2012).

Aortic sclerosis is classified as acquired or congenital. Acquired AS happens when there is calcification of the valve leaflets. The calcification causes narrowing of the aortic valve opening. AS occurs in approximately 16% of patients aged 65 and older and is described as mild, moderate, or severe (Bonow et al., 2012). Rheumatic fever that results from a group A streptococcal bacteria can also cause damage to the aortic valve, resulting in AS. Congenital AS happens when a person is born with two aortic valve leaflets (bicuspid). Normally the aortic valve has three leaflets (tricuspid). Blood flow across a bicuspid aortic valve has increased turbulence compared with that of a tricuspid valve. This turbulence causes damage to the valve leaflets, which leads to calcification and scarring, leading to AS.

Signs and Symptoms

The signs and symptoms of AS are dependent on the amount of stenosis. Most patients with mild to moderate AS do not have symptoms. Most symptoms present when there is severe AS and include shortness of breath with activity, chest pain, and dizziness or fainting. The presentation may vary, especially in older patients. They may present with fatigue, decreased tolerance to exertion, HF, or what they may perceive as a side effect of a medication, such as syncope after taking nitrates (Grimard & Larson, 2008).

The classical sign of AS is a harsh murmur heard best at the second right intercostal space and may radiate to the carotids. Other possible exam findings include delayed carotid upstroke and decreased second heart sound. Older patients may have a less intense murmur, or it may radiate to the apex (Grimard & Larson, 2008).

Diagnostic Testing

An ECG, while not diagnostic for AS, will often show evidence of LVH. Chest X-ray is another noninvasive procedure that aids in the diagnosis of AS. It is nondiagnostic, but can show a calcified aortic valve. An enlarged left atrium and ventricle may also be visible in patients who have had AS for a long time. A chest X-ray can also show whether the patient has HF.

Echo is the noninvasive test to evaluate for AS. Echo is an aid in diagnosing AS as well as in determining the severity of AS. An echo allows evaluation of the heart structure, including valves and their function, LV function, EF, and wall thickness. An echo should be repeated on the basis of guidelines published by the ACC. The rate of progression is not predictable, so asymptomatic patients with AS need frequent monitoring to assess for progression of AS (Bonow et al., 2006).

Cardiac catheterization is an invasive procedure and the definitive test for the diagnosis and degree of AS. This procedure can directly measure pressures in the left ventricle and aortic valve.

Cardiac catheterization is recommended before patients undergo an AV replacement to assist in determining the nature of the valve as well as uncovering patients at risk for CAD. When there is a discrepancy in clinical findings and noninvasive testing, a cardiac catheterization should be done to assess the degree of AS (Bonow et al., 2006).

Management of Aortic Stenosis

There is no medication management effective in the treatment of AS. However, the treatment of comorbid conditions such as CAD and evaluation of risk factors that increase the likelihood of AS should be done.

Aortic valve replacement (AVR) is the definitive treatment for AS. The aortic valve is replaced with a mechanical valve or a tissue valve. Mechanical valves are made from metal and are durable but have a risk of clots forming at the valve. To prevent this, patients are prescribed warfarin. In the past, AVR required open heart surgery; however, now transcatheter aortic valve implantation (TAVI) can be performed. This procedure involves valve replacement done via the femoral artery or transapical. TAVI is usually done on patients who are at high risk for open heart surgery. AVR should be considered in older patients who have symptoms, but various other factors should also be considered, including comorbid conditions and patient's expectations and wishes (Bonow et al., 2006).

Balloon valvuloplasty uses a balloon catheter that is placed through the femoral or brachial artery to the aortic valve. The balloon is inflated to increase the opening of the aortic valve. The ACC/AHA does not recommend aortic valve balloon valvuloplasty as a substitute for AVR. However, it may be considered reasonable as a bridge to AVR and considered for palliative treatment for patients who cannot undergo AVR owing to comorbid conditions (Bonow et al., 2006).

Summary

AS causes the heart to work harder and over time can lead to weakening of the heart. This happens because the aortic valve opening is narrowed, causing obstruction of blood flow. AS is classified as acquired or congenital. Acquired AS happens when there is calcification of the aortic valve, causing narrowing of the aortic valve opening. AS occurs in approximately 16% of patients aged 65 and older and is described as mild, moderate, or severe (Bonow et al., 2012). Group A streptococcal infection that causes rheumatic fever can cause damage to the aortic valve, resulting in AS. Congenital AS happens when a person is born with two aortic valve leaflets (bicuspid). Normally the aortic valve has three leaflets (tricuspid). Blood flow across a bicuspid aortic valve has increased turbulence than a tricuspid valve. This turbulence causes damage to the valve leaflets that leads to calcification and scarring, leading to AS.

Commonly, patients who have mild to moderate AS do not have symptoms. When AS is severe, patients often present with shortness of breath with activity, chest pain, and dizziness or fainting. Presentation may vary, especially in the older patient, who may complain of fatigue, exertion intolerance, HF, or suspected side effect of a medication, such as syncope after taking nitrates (Grimard & Larson, 2008). Approximately 50% of patients with severe AS have CAD (Bonow et al., 2012).

Diagnostic testing for AS can include ECG, echo, chest X-ray, and cardiac catheterization. If there is a discrepancy in clinical findings and noninvasive testing, a cardiac catheterization should be done to assess the degree of AS (Bonow et al., 2006). There is no medication to treat AS. The treatment of comorbid conditions such as CAD and evaluation of risk factors that increase the likelihood of AS should be undertaken. The definitive treatment for AS is AVR; however, various other factors should also be considered, including comorbid conditions and patient's expectations and wishes (Bonow et al., 2006).

DYSLIPIDEMIA

Cholesterol is produced by the liver and found in all cells of the body. Cholesterol has many important functions in the body, which include maintaining and building cell membranes, producing estrogens, androgens, and aldosterone hormones, synthesizing vitamin D, aiding in the production of bile, insulating nerve fibers, and aiding in the metabolism of fat-soluble vitamins (Murphy, 2011).

Cholesterol travels through the bloodstream on protein-covered molecules called lipoproteins. Lipoproteins are characterized by their density, and the most important ones are low-density lipoprotein (LDL), high-density lipoprotein (HDL), very low-density lipoproteins (VLDL), and triglycerides (Murphy, 2011).

LDL transports cholesterol, which is often referred to as the "bad" cholesterol because it plays a significant role in depositing cholesterol in the arteries. LDL makes up approximately 60% to 70% of the total cholesterol. LDL carries cholesterol from the liver to the cells in the rest of the body. When there is too much LDL, it deposits it in the artery walls. This buildup can cause plaque to form and over time limit arterial blood flow. This buildup of plaque is called atherosclerosis. Increased LDL increases the risk of CVD (Murphy, 2011). The treatment goal of the LDL level varies regarding patient's history. The National Cholesterol Education Program (NCEP) Expert Panel on Detection, Evaluation, and Treatment of High Blood Cholesterol in Adults (Adult Treatment Panel III) (2004) has posted guidelines.

HDL is often referred to as the "good" cholesterol. HDL takes away cholesterol from cells and back to the liver, where it is excreted from the body. HDL makes up approximately 20% to 30% of the total cholesterol. The goal level of HDL is greater than 40 mg/dl (Murphy, 2011). Evidence suggests that HDL protects against the development of atherosclerosis. When a low HDL is present, it often indicates the presence of other atherogenic risk factors (NCEP, 2002).

Triglycerides are made up of fatty acids and come from the liver or fats in our food. Triglycerides are removed from the blood by the liver and are packaged into VLDL, which are hard to move through the bloodstream and contribute to the buildup of plaque and thus atherosclerosis. The goal level of triglycerides is less than 150 mg/dl (Murphy, 2011). In the past, management of LDL has been the primary focus in the role of atherogenesis; however, evidence shows that VLDL and HDL are also important (NCEP, 2002).

Type and Risk Factors

Lifestyle and heredity affect cholesterol levels. Total cholesterol, LDL, HDL, VLDL, and triglycerides are all important players in the risk for CVD. An alteration in lipoproteins increases the risk of CVD. Abnormal lipoprotein metabolism is called dyslipidemia and is classified as primary or secondary (Murphy, 2011). For the purpose of this chapter, the focus will be on secondary dyslipidemia and its management.

Primary dyslipidemia is considered a genetic defect in lipid metabolism. Some of the genetic defects include familial hypercholesterolemia and familial defective apolipoprotein B-100. There is a defect in the production or balance of cholesterol (Murphy, 2011).

Secondary dyslipidemia is considered an acquired defect in lipoprotein metabolism (Murphy, 2011). Modifiable risk factors for secondary dyslipidemia include diet high in saturated fat, physical inactivity, hypothyroidism, diabetes, renal disease, liver disease, and obesity. In addition, some medications such as antihypertensives, estrogen, and antipsychotics can adversely affect lipoproteins (Murphy, 2011).

Screening for Dyslipidemia

The lipid profile is a blood test that measures total cholesterol, HDL, LDL, and triglycerides. The test is used for screening for dyslipidemia as well as the risk for CVD. In 2008, the U.S. Preventative Services Task Force (USPSTF) published guidelines regarding screening for lipid disorders in adults. These guidelines (Table 4.6) are used for patients who are 20 years old or older and have not previously been diagnosed with dyslipidemia.

As discussed above, a standard lipid test measures total cholesterol, LDL, HDL, and triglycerides. A more advanced lipid test called a lipoprotein assay measures lipoprotein particle size, density, and core lipid composition. They are not routinely used in primary care, but are used in lipid clinics, research studies, and often by cardiologists. At this time, NCEP ATPIII guidelines recommend a standard lipid panel and targeting treatment based on LDL, HDL, and triglyceride levels (Mora, 2009). However, new NCEP guidelines are expected in 2013 that will address lipoprotein assay and give recommendations for testing.

Dyslipidemia Management

Specific guidelines were published by the NCEP's Expert Panel on Detection Evaluation and Treatment of High Cholesterol in Adult National Heart in 2001. Updates were made in 2004 after five major clinical trials were conducted and provided data end points that showed the benefits of cholesterol-lowering therapy. New updates are expected in 2013.

Management of dyslipidemia begins with therapeutic lifestyle changes (TLC). NCEP (2004) published TLC recommendations, and Murphy (2011) discussed the following suggestions to help with TLC (O'Riordan, 2004):

- Reduction of saturated fats and cholesterol: Eat lean cuts of meat and remove visible fat before cooking, low-fat dairy products, avoid salad dressings, mayonnaise, and margarines, read food labels, and avoid fast food.
- Increasing physical activity: Start by walking at least 30 minutes a day, and this will need to increase or be altered as endurance increases.
- Increase plant stanols/sterols and increase in soluble fiber in the diet: These bind to cholesterol and help the body excrete it.
- Weight loss: Start with increasing physical activity and reduction in saturated fats.

TABLE 4.6 · Screening Guidelines for Lipid Testing

- Baseline screening for men aged 35 and older even without risk factors for CVD
- Baseline screening for women aged 45 and older even with risk factors for CVD
- Men aged 20 to 35 if they are at increased risk of CVD
- Women aged 20 to 45 if they are at increased risk of CVD
- No recommendations were made for or against routine screening for lipid disorders in men aged 20 to 35, or in women aged 20 and older who are not at increased risk for CVD

From United States Preventative Task Force. (2008). Screening for lipid disorders in adults. Retrieved from http://www.uspreventiveservicestaskforce.org/uspstf/uspschol.htm

Patients should be referred to a dietician for nutritional guidance and intervention (National Heart Lung and Blood Institute). When TLC alone is not enough for cholesterol control, medications are initiated. TLC should still be done in conjunction with medications. Tables 4.7 and 4.8 provide an outline of medications that can be used as cholesterol-lowering agents.

HMG CoA reductase inhibitors (statins) block the liver enzyme that controls the production of LDL. Statins are the most successful at lowering LDL. Reduction in LDL levels decreases the likelihood of plaque development. Statins are generally well tolerated by patients. Approximately 0.5% to 2.0% of patients on statin have elevated hepatic transaminases (Cleeman et al., 2002). Baseline liver function test should be gotten before initiation of statin therapy and then again every 3 months to ensure there is no increase in hepatic transaminase levels (Murphy, 2011). Myalgias are also a potential side effect of statins. This can be a sign of muscle breakdown known as rhabdomyolysis (Murphy, 2011). For patients who complain of myalgias or myopathy, a total creatine kinase can be drawn, and if elevated, statin use may need to be reconsidered. Also, other medications that could interact with statin medications should be considered (Sinzinger et al., 2002).

Bile acid sequestrants work to reduce LDL levels by preventing reabsorption in the ileum. These medications work in the intestine to bind to the bile acids in the intestine. Triglycerides levels are also lowered by these medications. The most common side effects are GI side effects such as diarrhea and nausea. These medications should be taken with meals. They can also potentially bind other medications and decrease their bioavailability (Murphy, 2011).

Nicotinic acids decrease LDL and triglycerides as well as increase HDL. They reduce the hepatic synthesis of triglycerides by inhibiting movement of free fatty acids from peripheral tissues. Increase in HDL is a result of the decrease in triglycerides and LDL. The most common side effect of these medications is flushing that is caused by an increase in prostaglandins. These side effects can be treated or a reduction in flushing can occur by taking 325 mg of aspirin 30 minutes before taking the medication. These medications may also increase the risk of gout, elevate glucose levels, and affect liver function. Baseline glucose and liver function tests should be obtained and monitored every 6 months while taking these medications (Murphy, 2011).

Fibric acids lower triglycerides and LDL and increase HDL levels. They work by increasing the removal of triglycerides and prevent the production of VLDL. The most common side effects of

TABLE 4.7 · ATP III LDL Cholesterol Cutoffs for Lifestyle Interventions and Drug Therapy in Different Risk Categories

Risk Category	LDL Cholesterol Goal	Initiate Therapeutic Lifestyle Changes	Consider Drug Therapy
High risk: CHD or CHD risk equivalents (10-year risk >20%)	<100 mg/dl (with an optional goal of <70 mg/dl)	>100 mg/dl	>100 mg/dl (consider drug options if LDL-C <100 mg/dl)
Moderately high risk: two or more risk factors (10-year risk 10%–20%)	<130 mg/dl (with an optional goal of <100 mg/dl)	>130 mg/dl	>130 mg/dl (consider drug options if LDL-C 100–129 mg/dl)
Moderate risk: two or more risk factors (10-year risk <10%)	<130 mg/dl	>130 mg/dl	>160 mg/dl
Low risk: <1 risk factor	<160 mg/dl	>160 mg/dl	>190 mg/dl (consider drug options if LDL-C 160–189 mg/dl)

From Grundy, S. M., Cleeman, J. I., Bairey Merz, C. N., Brewer, H. B, Jr., Clark, L. T., Hunninghake, D. B., ... Stone, N. J. (2004). Implications of recent clinical trials for the National Cholesterol Education Program Adult Treatment Panel III guidelines. *Circulation, 110*(2), 227–239, with permission.

TABLE 4.8 · Drug Class, Agents Lipid/Lipoprotein Side Effects Contraindications Clinical Trial and Daily Doses Effects Results

Drug Class, Agent, and Daily Dose	Lipid/Lipoprotein Effect	Side Effects	Contraindications	Clinical Trial Results
HMG CoA reductase inhibitors (statins)[a]	LDL ↓18%–55% HDL ↑5%–15% TG ↓7%–30%	Myopathy Increased liver enzymes	**Absolute:** ■ Active or chronic liver disease. **Relative:** ■ Concomitant use of certain drugs[b]	Reduced major coronary events, CHD deaths, need for coronary procedures, stroke, and total mortality
Bile acid sequestrants[c]	LDL ↓15%–30% HDL ↑3%–5% TG No change or increase	Gastrointestinal distress Constipation Decreased absorption of other drugs	**Absolute:** ■ Dysbetalipoproteinemia ■ TG >400 mg/dl **Relative:** ■ TG >200 mg/dl	Reduced major coronary events and CHD deaths
Nicotinic acid[d]	LDL ↓5%–25% HDL ↑15%–35% TG ↓20%–50%	Flushing Hyperglycemia Hyperuricemia (or gout) Upper GI distress Hepatotoxicity	**Absolute:** ■ Chronic liver disease ■ Severe gout **Relative:** ■ Diabetes ■ Hyperuricemia ■ Peptic ulcer disease	Reduced major coronary events and possibly total mortality
Fibric acids[e]	LDL ↓5%–20% (may be increased in patients with high TG) HDL ↑10%–20% TG ↓20%–50%	Dyspepsia Gallstones Myopathy Unexplained non-CHD deaths in WHO study	**Absolute:** ■ Severe renal disease ■ Severe hepatic disease	Reduced major coronary events

[a]Lovastatin (20 to 80 mg), pravastatin (20 to 40 mg), simvastatin (20 to 80 mg), fluvastatin (20 to 80 mg), atorvastatin (10 to 80 mg), and cerivastatin (0.4 to 0.8 mg).
[b]Cyclosporine, macrolide antibiotics, various antifungal agents, and cytochrome P-450 inhibitors (fibrates and niacin should be used with appropriate caution).
[c]Cholestyramine (4 to 16 g), colestipol (5 to 20 g), and colesevelam (2.6 to 3.8 g).
[d]Immediate-release (crystalline) nicotinic acid (1.5 to 3 g), extended-release nicotinic acid (Niaspan) (1 to 2 g), and sustained-release nicotinic acid (1 to 2 g).
[e]Gemfibrozil (600 mg b.i.d.), fenofibrate (200 mg), and clofibrate (1,000 mg b.i.d.).
From National Institute of Health, National Heart, Lung, and Blood Institute. (2001). Detection, evaluation, and treatment of high blood cholesterol in adults (Adult Treatment Panel III). Executive summary. Retrieved from http://www.nhlbi.nih.gov/guidelines/cholesterol/atp3xsum.pdf

these medications are dyspepsia, nausea, vomiting, diarrhea, and flatulence. Liver toxicity is also a potential side effect. As with other cholesterol medications, baseline liver function test should be obtained and repeated every 3 months while taking these medications (Murphy, 2011).

Dose consideration for statin therapy must be a primary consideration in older patients, particularly those over 80, due to the risk for myopathy. Many older patients have a small body frame, are frail, have multiple comorbidities, and are taking other medications. Many may have chronic musculoskeletal aches and pains, which can make it more difficult to make a distinction between myopathy and chronic complaints. Also, cognitive impairment can make it difficult for patients to discuss their complaints of myopathy. Evaluation of myopathic symptoms in older patients may be done with simple assessment of muscle strength. It is important to note that for patients 75 years and older, the ideal lipid levels have not been absolutely established. The lowest effective dose of lipid-lowering medications should be used in older patients to prevent complications (Tables 4.7 and 4.8) (Bonow et al., 2012).

Summary

Cholesterol is produced by the liver and found in all cells of the body and has many important bodily functions. Cholesterol travels through the bloodstream on lipoproteins. Lipoproteins are characterized by their density, and the most important ones are LDL, HDL, VLDL, and triglycerides (Murphy, 2011).

This section focused on secondary dyslipidemia, which is considered an acquired defect in lipoprotein metabolism. A diet high in saturated fat, physical inactivity, hypothyroidism, diabetes, renal and liver disease, and obesity are risk factors for secondary dyslipidemia (Murphy, 2011).

Lipid profile testing measures total cholesterol, HDL, LDL, and triglycerides and is used for screening for dyslipidemia and risk for CVD. Guidelines for management of dyslipidemia were published in 2001 by NCEP and updated in 2004. Management of dyslipidemia begins with TLC. Recommendations for TLC include reduction in saturated fat, increase in physical activity, weight reduction, and an increase in soluble fiber (NCEP, 2004).

Cholesterol-lowering medications should be initiated when TLC alone does not result in recommended goal levels. Several different cholesterol-lowering medications are available. Statins are the most successful in lowering LDL of all the cholesterol-lowering medications. Bile acid sequestrants lower LDL and triglyceride levels. Nicotinic acids decrease LDL and triglycerides as well as increase HDL levels. Fibric acids lower triglycerides and LDL and increase HDL levels. Baseline liver function test should be obtained prior to initiation of these medications and every 3 months while on these medications.

Owing to many reasons such as small body frame, frailty, comorbidities, conditions requiring multiple medications, and possible cognitive impairment, the lowest dose of cholesterol-lowering medications should be used. The lowest effective dose of lipid-lowering medications should be used in older patients to prevent complications (Bonow et al., 2012).

REFERENCES

Alexander, K. P., Newby, L. K., Armstrong, P. W., Cannon, C. P., Gibler, W. B., Rich, M. W., … Ohman, E. M. (2007). Acute coronary care in the elderly, part II: ST segment-elevation myocardial infarction: a scientific statement for healthcare professionals from the American Heart Association Council on Clinical Cardiology: in collaboration with the Society of Geriatric Cardiology. *Circulation, 115*(19), 2570.

American College of Cardiology & American Heart Association. (1997). ACC/AHA guidelines for exercise testing: executive summary. *Circulation, 96,* 345–354.

Anderson, J. L., Adams, C. D., Antman, E. M., Bridges, C. R., Califf, R. M., Casey, D. E., … Wright, R. S. (2007, October). American College of Cardiology/American Heart Association (ACC/AHA) pocket guideline, based on the ACC/AHA 2007 guideline revision. Management of patients with unstable angina/non–ST-elevation myocardial infarction. (2007). Retrieved from http://www.acc.org.ualoityandscience/clinical/pdfs/UA_NSTEMI_Final_pcoketguide.pdf

Antonopoulos, M. S., Lee, J. N., & Chang, A. V. (2007). Ranolazine (Ranexa): A first-in-class therapy for stable angina. *Pharmacy and Therapeutics, 32*(9), 488–493.

Bonow, R. O., Carabello, B. A., Chatterjee, K., De Leon, Jr., A. C., Faxon, D. P., Freed, M. D., … Riegel, B. (2006). ACC/AHA 2006 guidelines for the management of patients with valvular heart disease: A report of the American College of Cardiology/American Heart Association Task Force on Practice Guidelines (writing committee to revise the 1998 guidelines for the management of patients with valvular heart disease) developed in collaboration with the Society of Cardiovascular Anesthesiologists endorsed by the Society for Cardiovascular Angiography and Interventions and the Society of Thoracic Surgeons. *Journal of the American College of Cardiology, 48,* 1–148.

Bonow, R. O., Mann, D. L., Zipes, D. P., & Libby, P. (2012). *Braunwald's heart disease* (9th ed.). Philadelphia, PA: Elsevier.

Botta, D. M. (2011, March). Heart transplantation. Retrieved from http://www.emedicine.medscape.com/article/420816-overview#showall

Brater, D.C., (2000) Diuretic Therapy in congestive Heart Failure. *Congest. Heart Fail.* 6(4),197–201.

Bullock, B. L. (1996). *Pathophysiology: Adaptations and alterations in function* (4th ed.). Philadelphia, PA: Lippincott.

Campbell-Scherer, D. L., & Green, L. A. (2009). ACC/AHA guideline update for the management of ST-segment elevation myocardial infarction. *American Family Physician, 79*(12), 1080–1086.

Centers for Disease Control and Prevention. (2010). Heart disease facts. Retrieved from http://www.cdc.gov/Heart Disease/facts.htm

Chapman, D. P., & Perry, G. S. (2008). Depression as a major component of public health for older adults. *Preventing Chronic Disease, 5*(1), 1–9.

Cleeman, J. I., Lenfant, C., Pasternak, R. C., Smith, S. C., Bairey-Merz, N., & Grundy, S. M. (2002). ACC/AHA/NHLBI clinical advisory on the use and safety of statins. *Journal of the American College of Cardiology, 40*(3), 567–572.

Colucci, W. S. (2009, June). Overview of the therapy of heart failure due to systolic heart dysfunction. Retrieved from http://www.uptodate.com/contents/overview-of-the-therapy-due-to-systolic-dysfunction?source=search_results&selectedTitle=2%7E150

Colucci, W. S. (2011, January). Treatment of acute decompensated heart failure: Components of therapy. Retrieved from http://www.uptodate.com/contents/treatment-of-acute-decompensated-heart-failure-compenents-of-therapy?source=search_results&selectedTitle=3%7E150

Dhar, S., Koul, D., & D'Alonzo, G. E. (2008). Current concepts in diastolic heart failure. *Journal of the American Osteopathic Association, 108*(4), 203–209.

Diagnostic and Interventional Cardiology. (2008). ACC, AHA, HRS give 2008 guidelines for device-based therapy. Retrieved from http://www.dicardiology.com/article/acc-aha-hrs-give-2008-guidelines-device-based-therapy

Dor, V., Sabatier, M., Montiglio, F., Civaia, F., & DiDonato, M. (2004). Endoventricular patch reconstruction of ischemic failing ventricle. A single center with 20 years experience, advantages of magnetic resonance imaging assessment. *Heart Failure Reviews, 9*(4), 269–286.

Dua, A., Dang, P., Shaker, R., Varadarajan, P., & Pai, R. G. (2011). Barriers to surgery in severe aortic stenosis patients with class I indications for aortic valve replacement. *Journal of Heart Valve Disease, 20*(4), 396–400.

Falvey, J., & Blaxall, B. C. (2009). *Manual of heart failure management* (1st ed.). New York, NY: Springer.

Faris, R. F., Flather, M. D., Purcell, H., Poole-Wilson, P. A., & Coats, A. J. (2006). Diuretics for heart failure. *Cochrane Database of Systematic Reviews,* (1), CD003838.

Font, M. A., Krupinski, J., & Arboix, A. (2011). Antithrombotic medication for cardioembolic stroke prevention. *Stroke Research and Prevention, 2011,* 1–23.

Forman, D. E., Rich, M. W., Alexander, K. P., Zeiman, S., Maurer, M. S., Najjar, S. S., . Wenger, N. K. (2011). Cardiac care for older adults. *Journal of the American College of Cardiology, 57*(18), 1801–1810.

Fraker, T. D., Jr., Fihn, S. D., et al. (2007). 2007 chronic angina focused update of the ACC/AHA 2002 guidelines for the management of patients with chronic stable angina: A report of the American College of Cardiology/American Heart Association Task Force on Practice Guidelines Writing group to develop the focused update of the 2002 guidelines for the management of patients with chronic stable angina. *Journal of the American College of Cardiology, 50*(23), 2264.

Fuster, V., Ryden, L. E., Cannom, D. S., Crijns, H. J., Curtis, A. B., Ellenbogen, K. A., … Wann, L. S. (2011). 2011 ACCF/AHA/HRS focused updates incorporated into the ACC/AHA/ESC 2006 guidelines for the management of patients with atrial fibrillation: A report of the American College of Cardiology Foundation/American Heart Association Task Force on Practice Guidelines developed in partnership with the European Society of Cardiology and in collaboration with the European Heart Rhythm Association and the Heart Rhythm Society. *Journal of the American College of Cardiology, 57*(11), e101–e198.

Gage, B. F., van Walraven, C., Pearce, L., Hart, R. G., Koudstall, P. J., Boode, B. S., & Petersen, P. (2004). Selecting patients with atrial fibrillation for anticoagulation: Stroke risk stratification in patients taking aspirin. *Circulation, 110*(16), 2287–2292.

Gangemi, J. J., & Hicks, G. C. (2009). *Surgical options in the treatment of heart failure.* New York, NY: Springer.

Goodacre, S., & Irons, R. (2002). ABC of electrocardiography: Atrial arrhythmias. *British Medical Journal, 324*(7337), 594–597.

Grimard, B. H., & Larson, J. M. (2008). Aortic stenosis: Diagnosis and treatment. *American Family Physician, 78*(6), 717–724.

Gring, C. N., & Francis, G. S. (2004). A hard look at angiotensin receptor blockers in heart failure. *Journal of the American College of Cardiology, 44*(9), 1841–1846.

Henzlova, M. J., Cerqueira, M. D., Hansen, C. L., Taillefer, R., & Yao, S. S. (2009). ASNC imaging guidelines for nuclear cardiology procedures: Stress protocols and tracers. Retrieved from http://www.asnc.org/imageuploads/imaging-guidelinesstressprotocols021109.pdf

Hobbs, R., & Boyle, A. (2010, August). Center for continuing education: Disease management project. Retrieved from http://www.clevelandclinicmeded.com/medicalpubs/diseasemanagement/cardiology/heartfailure/

Horwich, T. B., MacLellan, W. R., & Fonarow, G. C. (2004). Statin therapy is associated with improved survival in ischemic and non-ischemic heart failure. *Journal of the American College of Cardiology, 43*(4), 642–648.

Hunt, S. A., Abraham, W. T., Chin, M. H., Feldman, A. M., Francis, G. S., Ganiats, T. G., … Yancy, C. W. (2009). 2009 focused update incorporated into the American College of Cardiology/American Heart Association 2005 Guidelines for the diagnosis and management of heart failure in adults: A report of the American College of Cardiology Foundation/American Heart Association Task Force on Practice Guidelines: developed in collaboration with the International Society for Heart and Lung Transplantation. *Circulation, 119*(14), e391–e479.

Kesselheim, A. S., Fischer, M. A., & Avorn, J. (2006). The rise and fall of Natrecor for congestive heart failure: Implications for drug policy. *Health Affairs, 25*(4), 1095–1102.

Kleinpell, R. M., & Avitall, B. (2005). Telemanagement in chronic heart failure: A review. *Disease Management Health Outcomes, 13*(1), 43–52.

Kumar, A., Meyerrose, G., Sood, V., & Roongsritong, C. (2006). Diastolic heart failure in the elderly and the potential role of aldosterone antagonists. *Drugs & Aging, 23*(4), 299–308.

Kushner, F. G., Hand, M., Smith, S. C., King, S. B., III, Anderson, J. L., Antman, E. M., … Williams, D. O. (2009). 2009 focused updates: ACC/AHA guidelines for the management of patients with ST - elevation myocardial infarction (updating the 2004 guideline and 2007 focused update) and ACC/AHA/SCAI guidelines on percutaneous coronary intervention (updating the 2005 guideline and 2007 focused update): A report of the American College of Cardiology Foundation/American Heart Association Task Force on practice guidelines. *Journal of the American College of Cardiology, 54*(23), 2205–2241.

Leclercq, C. (2007). New guidelines for cardiac resynchronization therapy: Simplicity or complexity for the doctor? *Heart, 93*, 1017–1019.

Mora, S. (2009). Advanced lipoprotein testing and subfractionation are not (yet) ready for routine clinical use. *Circulation, 119*(17), 2396–2404.

Murphy, K. (2011). Cholesterol: The good, the bad, and the ugly. Retrieved from http://www.NursingMadeIncredibly Easy.com

Murphy, S. A., Cannon, C. P., Wiviott, S. D., McCabe, C. H., & Braunwald, E. (2009). Reduction in recurrent cardiovascular events with intensive lipid lowering statin therapy compared with moderate lipid lowering statin therapy after acute coronary syndromes from the PROVE IT-TIMI 22 (Pravastatin or Atorvastatin Evaluation and Infection Therapy-Thrombolysis in Myocardial Infarction 22) trial. *Journal of the American College of Cardiology, 54*(25), 2358.

National Cholesterol Education Program Expert Panel on Detection, Evaluation, and Treatment of High Blood Cholesterol in Adults (Adult Treatment Panel III). (2002). Third report of the National Cholesterol Education Program (NCEP) Expert Panel on Detection, Evaluation, and Treatment of High Blood Cholesterol in Adults (Adult Treatment Panel III) final report. *Circulation, 106*, 3143–3421.

National Cholesterol Education Program Expert Panel on Detection, Evaluation, and Treatment of High Blood Cholesterol in Adults (Adult Treatment Panel III) Executive Summary. (2004). Retrieved from http://www.nhlbi.nih.gov/guidelines/cholesterol/atp3xsum.pdf

O'Riordan, M. (2004). Update to the NCEP ATP III guidelines recommends aggressively treating LDL cholesterol levels in high-risk patients. Retrieved from http://www.theheart.org/article/148997.do

Otto, C. M. (2004). Why is aortic sclerosis associated with adverse clinical outcomes? *Journal of the American College of Cardiology, 43*, 176–178.

Panteghini, M. (2002). Acute coronary syndrome. *Chest, 122*, 1428–1435.

Paulus, W. J., Sanderson, J. E., Rusconi, C., Flachskampf, F. A., Rademakers, F. E., Marino, P., … Brutsaert, D. L. (2007). How to diagnosis heart failure: A consensus statement on the diagnosis of heart failure with normal left ventricular ejection fraction. *European Heart Journal, 28*, 2539–2550.

Peterson, J. W., & Felker, G. M. (2008). Inotropes in the management of acute heart failure. *Critical Care Medicine, 36*(1), 106–111.

Phillips, C. O., Wright, S. M., Kern, D. E., Signa, R. M., & Rubin, H. R. (2004). Comprehensive discharge planning with post discharge support for older patients with congestive heart failure. *Journal of the American Medical Association, 291*(11), 1358–1367.

Reeder, G. S., & Kennedy, H. L. (2011). Criteria for diagnosis of acute myocardial infarction. Retrieved from http://www.uptodate.com/contents/criteria-for-the-diagnosis-of-acute-myocardial-infarction?source=search_result&search=myocardial+infarction&selectedTitle=2~150

Ridker, P. M., Cook, N. R., Lee, I., Gordon, D., Gaziano, M., Manson, J. E., … Buring, J. E. (2005). A randomized trial of low-dose aspirin in the primary prevention of cardiovascular disease in women. *New England Journal of Medicine, 352*, 1293–1304.

Samala, R. V., Navas, N., Saluke, E., & Ciocon, J. O. (2011). Heart failure in frail, older patients: We can do "more". *Cleveland Clinic Journal of Medicine, 78*(12), 837–845.

Shamsham, F., & Mitchell, J. (2000). Essentials of the diagnosis of heart failure. Retrieved from http://www.aafp.org/afp/2000/0301/p1319.html

Shekelle, P. G., Rich, M. W., Morton, S. C., Atkinson, S. W., Tu, W. Maglione, M., ... Warner Stevenson, L. (2003). Efficacy of angiotensin-converting enzyme inhibitors and beta-blockers in the management of left ventricular systolic dysfunction according to race, gender, and diabetic status: A meta-analysis of major clinical trials. *Journal of the American College of Cardiology, 41*(9), 1529–1538.

Sheridan, S., Pignone, M., & Mulrow, C. (2003). Framingham-based tools to calculate the global risk of coronary heart disease: A systemic review of tools for clinicians. *Journal of General Internal Medicine, 18*(12), 1039–1052.

Simon, S. R., Black, H. R., Moser, M., & Berland, W. E. (1992). Cough and ACE inhibitors. *Archives of Internal Medicine, 152*(8), 1698–1700.

Sinzinger, H., Wolfram, R., & Peskar, B. A. (2002). Muscular side effects of statins. *Journal of Cardiovascular Pharmacology, 40*(2), 163–171.

Sterns, R. H., & Colucci, W. S. (2010). Use of diuretics in patients with heart failure. Retrieved from http://www.uptodate.com/contents/use-of-diuretics-in-patients-with-heart-failure?view=print

Stiles, S. (2007). Mesh cardiac support devices promotes long-term reverse remodeling. Retrieved from http://www.theheart.org/article/834557.do

Strippoli, G. F., Craig, M., Deeks, J., Schena, F. P., & Craig, J. C. (2004). Effects of angiotensin converting enzyme inhibitors and angiotensin II receptor antagonists on mortality and renal outcomes in diabetic nephropathy: Systematic review. Retrieved from http://www.bmj.com/content/329/7470/828.full.pdf

Trochelman, K., Albert, N., Li, J., & Lin, S. (2010). Signs and symptoms of heart failure: Are you asking the right questions? *American Journal of Critical Care, 19*(5), 443–452.

U.S. Department of Health & Human Services. (2011, June 1). What is atherosclerosis? Retrieved from http://www.nhlbi.nih.gov/health/health-topics/topics/atherosclerosis/

U.S. Department of Health & Human Services. (2011a, February). What are coronary heart disease risk factors? Retrieved from http://www.nhlbi.nih.gov/health/health-topics/topics/hd/

U.S. Department of Health & Human Services. (2011b, June 1). What are the signs and symptoms of angina? Retrieved from http://www.nhlbi.nih.gov/health/health-topics/topics/angina/signs.html

U.S. Preventive Services Task Force. (2008). Screening for lipid disorders in adults. Retrieved from http://www.uspreventiveservicestaskforce.org/uspstf/uspschol.htm

Virginia Department of Health. (2005). Cardiovascular disease in Virginia: A report from the Virginia cardiovascular health project. Retrieved from http://www.vdh.virginia.gov

White, M. M., Howie-Esquivel, J., & Cadwell, M. A. (2010). Improving heart failure symptom recognition: A diary analysis. *Journal of Cardiovascular Nursing, 25*(1), 7–12.

Zile, M. R., & Colucci, W. S. (2011). Treatment and prognosis of diastolic heart failure. Retrieved from http://www.uptodate.com/contents/treatment-and-prognosis-of-diastolic-heart-failure?source=see_link

CHAPTER 4: IT RESOURCES

Websites

American Heart Association
    http://www.heart.org/HEARTORG/
American College of Cardiology
    http://www.cardiosource.org/
National Cholesterol Education Program
    http://www.nhlbi.nih.gov/about/ncep/
United States Department of Health and Human Services
    http://www.hhs.gov/
Virginia Department of Health
    http://www.vdh.state.va.us/
The following websites come from the U.S. National Library of Medicine and specifically
    PubMed Health.

Defines coronary heart disease and provides figures/images, causes, risk factors, tests, treatments, prognosis, prevention and references
http://www.ncbi.nlm.nih.gov/pubmedhealth/PMH0004449/

Defines high blood cholesterol levels (dyslipidemia) and provides figures/images, causes, risk factors, tests, treatments, prognosis, prevention and references
http://www.ncbi.nlm.nih.gov/pubmedhealth/PMH0001440/

Defines heart failure and provides figures/images, causes, risk factors, symptoms, tests, treatments, prognosis, prevention and references
http://www.ncbi.nlm.nih.gov/pubmedhealth/PMH0001211/

Defines aortic stenosis and provides figures/images, causes, risk factors, symptoms, tests, treatments, prognosis, complications, prevention and references
http://www.ncbi.nlm.nih.gov/pubmedhealth/PMH0001230/

WebMD—High Blood Pressure and Stroke
http://www.webmd.com/hypertension-high-blood-pressure/guide/
hypertension-high-blood-pressure-stroke%20

PDF Documents

Mayo Clinic—Cardiovascular Research 2008–2009
http://www.mayoclinic.org/mcitems/mc5700-mc5799/mc5751-16.pdf

Videos

Coronary Artery Disease Overview (2008)
The following video, from AnswerTV.com, provides an overview of Coronary Artery Disease. (6:48 minutes)
http://youtu.be/SjRPxGNOtjM

Dyslipidemia (Understanding Disease: Cardiovascular Medicine) (2012)
Get the facts on Dyslipidemia with this 100%-accurate animated video. Part of Focus Apps' Understanding Disease: Cardiovascular Medicine series, the Dyslipidemia app demonstrates how the elevation of plasma, cholesterol, and triglycerides (or low HDL levels) results in dyslipidemia. Explore the treatments for this condition as well as lifestyle changes that are necessary to prevent or control it. (2:52 minutes)
http://youtu.be/NklmCp8pyDM

Dyslipidemia (2012)
The LoCicero Medical Group's Elizabeth Remo Platt (ARNP) discusses Dyslipidemia—a lipid disorder caused by elevated cholesterol and triglycerides. (6:50 minutes)
http://youtu.be/ADRt08fq_A8

3D Medical Animation Congestive Heart Failure Animation (2010)
This video is one of ASK Visual Science most complex animations to date. With a total run-time of over 8 minutes across three modules, the program incorporated over 50 separate models, from the molecular (Angiotensin I, BNP, Endothelin), to the microscopic (red blood cells, platelets, endothelial cells), to whole organs (heart, lungs, kidney, liver, vascular system) and even a whole body. (3:41 minutes)
http://youtu.be/3YddwXPWVSc

Congestive Heart Failure (2008)
  Animation on congestive heart failure pathophysiology. (2:01 minutes)
  http://youtu.be/JXA6LjmKsaU
Understanding Heart Disease (2007)
  Heart disease affects more than 20 million Americans. Let's explore the various forms that
  heart disease can take. Watch More Health Videos at Health Guru: http://www.healthguru
  .com/?YT (2:56 minutes)
  http://youtu.be/3cW8__wFXDA
Atrial Fibrillation Symptoms and Treatments (2009)
  NorthShore University HealthSystem Cardiac Electrophysiologists Wes Fisher, MD,
  Jose Nazari, MD and Alex Ro, MD discuss atrial fibrillation. Atrial fibrillation is an
  irregular heart rhythm (arrhythmia) that starts in the upper parts (atria) of the heart.
  (9:00 minutes)
  http://youtu.be/BZ1vMLPrHnk
Atrial Fibrillation, Part 1—Fletcher Allen Health Care, Vermont
  Peter Spector, MD, a nationally renowned expert in heart rhythm disorders, discusses atrial
  fibrillation—an irregular heart beat—and a procedure used to correct this condition known
  as cardiac ablation. (9:26 minutes)
  http://youtu.be/vneiHyvTyZk
What Is Atrial Fibrillation? (2011)
  Heart and Stroke Foundation researcher Dr. Paul Dorian explains the causes and risk factors
  of atrial fibrillation, and how it differs from heart disease, using illustrations and animation.
  (3:55 minutes)
  http://youtu.be/onoVr3dVVic
Four videos geared towards health care professionals. The purpose of these videos is to
  provide information on aortic stenosis, its symptoms, diagnosis and treatment for primary
  care physicians.
  What Is Aortic Stenosis? (2008) (2:48 minutes)
  http://youtu.be/iul0k3Moc7I
Recognizing Aortic Stenosis Symptoms (2008) (6:03 minutes)
  http://youtu.be/4W6WVM7E4w0
Screening for Aortic Stenosis (2008) (4:52 minutes)
  http://youtu.be/R76dP8vyNu0
Treating Aortic Stenosis (2008) (5:41 minutes)
  http://youtu.be/VcM-vkBapUM
Tests and Procedures—Stress Echocardiogram (2009)
  Explains what a Stress Echocardiogram is and what to expect. (5:23 minutes)
  http://youtu.be/CHsUNn0Lnfk
Stress Echocardiography Test (2010)
  This patient education video is for patients who plan to undergo a *stress echocardiogram*.
  Included are the following sections: The Heart, Heart Diseases and Echo, How Echo Works,
  During a Stress Echo, After an Echo, Risks. (4:13 minutes)
  http://youtu.be/hBtPJZduzMA

From Google Videos

Coronary artery disease videos
http://www.google.com/search?q=coronary+artery+disease&hl=en&qscrl=1&nord=1&rlz=1
T4ADFA_enUS417US433&tbm=vid&source=lnms&ei=p-lDT5WsBOXL0QGytdzEBw&sa=
X&oi=mode_link&ct=mode&cd=4&ved=0CDMQ_AUoAw&biw=1024&bih=661

Dyslipidemia videos
http://www.google.com/search?q=dyslipidemia&hl=en&qscrl=1&nord=1&rlz=1T4ADFA_en
US417US433&tbm=vid&source=lnms&ei=LupDT46nI6bV0QG2pdnSDw&sa=X&oi=m
ode_link&ct=mode&cd=4&ved=0CDMQ_AUoAw&biw=1024&bih=661

Heart failure videos
http://www.google.com/search?q=heart+failure&hl=en&qscrl=1&nord=1&rlz=1T4ADFA_en
US417US433&tbm=vid&source=lnms&ei=pepDT-7mJ6b20gGft-GqBw&sa=X&oi=mode_
link&ct=mode&cd=4&ved=0CDMQ_AUoAw&biw=1024&bih=661

Atrial fibrillation videos
http://www.google.com/#q=atrial+fibrillation&source=lnms&tbm=vid&sa=X&ei=_
r-jUbO0GaLF0QHrvICQBQ&ved=0CAoQ_AUoBA&bav=on.2,or.r_qf.&bvm=
bv.47008514,d.dmQ&fp=51e90cf71e3aef05&biw=1024&bih=564

Aortic stenosis videos
http://www.google.com/search?q=aortic+stenosis&hl=en&qscrl=1&nord=1&rlz=1T4A
DFA_enUS417US433&tbm=vid&prmd=imvns&source=lnms&ei=AexDT7GtA8TG0AHs-Z
G2Bw&sa=X&oi=mode_link&ct=mode&cd=4&ved=0CDMQ_AUoAw&biw=1024&bih=661

Myocardial ischemia videos
http://www.google.com/search?q=myocardial+infarction&hl=en&qscrl=1&nord=1&
rlz=1T4ADFA_enUS417US433&tbm=vid&source=lnms&ei=5eVDT-fyC6XI0AHU_
Oi6Bw&sa=X&oi=mode_link&ct=mode&cd=4&ved=0CDEQ_AUoAw&biw=1024&bih=661
#hl=en&qscrl=1&nord=1&rlz=1T4ADFA_enUS417US433&tbm=vid&sclient=psy-ab&q=M
yocardial+ischemia&pbx=1&oq=Myocardial+ischemia&aq=f&aqi=g3&aql=&gs_sm=3&gs_
upl=74668l78226l0l79180l2l2l0l0l0l0l0l178l256l1.1l2l0&bav=on.2,or.r_gc.r_pw.r_qf.,cf.osb&fp
=6893b15720e5ec6e&biw=1024&bih=661

Myocardial infarction
http://www.google.com/search?q=myocardial+infarction&hl=en&qscrl=1&n
ord=1&rlz=1T4ADFA_enUS417US433&tbm=vid&source=lnms&ei=5eVDT-
fyC6XI0AHU_Oi6Bw&sa=X&oi=mode_link&ct=mode&cd=4&ved=0CDEQ_
AUoAw&biw=1024&bih=661

Atherosclerosis videos
http://www.google.com/search?q=atherosclerosis&hl=en&qscrl=1&nord=1&rlz=1T4ADFA_
enUS417US433&tbm=vid&source=lnms&ei=FOdDT4m6NaL30gHvq7S9Bw&sa=X&oi=
mode_link&ct=mode&cd=4&ved=0CDMQ_AUoAw&biw=1024&bih=661

Angina videos
http://www.google.com/search?q=angina&hl=en&qscrl=1&nord=1&rlz=1T4ADFA_enU
S417US433&tbm=vid&source=lnms&ei=2edDT7aBDLGQ0QGauv3yBw&sa=X&oi=m
ode_link&ct=mode&cd=4&ved=0CDMQ_AUoAw&biw=1024&bih=661

Images from Google Images

Coronary artery disease images
http://www.google.com/search?q=coronary+artery+disease&hl=en&qscrl=1&nord=1&rlz=1
T4ADFA_enUS417US433&tbm=isch&source=lnms&ei=nOlDT8L2MaXV0QHNh_32Ag&sa
=X&oi=mode_link&ct=mode&cd=2&sqi=2&ved=0CD4Q_AUoAQ&biw=1024&bih=661

Dyslipidemia images
http://www.google.com/search?q=dyslipidemia&hl=en&qscrl=1&nord=1&rlz=1T4ADFA_en
US417US433&tbm=isch&source=lnms&ei=LepDT7WWGojn0QHdxp3ABw&sa=X&oi=m
ode_link&ct=mode&cd=2&ved=0CCgQ_AUoAQ&biw=1024&bih=661

Heart failure images
http://www.google.com/search?q=heart+failure&hl=en&qscrl=1&nord=1&rlz=1T4ADFA_en
US417US433&tbm=isch&source=lnms&ei=oepDT6PECuf40gGtuuWvBw&sa=X&oi=m
ode_link&ct=mode&cd=2&sqi=2&ved=0CD8Q_AUoAQ&biw=1024&bih=661

Atrial fibrillation images
http://www.google.com/search?q=atrial+fibrillation&hl=en&qscrl=1&nord=1&rlz=1T4A
DFA_enUS417US433&tbm=isch&source=lnms&ei=DutDT5CuHvKO0QHVl4DVBw&sa=X
&oi=mode_link&ct=mode&cd=2&sqi=2&ved=0CD8Q_AUoAQ&biw=1024&bih=661

Aortic stenosis images
http://www.google.com/search?q=aortic+stenosis&hl=en&qscrl=1&nord=1&r
lz=1T4ADFA_enUS417US433&prmd=imvns&source=lnms&tbm=isch&ei=q-
tDT_a1C4Pf0QG7x5XIBw&sa=X&oi=mode_link&ct=mode&cd=2&sqi=2&ved=0C
CQQ_AUoAQ&biw=1024&bih=661

Myocardial ischemia images
http://www.google.com/search?q=Myocardial+ischemia&source=lnms&tbm=isch&sa=X&ei
=RsCjUfHsOojI0gGHtoHoCQ&ved=0CAcQ_AUoAQ&biw=1024&bih=564

Myocardial infarction images
http://www.google.com/search?q=Myocardial+infarction&source=lnms&tbm=isch&sa=X&ei
=a8CjUfuvHpLJ0gGjroGgBQ&ved=0CAcQ_AUoAQ&biw=1024&bih=564

Atherosclerosis images
http://www.google.com/search?q=atherosclerosis&hl=en&qscrl=1&nord=1&rlz=1T4ADFA_
enUS417US433&tbm=isch&source=lnms&ei=EudDT7DBLYnu0gHwoaiyBw&sa=X&oi=m
ode_link&ct=mode&cd=2&ved=0CDYQ_AUoAQ&biw=1024&bih=661

Angina images
http://www.google.com/search?q=angina&hl=en&qscrl=1&nord=1&rlz=1T4ADFA_enUS41
7US433&tbm=isch&source=lnms&ei=0-dDT4-nLcSr0AGSit3gBw&sa=X&oi=mode_link&ct
=mode&cd=2&sqi=2&ved=0CDgQ_AUoAQ&biw=1024&bih=661

Myocardial ischemia image from the Mayo Clinic:
http://www.mayoclinic.com/health/medical/IM03129

Skin Cancer

Faye Lyons, RN, DNP-C

INTRODUCTION

Skin, the largest organ in the body, has multiple functions. The skin protects the body's tissues and internal organs, serves as a barrier against injury, infection, and ultraviolet (UV) rays, helps regulate body temperature, and acts as a receptor for sensation (Arora & Attwood, 2009). It is the skin that receives the largest insults from the environment and displays the sign of aging. The outermost layer of the skin is called the *epidermis*. The epidermis is only about 20 cells deep, or as thick as a sheet of paper. The eyelids have an epidermal thickness of 0.05 mm, and the palms/soles of the feet have an epidermal thickness of 1.5 mm. The *dermis* ranges in thickness from 1-4 mm (about 1/32" [0.8 mm] to 1/8" [3.2 mm]) and contains tiny blood and lymph vessels. *Melanocytes* are a layer of cells between the epidermis and the dermis that produce a brown-black pigment (melanin) that determines skin and hair color (Habif, 2004).

Skin cancer is the most common form of cancer in the United States. More than 3.5 million skin cancers are diagnosed annually. Yearly, there are more new cases of skin cancer than cancers of the breast, prostate, lung, and colon combined (Skin Cancer Facts). Malignant neoplasms are strongly age-associated for the skin, for which there is an almost 20-fold increase in incidence in those aged 70 years or older when compared with those aged 35 to 40 years (Gilchrest, 2007).

The most common types of skin cancer are basal cell carcinoma (BCC), squamous cell carcinoma (SCC), and melanoma (Skin Cancer Facts). Skin cancers are divided into two major groups: (1) nonmelanoma, which includes BCC and SCC and (2) melanoma, the deadliest form of skin cancer. Thirteen million people are living with a history of nonmelanoma skin cancer, typically diagnosed as BCC and SCC. It is predicted that one in five Americans will develop BCC or SCC in their lifetime (Urist & Soong, 2007).

The estimated annual cost of skin cancer in 2004 was $39.3 billion, to include $29.1 billion in direct medical costs (costs of health services and products) and $10.2 billion in lost productivity costs (defined as costs related to consumption of medical care, impaired ability to work, and lost future earning potential because of premature death). On the basis of a practice of willingness to pay for symptom relief, the additional economic burden of skin disease on quality of life was an estimated $56.2 billion. Therefore, the total economic burden of skin disease to the US public in 2004 was approximately $96 billion (Bickers et al., 2006).

PATHOPHYSIOLOGY/PRESENTATION OF SKIN CANCERS

Advances in molecular genetics have provided important new insights into the understanding of nonmelanoma skin cancer. Cancer of the skin is caused by defects in the normal genetic code. These defects are classified as either germline mutations (those caused by inherited mutations) or somatic mutations (those caused by acquired mutations) (Wood et al., 2008).

Tumor suppressor genes and oncogenes are two basic classes of genes that undergo mutations leading to skin cancer. In BCC, the patched gene is affected, whereas in SCC the p53 gene is involved. Oncogenes also contribute to skin cancer formation. These genes are growth-signaling molecules that once altered can lead normal cells to become malignant (Wood et al., 2008).

BASAL CELL CARCINOMA

BCC, a disease of sun exposure, is the most common type of skin cancer in older adults. An estimated 2.8 million are diagnosed with BCC annually in the United States. This cancer accounts for approximately 75% of all nonmelanoma skin cancers. BCC is typically a disease of older, light-skinned individuals because of long-term sun exposure (Arora & Attwood, 2009). A 2003 review by Housman et al. examined the effect of treating nonmelanoma skin cancer in Medicare patients. Although skin cancers may not be as costly as other cancers (breast, lung, colorectal, or prostate cancers), the cost was significant when evaluating the morbidity and mortality as compared with other cancers. BCC is rarely fatal, but can be disfiguring if allowed to go untreated (Nolen et al., 2011). Metastases can occur and is associated with advanced patient age and neglected large lesions (Urist & Soong, 2007).

BCC starts in the lowest part of the epidermis, in round cells called basal cells. Upon histologic examination, most BCC arise in the basal keratinocytes of the epidermis and along the adnexal structures (hair follicles, sweat glands). UVB radiation damages deoxyribonucleic acid (DNA) and its repair system and alters the immune system. BCC appears to require the surrounding stroma to support its growth. BCC is not capable of spreading through blood vessels or lymphatics. The course of BCC is unpredictable; it can remain small for years, particularly in the older adult, or it may grow rapidly in bursts to expand the tumor (Habif, 2004).

Basal cells arise from mutations that activate the hedgehog signaling pathway, which controls cell growth. The affected genes are called Sonic Hedgehog, Patched 1, and Smothened genes. Inactivation of the Patched 1 gene is most common (James et al., 2006).

The sonic hedgehog (Shh) pathway has been implicated in both heredity (germline mutation) and sporadic (somatic mutation) cases of BCC. In the Shh pathway, the transmembrane protein receptor for Shh, called Patch 1 (Ptch 1), binds and stops another transmembrane protein called smothened (Smoh). The Smoh is responsible for growth, and when bound to Ptch 1, growth is kept in balance. However, when the soluble lipoprotein Shh binds with Ptch 1, this pattern is disrupted. Smoh is then activated, and unregulated growth of abnormal cells occurs (Wood et al., 2008).

The most common forms of BCC are *nodular*, *superficial*, and *sclerosing* or *morpheaform* (Arora & Attwood, 2009):

- *Nodular* is the most common form of BCC and is most likely to occur on the hand and neck. Nodular BCC generally begins as a small, dome-shaped, pink or pearly papule with a translucent appearance.
- *Superficial* is most commonly found on the trunk. It can also be seen on the extremities and is found least often on the head and neck. The thickness of the dermis on the back may serve as a barrier and may be the reason why superficial BCCs predominate in this region. It presents as a well-circumscribed, translucent or bright pink-to-red patch, which may contain irregular telangiectasia.
- *Sclerosing* or *morpheaform* is the least likely form of BCC. It tends to occur on the head and neck and is sometimes found on the trunk. It appears as a hypopigmented, vague variation in skin texture with a decreased ability to appreciate pore.

A basal cell is characterized by (Nolen et al., 2011) the following:

- A round area of thickened skin that does not change color or cause pain or itching.
- The lesion spreads out very slowly and develops a slightly raised edge, which may be translucent and smooth.
- The center will eventually become ulcerated and be covered with a thin skin, which can become sore and open.
- A form known as aggressive-growth BCC looks like a scar with a hard base. This type can spread quickly and needs to be treated aggressively (Figs. 5.1 to 5.4).

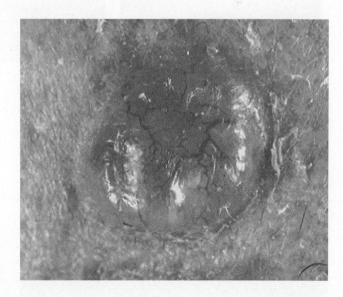

FIGURE 5.1. Nodular basal cell carcinoma. (From Nolen, M. E., Beebe, V. R., King, J. M., et al. [2011]. Nonmelanoma skin cancer: Part 1. *Journal of Dermatology Nurses Association, 3* [5], 260–281, with permission.)

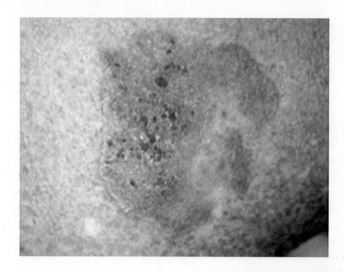

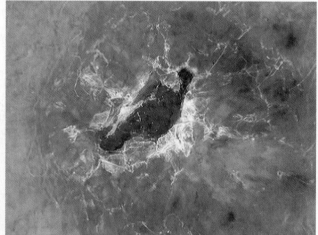

FIGURE 5.2. Superficial basal cell carcinoma. (From Nolen, M. E., Beebe, V. R., King, J. M., et al. [2011]. Nonmelanoma skin cancer: Part 1. *Journal of Dermatology Nurses Association, 3* [5], 260–281, with permission.)

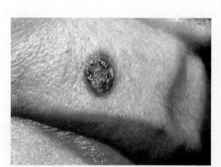

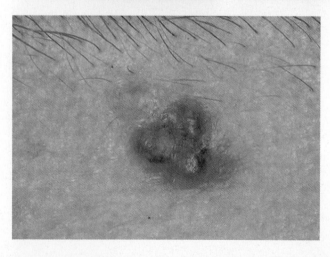

FIGURE 5.3. Pigmented basal cell carcinoma. (From Nolen, M. E., Beebe, V. R., King, J. M., et al. [2011]. Nonmelanoma skin cancer: Part 1. *Journal of Dermatology Nurses Association, 3*[5], 260–281, with permission.)

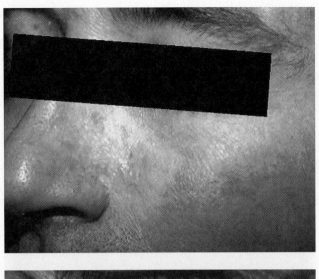

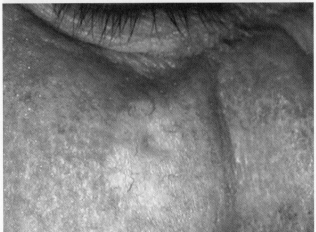

FIGURE 5.4. Morpheaform basal cell carcinoma. (From Nolen, M. E., Beebe, V. R., King, J. M., et al. [2011]. Non-melanoma skin cancer: Part 1. *Journal of Dermatology Nurses Association, 3* [5], 260–281, with permission.)

SQUAMOUS CELL SKIN CANCER

Every year in the United States, there are more than 700,000 new cases of SCC diagnosed, which results in approximately 2,500 deaths. SCCs are at least twice as frequent in men as in women, rarely appear before age 50, and are most common in individuals in their 70s (Nolen et al., 2011).

Common causes of SCC include sunlight, susceptible phenotype, compromised immunity, environmental conditions, and diseases (Urist & Soong, 2007). SCC develops from flat, scalelike skin cells called keratinocytes, which lie under the top layer of the epidermis. Many skin cancers contain changes in one or two genes. When the gene known as PTCH is damaged, cell growth is stimulated. If the damage involves the TP53 gene, then the normal death of damaged cells does not occur, and abnormal cells grow and become tumors (Nolen et al., 2011).

The protein P53 is encoded by the TP53 gene on chromosome 17p and is an important regulator of cell growth, DNA repair, and cell death. P53 mutations are induced by UV light. TP53 acts as a tumor suppressor gene or will function in a dominant-negative role, which causes abnormal mutant p53 protein to bind with normal p53 molecules and disrupt their function. Inactive p53 gene plays an important role in the development of SCC. The loss of the tumor suppressor ability of p53 and the ability of UV radiation to affect induction of cell death by p53 lead to tumor formation (Wood et al., 2008).

There are two main types of SCC (Nolen et al., 2011):

1. *SCC in situ* is the earliest form of SCC. The cancer has not invaded the surrounding tissue. Cancers will appear as large reddish patches that are scaly and crusted.
2. *Invasive SCC* is highly likely to spread (metastasize). The skin cancer lesions can grow rapidly over a few months. Eventually they become ulcerated, which can increase the likelihood of the cancer spreading (Figs. 5.5 to 5.8).

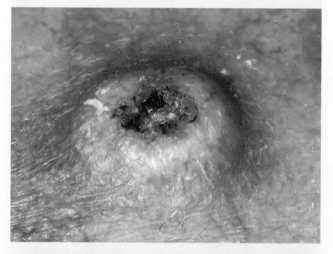

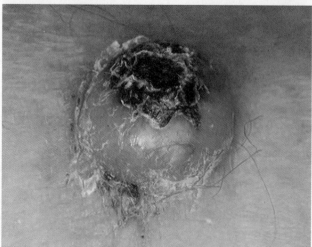

FIGURE 5.5. Keratoacanthoma. (From Nolen, M. E., Beebe, V. R., King, J. M., et al. [2011]. Nonmelanoma skin cancer: Part 1. *Journal of Dermatology Nurses Association, 3* [5], 260–281, with permission.)

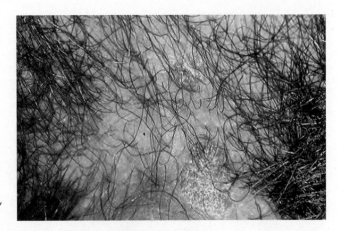

FIGURE 5.6. Bowenoid papulosis. (From Nolen, M. E., Beebe, V. R., King, J. M., et al. [2011]. Nonmelanoma skin cancer: Part 1. *Journal of Dermatology Nurses Association, 3* [5], 260–281, with permission.)

Most SCCs occur in sun-exposed areas, especially on the head and upper extremities. SCCs typically present as enlarging bumps that may have an irregular or reddened surface. The classic appearance is a skin depression with raised edges that are typically more indurated and inflamed than BCC and often crust or ooze (Arora & Attwood, 2009).

MALIGNANT MELANOMA

Melanoma, similar to other adult-onset cancers, is a complex, diverse cancer. Incidence rates differ between genders, ages, ethnic groups, and regions (Tucker, 2009). The incidence of melanoma is increasing faster than any other cancer type. One person dies of melanoma every 62 minutes (American Cancer Society, 2011). One in 55 people will be diagnosed with melanoma during their lifetime. Data from the National Cancer Institute (NCI) estimate that 62,480 new cases

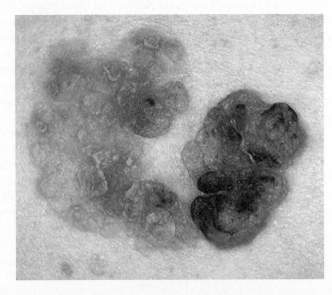

FIGURE 5.7. Squamous cell carcinoma, in situ. (From Nolen, M. E., Beebe, V. R., King, J. M., et al. [2011]. Nonmelanoma skin cancer: Part 1. *Journal of Dermatology Nurses Association, 3* [5], 260–281, with permission.)

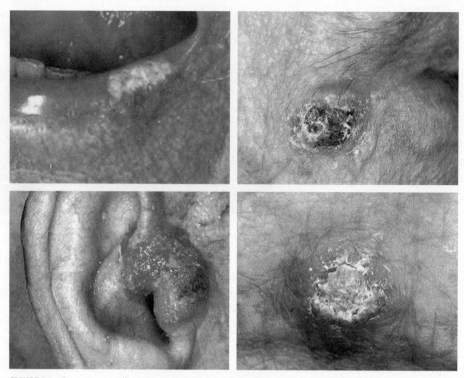

FIGURE 5.8. Squamous cell carcinoma, invasive. (From Nolen, M. E., Beebe, V. R., King, J. M., et al. Nonmelanoma skin cancer: Part 1. [2011]. *Journal of Dermatology Nurses Association, 3* [5], 260–281, with permission.)

of melanoma of the skin are diagnosed in the United States each year (34,950 men and 27,530 women) (Doben & Macgillivray, 2009). Melanoma is the most common form of cancer for young adults 25 to 29 years old and the second most common form of cancer for young people 15 to 29 years old (American Academy of Dermatology, 2011).

Melanoma trends in the United States were examined using data from the Surveillance Epidemiology, and End Results (SEER) Program (a NCI program that collects cancer and survival data from approximately 26% of the US population) and it was found that from 1973 to 1997, rates of melanoma doubled among females and tripled among males (Hawryluk & Fisher, 2011). As on January 1, 2008, in the United States, there were approximately 822,770 men and women alive who had a history of melanoma of the skin (National Cancer Institute, Surveillance Epidemiology and End Results, 2010).

Fortunately, approximately 80% of melanomas are diagnosed at early localized stages, and surgery alone is curative (Rubin, 2010). The American Cancer Society estimates that currently about 120,000 new cases of melanoma in the United States are diagnosed each year. In 2010, about 68,130 of these were invasive melanomas, with about 38,870 in males and 29,260 in females (Skin Cancer Foundation, 2011c). It is estimated that 123,590 new cases of melanoma will be diagnosed in the United States in 2011—53,360 noninvasive (in situ) and 70,230 invasive, with nearly 8,790 resulting in death (Skin Cancer Facts, 2011c).

In embryo, melanocytes are cells that migrate to multiple sites in the body, and are responsible for the color of the skin and nevi development. Melanocytes position themselves along the basement membrane of the dermoepidermal junction. These cells are vulnerable to cancer-causing stimuli, and this results in malignant transformation to become melanoma (Urist & Soong, 2007).

Melanomas exhibit two growth stages, the radial and the vertical phases. In the radial growth phase, reproduction of malignant melanocytes is confined to the epidermis and the upper dermis. In the vertical growth phase, malignant melanocytes form nests or nodules in the dermis (Armstrong et al., 2012; Swetter & Geller, 2011).

Several cancer staging systems are used worldwide; the most common staging system is the tumor-node-metastasis (TNM) classification endorsed by the American Joint Committee on Cancer (AJCC). The TNM system classifies melanoma by the size and extent of the primary tumor (T), the involvement of regional lymph nodes (N), and the presence or absence of distant metastasis (M) (Table 5.1). This system of classifying cancer by TNM status determines clinical stage I, II, III, or IV of the melanoma (Table 5.2).

The latest edition, called *Cancer Staging Manual,* is effective for cancer cases diagnosed on or after January 1, 2010. This seventh edition includes evidence-based revisions that further clarify the TNM classifications and stage grouping criteria, reflecting an improved understanding of the disease. These recommendations are based on a multivariate analysis of approximately 38,000 patients with melanoma—30, 946 with stages I, II, and III melanoma and the remainder with stage IV melanoma (Rubin, 2010).

Survival rates decline as tumor thickness increases (Swetter & Geller, 2011). When melanoma is detected early, before the tumor has penetrated the skin, the survival rate is about 99%. The survival rate decreases to 15% for advanced disease (Skin Cancer Facts, 2011c). The 5-year survival rate for people with a melanoma diagnosis is dependent on the stage of the neoplasm. There are five stages: Stage 0 is in situ melanoma, stage I or II is localized cutaneous disease, stage III is regional nodal disease, and stage IV is distant metastatic disease (Duncan, 2009). The 5-year survival data for lesion thickness smaller than 0.76 mm is 96% and those between 0.76 and 1.49 mm is 87%; however, these figures decline 10% for each 1 mm in depth. Therefore, older adult patients have a worse prognosis than younger ones (Gilchrest, 2007).

TABLE 5.1 · American Joint Committee on Cancer TNM System

| T stands for **tumor**. The T category is assigned a number (0–4) on the basis of the tumor's thickness (*Breslow measurement*). It may be assigned a small "a" or "b" on the basis of ulceration (the epidermal layer of skin is absent) and mitotic rate (number of cells that are in the process of dividing in a specified amount of tissue). **Breslow measurement for T staging:** **T1:** 1.0 mm or less **T2:** 1.1–2.0 mm **T3:** 2.1–4.0 mm **T4:** >4.0 mm | N stands for spread to nearby **lymph nodes**. The N category is assigned a number (0–3) on the basis of whether the melanoma cells have spread to the lymph nodes or in the lymphatic channels connecting the lymph nodes. It may be assigned a small "a," "b," or "c." **Clinical staging** is based on what is found on physical exam, biopsy/removal of the main melanoma, imaging test, and biopsy of lymph nodes. **Pathologic staging** is determined after the lymph node biopsy. | **M** is for metastasis, if the melanoma has spread to distant organs. |

(Continued)

TABLE 5.1 • American Joint Committee on Cancer TNM System *(Continued)*

TX: Primary tumor cannot be assessed.

T0: No evidence of primary tumor.

Tis: Melanoma **in situ**

T1a: The melanoma is ≤1.0 mm, without ulceration, and mitotic rate is <1/mm^2.

T1b: The melanoma is ≤1.0 mm thick, it is ulcerated, and/or the mitotic rate is ≥1/mm^2.

T2a: The melanoma is between 1.01 and 2.0 mm without ulceration.

T2b: The melanoma is between 1.01 and 2.0 mm with ulceration.

T3a: The melanoma is between 2.01 and 4.0 mm without ulceration.

T3b: The melanoma is between 2.01 and 4.0 mm with ulceration.

T4a: The melanoma is thicker than 4.0 mm without ulceration.

T4b: The melanoma is thicker than 4.0 mm with ulceration.

Clinical staging of the lymph **nodes**, which is done without the sentinel node biopsy.

NX: Regional lymph nodes cannot be assessed.

N0: No spread to nearby lymph nodes.

N1: Spread to one nearby lymph node.

N2: Spread to two or three nearby lymph nodes or spread of melanoma to nearby skin or toward a nearby lymph node area.

N3: Spread to four or more lymph nodes, or spread to lymph nodes that are grouped together, or spread of melanoma to nearby skin or toward a lymph node area and into lymph node.

Pathologic stage is determined after the lymph node biopsy.

Any Na (N1a or N2a) means that the melanoma is in the lymph node(s), but it can only be visualized through a microscope (microscopic spread).

Any Nb (N1b or N2b) means that the melanoma is in the lymph node(s) and was visualized on imaging or palpated by clinician before removal (macroscopic spread).

N2c means the melanoma has spread to small areas of skin in the form of satellite tumors or has spread to skin lymphatic channels around the tumor.

M0: No distant metastasis.

M1a: Metastasis to skin, subcutaneous tissue, or lymph nodes, with a normal blood LDH level.

M1b: Metastasis to the lungs, with normal LDH levels.

M1c: Metastasis to other organs, or distant spread to any site. LDH levels in the blood are elevated.

From American Cancer Society (2012). Retrieved from http://www.cancer.org/cancer/skincancer-melanoma/DetailedGuide/melanoma-skin-cancer-staging

Historically, the presence of nodal involvement has been determined by standard hematoxylin and eosin-stained sectioning; however, with the increasing availability of immunohistochemical (IHC) staining to detect melanoma-associated antigens, it is now possible to consistently detect nodal metastases in just a few collective cells (0.1 mm or less), an extremely low volume of tumor. Although it is recommended that both hematoxylin and eosin and IHC be performed, the AJCC considers IHC alone acceptable to determine the presence of microscopic nodal metastases, as long as the diagnosis is based on at least one melanoma-associated marker (such as HMB-45, Melan-A/MART 1) and the cells have malignant morphologic features that can be detected in the IHC-stained slides (Rubin, 2010).

Five principle histologic types of melanoma are observed (Armstrong et al., 2012; Arora & Attwood, 2009; Doben & Macgillivray, 2009; Swetter & Geller, 2011):

1. *Superficial spreading* appears as a plaque that is a few millimeters to several centimeters in diameter, with irregular borders and varied colors. Malignant melanocytes spread throughout

TABLE 5.2 · American Joint Committee on Cancer Stage Grouping

Stage Grouping		
Stage 0	**Tis, N0, M0:** Melanoma in situ	
Stage IA	**T1a, N0, M0:** Melanoma is <1.0 mm. It is not ulcerated and the mitotic rate is <1/mm². There is no lymph node or distant organ involvement.	
Stage IB	**T1b or T2a, N0, M0:** Melanoma is <1.0 mm. There is ulceration or has a mitotic rate of at least 1/mm², or is between 1.01 and 2.0 mm and is not ulcerated. There is no lymph node or distant organ involvement.	
Stage IIA	**T2b or T3a, N0, M0:** Melanoma is between 1.01 and 2.0 mm. There is ulceration, or it is between 2.01 and 4.0 mm and is not ulcerated. There is no lymph node or distant organ involvement.	
Stage IIB	**T3b or T4a, N0, M0:** Melanoma is between 2.01 and 4.0 mm and is ulcerated, or is >4.0 mm and is not ulcerated. There is no lymph node or distant organ involvement.	
Stage IIC	**T4b, N0, M0:** Melanoma is >4.0 mm and is ulcerated. There is no lymph node or distant organ involvement.	
Stage IIIA	**T1a–T4a, N1a or N2a, M0:** Melanoma can be of any thickness, but is not ulcerated. It has spread to one to three lymph nodes near the affected skin area, but there is no lymphadenopathy and the melanoma is found only when they are viewed under the microscope. There is no distant organ spread.	
Stage IIIB	**One of the following applies:**	**T1b–T4b, N1a or N2a, M0:** Melanoma can be of any thickness and is ulcerated. It has spread to one to three lymph nodes near the affected skin area, but there is no lymphadenopathy and the melanoma is found only when the nodes are viewed under a microscope. There is no distant spread.
		T1a–T4a, N1b or N2b, M0: Melanoma can be of any thickness, but is not ulcerated. It has spread to one to three lymph nodes near the affected skin area. There is lymphadenopathy. There is no distant spread.
		T1a–T4a, N2c, M0: Melanoma can be of any thickness, but is not ulcerated. It has spread to areas on nearby skin or lymphatic channels around the original tumor, but the nodes do not contain melanoma. There is no distant spread.
Stage IIIC	**One of the following applies:**	**T1b–T4b, N1b or N2b, M0:** Melanoma can be of any thickness and is ulcerated. It has spread to one to three lymph nodes near the affected skin area. There is lymphadenopathy. There is no distant spread.
		T1b–T4b, N2c, M0: Melanoma can be of any thickness and is ulcerated. It has spread to small areas of nearby skin or lymphatic channels around the original tumor, but the nodes do not contain melanoma. There is no distant spread.
		Any T, N3, M0: Melanoma can be of any thickness and may be ulcerated. It has spread to four or more nearby lymph nodes, or to nearby lymph nodes that are grouped together, or it has spread to nearby skin or lymphatic channels around the original tumor and to nearby lymph nodes. There is lymphadenopathy because of the melanoma. There is no distant spread.
Stage IV	**Any T, any N, M1 (a, b, or c):** Melanoma has spread beyond the original area of skin and nearby lymph nodes to other organs such as lung, liver, or brain, or to distant areas of skin, subcutaneous tissue, or distant lymph nodes. At this stage, lymph nodal spread or thickness is considered, but typically the melanoma is thick and has also spread to the lymph nodes.	

From American Cancer Society. (2012). Retrieved from http://www.cancer.org/cancer/skincancer-melanoma/DetailedGuide/melanoma-skin-cancer-staging.

the layers of the epidermis as single cells or nests. Dermal invasion is seen in the vertical growth phase.

2. *Lentigo maligna* begin as a nonpalpable tan or brown macule, enlarging gradually over many years. Dermal invasion is noted by palpable areas. A dermal nodule indicates a vertical growth phase.

3. *Acral lentiginous* arise on the palmar, plantar, subungual, and mucosal surfaces of the body.

4. *Nodular* are vertical-growth-phase melanomas. They present as dark, sometimes ulcerated pigmented nodules. On histology, there is a nodule of neoplastic cells in the dermis, with no adjacent radial growth phase.

5. *Desmoplastic* is a rare, aggressive subtype of melanoma that has a tendency to invade perineural areas and reoccur. Desmoplastic melanomas frequently occur on the head and neck of older men in their sixth and seventh decades of life and are often deep at the time of diagnosis owing to the difficulty of clinical diagnosis with these atypical and often unpigmented lesions.

The common sites for malignant melanoma for men are the head, neck, and torso, and women tend to have melanoma on the arms and legs. The less common sites for melanoma include fingers, genitals, lips, palms, soles of feet, and under fingernails or toenails (Markovic et al., 2007).

Although melanoma has been reported to metastasize anywhere in the body, the most common areas are the lung, liver, bone, and brain (Urist & Soong, 2007).

SCREENING AND RISK FACTORS

Some studies have shown that people with BCC or SCC may be at higher risk for a second cancer, including melanoma, cancer of the lip, salivary glands, larynx, lungs, breast, kidney, and non-Hodgkin lymphoma. Those at higher risk for such cancers are men and those diagnosed before age 60 with a BCC. Patients should be followed at 3- to 6-month intervals because there is a 36% to 50% chance of developing a second BCC or SCC within 5 years (Leber et al., 1999).

The lifetime risk of developing invasive melanoma for a person in 1935 was estimated at 1 in 1,500 compared with 2010 risk estimates of 1 in 39 for Caucasian men and 1 in 58 for Caucasian women. The incidence rates are increasing most for older individuals, doubling during a 25-year period (1983 to 2007) for men aged 60 to 64 and quadrupling for men aged 75 to 79. Although the diagnosis of early-stage melanoma has improved, the incidence of advanced melanoma has been increasing for men over age 65 (Geller & Swetter, 2012).

The following factors increase the risk for a person to develop skin cancer:

■ **Age over 40**—The incidence of nonmelanoma skin cancer increases with age. Recent evidence suggests that the incidence of BCC is increasing in Americans younger than 40 years old owing to the use of tanning beds and increased sun exposure (Nolen et al., 2011). The risk for melanoma increases with age; however the role of aging is not clear. With increasing age there is an increased risk for the initiation of new tumors, either through exposure to UV radiation or through the decreasing ability of individual cells to repair DNA damage. As a person ages, they lose Langerhans cells that help fight off early skin cancers (Urist & Soong, 2007).

Melanoma is most common in people over 40, with an average age at diagnosis of 57 years. In 2010, approximately 0.7% of people were diagnosed with melanoma under age 20; 7.1% between 20 and 34; 11.2% between 35 and 44; 18.6% between 45 and 54; 20.9% between 55 and 64; 18.1% between 65 and 74; 16.9% between 75 and 84; and 6.4% for age 85 and older

(National Cancer Institute, Surveillance Epidemiology and End Results, 2010). Superficial spreading melanoma affects females commonly on lower-extremity sites and at an early onset in age, but men are often affected with lentigo maligna melanomas on the head and neck or upper-extremity site at a late onset in age (Tucker, 2009).

- **Being male**—Men have a 30% higher incidence of having nonmelanoma skin cancer than women (Nolen et al., 2011). Men are more likely to have invasive and fatal melanoma than women, although some research suggests that the reason for the higher rates is that men do not get suspicious lesions evaluated before they become dangerous. The rate in women levels off somewhat at age 50; researchers think menopause potentially could have a protective effect (Markovic et al., 2007). From 1975 to 1989, the overall melanoma mortality that increased since then has stabilized: The mortality rates for men from 1975 to 1990 increased, but then flattened from 1990 to 2005. In 2005, the compiled age-adjusted mortality rate for men was 3.9 per 100,000, and for women was 1.7 per 100,000 (Tucker, 2009).
- **Chronic or severe skin problems**—Genetic disorders, including xeroderma pigmentosum and albinism, are associated with increased risk for many types of skin cancer. A history of chronic conditions of the skin such as burn scars (Marjolin ulcer), draining sinuses, infections, and ulcers are often associated with the development of SCCs (Urist & Soong, 2007). More than two thirds of all SCCs that occur in African Americans are in preexisting inflammatory conditions (hidradenitis suppurative, cutaneous lupus), burn injuries, or trauma, and these lesions are usually more aggressive (Leber et al., 1999).
- **Diseases**—Impaired immunity, especially cell-mediated immunity, is a well-documented cause of SCCs of the skin. The largest group of chronically immunosuppressed patients is those who underwent organ transplantation (Nolen et al., 2011; Urist & Soong, 2007). Twenty years posttransplantation, the occurrence of BCC and SCC is as high as 80%. BCC occurs approximately 10 times more often and SCC occurs 65 to 250 times more frequently in the immunosuppressed patient than in the general population. Malignancies of all types are more common in heart transplant recipients, probably because of the greater degree of immunosuppression required to prevent organ rejection (Nolen et al., 2011). Anybody with a depressed immune system (e.g., HIV, cancer patients) should have regular skin checks.

Melanoma has developed in patients who received solid organ transplants from donors who had the disease. Persons who have had non-Hodgkin lymphoma are at a higher risk for melanoma, and persons who have HPV (human papillomavirus) are at a higher risk of developing SCC in the genital and anal areas and around fingernails. Women who have a history of endometriosis have a 60% increased risk of developing melanoma (American Cancer Society, 2011).

A strong association between Parkinson disease and melanoma has been suspected and was perhaps based on the fact that both diseases involve cells that metabolize tyrosine via dopaquinone intermediates (Hawryluk & Fisher, 2011). Levodopa serves as a substitute for tyrosine hydroxylase, and might therefore accelerate melanoma tumor growth, but data are inconclusive for this (Gao et al., 2009). A family history of melanoma does not increase one's risk of developing Parkinson disease, but a diagnosis of Parkinson disease does increase one's risk of developing melanoma (Hawryluk & Fisher, 2011; Liu et al., 2011). Inzelberg et al. (2011) found in a 5-year limited-duration epidemiologic survey that the prevalence of melanoma in a group of Israeli Parkinson disease patients was higher than expected from existing data on the general Israeli population. The occurrence of melanoma did not appear to be related to the use of levodopa.

■ **Exposure to chemicals or radiation**—Occupational and environmental exposure to arsenic, organic hydrocarbon, ionizing radiation, and cigarette smoke has been associated with increasing risk for SCCs. Exposure to radiation and some chemicals (vinyl chloride, polychlorinated biphenyls, and petrochemicals) in health-care or industrial settings may increase the risk of melanoma (Leber et al., 1999; Urist & Soong, 2007). Airline pilots have been found to have an increased risk for melanoma possibly because of excessive exposure to ionizing radiation at high altitudes, or because they have more opportunity to spend time in sunny regions (Hawryluk & Fisher, 2011). Ionizing radiation exposure, either as a treatment for a disease state, such as acne, or as an accidental environmental exposure, as was seen in World War II, is associated with increased risk of nonmelanoma skin cancer. Radiologists whose hands were exposed to ionizing radiation while treating these patients developed SCC in areas where radiation dermatitis had occurred (Nolen et al., 2011). Treatment with chemoradiation creates a higher risk for BCCs and SCCs. Patel et al. (2010) found that patients who received chemoradiation and developed chronic radiation dermatitis did develop skin cancer of the face (98.4%) and scalp (1.6%).

■ **Geography**—States such as California and Hawaii have twice the incidence of nonmelanoma skin cancer than the Midwestern states because of increased sun exposure. Northern European countries, such as Finland, have lower incidence rates, and Australia has the highest incidence of BCC in the world (Nolen et al., 2011).

■ **Heavy Metals**—Arsenic, a heavy metal and naturally occurring element, is formed in the earth along with other ores, and is associated with increased risk of SCC. Human exposure to arsenic occurs from natural sources, such as well water. It is commonly seen in agricultural workers and exterminators and is found in the pesticide Paris green. It can be found in drinking water when arsenic leeches out of soil and rocks or the drinking water is contaminated by industrial sources (Nolen et al., 2011). Mining, metallurgy, decorative-glass making, and pressure-treated wood are all sources of arsenic exposure. In the past, arsenical preparations such as Fowler's solution (potassium arsenite) were used to treat syphilis and other conditions. Individuals may be exposed to arsenic by breathing sawdust or smoke from arsenic-treated wood, by living in an area with high levels of arsenic in rock, or by working in a job in which arsenic is used or made (Nolen et al., 2011).

■ **High mole count**—Individuals with a large number of nevi have a strong risk factor for the development of melanoma. Studies have shown that persons with a higher mole count, which is often counted on the back (greater than 40 on the back can be considered high), are at a greater risk for melanoma (Berwick et al., 2009). About 30% of the population has a history of dysplastic (abnormal) moles, which increases the risk of developing melanoma (Markovic et al., 2007).

Clinically, the number of dysplastic nevi is associated with increased risk of melanoma. One dysplastic nevus creates a 2-fold risk, whereas 10 or more dysplastic nevi induce a 12-fold increased risk of melanoma. Having many small nevi imparts an approximately twofold increased risk, and the presence of both small and large nondysplastic nevi results in a fourfold risk. Congenital nevi are not associated with melanoma risk; however, giant pigmented congenital nevi confer substantial melanoma risk (Goodson & Grossman, 2009; Hawryluk & Fisher, 2011).

■ **Medications that affect the immune system**—Potential skin cancer risks have been associated with the eczema drugs pimecrolimus (Elidel) and tacrolimus (Protopic) in a small number of people (O'Connor, 2010). Immunosuppressive drugs such as azathioprine, cyclosporine, and prednisone have been linked to a greater than 50% increase in the risk for SCC (Nolen et al., 2011). Persons who take TNF-alpha blockers to treat rheumatoid arthritis and other autoimmune diseases are at increased risk of developing melanoma and other nonmelanoma skin cancers (Amari et al., 2011).

- **Personal or family history of skin cancer**—Individuals with a family history, particularly first-degree relatives, of melanoma have twice the risk of developing melanoma as those without a family history (Berwick et al., 2009). Those persons who have had melanoma have an 11.4% risk for a second primary melanoma. This percentage is higher in older men and in those whose first melanomas appeared on the upper body and face (Hawryluk & Fisher, 2011).
- **Phenotype characteristics**—Phenotype is independently important as a risk factor for the development of skin cancers: light hair color (blonde and red-haired), light eye color (blue), and light skin color, including skin that freckles easily (Berwick et al., 2009; Nolen et al., 2011). Phenotype is not a high risk marker for the development of BCC, but is a high risk for SCC. However, the inability to tan is a high risk marker for the development of BCC (Habif, 2004).
- **Smoking**—Smoking generates free radicals and oxidative stress, and reduces the body's antioxidant defenses. Free radicals seem to play an important role in the etiology of BCC and SCC. Although free radicals are also involved in the etiology of melanoma, elastosis of the skin seems to overcome the direct effect of free radical production in the etiology of melanoma. Smoking increases skin aging, including elastosis (Grant, 2008).
- **UV radiation**—UVA is a long wavelength (320 to 400 nm) and accounts for 95% of UV radiation. It penetrates deep into the skin, can penetrate glass and clouds, and is present during all daylight hours, year-round. In the past, this wavelength was not thought to be a major factor in the development of skin cancer, but recent studies support the fact that UVA causes more DNA damage than UVB (Nolen et al., 2011).

  UVB is a shorter wavelength (290 to 320 nm) and penetrates the epidermal layer of the skin. It is responsible for burning, some tanning, and acceleration of skin aging. UVC (100 to 290 nm) is the shortest wavelength and is filtered by the ozone layer; therefore, it does not reach the earth's surface (Nolen et al., 2011).

  In all races, BCC is usually linked to UV light exposure. Information from the Singapore Cancer Registry suggests that UV exposure plays a role in skin cancer development among fair-skinned Asian populations (Koh et al., 2003). A Hawaiian study showed that the incidence of BCC and SCC was at least 45 times higher in the Japanese populations of Kauai, Hawaii (high UV exposure), than among the Japanese population in Japan (a temperate climate) (Chuang et al., 1995).

  Increased risk factors for nonmelanoma skin cancers include UV light exposure, radiation therapy, albinism, trauma, burn scars (particularly among Asian Indians), other chronic scarring processes (discoid lupus), arsenic exposure, solid organ transplantation, and genetic skin conditions (Skin Cancer Foundation, 2011). When further penetration of UV light is enhanced by the administration of *Oxsoralen* through a treatment known as PUVA (psoralen and ultraviolet-A light treatment), the risk of developing BCC and SCC increases (Nolen et al., 2011).

  UV radiation is a proven human carcinogen. Many individuals are unaware that different patterns of sun exposure have different effects on the development of melanoma. For example, chronic sun exposure, which is received daily during outdoor work, does not increase the risk of melanoma, but intermittent sun exposure and large doses of UV radiation are major contributors to developing melanoma (Berwick et al., 2009).

  Currently, tanning beds are regulated by the Food and Drug Administration (FDA) as Class I medical devices, the same designation given to elastic bandages and tongue depressors (Skin Cancer Foundation, 2011d). However, the International Agency for Research on Cancer (IARC, 2011), an affiliate of the World Health Organization (WHO), classifies UV tanning devices as Group 1, which includes the most dangerous cancer-causing substances such as plutonium, cigarettes, and solar UV radiation (Ghissassi et al., 2009). Skin exams should be done yearly on patients who have had a history of UV exposure or family history of skin cancers.

TREATMENTS

Antioxidants are chemicals or drugs that help prevent cell damage from unstable molecules called free radicals. Antioxidants that protect the skin include vitamins C and E, and coenzyme Q10 (CoQ10). Topical antioxidants that help to improve wrinkles and sun-damaged skin are selenium and vitamins E and C. However, most available brands contain very low concentrations of these antioxidants that are not well absorbed by the skin, so the effect is usually short-term. There is no evidence that these topical antioxidants prevent skin cancer. Another natural treatment is *Ingenol mebutate*, which is a gel that is extracted from the *Euphorbia peplus* plant. This extract breaks down the lesion and has antitumor activity by stimulating antibodies. It is not intended for the face (Ridky, 2007).

Nonmelanoma Skin Cancer

A number of options are available for treating nonmelanoma skin cancer, including surgery, electrodessication and curettage (ED&C), cryosurgery, photodynamic therapy (PDT), radiation, intralesional injections, topical 5-fluorouracil (5-FU; Efudex), and topical immunotherapy with imiquimod (Aldara), which has been proved to prevent skin cancer in certain people (Table 5.3). This medication prompts the immune system to fight off foreign substances, including cancer cells. Other chemopreventive drugs under investigation for the prevention of skin cancers are nonsteroidal anti-inflammatory drugs and retinoids. Treatment is usually dependent on the likelihood of recurrence after treatment, and patient factors such as physical or functional limitations that may affect the ability of patients to tolerate surgery, manage wound care, apply topical therapies, or return for follow-up impact the choice of treatment (Ridky, 2007).

ED&C is one of the most widely used methods for the treatment of BCCs and SCCs. Electrodessication uses electrical current to produce superficial tissue destruction. Another treatment that is utilized is cryosurgery, which is a cost-effective and useful tool used in the treatment of superficial BCCs and SCCs (Chartier & Aasi, 2011; Chartier & Stern, 2011; Galiczynski & Vidimos, 2011; James et al., 2006).

Intralesional therapies that include interferons, 5-FU, or bleomycin are used frequently for the management of BCC. There is limited data on the use of intralesional therapies; however, the case reports available suggest that these therapies are highly effective for the treatment of BCC (Chartier & Aasi, 2011).

PDT is a newer management option that has been utilized for the treatment of BCC. PDT uses light and porphyrins (5-aminolevulinic acid) to cause tumor destruction. The acid is applied to the tumor site and the use of the light therapy activates the acid to penetrate the area and cause cell death. Although PDT has been approved for the treatment of BCC in European countries, US FDA approval has not been granted for the treatment of BCC (Chartier & Aasi, 2011).

Most BCCs and SCCs are treated with surgery or radiation. Research has shown that surgery has the best results, but because of cosmetic effects, many patients opt for radiation (Arora & Attwood, 2009; Gilchrest, 2007). Radiation therapy is an option for patients who are poor candidates for surgical intervention or the BCC has a high risk of recurrence (Chartier & Aasi, 2011).

The American Academy of Dermatology has divided SCC tumors into three groups on the basis of depth: Lesions less than 4 mm deep are suitable for local excision, those lesions 4- to 8-mm

TABLE 5.3 · Treatment Options for BCC, SCC, and MM

	Superficial BCC/SCC	BCC	SCC	Malignant Melanoma
Efudex (topical 5-FU)Grade 2C	×			
Grade 2C				
Imiquimod (Aldara)	×	×	×	
Intralesional agents (bleomycin, 5-FU, interferon) Grade 2C	×	×		
Liquid nitrogen (cryotherapy)	×		×	
ED&CGrade 2C	×	×	×	
Surgical excision		×	×	×
Mohs surgery		×	×	×
Radiation		×	×	×
Photodynamic treatment				

From Chartier, T. K., & Aasi, S. Z. (2011, June 9). Treatment and prognosis of basal cell carcinoma. *UpToDate*. Retrieved from http://www.uptodate.com/contents/treatment-and-prognosis-of-basal-cell-carcinoma.

From Chartier, T. K., & Stern, R. S. (2011, February 8). Treatment and prognosis of cutaneous squamous cell carcinoma. *UpToDate*. Retrieved from http://www.uptodate.com/contents/treatment-and-prognosis-of-cutaneous-squamous-cell-carcinoma.

From Stone, M. (2011, September). Initial surgical management of melanoma of the skin and unusual sites. *UpToDate*. http://www.uptodate.com/contents/initial-surgical-management-of-melanoma-of-the-skin.

deep should undergo surgical excision, and lesions greater than 8 mm may require multimodality treatment with surgical excision, radiation, and possibly chemotherapy. The suggested margins for low-risk tumors less than 2 cm is 4 mm, and those greater than 2 cm should have 6-mm margins (Arora & Attwood, 2009).

Mohs micrographic surgery was developed by Dr. Frederick Mohs at the University of Wisconsin in 1936. He recognized that microscopically observing the surgical margins during excision would result in the overall clearance of the tumor and in lower rates of recurrence. Mohs surgical excision is a tissue-sparing technique that employs frozen-section control of 100% of the surgical margin. The evaluation of the surgical margin uses horizontal sections (not vertical as used in standard surgical excision), combined with precise mapping, which allows for the highest cure rates of skin lesions (James et al., 2006; Nolen et al., 2011).

Melanoma

Surgery is the primary treatment for all stages of melanoma. Mohs micrographic surgery is usually the technique utilized. The amount of tissue removed depends on the size, depth, and degree of invasion: Melanomas in situ require 0.5-cm margin of normal tissue (Grade 2C). Stage 1 lesions that are less than 1 mm deep require the smallest surgical cut; usually with 1 cm off each side and downward from the original lesion (Grade 1B). For melanomas that are 2 mm or thicker, a margin of 2 cm is important for reducing the risk of reoccurrence (Grade 2B). For melanomas greater than 4 mm thick, a 2-cm margin of normal tissue is recommended. There is no evidence that wider margins decrease the incidence of recurrence or improve overall survival (Grade 2C). Thicker lesions will require deeper cuts, which may require skin grafts. Lymph node testing and removal is required if there is evidence that the melanoma has spread to nearby nodes. Although melanoma cells tend to be more resistant to its effects, radiation may be used to help relieve the pain and discomfort caused by cancer that has spread or reoccurred (Urist & Soong, 2007).

Melanoma remains one of the most drug-resistant tumors perhaps in part due to the innate intratumoral differences (Duncan, 2009). Historically, the survival rate for metastatic melanoma has been bleak, with few patients achieving complete or prolonged responses to therapy. Late-stage melanoma patients have very few treatment options for their cancer. The overall median survival for patients with stage IV melanoma is less than a year, with approximately 10% long-term survivors (Chapman, 2011).

The treatment for metastatic melanoma includes several FDA-approved drugs. One is a chemotherapy drug, Dacarbazine (DTIC), a drug given intravenously, with varied response rates of 10% and 25%. Another FDA-approved drug that is often discussed as a treatment option is interleukin-2, an agent that boosts the immune system in its own special way, by activating T cells. The response rates are 15% initially, but only 5% have a prolonged response. Recently, a new agent, an anti-CTLA-4 antibody known as Ipilimumab (Yervoy), has shown increased survival rates (Rubin, 2010). This new drug is showing significant promise in clinical trials of patients with late-stage melanoma. Another new agent, Vemurafenib (Zelboraf), was the second drug approved for metastatic melanoma. These two drugs work differently to treat melanoma, and currently there are clinical trials to combine the treatment of these drugs (Chapman, 2011). Vemurafenib was successful in shrinking the tumors of 81% of patients who had the gene defect that is present in 40% to 60% of melanomas (Skin Cancer Foundation, 2011).

CULTURAL CONSIDERATIONS

The US Census Bureau projects that in the next 10 years, 50% of the US population will comprise Hispanics, Asians, and African Americans. Therefore, raising awareness of skin cancer in people of color is crucial (Skin Cancer Foundation, 2011).

In African American skin, melanin provides sun protection factor (SPF) approximately equivalent to 13.4, compared with 3.4 in white skin. Skin cancer comprises only 2% to 4% of all cancers in Chinese and Japanese Asians and 1% to 2% in African Americans and Asian Indians (Gloster & Neal, 2006). This discrepancy is why skin cancer is the most common type of malignancy in the United States among Caucasians; however, skin cancer in people of color is often associated with greater morbidity and mortality (Gloster & Neal, 2006; Halder, 2003).

In Caucasians, Hispanics, Chinese, and Japanese Asians, BCC is the most common skin malignancy and SCC is the second most common. In African Americans and Asian Indians, this is reversed, with SCC being the most common skin malignancy and BCC the second most common (Gloster & Neal 2006; Leber et al., 1999; Nolen et al., 2011). One study showed that when Hispanic patients develop BCC, they are likely to have multiple lesions at one time (Halder, 2003). African American persons who have scarring or chronic inflammation can develop aggressive SCC, which has the tendency to metastasize and cause death (Skin Cancer Foundation, 2011).

Global data for melanoma is available from the WHO, which states that the incidence of melanoma has been increasing over the past decades, with 132,000 melanomas occurring globally each year (due to UV radiation).

Melanoma is the third most common type of skin cancer among all racial groups. According to the American Cancer Society (2011), the lifetime risk of getting melanoma is about 2%

(1 in 50) for whites, 0.1% (1 in 1,000) for African Americans, and 0.5% (1 in 200) for Hispanics. Although UV light plays a role in the etiology of melanoma in Caucasians, the primary risk factor for melanoma in people of color is inconclusive (Gloster & Neal, 2006).

There are differences in melanoma incidence and mortality dependent upon ethnicity. The SEER data shows the highest incidence among Caucasians (19.1 females and 29.7 males per 100,000), followed by Hispanics (14.7 females and 4.4 males per 100,000), American-Indians/Alaska Natives, Asian/Pacific Islanders, and African Americans (1.0 female and 1.1 males per 100,000) (Hawryluk & Fisher, 2011). For all races, death rates for melanoma showed 4.0 per 100,000 for men and 1.7 per 100,000 for women (National Cancer Institute, Surveillance Epidemiology and End Results, 2010).

The incidence of melanoma in people of European descent has also increased worldwide. Incidence rates in central Europe were similar to those in the United States between 1970 and 2000. In France, the incidence rate between 1980 and 2005 increased by 3.1% in men and 2.25% in women. Population-based data from Canada during the last 50 years indicate an ongoing increase in melanoma incidence for older men and women (aged 60 and older) and a slightly decreasing rate for individuals 40 years and younger. In Australia and New Zealand, where incidence rates are the highest in the world (40 to 60 cases per 100,000 inhabitants), melanoma incidence has nearly doubled every 10 years (Geller & Swetter, 2012; Hawryluk & Fisher, 2011).

PREVENTION

In 2011, the Center for Drug and Evaluation and Research announced new sunscreen rules (Skin Cancer Foundation, 2011d):

- Broad-spectrum sunscreens (block UVA and UVB radiation) with an SPF of 15 or higher will be able to state, "if used as directed with other sun protection measures, this product reduces the risk of skin cancer and early skin aging, as well as helps prevent sunburn." Sunscreen manufacturers have never before been able to make such a claim.
- Broad-spectrum sunscreens with SPFs of 2 to 14 must display a warning that the product has not been shown to help prevent skin cancer or early skin aging.
- The terms "sweat proof" and "waterproof" are no longer allowed on sunscreen labels. However, sunscreens may claim to be "water-resistant," but must specify whether they protect the skin for 40 or 80 minutes of swimming or sweating, based on standard testing.
- A company cannot claim that its sunscreen products provide sun protection for more than 2 hours without submitting test results to the FDA.

UV protection can be provided by the clothes that are worn, such as clothes that are of bright or dark colors (red or black). These colors absorb more UV radiation than white or pastel shades. Also, synthetic fibers (polyester) offer more protection than materials like refined cottons or crepe. On cooler days, tightly woven or closely knitted fabrics, like denim, and denser fabrics, like heavyweight flannel, will absorb less UV light than thinner materials (Skin Cancer Foundation, 2011d).

Sun-protective garments should have an ultraviolent protection factor (UPF) label. This indicates what fraction of the sun's UV rays can penetrate the fabric. For example, a shirt with a UPF of 50 will let 1/50th of the sun's UVR reach the skin. The Skin Cancer Foundation recommends clothing with a UPF of 30+ (Skin Cancer Foundation, 2011d).

Recommendations for extra precautions are (1) avoiding reflective surfaces such as water, sand, concrete, and white-painted surfaces; (2) remembering that cloudy, hazy days can intensify the UVB exposure; (3) UV intensity depends on the angle of the sun, not the heat or brightness, so dangers are greater the closer to the start of summer; (4) skin burns faster at higher altitudes (one study suggested that an average-complexioned person burns in 6 minutes at 11,000' (3352.8 m) at noon compared with 25 minutes at sea level); and (5) avoiding sun lamps, tanning beds, and tanning salons. The machines use mostly high-output UVA rays (Lautenschlager et al., 2007).

PATIENT EDUCATION

Look for the following signs of possible skin cancer (American Academy of Family Physicians (2013)):

- *Asymmetry (A):* Skin cancers usually grow in an irregular, uneven way.
- *Border (B):* Moles with jagged or smudged edges may signal that the cancer is growing or spreading.
- *Color (C):* One of the earliest signs of melanoma is the appearance of various colors in a mole.
- *Diameter (D):* A diameter of 6 mm or larger should be examined.
- *Evolution (E):* A lesion that has changed in size, color, or appearance should be examined.

Keep in mind that the most important warning sign of melanoma is a new or changing skin lesion, regardless of its size and color. Changes that occur over a short time (particularly over a few weeks) are most concerning. Anyone with risk factors for skin cancer should check their entire body once a month. People who regularly check moles on their skin may have a lower risk of developing melanoma (Markovic et al., 2007).

Everyone, especially those at risk for developing skin cancers, should have a full-body skin exam yearly. People who have had melanoma should be checked every 3 to 6 months until they reach their third anniversary. By this time, 75% of patients at risk for metastasis will have had a reoccurrence (Urist & Soong, 2007). A baseline chest radiograph should be done after biopsy confirmation of all melanomas, annually for patients whose lesions are less than 3 mm thick, and every 6 months for the first 5 years if lesions are greater than 3 mm thick (Buzaid et al., 2012; Leber et al., 1999).

The Basic Skin Cancer Triage (BSCT) Web-based curriculum outlines a formal physical examination procedure utilizing a standard sequence of "down and back" (down the anterior body, then back up the posterior body). The BSCT curriculum was developed by a team of experts from the fields of education, psychiatry, and dermatology. The guiding principles underlying the BSCT were derived from similar successful preventative measures such as those used in smoking cessation. These principles involve addressing providers' predisposing attitudes and beliefs, and the extent of their knowledge, skills, and resources. The curriculum was designed to increase the ability of primary care physicians to accurately and confidently triage skin lesions and to counsel patients on skin cancer issues (Mikkilneni et al., 2001).

REFERENCES

Amari, W., Zeringue, A. L., McDonald, J. R., Caplan, L., Eisen, S. A., & Ranganathan, P. (2011). Risk of non-melanoma skin cancer in a national cohort of veterans with rheumatoid arthritis. *Rheumatology, 50*, 1431–1439.

American Academy of Dermatology. (2011). Melanoma [Fact sheet]. Retrieved from http://www.aad.org/media-resources/stats-and-facts/conditions/melanoma

American Academy of Family Physicians.(2013) Patient Education. Skin Cancer @www.mdconsult.com/das/patient/body/425829480-5/1479153990/10062/69902.html

American Cancer Society. (2011). What are the key statistics about melanoma skin cancer? Retrieved from http://www.cancer.org/Cancer/skincancer-melanoma/DetailedGuide/melanoma-skin-cancer-key-statistics

American Cancer Society. (2012). How is melanoma skin cancer staged? Retrieved from http://www.cancer.org/cancer/skincancer-melanoma/DetailedGuide/melanoma-skin-cancer-staging

Armstrong, A. W., Liu, V., & Mihm, M. C. (2012). Pathologic characteristics of melanoma. *UpToDate*. Retrieved from http://www.uptodate.com/contents/pathologic-characteristics-of-melanoma

Arora, A., & Attwood, J. (2009). Common skin cancers and their precursors. *Surgical Clinics of North America*, *89*, 703–712.

Berwick, M., Erdei, E., & Hay, J. (2009). Melanoma epidemiology and public health. *Dermatologic Clinics*, *27*, 205–214.

Bickers, D. R., Lim, H. W., Margolis, D., Weinstock, M. A., Goodman, C., Faulkner, E., & Dall, T. (2006). The burden of skin diseases: 2004 a joint project of the American Academy of Dermatology Association and the Society for Investigative Dermatology. *Journal of the American Academy of Dermatology*, *55*(3), 490–500.

Buzaid, A. C., Gershenwald, J. E., & Ross, M. I. (2012, May 11). Staging work-up and surveillance after treatment of melanoma. *UpToDate*. Retrieved from http://uptodate.com/contents/staging-work-up-nd-surveillance-after-treatment-of-melanoma

Chapman, P. B. (2011). How zelboraf (vemurafenib), a new FDA-approved therapy, extends life for patients with metastatic melanoma. *The Melanoma Letter*, *29*(2), 2–6.

Chartier, T. K., & Aasi, S. Z. (2011, June 9). Treatment and prognosis of basal cell carcinoma. *UpToDate*. Retrieved from http://www.uptodate.com/contents/treatment-and-prognosis-of-basal-cell-carcinoma

Chartier, T. K., & Stern, R. S. (2011, February 8). Treatment and prognosis of cutaneous squamous cell carcinoma. *UpToDate*. Retrieved from http://www.uptodate.com/contents/treatment-and-prognosis-of-cutaneous-squamous-cell-carcinoma

Chuang, T. Y., Reizner, G. T., Elpern, D. J., Stone, J. L., & Farmer, E. R. (1995). Nonmelanoma skin cancer in Japenese Ethnic Hawaiians in Kauai, Hawaii: An incidence report. *Journal of the American Academy of Dermatology*, *33*, 422–426.

DermNet. (n.d.). Basal cell and squamous cell images. Retrieved from http://www.dermnetnz.org

Doben, A. R., & Macgillivray, D. C. (2009). The classification of cutaneous melanoma: Malignant melanoma. *Surgical Clinics of North America*, *89*, 713–725.

Duncan, L. M. (2009). The classification of cutaneous melanoma. *Hematology/Oncology Clinics of North America*, *23*, 501–513.

Duthie, E. H., Katz, P. R., & Malone, M. (2007). *Practice of geriatrics* (4th ed.). Philadelphia, PA: Saunders.

Engkilde, K., Thyssen, J. P., Menne, T., & Johansen, J. D. (2011). Association between cancer and contact allergy: A linkage study. *British Medical Journal Open*, *1*, 1–5.

Galiczynski, E. M., & Vidimos, A. T. (2011). Nonsurgical treatment of nonmelanoma skin cancer. *Dermatologic Clinics*, *29*, 297–309.

Gao, X., Simon, K. C., Han, J., Schwarzchild, M. A., & Ascherio, A. (2009). Family history of melanoma and Parkinson disease risk. *Neurology*, *73*(16), 1286–1291.

Geller, A. C., & Swetter, S. (2012, May 11). Screening and early detection of melanoma. *UpToDate*. Retrieved from http://www.uptodate.com/contents/screening-and-early-detection-of-melanoma

Ghissassi, E. L., Baan, R., Straif, K., Grosse, Y., Secretan, B., Bouvard, V., & Cogliano, V. (2009). A review of human carcinogens—Part D: Radiation. *Lancet Oncology*, *10*(8), 751–752.

Gilchrest, B. A. (2007). Skin disorders. In E. H. Duthie, P. R. Katz, & M. Malone (Eds.), *Practice of geriatrics* (4th ed., pp. 531–546). Philadelphia, PA: Saunders.

Gloster, H. M., & Neal, K. (2006). Skin cancer in skin of color. *Journal of American Academy of Dermatology*, *55*, 741–760.

Goodson, A. G., & Grossman, D. (2009). Strategies for early melanoma detection: Approaches to the patient with nevi. *Journal of the American Academy of Dermatology*, *60*, 719–735.

Grant, W. B. (2008). Skin aging from ultraviolet irradiance and smoking reduces risk of melanoma: Epidemiological evidence. *Anticancer Research*, *28*(6B), 4003–4008.

Habif, T. P. (2004). *Clinical dermatology* (4th ed.). Philadelphia, PA: Mosby.

Halder, R. M. (2003). Skin cancer and photo aging in ethnic skin. *Dermatology Clinic*, *21*, 725–732.

Hawryluk, E. B., & Fisher, D. E. (2011). Melanoma epidemiology, risk factors, and clinical phenotypes. In A. W. Armstrong (Ed.), *Advances in malignant melanoma—Clinical and research perspectives* (pp. 3–28). Retrieved from http://www.intechopen.com/articles/show/title/melanoma-epidemiology-risk-factors-and-clinical- phenotypes

Housman, T. S., Feldman, S. R., Williford, P. M., Fleischer, A. B., Jr., Goldman, N. D., Acostamadiedo, J. M., & Chen, G. J. (2003). Skin cancer is among the most costly of all cancers to treat for the Medicare population. *Journal of the American Academy of Dermatology*, *48*(3), 425–429.

International Agency for Research on Cancer. (2011). Agents classified by the IARC monographs. Retrieved from http://monographs.iarc.fr/ENG/Classification/ClassificationsAlphaOrder.pdf

Inzelberg, R., Rabey, J. M., Melamed, E., Djaldetti, R., Reches, A., Badarny, S., ... Giladi, N. (2011). High prevalence of malignant melanoma in Israeli patients with Parkinson's disease. *Journal of Neural Transmission, 118*, 1199–1207.

James, W. D., Berger, T. G., & Elston, D. M. (2006). Andrew's diseases of the skin. *Clinical dermatology* (10th ed.). Philadelphia, PA: Saunders.

Koh, D., Wang, H., Lee, J., Chia, K. S., Lee, H. P., & Goh, C. L. (2003). Basal cell carcinoma, squamous cell carcinoma and melanoma of the skin: Analysis of the Singapore cancer registry data 1968–1997. *British Journal of Dermatology, 148*, 1161–1166.

Lautenschlager, S., Wulf, H. C., & Pittelkow, M. R. (2007). Photoprotection. *Lancet, 370*, 528–537.

Leber, K., Perron, V. D., & Sinni-McKeehen, B. (1999). Common skin cancers in the United States: A practical guide for diagnosis and treatment. *Nurse Practitioner Forum, 10*(2), 106–112.

Liu, R., Gao, X., Lu, Y., & Chen, H. (2011). Meta-analysis of the relationship between Parkinson's disease and melanoma. *Neurology, 76*, 2002–2009.

Markovic, S. N., Erickson, L. A., Rao, R. D., Weenig, R. H., Pockaj, B. A., Bardia, A., ... Cameron, J. S. (2007). Malignant melanoma in the 21st century, Part 1: Epidemiology risk factors, screening, prevention, and diagnosis. *Mayo Clinic Proceedings, 82*(3), 364–380.

Melanoma. (n.d.). Retrieved from http://www.melanoma.org

Melanoma images. (n.d.). Retrieved from http://www.pic.search.com/pictures/health

Mikkilneni, R., Weinstock, M. A., Goldstein, M. G., Dube, C. E., & Rossi, J. S. (2001). Impact of the basic skin cancer triage curriculum on providers' skin cancer control practices. *Journal of General Internal Medicine, 16*, 302–307.

Moody, M. N., Landau, J. M., Holzer, A., & Goldberg, L. H. (2011). Non-surgical treatment of skin cancers and precancers. *Skin Cancer Foundation Journal, 29*, 52–54.

National Cancer Institute, Surveillance Epidemiology and End Results. (2010). SEER stat fact sheets: Melanoma of the skin. Retrieved from http://seer.cancer.gov/statfacts/html/melan.html

Nolen, M. E., Beebe, V. R., King, J. M., Bryn, N., & Limaye, K. M. (2011). Nonmelanoma skin cancer, Part 1. *Journal of the Dermatology Nurses' Association, 3*(5), 260–283.

O'Connor, N. R. (2010). FDA boxed warnings: How to prescribe drugs safely. *American Family Physician, 81*(3), 298–303.

Patel, C. B., Rashid, R. M., & Nguyen, T. H. (2010). Management of extensive squamous cell carcinoma on the site of radiation-induced dermatitis with severe fibrosis: A case report. *Journal of Radiotherapy in Practice, 9*, 125–128.

Piris, A., & Mihm, M. C. (2009). Progress in melanoma histopathology and diagnosis. *Hematology and Oncology Clinic of North America, 23*, 467–480.

Ridky, T. W. (2007). Nonmelanoma skin cancer. *Journal of the American Academy of Dermatology, 57*, 484–501.

Rubin, K. M. (2010). Melanoma staging: A review of the revised American joint committee on cancer guidelines. *Journal of the Dermatology Nurses' Association, 2*(6), 254–259.

Skin Cancer Foundation. (2011a). Retrieved from http://www.skincancer.org

Skin Cancer Foundation. (2011b, Fall). Breakthrough melanoma drug approved: First in a new class of "targeted" treatments. *Sun & Skin News, 28*(3), 1–2.

Skin Cancer Foundation. (2011c, May). Skin cancer facts. Retrieved from http://www.skincancer.org/skin-cancer-facts

Skin Cancer Foundation. (2011d, June–August). FDA issues new sunscreen labeling rules. *Sun & Skin News, 28*(2). Retrieved from http://www.skincancer.org/publications/sun-and-skin-news/summer-2011-28-2/New-FDA-Rules

Stone, M. (2011, September). Initial surgical management of melanoma of the skin and unusual sites. *UpToDate*. Retrieved from http://www.uptodate.com/contents/initial-surgical-management-of-melanoma-of-the-skin

Swetter, S., & Geller, A. (2011, May). Skin examination and clinical features of melanoma. *UpToDate*. Retrieved from http://www.uptodate.com/contents/skin-examination-and-clinical-features-of-melanoma

Tucker, M. A. (2009). Melanoma epidemiology. *Hematology/Oncology Clinics of North America, 23*, 383–395.

Tung, R., & Vidimos, A. (2010). Nonmelanoma skin cancer. In W. D. Carey (Ed.), *Cleveland Clinic: Current clinical medicine* (2nd ed.). Philadelphia, PA: Saunders. Retrieved from http://www.expert.com

Urist, M. M., & Soong, S. (2007). Melanoma and cutaneous malignancies. In D. Townsend, M. Beauchamp, & M. Evers (Eds.), *Sabiston textbook of surgery* (18th ed., pp. 767–785). Philadelphia, PA: Saunders.

U.S. Food and Drug Administration. (2011). Learn if a medical device has been cleared by FDA for marketing. Retrieved from http://www.fda.gov/medicaldevices/resourcesforyou/consumers/ucm142523.htm

Wood, G. S., Gunkal, J., Stewart, D., Gordon, E., Bagheri, M. M., Gharia, M., & Snow, S. N. (2008). Nonmelanoma skin cancers: Basal cell and squamous cell carcinomas. In M. D. Abeloff, J. O. Armitage, J. E. Niederhuber, M. B. Kastan, & W. G. Mckenna (Eds.), *Abeloff's clinical oncology* (pp. 1253–1270). Philadelphia, PA: Churchill Livingstone Elsevier.

World Health Organization. (2011). Ultraviolet radiation and the INTERSUN programme. Retrieved from http://www.who.int/uv/en/

CHAPTER 5: IT RESOURCES

Websites

American Cancer Society
   www.cancer.org

American Academy of Dermatology
   www.aad.org

American Society for Dermatologic Surgery
   www.asds.net

Melanoma Patients' Information Page
   www.mpip.org

National Cancer Institute
   www.cancer.gov

National Comprehensive Cancer Network
   www.nccn.org

The Skin Cancer Foundation
   www.skincancer.org

UV index information
   www.epa.gov/sunwise/uvindex.html

Interactive Skin Cancer Library
   http://www.cancer.org/Cancer/news/Features/interactive-skin-cancer-presentation

Skin Cancer—Melanoma
   http://www.cancer.org/cancer/skincancer-melanoma/index

Skin Cancer—Basal and Squamous Cell
   http://www.cancer.org/cancer/skincancer-basalandsquamouscell/index

Skin Cancer Treatments and Drugs—Mayo Clinic
   http://www.mayoclinic.com/health/skin-cancer/DS00190/DSECTION=treatments-
   and-drugs

Skin Cancer Prevention—Mayo Clinic
   http://www.mayoclinic.com/health/skin-cancer/DS00190/DSECTION=prevention

Skin Cancer Prevention and Early Detection
   http://www.cancer.org/Cancer/SkinCancer-Melanoma/MoreInformation/
   SkinCancerPreventionandEarlyDetection/index

Videos

3D Skin Cancer Library
   An interactive learning experience that explains the causes, conditions, and treatment options
   for Skin Cancer, including: Skin Self-Exam, Actinic Keratosis, Skin Cancer, Mohs Surgery,
   How Sunscreen Works, and Sunburns.
   http://www.skincancer.org/skin-cancer-information/videos/sunscreen-video

Examining Skin Growths (Skin Cancer #1) (2007)
   You know that something strange has cropped up on your body, but what it is has you
   clueless. Check out this video for help! (3:14 minutes)
   http://www.youtube.com/watch?v=DsznOhIs-6E

CareFlash website
  Contains various free, plainly narrated, multilingual videos and includes the transcript and
  embed links.
  http://www.careflash.com/video/skin-cancer?lc=en
Nodular Basal Cell Carcinoma (2010)
  Dr. Shane Chapman, MD, discusses Skin Cancer Nodular Basal Cell Carcinoma (4 minutes)
  http://youtu.be/y7bXnVerYjM
Superficial Cell Carcinoma (2010)
  Dr. Shane Chapman, MD, discusses Skin Cancer Basal Cell Carcinoma Superficial Basal Cell
  Carcinoma (1 minute)
  http://youtu.be/Q9rQ4yHT9TM
Sclerosing or Mopheaform Basal Cell Carcinoma (2010)
  Dr. Shane Chapman, MD, discusses Sclerosing or Morpheaform Basal Cell Carcinoma
  (1 minute)
  http://youtu.be/rqdBrudAb8s
Skin Cancer Superficial Spreading Melanoma (2010)
  Dr. James L. Campbell Jr., MD, discusses Skin Cancer Superficial Spreading Melanoma (2:02 minutes)
  http://youtu.be/iIqHVtwNO-I
Lentigo Maligna Melanoma (2010)
  Dr. James L. Campbell Jr., MD, discusses Skin Cancer Lentigo Maligna Melanoma (1:29 minutes)
  http://youtu.be/se_6ZBxnJ-Y
Acral-Lentiginous Melanoma (2010)
  Dr. James L. Campbell Jr., MD, discusses Skin Cancer Acral-Lentiginous Melanoma (1:25 minutes)
  http://youtu.be/J-YBS87X328
Skin Cancer Nodula Melanoma (2010)
  Dr. James L. Campbell Jr., MD, discusses Skin Cancer Nodular Melanoma (1:34 minutes)
  http://youtu.be/hwDeahZEcFE

Images

Melanoma Photos
  http://www.webcrawler.com/info.wbcrwl.303/web/melanoma%20photos
Search engine page with various links to pictures of melanoma in different stages.
Photos of Malignant Melanoma
  http://www.dermnet.com/images/Malignant-Melanoma
Image collection of Skin Problems, including Basal and Squamous Cell Carcinoma
  http://www.medicinenet.com/script/main/art.asp?articlekey=109865
Google images for Superficial Cell Carcinoma
  http://www.google.com/search?q=superficial+cell+carcinoma&source=lnms&tbm=isch&sa=
  X&ei=elunUZDwCOzh0wHj6ICYAg&ved=0CAcQ_AUoAQ&biw=1011&bih=220
Google images for SCC in Situ
  http://www.google.com/search?q=scc+in+situ&source=lnms&tbm=isch&sa=X&ei=Q1unUa
  XrG_O60QGCkoHYDA&sqi=2&ved=0CAcQ_AUoAQ&biw=1011&bih=220
Google images for Invasive SCC
  http://www.google.com/search?q=invasive+scc&source=lnms&tbm=isch&sa=X&ei=KVunU
  YmWC8O80gHIvoG4Dg&ved=0CAcQ_AUoAQ&biw=1011&bih=220

Gastrointestinal Disease

Andrea D. Harrelson, FNP-BC
Brent S. Williams, MD
Deborah D. Cox, FNP-C

INTRODUCTION

Although gastrointestinal (GI) problems are among the most frequent complaints of older adults, they often present with atypical symptoms. Many older patients do not discuss their symptoms of reflux because it is believed this is normal "at their age," or discuss flatulence because they are embarrassed, and also may have relied on laxatives for years and do not discuss constipation. Thus, the GI system becomes a puzzle in assessment for the clinician to investigate the symptoms for causation.

Many changes do occur in the upper and lower GI tract as one ages. Oral mucosa is dry with less sensitivity to taste as well as gum disease may be prevalent in some older adults. Esophageal sphincter pressure is lower with a decrease in GI motility. This can lead to reflux, flatulence, abdominal discomfort, and constipation (Mauk, 2014). These normal age-related changes, when the patient presents with increased symptoms, must be assessed and other causes ruled out.

In this chapter, we will discuss GI disorders and how they relate to the older adult. We will concentrate on gastroesophageal reflux disease (GERD), irritable bowel syndrome (IBS), diverticulitis/diverticulosis, and constipation. In addition, each disorder's symptomatology, complications, treatments, and goals of therapy will be addressed.

GASTROESOPHAGEAL REFLUX DISEASE

Definition

GERD is the most common esophageal disease in the older adult. It is defined as the symptoms that result from mucosal damage produced by the abnormal reflux of gastric contents into the esophagus.

GERD is typically caused by changes in the barrier between the stomach and the esophagus, producing an abnormal relaxation of the lower esophageal sphincter (LES) (DeVault & Castell, 2005). According to Beers and Berkow (2000), aging has only minor effects on esophageal motor and sensory function in healthy persons. However, it is suggested that upper esophageal pressure decreases in the older adult, as does the amplitude of secondary peristalsis; LES pressure does not seem to change.

Epidemiology

GERD affects up to one third of adults. It is the most common esophageal disease in the older adult, affecting 59% of adults over the age of 65. Erosive esophagitis is present in approximately 50% to 65% of patients with GERD, and in the primary care setting in the United States, as many as 20% of older patients report acid reflux (Pilotto et al., 2005). In a Japanese study, the prevalence of reflux esophagitis in patients aged above 70 years was more than triple the prevalence in patients younger than 39 years (Pilotto et al., 2005).

Symptomatology and Clinical Presentation

The presentation of GERD in older adults is somewhat different than that of younger adults. These patients have unique characteristics that influence the management and overall goals of treatment. The most common and atypical symptoms of GERD among all populations are discussed below.

The most common symptoms in young adults are burning pain in the epigastric area, which may radiate into the oropharynx (heartburn), sour taste in the mouth, frequent belching and/or flatulence, dysphagia, early satiety, and regurgitation of gastric contents (Lynch, 2003). See Table 6.1 for extraesophageal (atypical) symptoms typically seen in older adults.

The most common symptoms of GERD are heartburn and acid regurgitation (Chait, 2005). Generally, these symptoms do not change with age, except for heartburn. Remarkably, the frequency of severe heartburn seems to decline with age, possibly because of the decrease in esophageal pain perception and atrophic gastritis. In addition, heartburn severity does not seem to reliably indicate the severity of erosive esophagitis (Johnson & Fennety, 2004).

TABLE 6.1 • Extraesophageal (Atypical) Symptoms

Ear, Nose, and Throat	Pulmonary	Miscellaneous
Hoarseness	Asthma	Noncardiac chest pain
Cough	Bronchitis	Vomiting
Globus sensation	Bronchiectasis	Anorexia
Persistent pharyngitis	Aspiration pneumonia	
Otitis media	Idiopathic pulmonary fibrosis	
Laryngitis		
Sinusitis		
Vocal cord granulomas		
Laryngeal cancer		

Dysphagia is another significant symptom that is increased in the older patient. It may be related to several disease states more common in the older adult, such as Parkinson disease, cerebrovascular disease, and diabetes. In patients with GERD, it usually occurs in the setting of long-standing GERD and is progressive from dysphagia with solids to, when severe, dysphagia with liquids. Dysphagia may foretell a more severe problem, such as severe peristaltic dysfunction, peptic stricture, or cancer.

As with many conditions, symptoms of GERD may be atypical and extraesophageal such as atypical chest pain that can simulate angina; ear, nose, and throat (ENT) manifestations such as globus sensation, laryngitis, and dental problems; and pulmonary problems such as chronic cough, asthma, and pulmonary aspiration (Chait, 2005). Atypical noncardiac chest pain from GERD may be very difficult to distinguish from angina. Chest pain has been related to GERD in up to 60% of cases, with 50% being related to reflux injury and 10% to esophageal motility. Remarkably, some patients may only present with a chronic cough, making this condition extremely difficult to diagnose.

Complications

Complications of GERD are much more common in the older adult. Up to 20% of patients seeking medical attention for GERD in the United States suffer from related complications. The most common type of complication of GERD is esophagitis. When left untreated, this could progress to severe ulceration and hemorrhage. Esophageal stricture, or narrowing of the esophagus, occurs in up to 10% of patients who have reflux esophagitis, especially in older men and are associated with the use of nonsteroidal anti-inflammatory drugs (NSAIDs) (Chait, 2005). There are many medications that have been associated with GERD (Wells, 2010); Table 6.2 lists some of the more commonly used medications seen in older adults that are associated with GERD.

GERD complications may vary from the minor problems of esophagitis to major problems such as recurrent pulmonary aspiration, Barrett esophagus, and esophageal cancer. Barrett

TABLE 6.2 · Common Medications Associated with GERD

Medications Associated with Decreased LES tone
Calcium channel blockers
β-Blockers
Anticholinergics
Benzodiazepines
Theophylline
Nitrates
Barbiturates
Narcotic analgesics
Medications Associated with Injury to the Esophageal Mucosa
NSAIDs
Bisphosphonates
Potassium supplements

esophagus occurs in approximately 10% to 15% of patients with GERD symptoms and is more common in older white males over the age of 60 (Chait, 2005). It is a premalignant condition highly associated with the development of adenocarcinoma of the esophagus and the gastric cardia. Adenocarcinoma of the esophagus is now the most common form of esophageal cancer and among the fastest growing carcinomas by incidence in the United States. The incidence of adenocarcinoma in patients with Barrett esophagus is approximately 1% per year, and is typically present in the seventh or eighth decade of life with weight loss and dysphagia (Chait, 2005).

Social and Economic Impact

The economic burden of GERD is substantial, with approximately $10 billion per year in direct costs alone. In 2004, GERD was responsible for more than 5.5 million outpatient clinic visits. In the same year, 8 million prescriptions were filled for the treatment of GERD with costs totaling greater than $10 million, including over-the-counter (OTC) preparations (Wells, 2010).

Pathophysiology

There are a number of abnormalities that appear to play a pathogenic role in GERD, and they are often more severe in the older adult. These include a defective antireflux barrier, abnormal esophageal clearance, reduced salivary production, altered esophageal mucosal resistance, and delayed gastric emptying (Chait, 2005). Injury to the esophagus is due primarily to gastric acid and pepsin. Additionally, over time, reflux of gastric contents results in esophageal damage. The reflux barrier may be impaired by alterations in LES tone, including alterations caused by medications or the presence of hiatal hernia. Although LES dysfunction has never been shown to increase with age, these patients take medications that can alter LES more frequently and have higher incidences of hiatal hernias (see Table 6.3). The LES is the antireflux barrier. Abnormalities that make it dysfunctional promote acid reflux and the constellation of GERD problems. The most common cause of reflux episodes is transient LES relaxations; the drop in LES pressure is not accompanied by swallowing. Incompetence of the LES is typically more prevalent in the older adult (Chait, 2005).

Esophageal acid clearance can be impaired owing to disturbances of esophageal motility and saliva production. There is a significant decrease in the amplitude of peristaltic contraction and an increase in the frequency of nonpropulsive and repetitive contractions compared with younger individuals. Salivary production is slightly decreased with age, with a significantly decreased salivary bicarbonate response to acid perfusion of the esophagus. Medications taken for comorbidities can affect not only the LES, but the esophageal motility as well (Chait, 2005).

TABLE 6.3 • Risk Factors Associated with GERD

Controllable	Fixed
Smoking	Age
Obesity	Diabetes
Diet	Asthma
	Neurologic disorders (e.g., Parkinson)
	Hiatal hernia

The role of delayed gastric emptying is less defined in older adult patients with GERD. However, medications used in disease states more commonly seen in these patients may make these factors more important in the aging population. Medications such as NSAIDs, potassium supplements, and bisphosphonates are often used and have been shown to cause direct injury to the esophageal mucosa (see Table 6.2). Gastric acid secretion does not decrease with age alone. However, factors that lead to atrophic gastritis, such as *Helicobacter pylori*, reduce gastric acid. Such factors in association with the age-related decrease in esophageal pain perception may explain the phenomenon of reduced heartburn symptom severity as patients grow older (Chait, 2005).

Risk Factors

A number of risk factors have been suggested for GERD, some of which may be more common in the older adult. Studies show there is a significant association between monozygotic twins who share a parental history of reflux disease, thus indicating that there is a genetic component to the development of GERD. Other identified risk factors include increased body mass index (BMI), use of certain medications, and smoking (Wells, 2010). See Table 6.3 for more information on risk factors associated with GERD.

Although age has not been shown to be an independent risk factor, older patients are more likely to possess other risk factors. Older adults are known to take more medications that are associated with GERD when compared with younger populations and are more likely to have hiatal hernias, as well as neurologic and respiratory diseases associated with GERD (Wells, 2010).

Treatment

Lifestyle Modification

Although treatment of GERD in older patients is essentially the same as in adults, a more aggressive approach to treatment may often be necessary in this group owing to a higher incidence of complications. The treatment goals for GERD include elimination of symptoms, healing of esophagitis, managing or preventing complications, and maintaining remission. The vast majority of patients can be treated successfully with noninvasive methods of lifestyle modification and medication (see Table 6.4) (Chait, 2005).

Although lifestyle modification remains a cornerstone of therapy in GERD, it may not be sufficient to control symptoms, especially in those with complications. Patients should try to elevate the head of their beds before going to sleep, avoid eating within 3 hours of bedtime, stop smoking

TABLE 6.4 • Lifestyle Modifications for the Treatment of GERD
Elevation of the head of the bed or use of a foam wedge
Decreased fat intake
Smoking cessation
Weight loss
Avoiding recumbency for 3 hours postprandially
Avoidance of alcohol and caffeine

tobacco, change their diet to decrease fat and volume of meals, and to avoid dietary irritants such as alcohol, peppermint, onion, citrus juice, coffee, and tomatoes.

Medications

A number of pharmacologic options are available for the treatment of GERD. Theoretically, these agents target the dysmotility component of GERD (i.e., promotility agents) or, more commonly, they decrease the acid production in the stomach to decrease the caustic consequences of refluxed contents (i.e., acid-suppressing or neutralizing agents). These agents include OTC antacids and antireflux agents, promotility agents (e.g., metoclopramide), histamine receptor type 2 (H_2) antagonists, and proton pump inhibitors (PPIs) (Wells, 2010).

OTC antacids and H_2-blockers on an as-needed basis may be helpful for those individuals who have mild disease. However, for patients with daily symptoms or complications, prescription agents must be used for more effective therapy, at least until symptoms are initially controlled.

Motility agents, such as, metoclopramide, erythromycin, and bethanechol, have helped some in improving LES tone and esophagogastric motility in select patients. For patients with diabetes, metoclopramide has been used with moderate success in improving gastric emptying and reducing GERD symptoms. However, metoclopramide must be used with caution owing to side effects such as muscle tremors, spasms, agitation, insomnia, drowsiness, and tardive dyskinesia (Chait, 2005).

H_2-receptor antagonists, including ranitidine, famotidine, and nizatidine, are very helpful in patients with GERD, by providing adequate acid suppression and symptom relief (see Table 6.5). They are remarkably similar in their action and equally effective at equivalent doses. However, high doses of up to four times daily may be necessary in some patients. Although they are safe

TABLE 6.5 • Histamine Receptor Antagonists

Available Histamine Type 2 Receptor Antagonists and Dosages

Agent	Maximum Approved Adult Daily Dosage	Available Dosages
Cimetidine (Tagamet)	800 mg q.h.s., 400 mg b.i.d., or 300 mg q.i.d.	200, 300, 400, 800 mg tablets
		300 mg oral suspension
		150 mg/ml for injection
Famotidine (Pepcid)	40 mg q.h.s. or 20 mg b.i.d.	20 and 40 mg tablets
		20 and 40 mg oral disintegrating tablets
		40 mg/ml oral suspension
		10 mg/ml for injection
Nizatidine (Axid)	300 mg q.h.s. or 150 mg b.i.d.	75, 150, 300 mg capsules
		15 mg/ml oral solution
Ranitidine (Zantac)	300 mg q.h.s. or 150 mg b.i.d.	15, 150, 300 mg tablets
		15 mg oral syrup
		25 mg effervescent tablets
		25 mg/ml for injection

agents in the older adult, reduced doses in persons with chronic kidney disease and renal insufficiency are necessary. Central nervous system side effects such as mental confusion, delirium, headache, and dizziness are more common in older adults. Cardiac side effects of sinus bradycardia, atrioventricular block, and prolongation of the QT interval, and hematologic side effects of anemia, neutropenia, and thrombocytopenia have increased frequency in the older adult, especially with comorbid conditions. However, most side effects are reversible with reduced dosage or withdrawal of the drug (Chait, 2005).

PPIs, such as esomeprazole, lansoprazole, omeprazole, and pantoprazole, represent the most effective therapy for GERD. PPIs provide superior acid suppression and effective symptom relief. These agents are particularly useful in older persons who often require more acid suppression owing to more severe disease or complications (Chait, 2005). The safety profile of PPIs is excellent. Although the renal clearance of PPIs is reduced in the older patient, no reduction in the dose of either omeprazole or lansoprazole is needed, including those with renal or hepatic dysfunction (Wells, 2010). Consistent with this theory, Calabrese agrees that PPIs are central in the management of GERD and are unchallenged with regard to their efficacy (Calabrese et al., 2007). They are considered safe and more effective than H_2-receptor antagonists for healing esophagitis and for preventing its recurrence using a long-term maintenance treatment. PPIs have minimal side effects, have very few drug interactions, and are considered safe for long-term treatment. Pantoprazole is well tolerated even for long-term therapy, and its tolerability is optimal. Although the majority of older adults have concomitant illnesses and receive other drugs, this does not adversely affect the efficacy of pantoprazole because of its pharmacokinetics, which are independent of patient age. Therefore, Calabrese recommends that low-dose maintenance of PPIs be used in older patients with GERD (Calabrese et al., 2007).

Although PPIs are considered the most powerful and most favorable class of antacid drugs, Denoon (2010) argues that PPIs are to be used for serious conditions only, not for mild cases of heartburn. According to Denoon, doctors tend to overprescribe PPIs, especially for hospitalized patients. It is this overprescribing that has a direct correlation with increased incidences of *Clostridium difficile* diarrhea in hospitalized patients. Those patients taking PPIs were more than three times as likely to develop *C. difficile* as those who were not taking this class of drugs. Consistent with this, a study conducted at the Boston Medical Center discovered that for those patients treated for *C. difficile* infections, 42% were more likely to have the infection return if they were taking PPIs. Consequently, it is suggested that the risk of getting *C. difficile* while in the hospital is higher for patients receiving PPIs.

Surgical Interventions

Although the vast majority of patients can be successfully managed with medical therapy, surgical interventions and endoscopic treatment of GERD may be warranted. Surgery is contemplated now with more frequency because of the ability to perform antireflux surgery laparoscopically. It is indicated in patients with intractable GERD, difficult-to-manage strictures, severe bleeding, nonhealing ulcers, recurrent aspiration, and GERD requiring large maintenance doses of PPIs or H_2-receptor antagonists. Given that there appears to be no more increase in postoperative morbidity or mortality as in younger adults with this type of surgery, healthy older patients should not be denied surgery on the basis of age alone. Careful patient selection with complete preoperative evaluation, including upper GI endoscopy, esophageal manometry, pH testing, and gastric emptying studies, should be done prior to surgery. Endoscopic therapy of GERD is evolving. The Stretta Procedure has been effective in reducing symptoms through its delivery of radiofrequency energy to the gastroesophageal junction. In addition, endoscopically suturing below the gastroesophageal junction has been used successfully to treat GERD (Chait, 2005). Endoscopy should be pursued in patients who do not respond to therapy, when there are symptoms suggestive of complicated disease (dysphagia, bleeding, anemia, or weight loss), and when the duration of symptoms is sufficient to place the patient at risk for Barrett esophagus, generally greater than 5 to 10 years (Wells, 2010). Furthermore, endoscopy should be used early in the evaluation of all older patients owing to the higher frequency of complicated disease concomitant with less severe symptoms (Wells, 2010).

Patient Education

The goal of treatment for GERD is the prevention of complications. If left untreated, GERD can lead to the development of precancerous cells, even life-threatening cancer. It is imperative that patients are educated on the prevention of such complications and understand the importance of reporting symptoms. The first line of treatment and thus prevention is lifestyle modifications. These include elevation of the head of the bed 2″ to 6″ or the use of a foam wedge to sleep, avoidance of spicy and fatty foods, tomato and citrus juices, chocolate, mints, coffee, tea, cola, and alcoholic drinks, smoking cessation, weight loss, eating smaller meals, avoiding recumbency for 3 hours postprandially, avoiding tight-fitting clothing, and bending down using the knees (Lynch, 2003; Wells, 2010).

The Physicians Committee for Responsible Medicine (PCRM, n.d.) suggests that coffee reduces the LES pressure, thereby permitting gastroesophageal reflux. In addition, the total amount of food consumed during a meal also appears to be related to reflux symptoms, perhaps because gastric distension triggers GERD symptoms. Reducing the meal size may therefore be a reasonable prevention strategy, particularly for patients who frequently experience delayed gastric emptying. It is further suggested that alcohol users have more than double the risk for GERD when compared with nonusers. Additionally, it was determined that those who consume high-fiber diets have a 30% lower risk for GERD.

If lifestyle modifications are unsuccessful, a stepwise approach is made in the treatment of GERD. OTC antacids are second line of treatment, followed by H_2-blockers and PPIs as surgical management is conserved for those suffering from serious complications and do not respond to previous treatment.

As stated earlier, the prevention of GERD complications is the overall goal of treatment. All health-care professionals must be alert to the extraesophageal manifestations typically presented in this population, and therefore educate patients to report increased, changing, or newly developed symptoms of GERD.

Cultural Considerations

According to Goodman (2011), men and women experience symptoms of GERD differently. In a recent study comparing gender and GERD symptoms, researchers surveyed nearly 3,000 Australian adults living in the community and more than 2,000 men and women who were having surgery to correct their GERD. Both women in the community and those who were having surgery complained of more frequent and severe heartburn than men. They also reported having more trouble swallowing solid foods and were more likely than men to be taking medication to treat their heartburn. However, when physicians evaluated the characteristics of patients who came in for surgery, they found that men actually had more physical manifestations of GERD. The men, who were about 7 years younger than the female surgical patients, were more likely to have weak valves in the esophageal sphincter. Men were also more likely to have esophagitis or Barrett esophagus. On the other hand, women were more likely to have a hiatal hernia, and were also more likely to be obese than their male counterparts. In line with this theory, the Arizona Center for Digestive Health (n.d.) proposes that men develop Barrett esophagus twice as often as women and Caucasian men are affected more than men of other races.

In relation to gender differences, the role of dietary factors in GERD remains debatable. It is noteworthy, however, that cultural differences are associated with differences in prevalence, suggesting a role for diet. The incidence of GERD is lower in China (5% incidence) and certain other countries than in Western countries, which may reflect differences in eating styles, food choices, and body weight (PCRM, n.d.).

Quality of Life

Since impairment of normal life consequent upon GERD symptoms, quality of life (QOL) is generally the primary motive of the patient to seek therapy, as he or she is most concerned with the relief of GERD symptoms. From the perspective of the patient, symptom relief is the most critical component in determining the success of treatment. The frequency and severity of common GERD-related symptoms correlate with an impairment of normal functioning and overall well-being. An adequate control of symptoms and a sustained reduction of symptoms to a level that does not significantly impair QOL is gold standard in the treatment of GERD (Calabrese et al., 2007).

GERD is a very common disease in both young and old patients and can markedly interfere with QOL. Although older adults appear to have fewer complaints, their disease is usually more severe and has more complication. It is crucial that advanced practice nurses, as well as other health-care professionals, remain vigilant to detect and manage GERD in older adults.

DIVERTICULOSIS/DIVERTICULITIS

Colonic diverticular disease is a disease primarily of the Western and industrialized world. Acquired diverticula form through the relative weakness in the muscle wall of the colon to form herniations or "outpouchings" of the colonic mucosa and submucosa (Salzman & Lillie, 2005). Diverticula are primarily located in the sigmoid colon, though they can occur throughout the large bowel. The term "diverticulosis" refers to the presence of more than one diverticulum or many diverticula of the intestine. The term "diverticulitis" refers to the inflammation of a diverticulum or diverticula, which may cause obstruction, perforation, or bleeding. The primary focus of this section will be on diverticulitis as it is the complication of diverticulosis that requires proper diagnosis and treatment.

Epidemiology/Demographics

The prevalence of diverticulosis is similar in men and women and increases with age (PCRM, n.d.)—approximately 10% of adults younger than 40 years and 50% to 70% among those aged 80 and older (Feroco et al., 1998; Tursi, 2004a). Diverticulosis is a disease of aging as 80% of persons suffering with the disease are 50 years of age or older (Ambrosetti et al., 1994). Although most patients with diverticular disease remain asymptomatic, as many as 15% to 20% have symptomatic diverticular disease (Salzman & Lillie, 2005). Three fourths of this group have crampy abdominal pain but no inflammation. The remaining one fourth, or approximately 5% of the

TABLE 6.6 • Forms of Diverticular Disease

Disease	Clinical Features	Management
Asymptomatic diverticulosis	Diverticula in the absence of symptoms	High-fiber diet
Symptomatic diverticulosis	Abdominal pain, ± changes in bowel habits	High-fiber diet, avoid NSAIDs
Mild diverticulitis	Abdominal pain, fever, leukocytosis, able to tolerate p.o. fluids	Oral antibiotics, clear liquid diet
Complicated diverticulitis	Abdominal pain, fever, leukocytosis, unable to tolerate p.o. fluids, ± evidence of complication	IV antibiotics, IV fluids, bowel rest, CT, colonoscopy after 4–6 weeks, ± surgical consult/percutaneous drainage

total population with diverticula, will develop inflammation or diverticulitis. Table 6.6 demonstrates the various forms of diverticular disease.

Diverticular disease presents a considerable clinical burden on the US population with over 300,000 admissions and 1.5 million days of inpatient care annually (Lo & Chu, 1996). Elective operations for diverticulitis rose 29% from 16,100 in 1998 to 22,500 in 2005 (Harford, 2012).

The highest prevalence of diverticular disease is seen in the United States, Europe, and Australia with the disease being rare in rural Africa and Asia. In Western countries, diverticular disease occurs primarily in the left colon (sigmoid), whereas in the Far East (Japan), diverticula occur predominantly in the right colon and tend to occur at younger ages (Farrell et al., 2011; Reisman et al., 1999).

Pathophysiology/Etiology

Diverticular disease is thought to be caused by several variables, including alterations in colon wall resistance or compliance leading to a reduced colonic diameter, disordered colonic motility, and diet. There are associations between diverticular disease and diets that are low in dietary fiber and high in refined carbohydrates (Burkitt et al., 1974). The deficiency of fiber contributes to diverticular formation as a low-fiber diet leads to less bulky stools, resulting in an alteration in colonic transit time and a reduced colonic diameter—especially in the sigmoid colon (Floch & White, 2006). A reduced colon diameter will lead to the formation of closed segments during contractions of the colon, resulting in increased intraluminal pressure. Other factors that have been associated with an increased risk of diverticular disease include constipation, obesity, smoking, and physical inactivity (Stollman & Raskin, 1999).

Alterations in the colon wall resistance or compliance are due to changes in the colon wall, which include increased elastin deposition in the muscle layers as well as increased collagen cross-linking. These changes make the colonic wall less compliant, leading to increased intraluminal pressure. As a result of this increased intraluminal pressure, the two innermost layers of the colon wall—the mucosa and submucosa—herniate through defects or "gaps" in the muscular muscularis layer of the colon wall where medium-sized perforating arteries also pass through (Harford, 2012). The diverticulum that results is considered a colonic pseudodiverticula (Truelove, 1966).

One or more diverticula may become infected or inflamed and lead to diverticulitis. Diverticulitis may result from several factors, including (1) an abrasion of the mucosa by inspissated stool, (2) changes in bacterial colonic microflora leading to low-grade chronic inflammation, (3) stasis or obstruction of the diverticulum by stool, and (4) local ischemia (Jacobs, 2007). The most commonly isolated organisms are anaerobes (bacteroides, fusobacterium, peptostreptococcus, and clostridium) and gram-negative aerobes, including *Escherichia coli* (Brook & Frazier, 2000). The risk of diverticulitis also increases with the use of NSAIDs, steroids, and opioids (Harford, 2012).

A diverticulum may become obstructed, perforate, bleed, or obstruct the colon. If perforation occurs, the infection may lead to pericolonic abscess or phlegmon formation, peritonitis, or fistula formation. Fistula formation occurs when the infection erodes into an adjacent structure such as the bladder or skin. High-grade colonic obstruction is a rare complication, but is likely due to stricture formation and/or colonic edema. These complications of diverticular disease are more common in immunocompromised patients and the older adult, especially the frail older adult.

Diagnosis and Screening

There are no official screening guidelines concerning diverticulosis. Diverticula are most often discovered incidentally during investigation of another condition or during investigation of a patient's specific diverticular symptoms, however severe they may be. The diagnosis is essentially one of exclusion in the patient who presents with lower abdominal pain. Plain film radiographs will only show free air, obstruction, or evidence of excessive stool in the colon. Diverticula can be detected on barium enema and abdominal computed tomography (CT) scans. Colonoscopy is the gold standard for identification of diverticula and is considered, by consensus expert opinion, to be standard in the exclusion of underlying colonic neoplastic disease in patients with symptomatic diverticular disease (Machicado & Jensen, 1997).

Clinical Presentation

Diverticulosis is most typically asymptomatic. Symptomatic diverticular disease is characterized by paroxysms of abdominal pain. The pain is often described as colicky in nature and often relieved by passing flatus or having a bowel movement. On physical examination, there is often localized tenderness in the left lower quadrant, although this finding may not be present. Constipation and even obstipation is more common than diarrhea. Other symptoms can include the following:

- Fever—high or low grade (may be absent in older adults)
- Constipation or obstipation (severe constipation)
- Nausea, vomiting, or diarrhea
- Anorexia
- Right-sided pain (mimicking appendicitis) in a patient with redundant sigmoid colon
- Recurrent urinary tract infections (UTIs), pneumaturia, or fecaluria with colovesical fistulas
- Severe diarrhea with enterocolonic fistulas
- Stool passing through vagina in colovaginal fistulas
- Rectal bleeding

A thorough problem-oriented physical exam is necessary to clarify the patient's condition and to guide in further evaluation of the patient. Prominent physical exam findings may include the following:

- Localized tenderness on abdominal exam (mainly left lower quadrant)
- Increased temperature (high or low grade)
- Palpable abdominal mass
- Systemic toxicity (severe cases)
- Abdominal distention

- Abdominal peritoneal signs—muscle guarding, tenderness, and rebound tenderness
- Bowel sounds decreased or normal early on, but later may be increased if there is obstruction
- Tenderness or mass on rectal exam—may indicate low-lying pelvic mass
- Rectal bleeding or positive fecal occult blood testing—may indicate other colon pathology

Differential Diagnosis

Acute appendicitis, inflammatory bowel disease, pelvic inflammatory disease, UTI, infectious colitis, and colon cancer are the primary considerations in patients who present with lower abdominal pain. Other conditions may mimic acute diverticulitis, which include the following:

- Inflammatory bowel disease—Crohn disease, ulcerative colitis
- Perforated colon cancer
- Ischemic colitis
- Infectious colitis
- Mesenteric appendagitis, omental torsion
- Gynecologic conditions such as pelvic inflammatory disease, ovarian torsion, ruptured ovarian follicle cyst, endometriosis, and ovarian tumor
- Appendicitis (on left side in situs inversus)
- IBS
- Pseudomembranous colitis (*C. difficile* infection)
- Large bowel obstruction
- Incarcerated hernia of small intestine
- Gall bladder disease
- Acute pancreatitis
- Ectopic pregnancy
- UTI (acute pyelonephritis)
- Nephrolithiasis

Evaluation (Workup)

Several lab tests and imaging studies are helpful in evaluating the patient suspected of having diverticulitis. Tests that are useful according to the American Society of Colon and Rectal Surgeons include (1) complete blood count (CBC), (2) urinalysis, and (3) plain abdominal X-rays, which may help to show edema, abscess (mass effect), pneumoperitoneum from perforated viscous, and signs of bowel obstruction. Leukocytosis is an indicator of inflammation and is often present in suspected left colonic diverticulitis. On the other hand, leukocytosis may be absent in older adults. Certain markers of systemic inflammation such as C-reactive protein and erythrocyte sedimentation rate may be suggestive.

The imaging study considered the gold standard is the CT scan of the abdomen. This should be included in the evaluation if diverticulitis is suspected. The CT scan combined with the clinical exam findings is useful in determining prognosis and treatment of the patient with diverticulitis. CT scan is also valuable in evaluating intraluminal and extraluminal colon pathology, pericolic tissue, and involvement of adjacent organs. It can rule out conditions such as appendicitis and gynecologic abnormalities. CT scan findings in diverticulitis may include pericolic fat infiltration, thickened fascia, muscular hypertrophy, and the "arrowhead sign" (colonic wall thickening with an arrowhead-shaped lumen pointing to inflamed diverticula) (Harford, 2012). It is important to note that in 10% of cases, CT scan cannot differentiate between diverticulitis and colon cancer because of thickened bowel wall. Expert opinion suggests that colonoscopy and sigmoidoscopy be performed once the acute process has resolved to rule out other diseases such as cancer and inflammatory bowel disease (Jacobs, 2007; Salzman & Lillie, 2005).

The use of barium enema in diverticulitis is limited because diverticulitis is an extraluminal process and should be avoided in suspected acute diverticulitis owing to the risk of colonic perforation and barium contamination of the peritoneum (Harford, 2012).

Treatment

The treatment of diverticulitis depends on several variables. These include findings on history and physical examination, lab findings, and imaging results. On the basis of these variables, diverticulitis can be divided into (1) mild or uncomplicated diverticulitis and (2) complicated diverticulitis. Mild diverticulitis involves inflammation of diverticula, whereas complicated diverticulitis is an acute process that can be associated with abscess, fistula formation, obstruction, or free intra-abdominal perforation leading to a peritonitis.

The Hinchey classification system of acute diverticulitis is helpful in classifying the severity of diverticulitis with its complications and in choosing treatment options and surgical strategy in more severe cases (Harford, 2012):

- Stage 0 Mild clinical diverticulitis (left lower quadrant abdominal pain, low-grade fever, leukocytosis, no imaging studies done)
- Stage I Confined pericolic or mesenteric inflammation or abscess (abscess may be palpable, fever, severe localized abdominal pain)
- Stage II Pelvic, retroperitoneal or distant intraperitoneal abscess—may be palpable (fever, systemic toxicity)
- Stage III Generalized purulent peritonitis (no communication with bowel lumen)
- Stage IV Generalized fecal peritonitis (open communication with bowel lumen)

Mild diverticulitis (stage 0 or stage I with inflammation) can be treated in an outpatient setting with clear liquids and oral antibiotics. Patients should avoid solid foods until the episode resolves. Antibiotic coverage should include gram-negative rods and anaerobes. Examples of antibiotic coverage may include amoxicillin/clavulanic acid (Augmentin), metronidazole (Flagyl) plus a quinolone, or metronidazole plus trimethoprim/sulfamethoxazole. Follow-up or reevaluation is recommended within 3 to 7 days to assess the patient's progress. If the patient is continuing to improve after 7 days, then the diet can be normalized and antibiotics can be discontinued. If such patients do not improve in the first 2 to 3 days, then hospitalization may be needed with the initiation of intravenous (IV) fluids, IV antibiotics, and bowel rest. Abdominal CT scan may need to be performed if not done so already.

Severe/complicated diverticulitis (stage I with abscess or stage II, III, or IV) usually must be hospitalized (Harford, 2012). These patients usually present with systemic toxicity, temperature greater than 101°F (38.3°C), vomiting, an abdominal mass, or signs of peritonitis. Treatment should include bowel rest, IV fluids, and IV antibiotics with the aim of avoiding urgent surgery. Examples of IV antibiotic therapy to cover anaerobes are metronidazole or clindamycin and aminoglycoside, quinolone, or third-generation cephalosporins for gram-negative rods. Combinations such as ampicillin/sulbactam (Unasyn) and ticarcillin/clavulanate (Timentin) have been advocated as single agents (Reisman et al., 1999). In these cases, abdominal CT scan should be done promptly.

Surgical consultation should be obtained promptly in cases involving (1) immunocompromised patients, (2) patients on chemotherapy, (3) failed antibiotic therapy, (4) recurrent episodes of diverticulitis, (5) transplant recipients, and (6) patients with complications such as stricture, fistula, or pericolonic abscess. Urgent surgery would be considered in patients with a ruptured abscess or perforation with fecal spillage. About 20% to 30% of patients who are hospitalized for the first time with diverticulitis require urgent or elective surgery (Harford, 2012).

Another management option is percutaneous drainage for patients with large diverticular abscess or a perforation complicated by abscess (Jacobs, 2007). This may negate the need for emergency surgery, thus allowing the option of elective surgery at a later date.

Complications

Complications of diverticular disease include abscess, fistula formation, perforation, and bowel obstruction. Abscess formation is fairly common with diverticulitis and in up to 10% of cases leads to fistula formation (Salzman & Lillie, 2005). Intestinal obstruction and perforation are rare complications, perforation being more common in patients taking NSAIDs and corticosteroids (Goh & Bourne, 2002).

Prognosis

After the resolution of the first episode of diverticulitis with medical therapy, about one third of patients will remain asymptomatic. Another third will have periodic abdominal cramps (painful diverticulosis), and the remaining third will subsequently have a second attack of diverticulitis. If surgery is performed, progression of diverticulosis in the remaining colon occurs in only 15% of patients.

Follow-up

Evaluation of the colon after recovery from the acute initial episode is recommended to confirm the diagnosis and also to exclude coexisting colon cancer. This evaluation can be done with colonoscopy or alternatively with barium enema X-ray.

Prevention

Prevention or reducing the risk of diverticular disease may be accomplished via the following: (1) dietary changes involving fiber, fat, and red meat, (2) use of Rifaximin on a monthly basis (Tursi, 2004b), (3) avoidance of NSAID medications, and (4) increased levels of physical activity. Dietary changes that appear to be beneficial include a diet high in insoluble fiber (fibrous fruits, legumes, nuts, leafy greens) and low in red meat and fat content. General recommendations include maintaining a high-fiber diet for life (18 to 30 g/day) after gradually increasing the fiber intake (to minimize flatulence and bloating). Fiber from fruits and vegetables may be preferable over cereal fiber. Avoidance of nuts and seeds has not been shown to reduce the risk for diverticulitis. NSAIDs should be avoided in patients with diverticular disease, as they have been associated with an increased risk of complications (Goh & Bourne, 2002; Morris et al., 2003).

CONSTIPATION

Constipation is one of the most common GI complaints in the United States. More than 4 million Americans report frequent constipation, and the diagnosis accounts for 2.5 million physician visits each year (Hsieh, 2005). Constipation is a frequent concern for elders and their health-care providers. It is a problem disproportionately affecting older adults with an estimated prevalence of 50% in community-dwelling elders and 74% in long-term-care facilities. Self-reported constipation has been associated with symptoms of depression, anxiety, and poor health perception (Rao & Go, 2010). Clinical constipation is related to morbidity in frail elders and sometimes leads to serious complications.

Presentation

There are varying definitions of constipation. The subjectivity of the definition means practitioners should always ask their patient about specific symptoms. Patients usually define constipation as any form of "difficult defecation," including hard stool, difficulty passing stool, strenuous straining, and nonproductive urge. Many health-care providers define constipation as less than three bowel movements per week (Rao & Go, 2010). The accepted norm for stool production is every day, but "normal" patterns vary widely among individuals. The frequency of normal stooling varies from three times a day to three times a week. The Rome criteria were developed by an international panel of experts to define constipation as objectively as possible. Rome III criteria (Table 6.7) are currently used widely to perform clinical research on constipation (Longstreth et al., 2006). The Rome criteria differentiate functional constipation from IBS with constipation. In order to be labeled with functional constipation, there must be more than two of the following symptoms: straining, lumpy or hard stools, sensation of incomplete evacuation, sensation of anorectal blockage, manual maneuvers to facilitate defecation, and less than three stools per week.

Pathophysiology

Constipation is not considered a normal part of the aging process even though it is common in people over the age of 65 years. Changes associated with aging such as decreased mobility, medication use, and dietary changes may be the contributing factors. Causal factors associated with constipation may be considered either primary or secondary. Primary constipation can be further delineated into three groups: normal transit constipation, slow transit

TABLE 6.7 • Rome III Criteria

Functional Constipation*	Irritable Bowel Syndrome

1. Must include two or more of the following:
  a. Straining during atleast 25% of defecations
  b. Lumpy or hard stools in atleast 25% of defecations
  c. Sensation of incomplete evacuations for atleast 25% of defecations
  d. Manual maneuvers to facilitate atleast 25% defecation (digital evacuation, support of the pelvic floor)
  e. Fewer than these defecations per week
2. Loose stools are rarely present without use of laxatives
3. Insufficient criteria for IBS-C
	IBS: Recurrent abdominal pain/discomfort ≥3 days/month for the past 3 months, associated with ≥2 of the following:
	1. Improvement with defecation
	2. Onset associated with change in stool frequency
	3. Onset associated with change in stool form
	IBS is subtyped by predominant stool pattern
	  ■ IBS-D: loose or watery stools <25% of defecations
	  ■ IBS-C: hard or lumpy stools ≥25% of defecations

* Criteria fulfilled in the last 3 months with symptom on set atleast 6 months prior to diagnosis.

constipation, and anorectal dysfunction (also called dyssynergic defecation) (Kurniawan & Simadibrata, 2011).

Normal transit constipation is the most common type; in this disorder, stool passes through the colon at a normal rate. In slow transit constipation, stool passage is delayed and may be associated with abdominal bloating and infrequent bowel movements. Slow transit constipation is theorized to be caused by abnormalities of the mesenteric plexus, defective cholinergic innervation, or ineffective noradrenergic neuromuscular transmission. Anorectal dysfunction is characterized by difficulty expelling stool from the anorectum and may be due to impaired rectal contraction, paradoxical anal contraction, or inadequate anal relaxation. Anorectal dysfunction is more common in women and theorized to be related to injury to the pelvic floor during childbirth (Hsieh, 2005).

Screening and Risk Factors

Secondary constipation may be caused by numerous medical and psychiatric conditions, which are listed in Table 6.8. Use of medications, both prescribed and OTC, commonly attributes to secondary constipation. Medications affecting the central nervous system, nerve conduction, and smooth muscle function are common culprits (Hsieh, 2005). Table 6.9 lists the medications commonly associated with secondary constipation.

TABLE 6.8 • Causes of Secondary Constipation

Endocrine and Metabolic Diseases	Psychological Conditions
Diabetes mellitus	Anxiety
Hypercalcemia	Depression
Hyperparathyroidism	Somatization
Hypothyroidism	
Uremia	**Structural abnormalities**
	Anal fissures, strictures, hemorrhoids
Myopathic conditions	Colonic strictures
Amyloidosis	Inflammatory bowel disease
Myotonic dystrophy	Obstructive colonic mass lesions
	Rectal prolapse or rectocele
Neurologic diseases	
Autonomic neuropathy	**Other**
Cerebrovascular disease	Irritable bowel syndrome
Hirschsprung disease	Pregnancy
Multiple sclerosis	
Parkinson disease	
Spinal cord injury, tumors	

TABLE 6.9 · Medications Associated with Secondary Constipation

Antacids[a]	Levodopa
Anticholinergics	Narcotics
Antidepressants	Nonsteroidal anti-inflammatory drugs
Antihistamines	Opioids
Calcium channel blockers	Psychotropics
Clonidine (Catapres)	Sympathomimetics
Diuretics	
Iron	

[a]Antacids containing aluminum or calcium.

Evaluation of Disease

Evaluation of constipation in the older patient should start with the practitioner asking the patient to define constipation. Are they unhappy with the frequency or consistency of bowel movements or are they having to go to extraordinary measures to evacuate?

Once constipation has been defined by the patient, the practitioner can somewhat tailor the history to the patient's complaints. Elders with intact cognition should be asked to keep a bowel diary for 1 week. The diary would include information such as number of bowel movements per day or week, character of stools produced, and symptoms associated with evacuation (pain prior to defecation, straining, manual maneuvers needed). Patients should be asked about feelings of anal blockage or incomplete evacuation, fecal or urinary incontinence, and history of hemorrhoids/anal deformities or surgeries. Prolonged straining or manual maneuvers (such as vaginal splinting) may indicate pelvic floor dysfunction. Fecal soiling of undergarments indicates either an impaction or chronic loose stools, which may be secondary to laxative overuse (Rao & Go, 2010).

Symptom onset should be evaluated; if symptoms are present since childhood, the problem may be congenital. Bowel habits recently altered might indicate mechanical obstruction. Alarm symptoms may include melena, copious bright red rectal bleeding, weight loss, fever, anorexia, and nausea or vomiting (Kurniawan & Simadibrata, 2011).

Social and family history should be explored. Does the patient live alone, with family, or in an institution? How much exercise do they get each day? The practitioner may need to explore the activities of daily living to ascertain the independence of the individual. Does family history include GI problems/cancers or other bowel diseases? Personal or familial history of psychiatric illness should be noted as well as any other systemic morbidities.

Every patient should be asked about prescription and OTC medications used, including those used to aid in defecation. Dietary habits need to be reviewed; special attention should be given to fluid and fiber intake, number of meals, and when they are consumed.

Physical examination should begin with assessment of the abdomen. Inspect skin on the abdomen for scars or other abnormalities; assess contour and symmetry of the abdomen. Auscultate abdominal quadrants, noting the character and frequency of bowel sounds. Hyperactive sounds are loud, high-pitched, rushing, tinkling, and may occur with early bowel obstruction, brisk diarrhea, and subsiding paralytic ileus. Hypoactive or absent sounds may indicate late bowel obstruction. Light and deep palpation is then performed to ascertain tenderness or distinguish masses (Jarvis, 1993).

Rectal examination is done with the patient in left lateral recumbent position. Perianal skin should be assessed for fissures, hemorrhoids, rectal prolapse, or masses. Stroking the quadrants of perineal skin with a cotton swab should invoke a reflex contraction of the external anal sphincter; absence of reflex may indicate neurologic impairment. Digital exam is performed to assess for structural abnormalities as well as internal sphincter tone (Jarvis, 1993).

Routine blood tests such as complete blood count, metabolic panel, and thyroid function tests can be used to rule out metabolic or pathologic disorders. An abdominal radiograph can help determine distribution of feces throughout the colon and rectum, and should be performed when fecal impaction or colonic dysmotility is suspected. Fecal loading in the descending and sigmoid colon indicates increased transit time (Kurniawan & Simadibrata, 2011).

Referral to specialty care can be made when constipation is refractory or when alarm signs are present. Specialty care diagnostics might include colonoscopy, colonic transit study, barium enema, anorectal manometry, or balloon expulsion test (Kurniawan & Simadibrata, 2011).

Treatment of Constipation

Constipation should be treated with least invasive means necessary. Perhaps an underlying illness needs better control or treatment, or maybe an offending medication can be stopped or changed. Patients using iron supplementation for anemia usually should take only 325 mg q.d. as evidence is not available to indicate higher doses. Opioid use is almost certain to cause constipation, and patients requiring opioids should be on prophylactic stool softeners or laxatives (Hsieh, 2005).

Nonpharmacologic Treatments and Prevention

Nonpharmacologic treatment should begin with review of the stool diary when applicable. Perhaps the patient just needs education that it is acceptable to have a bowel movement every other day. The diary may be helpful in identifying other barriers to treatment. Studies show that most people move their bowels at approximately the same time each day—usually after breakfast. This should be encouraged as colonic activity is greatest after waking and the gastrocolic reflex is stimulated by eating (Hsieh, 2005). Constipated elders should attempt a bowel movement twice a day after meals and should not strain more than 5 minutes (Rao & Go, 2010).

Foods rich in fiber (bran, fruit, vegetables, and nuts) have been shown to help alleviate constipation. Most Americans consume between 5 and 10 g of fiber each day; however, the recommended daily amount is 20 to 35 g. When adding dietary fiber, patients should add only 5 g extra per week as the additional fiber may cause bloating at first (Hsieh, 2005). Prunes have been shown to be superior to psyllium in managing mild to moderate constipation (Rao & Go, 2010).

There is not good clinical evidence to support that lack of hydration is a factor in constipation. There is, however, evidence to indicate that fewer meals and fewer calories are associated with constipation (Rao & Go, 2010). Decreased physical activity is associated with a twofold risk for constipation (Hsieh, 2005).

Pharmacologic Treatments

Fiber and laxatives improve bowel movement frequency as compared with placebo in adults, according to a systematic review. Data concerning the efficacy of individual treatments are limited secondary to the limited number of studies, small sample size, or methodologic flaws (Hsieh, 2005). A study in Norway concluded that "treatment of constipation in nursing homes was unsatisfactory and independent of treatment regimens" (Fosnes et al., 2011). There are very limited data on benefits and risks of laxatives and fiber preparations, especially as pertaining to the older adult (Hsieh, 2005).

Bulk-forming agents absorb water from the intestine, increase stool mass, and soften the stool. These laxatives are made from psyllium, pectin, guar, or cellulose. They are useful in patients with normal transit constipation, but may be detrimental in patients with anorectal dysfunction or slow transit constipation (Hsieh, 2005). These agents may cause fecaliths if insufficient fluid is consumed. Studies have reported reduced efficacy of some medications with these including warfarin, digoxin, potassium-sparing diuretics, salicylates, and antibiotics. Psyllium has the additional benefit of binding bile acids in the intestine, thereby lowering serum cholesterol (National Digestive Diseases Information Clearinghouse [NDDIC], 2011).

Emollient laxatives (stool softeners) allow water to enter the bowel by lowering surface tension. Stool softeners may be the laxative of choice for patients with anal fissures or hemorrhoids; however, they are not as effective in relieving constipation as psyllium. Stool softeners are ineffective in chronically ill elders (Hsieh, 2005).

Saline (or osmotic) laxatives draw water into the intestinal lumen by osmosis. These agents include magnesium hydroxide, magnesium citrate, and sodium biphosphate. These agents should be used carefully in patients with congestive heart failure or renal insufficiency as they may cause electrolyte imbalances (Hsieh, 2005).

Hyperosmotic laxatives include sorbitol, lactulose, glycerin (suppository form), and polyethylene glycol. A comparison study of 99 subjects with chronic constipation found polyethylene glycol superior to lactulose, causing less flatulence. A multicenter trial of 104 patients found lactulose more effective than senna, anthraquinone derivatives, or bisacodyl (Hsieh, 2005).

Stimulant laxatives (senna and bisacodyl) increase intestinal motility and secretion of water into the bowel. Bowel movements may be produced 8 to 12 hours after administration, but frail elders usually have a slower response time. These may cause cramping, and should not be given if obstruction is suspected. One study of 77 nursing home residents found a combination of senna and bulk agents to be more effective than lactulose at improving stool frequency and consistency (Hsieh, 2005).

Probiotics such as bifidobacterium and lactobacillus have recently gained a lot of attention. There is some evidence that these may improve colonic transit time in elders; however, their clinical relevance remains unclear (NDDIC, 2011).

Biofeedback, or pelvic floor retraining, is the main treatment for patients suffering from anorectal dysfunction. Recent studies show success rates from 50% to 90% in patients with chronic constipation (NDDIC, 2011). The decision for biofeedback or any invasive treatment is deferred to specialty care. The American Geriatrics Society (AGS) has distilled recommendations for treating chronic constipation into six steps, as shown in Table 6.10.

TABLE 6.10 • Management of Chronic Constipation

Step 1	Stop all constipating medications if possible.
Step 2	Increase dietary fiber to 6–25 g/day, increase fluid to ≥1,500 ml/day, and increase physical activity; or add bulk laxative if fluid ≥1,500 ml/day. If fiber exacerbates symptoms or not tolerated, go to step 3.
Step 3	Add an osmotic (sorbitol or polyethylene glycol).
Step 4	Add a stimulant laxative (senna or bisacodyl) two to three times per week. Alternative is saline laxative but avoid this if CrCl <30 ml/min.
Step 5	Tap water enema or saline enema two times per week.
Step 6	Oil retention enema for refractory constipation.

Cultural Considerations

The most important cultural consideration relates to the lack of fiber in the Western diet, which serves to increase the likelihood of chronic constipation. Diet change is not easy with older adults who live on fixed income and been used to a particular diet for many years.

REFERENCES

Ambrosetti, P., Robert, J. H., Witzig, J. A., Mirescu, D., Mathey, P., Borst, F., & Rohner, A. (1994). Acute left colonic diverticulitis: A prospective analysis of 226 consecutive cases. *Surgery, 115*(5), 46–50.

Arizona Center for Digestive Health. (n.d.). How GERD leads to Barrett's. Retrieved from http://www.azcdh.com/patient-education/

Beers, M. H., & Berkow, R. (2000). *The Merck manual of geriatrics* (3rd ed.). Whitehouse Station, NJ: Merck Sharp & Dohme.

Brook, I., & Frazier, E. H. (2000). Aerobic and anaerobic microbiology in intra-abdominal infections associated with diverticulitis. *Journal of Medical Microbiology, 49*(9), 827–830.

Burkitt, D., Walker, A., & Painter, N. (1974). Dietary fiber and disease. *Journal of the American Medical Association, 229*(8), 1068–1074.

Calabrese, C., Fabbri, A., & Di Febo, G. (2007). Long-term management of GERD in the elderly with pantoprazole. *Clinical Intervention in Aging, 2*(1), 85–92. Retrieved from http://www.ncbi.nlm.nih.gov

Chait, M. (2005). Gastroesophageal reflux disease in the elderly. *Practical Gastroenterology, 52,* 54–60. Retrieved from http://www.practicalgastroenterology.com

Denoon, D. J. (2010). C diff infections, fractures linked to acid reflux drugs. *WebMD News Archives.* Retrieved from http://www.webmd.com

Department of Health and Human Services, Administration on Aging. (2011). Aging statistics. Retrieved from http://www.aoa.gov

DeVault, K. R., & Castell, D. O. (2005). Updated guidelines for the diagnosis and treatment of gastroesophageal reflux disease. *American Journal of Gastroenterology, 100,* 190–200.

Farrell, R. J., Farrell, J. J., & Morrin, M. M. (2001). Diverticular disease in the elderly. *Gastroenterol Clinics of North America, 30*(2), 475–496.

Feroco, L. B., Raptopoulos, V., & Silen, W. (1998). Acute diverticulitis. *New England Journal of Medicine, 338,* 1521–1526.

Floch, M. H., & White, J. A. (2006). Management of diverticular disease is changing. *World Journal of Gastroenterology, 12,* 3225–3228.

Fosnes, G. S., Lydersen, S., & Farup, P. G. (2011). Effectiveness of laxatives in elderly—A cross sectional study in nursing homes. *BMC Geriatrics, 11,* 76.

Goh, H., & Bourne, R. (2002). Non-steroidal anti-inflammatory drugs and perforated diverticular disease: A case-control study. *Annals of the Royal College of Surgeons of England, 84,* 93–96.

Goodman, B. (2011). Men, women may experience acid reflux differently. *WebMD Health News.* Retrieved from http://www.webmd.com

Harford, W. V. (2012). Diverticulosis, diverticulitis, and appendicitis. In E. G. Nabel & D. D. Federman (Eds.), *ACP medicine*. Philadelphia, PA: Decker.

Hsieh, C. (2005). Treatment of constipation in older adults. *American Family Physician, 72*(11), 2277–2284.

Jacobs, D. (2007). Diverticulitis. *New England Journal of Medicine, 357*(20), 2057–2066.

Jarvis, C. (1993). *Pocket companion for physical examination and health assessment.* Philadelphia, PA: WB Saunders.

Johnson, D. A., & Fennety, M. B. (2004). Heartburn severity does not reliably indicate severity of erosive esophagitis. *Gastroenterology, 126,* 660–664.

Kurniawan, I., & Simadibrata, M. (2011). Management of chronic constipation in the elderly Indonesian. *Journal of Internal Medicine, 43*(3), 195–205.

Lo, C. Y., & Chu, K. W. (1996). Acute diverticulitis of the right colon. *American Journal of Surgery, 171,* 244–246.

Longstreth, G. F., Thompson, W. G., Chey, W. D., Houghton, L. A., Mearin, F., & Spiller, R. C. (2006). Functional bowel disorders. *Gastroenterology, 130,* 1480–1491.

Lynch, J. S. (2003). Can chronic hoarseness be a symptom of GERD? *Medscape Nurses, 5*(1). Retrieved from http://www.medscape.com

Machicado, G. A., & Jensen, D. M. (1997). Acute and chronic management of lower gastrointestinal bleeding: Cost effective approaches. *Gastroenterologist, 5,* 189–201.

Mauk, K. L. (2014). *Gerontological nursing: Competencies for care* (3rd ed.). Burlington, MA: Jones & Bartlett.

Morris, C. R., Harvey, I. M., Stebbings, W. S., Speakman, C. T., Kennedy, H. J., & Hart, A. R. (2003). Anti-inflammatory drugs, analgesics and the risk of perforated colonic diverticular disease. *British Journal of Surgery, 90,* 1267.

National Digestive Diseases Information Clearinghouse. (2013). Constipation. Retrieved from http://digestive.niddk.nih.gov/ddiseases/pubs/constipation/

Physicians Committee for Responsible Medicine. (n.d.). Gastroesophageal reflux disease. Retrieved from http://www.tcolincampbell.org

Pilotto, A., Franceschi, M., & Paris, F. (2005). Advance in the treatment of GERD in the elderly. *International Journal of Clinical Practice, 59*(10), 1204–1209. Retrieved from http://www.medscape.com

Rao, S. C., & Go, J. T. (2010). Update on the management of constipation in the elderly: New treatment options. *Clinical Interventions in Aging, 5,* 163–171.

Reisman, Y., Ziv, Y., Kravrovitc, D., Negri, M., Wolloch, Y., & Halevy, A. (1999). Diverticulitis: The effect of age and location on the course of disease. *International Journal of Colorectal, 14,* 250–254.

Salzman, H., & Lillie, D. (2005). Diverticular disease: Diagnosis and treatment. *American Family Physician, 72*(7), 1229–1234.

Stollman, N. H., & Raskin, J. B. (1999). Diverticular disease of the colon. *Journal of Clinical Gastroenterol, 29,* 241–242.

Truelove, S. C. (1966). Movements of the large intestine. *Physiological Reviews, 46,* 457–512.

Tursi, A. (2004a). Acute diverticulitis of the colon—Current medical therapeutic management. *Expert Opinion on Pharmacotherapy, 5,* 55–59.

Tursi, A. (2004b). Preventive therapy for complicated diverticular disease of the colon: Looking for a correct therapeutic approach. *Gastroenterology, 127,* 1865.

Wells, Q. (2010). Improving pharmaceutical care of the elderly patient with GERD. *Pharmacy Times.* Retrieved from https://securepharmacytimes.com

CHAPTER 6: IT RESOURCES

Websites

Rome III Disorders and Criteria
http://www.romecriteria.org/

Arizona Center for Digestive Health
http://www.azcdh.com/

Effects of Aging on the Digestive System
http://www.merckmanuals.com/home/digestive_disorders/biology_of_the_digestive_system/effects_of_aging_on_the_digestive_system.html

Diverticular Disease: What You Should Know
http://www.aafp.org/afp/2005/1001/p1241.html

Nutrition: Choosing Healthy, Low-Fat Foods
http://www.aafp.org/afp/2004/0215/p927.html

Gastrointestinal Disease
http://www.nysopep.org/Causes_Gastrointestinal.shtm

Gastroesophageal Reflux Disease in Older Adults: What Is the Difference?
http://www.clinicalgeriatrics.com/articles/Gastroesophageal-Reflux-Disease-Older-Adults-What-Is-Difference

Diagnosis and Management of Gastroesophageal Reflux Disease and Dyspepsia among Older Adults
http://www.medscape.com/viewarticle/579847

Senior GERD
http://www.aplaceformom.com/senior-care-resources/articles/senior-gerd

10 Things You Should Know About Avoiding Acid Reflux
   http://www.aarp.org/health/conditions-treatments/info-12-2010/ten_acid_reflux_tips.html
Gastroesophageal Reflux Disease—Special Considerations in Older Patients
   http://www.medscape.org/viewarticle/525128
Gastroesophageal Reflux Disease—Symptoms, Diagnosis, and Treatment
   http://www.aaaai.org/conditions-and-treatments/related-conditions/gastroesophageal-
   reflux-disease.aspx
Gastoesophageal Reflux Disease: Symptoms and Risk Factors
   http://www.tcolincampbell.org/courses-resources/article/gastro-
   esophageal-reflux-disease-symptoms-and-risk-factors/category/
   gastrointestinal-disorders/
Diverticulosis and Diverticulitis
   http://www.emedicinehealth.com/diverticulosis_and_diverticulitis/article_em.htm
Diverticulitis and the Elderly
   http://www.livestrong.com/article/258529-diverticulitis-the-elderly/
Diverticulosis and Diverticulitis
   http://www.betterhealth.vic.gov.au/bhcv2/bhcarticles.nsf/pages/
   Diverticulosis_and_diverticulitis
Diverticulitis—Merck Manual
   http://www.merckmanuals.com/home/digestive_disorders/diverticular_disease/
   diverticulitis.html
Hinchey Classification of Acute Diverticulitis
   http://www.kallus.com/er/diveriticulitis_hinchey.htm
Colonic Diverticular Disease
   http://www.clevelandclinicmeded.com/medicalpubs/diseasemanagement/gastroenterology/
   colonic-diverticular-disease/
Treatment of Constipation in Older Adults
   http://www.aafp.org/afp/2005/1201/p2277.html
Chronic Constipation in Older Patients
   http://www.mayoclinic.org/medicalprofs/constipation-older-adults-pudd0412.html

PDF Documents

Diverticular Disease
   http://eradiology.bidmc.harvard.edu/LearningLab/gastro/Gross.pdf
World Gastroenterology Organisation Practice Guidelines: Diverticular Disease
   http://www.worldgastroenterology.org/assets/downloads/en/pdf/guidelines/07_diverticular_
   disease.pdf
Rome III Diagnostic Criteria for Functional Gastrointestinal Disorders
   http://www.romecriteria.org/assets/pdf/19_RomeIII_apA_885-898.pdf
Preventing, Assessing and Managing Constipation in Older Adults
   http://www.nursingcenter.com/pdf.asp?AID=1467783
Pathophysiology of Constipation in Older Adults
   http://www.wjgnet.com/1007-9327/14/2631.pdf

Videos

(1/5) Optimal Diagnosis and Treatment of IBD in the Older Adult (2012) (17:20 minutes)
http://youtu.be/8jubbDt3cPc

(2/5) Optimal Diagnosis and Treatment of IBD in the Older Adult (2012) (5:23 minutes)
http://youtu.be/2PgWBB8vcko

A Call to Action: Optimal Diagnosis and Treatment of IBD in the Older Adult is a CME-certified online video activity featuring a series of conversations in which Drs. Seymour Katz, from the Albert Einstein College of Medicine, Darrell Pardi, from the Mayo Clinic, and Christina Surawicz, from the University of Washington School of Medicine discuss diagnosis and treatment of older patients with IBD and deliver information that will help clinicians to improve the IBD care they provide and achieve better outcomes for their older IBD patients.

Digestive System Disorders (2012) (1:49 minutes)
http://youtu.be/yQHx9WEfT-Y

Crohn's and Other GI Disorders (2013)
Dr. Tom Roselle and Dr. Scott Lamp discuss Crohn', Colitis, Inflammatory Bowel Disease and Gastrointestinal Disorders. (48:15 minutes)
http://youtu.be/VJD7-2nFcUQ

GERD—Focus on Health (2013) (33:34 minutes)
http://youtu.be/R389G5W6So0

Images

Google images for Gastrointestinal Diseases
http://www.google.com/search?q=gastrointestinal+diseases+and+older+adults&source=lnms&tbm=isch&sa=X&ei=IGejUYPVHtOz4APpjoDYDw&ved=0CAcQ_AUoAQ&biw=1011&bih=220

Google images for Diverticulitis
http://www.google.com/search?q=Diverticulitis+in+Older+Adults&source=lnms&tbm=isch&sa=X&ei=ZIOjUbPKA6fg0gGe1YCgDw&ved=0CAcQ_AUoAQ&biw=1024&bih=564

Google images for GERD Disease
http://www.google.com/search?q=GERD+disease+and+older+adults&source=lnms&tbm=isch&sa=X&ei=g4OjUa6yIYzE0AGF3oCIBg&ved=0CAcQ_AUoAQ&biw=1024&bih=564

Google images for Gastroesophageal Reflux Disease
http://www.google.com/search?q=gastroesophageal+reflux+disease+in+older+adults&source=lnms&tbm=isch&sa=X&ei=04OjUaWKGJC20QHxmoCwAQ&ved=0CAcQ_AUoAQ&biw=1024&bih=564

Neurologic Disorders

Shravan Kumar R. Gaddam, MD, CMD
Christopher D. Wood, DO

INTRODUCTION AND PREVALENCE

Stroke is the fourth leading cause of death (1 out of 18 deaths) in the United States and is a leading cause of disability (Fang et al., 2012). Stroke is caused by either a blockage in an artery that supplies blood to the brain or by the rupturing of a blood vessel in the brain, causing bleeding and cell death. When this occurs, it deprives the brain of oxygen, causing tissue death.

Although strokes are more common in men than women in most age groups, about 40% of stroke deaths occur in males and 60% in females (Pleis & Lethbridge-Cejku, 2007). Also, men generally have higher age-specific stroke incidence rates than women (based on age-specific rates calculated from strata defined by race/ethnicity), and this is true for ischemic as well as hemorrhagic strokes. The exceptions are those who are 35 to 44 years of age and those older than 85 years of age. African Americans are at a higher risk for stroke death than Caucasians. The risk of stroke approximately doubles for each decade of life over the age of 55 (Kissela et al., 2004; Sacco et al., 1998).

CLASSIFICATION AND DEFINITIONS

In the United States, 87% of all strokes are ischemic secondary to large artery atherosclerosis, cardioembolism, small-vessel occlusion, and other causes. Table 7.1 lists the potential conditions that can lead to a thrombotic or cardioembolic stroke. The remaining 13% of strokes are hemorrhagic owing to intracerebral or subarachnoid bleeding (Adams et al., 1993; Go et al., 2013).

A transient ischemic attack (TIA) is defined as a transient motor or sensory deficit that resolves completely within a 24-hour period with or without radiologic evidence of stroke. These patients are at high risk for a subsequent stroke and need a complete workup (Furie et al., 2011).

TABLE 7.1 · Causes of Ischemic Strokes

Thrombotic Causes	Embolic Causes
Aortic dissection	Arrhythmia (atrial fibrillation/flutter)
Arteritis/vasculitis	Artery-to-artery embolization
Atherosclerosis	Bacterial endocarditis
Fibromuscular dysplasia	Bioprosthetic or mechanical heart valve
Hypercoagulable disorders	Dilated cardiomyopathy
Malignancy	Deep venous thrombosis
Polycythemia vera	Heart failure with ejection fraction of <30%
Thrombocytosis	Iatrogenic
Vasoconstriction	Myocardial infarction within the past month
	Patent foramen ovale
	Rheumatic mitral or aortic valve disease
	Systemic hypoperfusion (secondary to sepsis or shock)

Ischemic strokes (Fig. 7.1) are defined by anoxia that results from occlusive disease secondary to thrombosis, embolic disease, or cerebral hypoperfusion. It is important to make an effort to determine the likely type of ischemic stroke as both the initial management as well as the therapy aimed at preventing further strokes will differ. Brain imaging is important in defining the location and extent of the injury. These studies, in addition to a careful history and physical examination, will assist the clinician with decision making.

Hemorrhagic strokes are defined by the anoxic damage to neurons in the central nervous system (CNS) that occurs secondary to bleeding, and are often secondary to a bleeding aneurysm. The bleeding can be intracerebral, subdural (Fig. 7.2), or subarachnoid. Clinically, these present with abrupt onset of focal symptoms and may have gradual worsening of symptoms, reflecting the increasing size of hematoma as well as surrounding brain edema. Nontraumatic intracranial hemorrhage (ICH) accounts for a disproportionate number of stroke-related deaths; mortality from this condition approaches 50% (Broderick et al., 2007). Its prevalence is higher in African Americans and is equal between genders, although there is both racial and gender heterogeneity in the hemorrhage location. The ICH score is a simple, validated predictor of outcome. Points are given for a low Glasgow Coma Scale (GCS) score, infratentorial origin, volume greater than 30 ml, the presence of intraventricular blood, and age greater than 80 years. Scores between 0 and 6 predict 30-day mortalities between 0% and near 100%. Clinicians should be familiar with regularly published guidelines for diagnosis and management of ICH.

Subarachnoid hemorrhage (SAH) is less common than ICH but causes similar mortality and substantial morbidity. Racial heterogeneity is similar to that of other cerebrovascular diseases; however, SAH is more common in women. The predictors of outcome include level of consciousness at admission, age, and amount of blood visualized on head computerized tomography (CT).

Nontraumatic SAH (Figs. 7.3 and 7.4) most commonly results from rupture of aneurysms of the Circle of Willis, for which aneurysms of the anterior and posterior communicating arteries are most

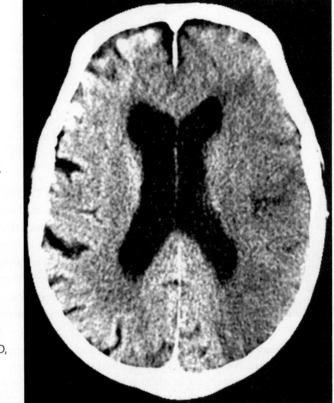

FIGURE 7.1. Acute CVA: Axial noncontrast CT image of the head obtained 12 hours after onset of stroke symptoms demonstrates a large area of relative hypodensity in the left frontal and parietal lobes with loss of the gray–white matter differentiation and effacement of left sulci. These findings are secondary to brain edema following left middle cerebral artery ischemic stroke. No hemorrhage is present. (CT image courtesy Carilion Clinic Radiology, Vishal M. Patel, MD, Department of Radiology, Carilion Clinic, Assistant Professor, Virginia Tech Carilion School of Medicine.)

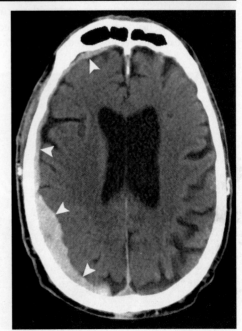

FIGURE 7.2. Acute SDH: Axial noncontrast CT image of the head demonstrates a crescentic high-density acute subdural hematoma on the right *(arrowheads)*; greatest in thickness in the parietal region where there is mass effect on the underlying brain. The sulci contain no subarachnoid blood products. (CT image courtesy Carilion Clinic Radiology, Vishal M. Patel, MD, Department of Radiology, Carilion Clinic, Assistant Professor, Virginia Tech Carilion School of Medicine.)

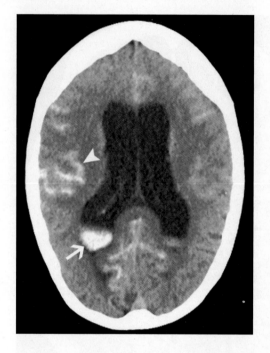

FIGURE 7.3. Acute SAH (1 of 2): Axial noncontrast CT image of the head demonstrates high-density acute subarachnoid blood filling the sulci *(arrowhead)* and acute intraventricular blood layering in the occipital horns of the lateral ventricle *(arrow)*. (CT image courtesy Carilion Clinic Radiology, Vishal M. Patel, MD, Department of Radiology, Carilion Clinic, Assistant Professor, Virginia Tech Carilion School of Medicine.)

frequently responsible. Hypertension and cigarette smoking are clear risk factors for aneurysmal rupture. A family history of ruptured intracranial aneurysms in first-degree relatives is also a risk factor for aneurysm. In addition to severe headache ("worst headache of my life"), the following suggest SAH and should prompt a thorough evaluation: rapid onset, photophobia, stiff neck, decreased level of consciousness, and focal neurologic signs. Up to 50% of patients with SAH present with a resolving headache caused by a so-called warning leak or sentinel hemorrhage. They may not exhibit focal signs because bleeding occurs outside the brain, except when an aneurysm bleeds into a focal

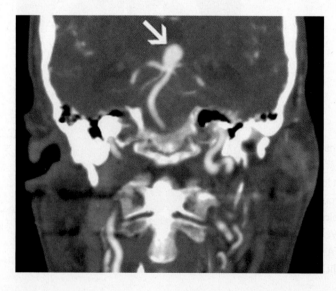

FIGURE 7.4. Acute SAH from basilar tip aneurysm (2 of 2): Coronal CT of the brain on the same patient following IV contrast demonstrates a large aneurysm arising from the tip of the basilar artery *(arrow)*. Rupture of the aneurysm led to the subarachnoid and intraventricular hemorrhage. (CT image courtesy Carilion Clinic Radiology, Vishal M. Patel, MD, Department of Radiology, Carilion Clinic, Assistant Professor, Virginia Tech Carilion School of Medicine.)

location such as the posterior communicating artery aneurysm compressing the third cranial nerve. Modern head CT has near-perfect sensitivity for diagnosis of SAH within 12 hours of symptom onset. If CT is negative and clinical suspicion remains high, lumbar puncture and examination of the cerebrospinal fluid for xanthochromia are necessary. Establishing the diagnosis early and consequent prompt aneurysm clipping can reduce long-term morbidity and mortality.

CULTURAL CONSIDERATIONS AND SOCIAL IMPACT

In 2010, it cost Americans about $73.7 billion for stroke-related medical costs and disability (Fang et al., 2012). Strokes are one of the leading causes of nursing home admissions and caregiver stress. Strokes can cause a wide range of problems, ranging from no symptoms to death. Other effects include weakness, visual loss, dysphagia, dysphasia, memory loss, delirium, and dementia.

ANATOMY

The effects of a stroke depend on the area of the brain that is affected and the extent of brain tissue involved. Therefore, it is important to understand the basics of neuroanatomy. Figures 7.5 and 7.6 show the Circle of Willis and vascular distribution of the brain by the various arteries. Figure 7.7 shows a normal brain CT with the white- and gray-matter differentiation.

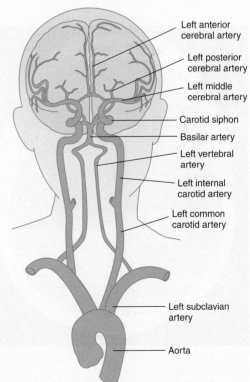

FIGURE 7.5. Circle of Willis. (From Waxman, S. G. [2009]. *Clinical neuroanatomy* [26th ed.]. New York, NY: McGraw-Hill, with permission.)

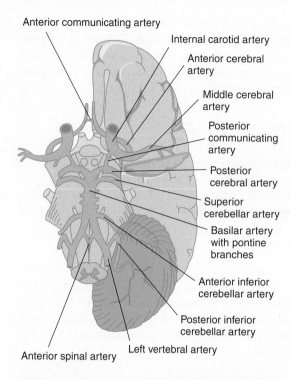

FIGURE 7.6. Vascular distribution of the brain. (From Waxman, S. G. [2009]. *Clinical neuroanatomy* [26th ed.]. New York, NY: McGraw-Hill, with permission.)

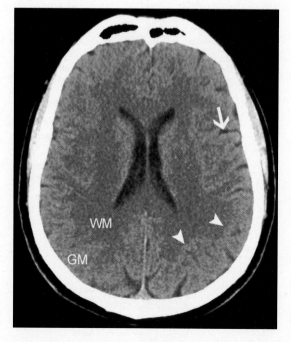

FIGURE 7.7. Normal brain picture: Axial noncontrast CT image of the head demonstrates a normal CT appearance of the brain. Cortical gray matter (GM) can be differentiated from subcortical white matter (WM) with a preserved gray–white matter interface *(arrowheads)*. Normal noneffaced low-density sulci *(arrow)* are observed. (CT image courtesy Carilion Clinic Radiology, Vishal M. Patel, MD, Department of Radiology, Carilion Clinic, Assistant Professor, Virginia Tech Carilion School of Medicine.)

DIFFERENTIAL DIAGNOSIS OF STROKE

There are a number of conditions, particularly in the older adult, that can present in a similar fashion to stroke and must be ruled out. These include seizures and especially the postictal state. One would see gradual improvements without focal neurologic signs. Systemic infections, syncope/presyncope or hypotension, and toxic metabolic disturbances generally respond to correction of the primary insult along with hydration. Tumors can present with a stroke syndrome with a mass noted on neuroimaging (Bernheisel et al., 2011).

Delirium or the acute confusional state can be medication-induced, owing to alcohol or other encephalopathy or secondary to an acute exacerbation of a chronic disease. While not as common in the older populations as in younger populations, migraines can present with focal neurologic deficits. Vertigo from ear disease can present like a posterior circulation stroke. Finally, functional or medically unexplained symptoms such as psychogenic disorders can take the form of a stroke syndrome.

RISK FACTORS

There are several risk factors for strokes, some of which are modifiable. It is important to control diseases that may increase the risk of strokes, such as diabetes mellitus and hypertension. Table 7.2 gives a list of modifiable and nonmodifiable risk factors for stroke.

TABLE 7.2 · Risk Factors

Disease States	Lifestyle Modifications
Hypertension	Tobacco use/exposure
Diabetes mellitus type 2	Heavy alcohol use
Metabolic syndrome	Substance abuse (cocaine)
Prediabetes	Physical inactivity
Atrial fibrillation	High dietary sodium intake
Hyperlipidemia	Hormone replacement therapy
Carotid artery stenosis	
Proteinuria	
Sleep apnea	
History of TIA/stroke	
History of vasculitis	

EVALUATION

It is very important to establish the exact time of onset of symptoms for determining eligibility for thrombolysis within the approved window period. Information from caregivers or family as to when the patient was last seen to be normal can be very helpful in making this determination. Many times, however, it is hard to ascertain the exact onset of symptoms, which makes thrombolysis therapy less useful.

There are various tools used currently that have been well-validated to classify stroke severity and its diagnosis. Table 7.3 lists some of the tools. Medical personnel, including first responders such as emergency medical personnel, need to quickly assess persons with suspected acute ischemic stroke. The National Institutes of Health Stroke Scale (NIHSS) was designed to be completed in 5 to 8 minutes. A high index of suspicion and urgent evaluation are keys to effectively evaluate and treat acute stroke. Reliably distinguishing between intracerebral hemorrhage and ischemic stroke can be done only by neuroimaging.

Depending on the symptomatology and clinical presentation, most strokes can be easily classified and the location of injury narrowed down. While a thorough physical examination is warranted, in the interest of time, imaging and laboratory evaluation often takes precedence, especially if acute stroke is suspected.

Common constellations of symptoms characterize ischemic strokes and can be deduced from the vascular supply to the brain. Table 7.4 lists the common neurologic findings of the major occlusive stroke syndromes. Two pairs of vessels supply blood to the brain: the internal carotid arteries and the vertebral arteries. These vessels, which carry 20% of the cardiac output, join and branch on the ventral surface of the brain to form the intracranial vessels and the Circle of Willis.

The anterior cerebral artery (ACA) supplies blood to the medial frontal and deep structures. Occlusion of the ACA is characterized by contralateral leg weakness, but isolated infarction of the ACA is uncommon. The middle cerebral artery (MCA) divides into two major trunks, and each trunk divides into five to seven branches that supply blood to the lateral hemisphere. Because the MCA supplies a large territory, MCA occlusion causes a clinical syndrome that includes contralateral hemiparesis and hemisensory deficit (in which the deficit in the face and arm is greater than the deficit in the leg), aphasia (if the dominant hemisphere is affected) or neglect (if the nondominant hemisphere is affected), contralateral visual field defect, deviation of gaze, dysarthria, and other cortical symptoms.

TABLE 7.3 • Selected Stroke Screening Tools

Cincinnati Prehospital Stroke scale (facial paralysis, arm drift, abnormal speech)
Face, Arm, Speech test (needs GCS of >6 and one of the following: facial paralysis, arm weakness, and speech impairment)
Los Angeles Prehospital Stroke care (sensitivity and specificity ranges between 80% and 90% in screening for stroke symptoms)
NIHSS scale (minimum score of 0, maximum score of 42, score of 15–20 shows high severity, 13-item scoring system, in cooperation with the following components: cranial nerves (visual), motor, sensory, cerebellar, inattention, language, LOC)

TABLE 7.4 • Clinical Features of the Major Cerebral Vascular Occlusive Syndromes

Artery	Major Clinical Features
Anterior cerebral artery	Contralateral leg weakness
Middle cerebral artery	Contralateral face + arm > leg weakness, sensory loss, visual field cut, aphasia/neglect
Posterior cerebral artery	Contralateral visual field cut
Basilar artery	Oculomotor deficits and/or ataxia with "crossed" sensory/motor deficits
Vertebral artery	Lower cranial nerve deficits and/or ataxia with "crossed" sensory deficits
Penetrators	Contralateral motor or sensory deficit without cortical signs

The two vertebral arteries unite to form the basilar artery. The major branches of the basilar artery are the anterior inferior cerebellar artery and the superior cerebellar artery, which supply parts of the pons and cerebellum. Occlusion of the vertebral arteries or basilar artery leads to a combination of signs and symptoms that depend on the level and extent of infarction. These signs and symptoms include so-called crossed facial and body sensory and motor signs, diplopia, facial numbness and weakness, vertigo, nausea and vomiting, tinnitus, hearing loss, ataxia, gait abnormality, hemiparesis, dysphagia, and dysarthria. The basilar artery terminates by dividing into two posterior cerebral arteries that supply the medial temporal lobe, the occipital lobe, and parts of the thalamus.

Occlusion of the posterior cerebral artery results in occipital infarction and therefore contralateral visual field loss. Such occlusion may also cause contralateral hemiparesis and behavioral changes.

After leaving the Circle of Willis, the vessels branch repeatedly and ultimately become end arteries. Occlusion of these penetrating vessels can manifest as isolated neurologic deficits. Pure motor hemiparesis, pure sensory loss, clumsy hand–dysarthria syndrome, and ataxic hemiparesis have moderate specificity for small-vessel or end-artery etiology (Kasner & Heather, 2010).

LABORATORY AND IMAGING IN THE INITIAL EVALUATION

Table 7.5 lists the recommended imaging and laboratory tests to be considered in the evaluation of the patient with a suspected acute stroke. For definitive diagnosis in the setting of acute stroke, emergent noncontrast head CT or magnetic resonance imaging (MRI) needs to be performed. Diffusion-weighted MRI of the brain can be useful for determining infarction size and confirming the presence of ischemic stroke if the diagnosis is in question (cerebral infarction often is not seen initially on CT imaging). Diffusion-weighted MRI is the most sensitive and specific modality for early detection of acute cerebral infarction.

Magnetic resonance angiography (MRA) is useful for characterization of vascular disease. It has higher sensitivity and specificity than ultrasonography for detecting carotid artery disease. In addition to measuring atherosclerotic carotid stenosis (a common cause of ischemic stroke), it may also help identify less common etiologies, such as arterial dissection, venous thrombosis, fibromuscular dysplasia, and vasculitis. However, MRA is significantly more expensive, and its

TABLE 7.5 · Laboratory and Imaging Test to Evaluate Stroke Patients

Initial evaluation in all patients

■ Noncontrast brain CT or brain MRI

■ Blood glucose

■ Serum electrolytes and renal function tests

■ Electrocardiography

■ Markers of cardiac ischemia

■ Complete blood count, including platelet count

■ Prothrombin time/international normalized ratio

■ Activated partial thromboplastin time

■ Oxygen saturation

Selected patients

■ Hepatic function tests

■ Toxicology screen

■ Blood alcohol level

■ Pregnancy test

■ Arterial blood gas (if hypoxemia suspected)

■ Chest radiography (if lung disease suspected)

■ Lumbar puncture (if subarachnoid hemorrhage suspected and head CT negative for blood)

■ Carotid Dopplers

■ Electroencephalography (if seizure suspected)

■ Echocardiography

■ Rare causes of ischemic stroke—check for protein C & S, anticardiolipin antibody test, antithrombin, prothrombin gene mutation, factor V Leiden, ESR, ANA, RPR, HIV, prothrombin gene mutation

use is limited in patients who have metallic implants, pacemakers, or severe claustrophobia, or who cannot tolerate contrast media (Wardlaw, 2004).

Carotid artery ultrasonography is an inexpensive and useful modality for identifying atherosclerotic carotid stenosis (Latchaw et al., 2009). Patients with greater than 70% carotid stenosis on the side of the neurologic deficit may have a reduced risk of future stroke if carotid endarterectomy (CEA) is performed, preferably within 2 weeks of the ischemic event (European Carotid Surgery Trialists' Collaborative Group, 1998; Rothwell et al., 2004). Patients with moderate ipsilateral stenosis (50% to 69%) may benefit from early endarterectomy, depending on patient-specific factors (e.g., age, sex, comorbidity, severity of initial symptoms), but the evidence is less clear. Surgical intervention has not been shown to benefit patients with ipsilateral carotid stenosis of less than 50% (Barnett et al., 1998).

There are no clear recommendations regarding the routine use of echocardiography in the evaluation of ischemic stroke. Although it is commonly performed in the initial diagnostic workup, its value may be limited when there is low suspicion for an embolic source. In patients with risk factors for embolic stroke, some studies have shown that transthoracic echocardiography alone can miss up to 32% of pertinent abnormalities, such as intracardiac thrombi that would require anticoagulation or structural lesions (e.g., patent foramen ovale) that may benefit from surgical repair (de Abreu et al., 2008). If a patient has any risk factor for embolic stroke and no pertinent abnormality is detected on transthoracic echocardiography, transesophageal echocardiography is recommended.

TREATMENT

Acute Treatment of Ischemic Stroke

Thrombolysis

Once a stroke has been appropriately diagnosed, the first step is to screen the patient to determine whether he/she is a candidate for thrombolysis. Table 7.6 lists the AHA/ASA (American Heart Association/American Stroke Association) inclusion and exclusion screening criteria for consideration of thrombolysis (Practice Advisory: Thrombolytic Therapy for Acute Ischemic Stroke, 1996). The first criterion is to know the time interval.

TPA (Tissue plasminogen activator) should be given only after blood pressure control to acceptable levels has been achieved. TPA should be administered at 0.9 mg/kg (maximum dose of 90 mg) over 60 minutes with 10% given as a bolus over 1 minute. If TPA is given, the patient should be monitored in an intensive care unit (ICU) setting and evaluated for worsening symptoms. Caregivers should be aware of the potential side effects including bleeding, angioedema (which may cause partial airway obstruction), and hemorrhagic conversion of an ischemic stroke. Larger infarcts are at higher risk for hemorrhagic conversion. Blood pressure should continue to be monitored and neurologic assessments made every 15 minutes while TPA is being administered, then every 30 minutes for the next 6 hours, then every hour for 24 hours post-treatment. An emergency head CT should be obtained if the patient develops a headache, hypertension, nausea, or vomiting. Placement of nasogastric tubes, indwelling bladder catheters, and intra-arterial pressure catheters should be delayed if TPA is given. A follow-up head CT should be obtained at 24 hours prior to starting anticoagulants or antiplatelets.

Intra-arterial thrombolysis may be an option for selected patients with a major stroke if identified within 6 hours of an occlusion of the MCA who are not otherwise candidates for IV thrombolysis. This treatment should only be given at a certified stroke center with a qualified interventional radiologist and immediate access to cerebral angiography.

Blood Pressure Regulation

After an ischemic stroke, an elevated blood pressure is acceptable to a certain degree. Permissive hypertension allows increased blood flow to the penumbra (the area of brain that surrounds the ischemic area). The penumbra may survive for several hours after the acute episode owing to collateral blood flow. The patient's home blood pressure medications are usually held and blood pressure is treated only if systolic blood pressure is greater than 220 mm Hg or diastolic blood pressure is greater than 120 mm Hg in ischemic strokes. Labetalol given IV, nitropaste, or

TABLE 7.6 · Guidelines for the use of rt-PA (Alteplase)

Inclusion criteria for IV rt-PA (Alteplase) treatment for ischemic stroke (AHA/ASA Class I, Level A)

- Ischemic stroke causing measurable neurologic deficit (caution if major deficits)

- Neurologic signs not clearing spontaneously

- Neurologic signs not minor and isolated

- Onset of symptoms <3 hours before treatment (but expanded to <4.5 hours for some patients in updated recommendations, see below)

Exclusion criteria for rt-PA treatment for ischemic stroke

- Symptoms suggestive of subarachnoid hemorrhage

- Head trauma or prior stroke within 3 months

- Myocardial infarction within 3 months

- Gastrointestinal or urinary tract hemorrhage within 21 days

- Major surgery within 14 days

- Arterial puncture at noncompressible site within 7 days

- History of ICH

- Systolic blood pressure ≥185 mm Hg and diastolic blood pressure ≥110 mm Hg

- Active bleeding or acute trauma (fracture)

- Taking oral anticoagulant and INR >1.7

- Receiving heparin within 48 hours and activated partial thromboplastin time (aPTT) not in normal range

- Platelet count <100,000 mm

- Blood glucose concentration <50 mg/dl (2.7 mmol/L)

- Seizure with postictal residual neurologic impairment

- Multilobar infarction on CT (hypodensity >1/3 cerebral hemisphere)

- Patient or family members not understanding risks and benefits of treatment

Inclusion criteria remain the same 3–4.5 hours after stroke onset but exclusion criteria expanded to, all exclusion criteria noted above, plus

- Age >80 years (DynaMed commentary—age ≥65 years suggested on the basis of subgroup analysis of ECASS III trial published after updated AHA/ASA recommendation)

- All patients taking oral anticoagulants (regardless of INR)

- NIH stroke scale score >25

- History of stroke and diabetes

From DynaMed in September 2012, Practice advisory: Thrombolytic therapy for acute ischemic stroke. Report of the Quality of Standards Subcommittee of the American Academy of Neurology. (1996). *Neurology, 47*, 835–839, with permission.

a nicardipine infusion are good options for acute blood pressure management. After 24 hours, a reasonable goal is to lower blood pressure by about 15%. Both low and very high blood pressures are associated with a poor outcome after a stroke (Anderson et al., 2008).

Carotid Endarterectomy

CEA is indicated in patients with recent TIA or ischemic stroke and ipsilateral severe (70% to 99%) carotid stenosis if performed by a surgeon with perioperative morbidity and mortality less than 6% (AHA/ASA Class I, Level A). The benefits of surgery are lower with ipsilateral moderate (50% to 69%) carotid stenosis (AHA/ASA Class I, Level B). Carotid artery angioplasty and stenting is an alternative to CEA (AHA/ASA Class I, Level B) in selected patients (Sacco et al., 2006).

Hemorrhagic Stroke

One of the key goals of initial treatment is to reverse coagulopathy, if present. Patients with ICH deteriorate over the first 24 to 48 hours as edema worsens and intracranial pressure (ICP) increases. An ICP monitor is to be considered in patients who are obtunded (those with GCS of less than 9). There are multiple strategies used to control ICP:

- Sedation with or without chemical neuromuscular paralysis, helpful in intubated patients.
- Osmotic diuretics are often used in the short term.
- Hyperventilation—lowers ICP by reducing cerebral blood flow through vasoconstriction but is a short-lived effect (6 to 12 hours).
- Surgical approaches—ventricular drainage, early evacuation of hematoma decreases the ICP.
- Steroids are not recommended.

Blood pressure management in ICH remains controversial because of the competing goals of limiting hemorrhage expansion and promoting cerebral perfusion. Intensive blood pressure lowering to a systolic target of 140 was well tolerated, reduced hematoma growth, and did not affect functional outcome at 90 days in a randomized trial (Anderson et al., 2008). The AHA guidelines recommend that mean arterial blood pressure be kept lower than 110 mm Hg in patients without elevated ICP.

Subarachnoid Hemorrhage

Definitive treatment of SAH involves localizing the aneurysm with cerebral angiography and early repair using either surgical or endovascular catheter-based techniques (Bederson et al., 2009). Disability-free survival at 1 year was better with endovascular coiling (Molyneux et al., 2002, 2005). Before aneurysm clipping or coiling, patients are mildly sedated and given stool softeners to reduce the risk of rebleeding. Anticonvulsants should be given at the first sign of seizures. Blood pressure should be gently controlled, although hypertension is related to rebleeding. Drastic reduction in blood pressure should be avoided. Common complications include rebleeding, hydrocephalus, and vasospasm. Treatment with Nimodipine and simvastatin are indicated and shown to improve outcomes. Any mental status changes should prompt emergency CT scan evaluation to look for signs of hydrocephalus, which is common and is treatable with ventricular drainage. Any evidence of vasospasm with accompanying focal neurologic signs should prompt therapy of hypertension and hypovolemia. Angioplasty is, at times, indicated.

Long-term Management and Prevention of Complications

Dysphagia

Dysphagia is a common complication of stroke, especially in the older adult. Dysphagia can result in aspiration, leading to pneumonia, poor nutrition, and dehydration. In order to reduce the risk of aspiration and pneumonia, all patients with stroke should have swallowing evaluated before initiating any oral intake. The initial swallowing screen should include observations of level of consciousness, postural control, and ability to mobilize oral secretions. After this assessment, a water swallow test is to be performed (DePippo et al., 1992).

Dysphagia may persist for many months and is a marker of poor prognosis associated with three to seven times increased risk of aspiration pneumonia. In addition, persistent dysphagia is an independent predictor of mortality after stroke. The reported recovery rates vary. Swallow may recover in greater than 80% of patients within 2 to 4 weeks of stroke onset. Of the remaining 20%, about 50% will not recover to normal swallow by 6 months after the stroke.

Percutaneous endoscopic gastrostomy (PEG) placement was associated with a lower probability of intervention failure compared with feeding by a nasogastric tube. There is no significant difference in mortality rates between comparison groups, and pneumonia irrespective of underlying disease (medical diagnosis). Thus, in conclusion, the mortality rates are the same in both interventions (Gomes et al., 2010).

Aspiration Precaution

Depending on the area of brain that is affected, aspiration is a common problem in stroke patients. Either a bedside nursing evaluation or a formal speech and language pathology (SLP) evaluation should be performed before oral intake is allowed. If a swallowing deficit is observed, the patient should remain NPO (nothing by mouth). A modified barium swallow study may be helpful to determine whether a modified food consistency is safe. If no safe oral intake can be given, a feeding nasogastric tube may be placed for nutrition. A discussion regarding a more permanent feeding tube may be needed if no improvement is seen over time.

The clinical features most predictive of aspiration risk include wet voice, weak voluntary cough, cough on swallowing, prolonged swallow, abnormal gag reflex, and reduced laryngopharyngeal sensation. Basal ganglia strokes might predispose patients to pneumonia owing to frequent aspiration during sleep (Nakagawa et al., 1997).

Venous Thromboembolism

Unfractionated heparin and low-molecular-weight heparin have been shown to reduce the incidence of venous thromboembolism after ischemic stroke (Coull et al., 2002; Hillbom et al., 2002). Evidence on sequential leg compression devices is lacking, but they are probably less effective than heparin-based products and should be used only when heparin is not an option. Current guidelines recommend a prophylactic dose of unfractionated or low-molecular-weight heparin for patients with restricted mobility after ischemic stroke, unless there is a specific contraindication to the therapy. Fondaparinux (Arixtra) is also an option for the prevention of venous thromboembolism after stroke.

Pressure Ulcers

Early mobilization, frequent turning and skin examinations, and use of alternating pressure mattresses should be considered to prevent skin damage after ischemic stroke. Assessing nutritional status with measurement of albumin, prealbumin, and cholesterol levels can aid in identifying patients at higher risk of wound formation (low levels indicate higher risk).

Infection

Patients with neurologic deficits leading to immobility are at a higher risk of pneumonia from atelectasis and aspiration. These patients should be mobilized early in the hospital stay and encouraged to use bedside incentive spirometry hourly to aid deep breathing and ease cough. Medications that reduce the level of consciousness or increase the risk of aspiration pneumonia (e.g., proton pump inhibitors) should be discontinued unless specifically indicated (Herzig et al., 2009). Urinary tract infections are common after stroke, and indwelling catheters should be avoided. Fever is independently linked to poor outcomes in patients with stroke. Although antipyretics have not been shown to improve neurologic outcomes, a workup for the source of any fever should be performed (Adams et al., 2007).

Delirium

Delirium, defined as an acute change in cognition and attention that fluctuates throughout the day, can develop after stroke, especially in older adults. Delirium can lead to increased length of hospitalization, high death rates, and limited functional capacity. Measures to reduce the risk of delirium after stroke include limiting anticholinergic and sedative medications, avoiding disturbances of the sleep–wake cycle, and preserving available sensory input.

Rehabilitation

Once a patient has been stabilized from the acute stroke, early initiation of therapy is essential for regaining function. An intensive rehabilitation program should be started during the inpatient period. It is important to remember to train caregivers as well during rehabilitation to reduce cost and improve both patient and caregiver psychosocial outcomes at 1 year.

Physical therapy may improve functional independence following a stroke, and a high-intensity in-home physical therapy program may have similar improvement in mobility as a standard outpatient program. Occupational therapy focuses on the preservation of the ability to perform activities of daily living (ADLs). There are many different modified devices to help patients perform tasks such as mobility, feeding, and other fine motor skills.

SLP is helpful in the prevention and treatment of both dysphagia and dysphasia. There are numerous tips to help with swallowing such as tucking the chin and swallowing twice with each bite. There are also additives that can be added to liquids to change the consistency. Speech language pathologists can help patients with word finding or receptive aphasia.

Secondary Prevention

Noncardioembolic Ischemic Stroke

Antiplatelet agents are recommended over anticoagulants (ACCP Grade 1A, AHA/ASA Class I, Level A, CSN Grade A) (Adams et al., 2007; Sacco et al., 2006). Aspirin in doses as low as 75 mg/day reduces the risk of vascular events in patients with previous stroke or TIA. Clopidogrel (Plavix) 75 mg once daily may be slightly more effective than aspirin at reducing ischemic events. The combination of aspirin 25 mg plus extended-release dipyridamole 200 mg (Aggrenox, Asasantin) twice daily is more effective than aspirin at reducing vascular events and appears similar to clopidogrel for prevention of recurrent stroke, but may have slightly more major hemorrhagic events. The combination of aspirin plus clopidogrel is currently not recommended for secondary stroke prophylaxis (ACCP Grade 1B, AHA/ASA Class III, Level A, CSN Grade B) owing to the increased risk of life-threatening or major bleeding (Adams et al., 2007; Sacco et al., 2006). However, a recent study looking at medical management compared with stenting for patients with intracranial arterial stenosis used aspirin plus clopidogrel and found it superior to stenting (Chimowitz et al., 2011). Other antiplatelet agents that may be as effective as aspirin with a lower risk of hemorrhage include cilostazol (Pletal) and triflusal (Aflen, Disgren, Grendis, Triflux). Anticoagulation therapy appears to increase adverse events without increased benefits compared with aspirin in patients with nonembolic stroke or TIA.

Cardioembolic Stroke

Anticoagulation is preferred over antiplatelet therapy in patients with atrial fibrillation; the recommendation is for long-term oral anticoagulation use with a target international normalized ratio (INR) of 2.5 (range 2 to 3) (ACCP Grade 1A, AHA/ASA Class I, Level A). When there are contraindications to anticoagulant therapy, aspirin 75 to 325 mg/day (ACCP Grade 1B, AHA/ASA Class I, Level A) is the recommended alternative. Anticoagulants reduce the risk of stroke and appear more effective than antiplatelet therapy (Wiebers et al., 2003). Statins should be considered as they reduce subsequent cerebrovascular events in adults with a history of stroke or TIA.

Intracranial Hemorrhage

Treatment of hypertension, smoking cessation, reduction of heavy alcohol use, and cocaine avoidance are the cornerstones of decreasing the risk of recurrent ICH.

Subarachnoid Hemorrhage

The risk of aneurysm rupture depends on the size, location, and prior SAH. For patients with no history of SAH, the risks of rupture in the first year are approximately 0.05% for aneurysms less than 7 mm, 2% for those 7 to 12 mm, 8% for those 13 to 25 mm, and 17% for those greater than 25 mm. Routine screening of patients with a history of SAH in a first-degree relative is not recommended (Chollet et al., 2011).

Long-term Follow-up

Long-term follow-up is essential for risk factor reduction and attention to the potential complications of stroke. There should be optimization of lipids and blood pressure and avoidance of tobacco use and heavy alcohol use. Depression is very common after stroke; the clinician should have a high index of suspicion. Antidepressants have not been shown to prevent poststroke depression, but are effective in the treatment. Counseling, support groups, or psychotherapy may reduce the incidence of depression after stroke.

Escitalopram (Lexapro) may reduce the incidence of depression and fluoxetine might reduce poststroke depression and improve motor function in patients receiving physical therapy after acute ischemic stroke (Chollet et al., 2011; Robinson et al., 2008). Therapeutic exercise may reduce poststroke depression symptoms.

Cognitive impairment is common after stroke, but there is insufficient evidence to guide optimal management other than prevention and treatment of comorbidities.

Vitamin D supplementation reduces the risk of falls in patients with a history of stroke, but exercise or bisphosphonates may not reduce the fall risk. Interventions that reduce the incidence of hip fracture in stroke patients include combination of folate and methylcobalamin (vitamin B_{12}) and possibly risedronate.

In summary, older adults are at greater risk than the general population for cerebrovascular accidents, and the rate increases with increasing age (Fig. 7.8). There is also a significant increase in comorbidities contributing to and complications secondary to stroke with increasing age. A multidisciplinary team approach including a Neurologist, Primary Care Physician, Speech and Language Pathologist, and Physical and Occupational Therapist working together is more likely to achieve a realistic and favorable outcome. Families and caregivers need to be

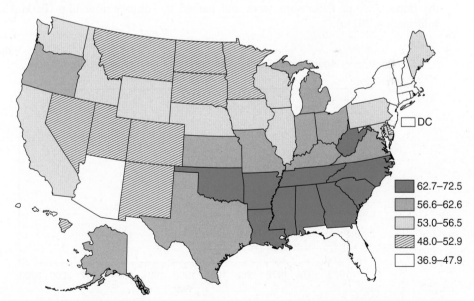

FIGURE 7.8. Age-adjusted death rates from stroke for persons aged ≥18 years and above—United States, 2007 to 2009. (From Gorina, Y., & Centers for Disease Control and Prevention. [2012]. Quick-Stats: Age-adjusted death rates from stroke for persons aged ≥18 years—United States, 2007–2009. *Morbidity and Mortality Weekly Report, 61*[13], 234. Retrieved from http://www.cdc.gov/mmwr/preview/mmwrhtml/mm6113a5.htm)

involved from early on in the diagnosis, management, and setting of goals. Realistic goals of care need to be established on the basis of reasonable goals of recovery, taking into consideration the patient's premorbid functional and mental capacity and any coexisting conditions. The patient's risk of falls needs careful review in determining the advisability of chronic anticoagulation therapy. The patient's ability to take adequate nutritional intake over a period of time needs to be reassessed. Finally, for those patients who require tube feedings, there should be trials of oral feeding to determine whether there are improvements in swallowing as time progresses.

PARKINSON DISEASE

Epidemiology/History

The annual US death rates for Parkinson disease increased during 1973 to 2003 as Parkinson disease became the 14th leading cause of death in the United States in 2003. Figure 7.9 demonstrates the increased age-adjusted death rate during the 30 years from 1973 to 2003. This increase might be attributable to multiple factors, including an aging population, greater awareness of the disease, and improved identification of cases (Hoyert et al., 2006).

Parkinson disease is a condition that has been known about since ancient times. It is referred to in the ancient Indian medical system of Ayurveda under the name Kampavata. In Western medical literature, it was described by the physician Galen as "shaking palsy" in AD 175. However, it was not until 1817 that a detailed medical essay was published on the subject by a London doctor, James Parkinson. A French neurologist named Charcot was the first to truly recognize the importance of Parkinson's work and named the disease after him (Parkinson's Disease Information, 2013a).

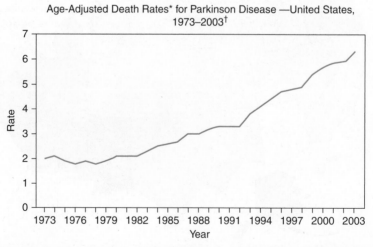

FIGURE 7.9. Age-adjusted death rates for Parkinson disease—United States, 1973 to 2003. (From Hoyert, D. L., Heron, M., Murphy, S. L., & Kung, H. C. [2006]. *Health e-stats. deaths: Final data for 2003.* Hyattsville, MD: U.S. Department of Health and Human Services, Center for Disease Control and Prevention. Retrieved from http://www.cdc.gov/nchs/products/pubs/pubd/hestats/finaldeaths03/finaldeaths03.htm)

Incidence of Parkinson Disease

The peak incidence is noted in the sixth and seventh decades of life with a preponderance in males versus females of 1.4:1. People in industrialized nations have a higher incidence of this disease, suggestive of environmental factors. In the United States, about 1 in 300 individuals will develop Parkinson disease (Parkinson's Disease Information, 2013a).

Pathophysiology/Causes

Parkinson disease is a progressive neurodegenerative disorder involving the nigrostriatal system primarily localized in midbrain and brain stem. In the normal brain, some nerve cells produce the chemical dopamine, which transmits signals within the brain to produce smooth movement of muscles. In patients with Parkinson disease, 80% or more of these dopamine-producing cells are damaged, dead, or otherwise degenerated. This causes the nerve cells to fire wildly, leaving patients unable to control their movements.

In addition to the neurotransmitter abnormalities in Parkinson disease, there is a loss of pigmentation and cellularity within the substancia nigra. The normal cells are replaced with Lewy bodies, which are eosinophilic inclusion bodies with aggregates of protein.

Currently, there is a lot of research concentrated on trying to identify and locate the genes (or combination of genes) that lead to Parkinson disease. To date, mutations have been found in four genes with abnormalities in five proteins that are associated with Parkinson disease. The five proteins are alpha-synuclein, parkin, ubiquintin carboxyl terminal hydrolase, SCA2, and DJ-1. These mutations have been found to have a role in abnormal protein processing in cells. Researchers have found that these mutations lead to cell death. This cell death extends to neurons that release dopamine (Parkinson's Disease Information, 2013b).

Striatal glutamate–dopamine imbalance may be important in the pathogenesis—excessive output from subthalamic nucleus and overactive subthalamo-pallidal glutamatergic pathway results in akinesia and rigidity. Neurotoxins have been investigated in the etiology of Parkinson disease, especially actions of methamphetamine and MPTP (1-methyl 1,4-phenyl 1,2,3,6-tetrahydropyridine). Their effect can be prevented by NMDA (N-methyl-D-aspartate)-receptor antagonists (Ossowska, 1994; Thomas, 1995).

Screening and Risk Factors

While Parkinson disease can occur in younger individuals, advancing age is the most consistent risk factor for the development of the disease. Men are more commonly affected than women. The genetic factors mentioned earlier indicate that there is a familial nature to the disease, even though the disease does not follow a purely familial inheritance pattern.

Other risk factors that have been noted or considered include declining estrogen levels, decreased levels of vitamin B_{12} and folate, and exposure to MPTP, heavy metals, especially manganese and iron, and carbon monoxide. Workers in steel alloy industries have a higher-than-expected prevalence (Dick et al., 2007). Repeated head trauma has been associated with Parkinson disease, with professional boxers having a higher-than-expected incidence of Parkinson disease (Bower et al., 2003). In case reports, head injury is documented to cause Parkinson disease through infarction of left caudate nucleus (Doder et al., 1999).

There are no particular screening tests or diagnostic tests to be done. When a patient presents with falls or tremor, the physical examination is the most important factor that will direct the clinician toward the diagnosis of Parkinson disease. Once the diagnosis is suspected, checking thyroid functions, vitamin B_{12}, and folate is warranted. There is no characteristic finding on CT, MRI, or CSF (Cerebrospinal fluid). PET (Positron emission tomography) and SPECT (Single-photon emission computed tomography) scanning were considered research tools when this chapter was written.

Cigarette smoking and caffeine intake have been associated with decreased risk of Parkinson disease (Checkoway et al., 2002; Gale & Martyn, 2003). It has been observed that patients on nonsteroidal anti-inflammatory drugs (NSAIDs) (Driver et al., 2011), calcium-channel blockers (Driver et al., 2008), and statins (Wahner et al., 2008) have a lower-than-expected risk of developing Parkinson disease.

Diagnosis/Clinical Findings

Parkinson disease often has an asymmetrical presentation and the diagnosis requires two out of three clinical findings (tremor, bradykinesia, and cogwheel rigidity). Table 7.7 lists the specific motor and nonmotor symptoms of Parkinson disease, and Table 7.8 the differential diagnosis criteria. About 30% of patients present with unilateral rigidity and bradykinesia without a resting tremor. It has been noted that patients who present with tremor have a more favorable prognosis than those who present with rigidity and gait disturbance. Levodopa responsiveness and the presence of progressive symptoms help in consolidating the diagnosis. Other characteristic findings are soft, monotonous speech (hypophonia), decreased blinking and masking of facial expression (masked faces), small handwriting (micrographia), drooling, difficulty arising from a low or soft chair, decreased spontaneous arm swing while walking, and flexion posture while standing and walking.

TABLE 7.7 · Symptoms of Parkinson Disease

Motor Symptoms	Nonmotor Symptoms
Tremor	Dementia
Bradykinesia	Dysphoria
Akinesia	Depression
Shuffling gait	Orthostasis—fluctuation in blood pressure
Masked facies	Temperature sensitivity—drenching sweats
Micrographia	Digestive problems—dysphagia
Flexed posture	Dysarthria—monotonous speech
Decreased arm swing	Sleep disturbance—daytime somnolence
Decreased blinking	REM sleep disturbances
Dysphagia	Skin changes—seborrheic dermatitis
	Balance—recurrent falls
	Sialorrhea

TABLE 7.8 · Diagnostic Criteria for Parkinson Disease

Criteria for diagnosis include bradykinesia and at least one of the following:

- ■ Muscular rigidity,
- ■ 4- to 6-mHz/sec resting tremor of low to medium amplitude (classic pin rolling/watch winding), and/or
- ■ Postural instability not caused by primary visual, vestibular, cerebellar, or proprioceptive dysfunction.

Disease Progression

The disease progression varies for each individual; however, mounting motor impairment leads to increasing functional impairment and disability. For the first few years, the onset of symptoms is insidious, usually starting in one upper limb with unilateral tremor and increased rigidity. This is followed by progression to the lower limb and sometimes to the opposite limb. Also, associated with this is an increase in tremor, rigidity, and reduced finger and hand dexterity.

Patients will then start to experience increasing difficulty with ADLs as the bradykinesia worsens. A flexed posture with decreased facial expression and a soft slurring of voice evolves. Initially, the gait may be normal in terms of stride length, but arm swing may be decreased unilaterally. As the disease progresses, neither arm swings during walking, resulting in the tendency to assume a flexion posture to maintain the sense of balance. Eventually, the stride length shortens and the gait becomes somewhat shuffling. The patient begins having difficulty with pivoting when changing direction. Finally, in more advanced stages of Parkinson disease, postural reflexes are impaired, and the patient has a tendency to fall spontaneously or with sling postural perturbations.

The nonmotor signs and symptoms in Parkinson disease include personality changes, apathy, depression, drug-induced psychosis, dementia, and anxiety. These nonmotor manifestations do not tend to respond to the typical pharmacologic therapies utilized but do affect significant proportions of patients with Parkinson disease. Dementia occurs in 30% to 50% of patients with long-standing Parkinson disease. Dementia is not a presenting sign of Parkinson disease, nor is it seen early in the course of the disease. Anxiety and depression develop in 30% of patients. Other nonmotor features of Parkinson disease are autonomic instability reflected by orthostatic hypotension, urinary incontinence, constipation, and episodes of drenching sweats. Seborrheic dermatitis of the face and forehead is often seen. Sleep disturbances, including insomnia, daytime sleepiness, vivid dreams, and rapid eye movement (REM) sleep behavior disorder are common. Erectile dysfunction is common in males.

Differential Diagnosis

When a patient presents with signs and symptoms suggestive of Parkinson disease, the clinician must look for other conditions and the secondary causes of Parkinsonism (see Table 7.9). The most common diagnosis when faced with the constellation of symptoms is idiopathic Parkinson disease. Drug-induced Parkinsonism is important to rule out as removal of the offending drug may result in improvement in signs and symptoms. The most common drugs that lead to Parkinsonism include the antipsychotics, metaclopramide, reserpine, prochloperazine, and valproic acid.

TABLE 7.9 · Differential Diagnosis of Parkinson Disease

- Idiopathic Parkinson disease
- Drug-induced Parkinsonism
- Vascular Parkinsonism
- Essential tremor
- Normal pressure hydrocephalus
- Parkinson-plus syndromes
  - Progressive supranuclear palsy
  - Multiple system atrophy (Shy–Drager syndrome)
  - Corticobasal degeneration
- Dementia with Lewy bodies

The Parkinson-plus syndromes are rare degenerative neurologic conditions that result in parkinsonian symptoms in addition to other differentiating signs and symptoms. Progressive supranuclear palsy has, in addition to classic parkinsonian signs, a vertical gaze abnormality and profound fall risk. Shy–Drager syndrome is marked by a profound and debilitating orthostatic hypotension.

Treatment

Drug Treatment

Currently, all pharmacologic treatments of Parkinson disease are based on attempts at eliminating or minimizing symptoms. There are no neuroprotective or disease-modifying pharmacologic therapies available. The medications each have significant adverse effects, making treatment frustrating. The medications do serve to improve and maintain function, thus allowing patients to continue in their daily activities with as little impairment as possible. Since all medications have significant adverse effects and seem to have a finite period of peak effectiveness, initiation of therapy should be postponed until symptoms become significant or troubling to the patient. If a patient has a minimal resting tremor in one hand and does not complain of any impaired function of that hand, there is little reason to initiate therapy.

People respond differently to the Parkinson disease drugs, so finding the right medication at the optimal dose for each individual takes time and patience. As the disease progresses, it is necessary to increase the dosage, and sometimes it is necessary to combine medications. There are six important classes of drugs used to treat Parkinson symptoms as well as one approved surgical option.

Levodopa. Levodopa or L-dopa remains the most commonly prescribed medication and the gold standard for the treatment of Parkinson disease. It was introduced in 1967 and held promise as a cure for Parkinson disease. It works simply by replacing the depleted dopamine with levodopa. Unfortunately, the adverse effects and waning effectiveness over time have limited its usefulness. Despite these limitations, L-dopa is the most important medication and is effective in nearly all patients with idiopathic Parkinson disease. In fact, because it is so highly effective, it is often employed in diagnosing the condition in addition to its use in treatment.

Most of the adverse effects are related to the toxicity of levodopa in periphery, especially gastrointestinal tract. This has resulted in the necessity to combine levodopa with carbidopa, a compound that inhibits the peripheral conversion of levodopa to its active metabolite, therefore assuring that a greater percentage of the levodopa crosses the blood–brain barrier, minimizing the gastrointestinal side effects.

Levodopa/carbidopa (Sinemet) is highly effective in helping with the motor symptoms of Parkinson disease. In most cases, it should be the initial medication prescribed when it is determined that the functional status is such that medication should be utilized. The usual starting dose is levodopa/carbidopa (Sinemet) 25/100 three times daily with modifications based on effect and side effects. Over time, there is an inevitable need to increase the dose. There are multiple formulations with a variety of combinations; there is a controlled release formulation of levodopa/carbidopa (Sinemet) that is particularly useful when taken at night and often serves to diminish the morning stiffness. Chronic use of L-dopa in Parkinson disease does not enhance the progression of disease pathology as far as can be determined by observations with substancia nigra neuronal counts and Lewy body densities (Parkkinen et al., 2011).

The most commonly encountered side effect of L-dopa is gastrointestinal intolerance with nausea, vomiting, and anorexia. A more complete list of the side effects can be found in Table 7.10. The first step in attempting to improve these symptoms is to take them with food. The one caution here is that the absorption of levodopa is greatly reduced in the presence of a high-protein meal. Therefore, it is best taken with light meals that are not high in protein content. If nausea persists, taking extra doses of Carbidopa helps prevent dopamine effects in the periphery. Finally, one might have to lower the dose and very slowly taper the dose up to effectiveness.

Patients who develop compulsive behavior will need to undergo a dose reduction with the possible addition of a second agent. Daytime sleepiness is often a symptom of depression or of poor nighttime sleep. Attempts at treating depression and improving the sleep hygiene should be tried. Melatonin and modafinil are not recommended.

The on–off phenomenon is a frightening but very common occurrence in patients after long-term treatment with L-dopa. It is characterized by unpredictable, abrupt fluctuations in motor state from when the medication is effective and symptoms are controlled ("on") to when parkinsonian symptoms worsen ("off"). These motor complications can be treated by adding a dopamine agonist, monoamine oxidase-B (MAO-B) inhibitor, or catechol-O-methyltransferase (COMT) inhibitor.

TABLE 7.10 · Levodopa/Carbidopa Adverse Effects

Nausea and vomiting
Hallucinations
Paranoia
Nightmares
Compulsive behavior
Drowsiness/daytime sleepiness
Long-term use results in dyskinesias (involuntary movements)
On–off phenomenon

As mentioned earlier, in most patients there is a wearing off in the effectiveness that occurs over time. This is initially managed with increasing the dose and dose frequency of the medication. Eventually, however, other side effects make further dose increases impossible, and other therapies should be employed.

Dopamine Agonists. Dopamine agonists directly stimulate dopamine receptors. They mainly work to reduce motor complications, and work best when they are not combined with any other drug. They are, however, often added to levodopa/carbidopa in an effort to improve the overall function and reduce the "on–off" phenomenon. There are several dopamine agonists on the market, including Ropinirole (Requip, Ropark, Adartrel), Bromocriptine (Parlodel, Cycloset), Pergolide (Permax, Pergotoliderived), Pramipexole (Mirapex), and Apomorphine (Apokyn).

Each of the above medications is used orally with the exception of Apomorphine, which is used subcutaneously. While they can be effective when used alone, they are often used early in an effort to delay the need for L-dopa. They are also effective when used in combination with L-dopa when motor effects and side effects become more problematic.

As with all medications used to treat Parkinson disease, these drugs have particularly troublesome adverse effects, including psychosis, edema, nausea and vomiting, fibrosis, and orthostatic hypotension. The side effects can sometimes be managed with changing the time and frequency of administration or by trying a different dopamine agonist. In the case of edema and orthostatic hypotension, patients should be educated on ways to reduce the impact of the effect. Psychosis and hallucinations are the adverse effect that most often results in having to abandon the dopamine agonists as a class in the treatment of that particular patient. Patients should be warned about the potential for dopamine agonists to cause impulse control disorder and excessive daytime somnolence. They should be informed of the implications of driving/operating machinery while on these medications.

Catecol-*O*-Methyltransferase Inhibitors. The COMT inhibitors are particularly useful in the treatment of Parkinson disease because they work by increasing the bioavailability of levodopa. Metabolic reactions allow only about 1% of administered levodopa taken in pill form to reach the brain. Adding COMT inhibitors reduces the metabolic actions that break down levodopa, including inhibiting an enzyme that degrades the drug, which leads to more levodopa entering the brain. Clinical trials have shown that L-dopa works for a longer time in the presence of a COMT inhibitor (Waters, 2000).

The currently available COMT inhibitors include Entacapone (Comtan) and Tolcapone (Tasmar). Entacapone is taken as a 200-mg tablet with each dose of levodopa/carbidopa, up to eight times per day. Tolcapone is taken as 100 to 200 mg three times a day. Liver function tests should be done every 2 to 4 weeks, and the drug should be discontinued if there is no benefit after 3 weeks of therapy.

There is a combination drug, Stalevo, which includes levodopa, carbidopa, and entacapone. There are multiple combinations available, with dosing recommended at up to eight times per day.

The adverse effects of this class of drugs include psychosis, diarrhea, abdominal pain, dry mouth, urine discoloration (entacapone), and orthostatic hypotension. In addition, when first introduced there may be accumulation of levodopa, resulting in dyskinesias. This should prompt the clinician to reduce the dose of L-dopa.

Monoamine Oxidase-B Inhibitors. Selegiline and Resagiline are the primary MAO-B inhibitors currently on the market. Monamine oxidase is one of the enzymes involved in the breakdown of dopamine, so these drugs are thought to work by preventing the metabolism of dopamine. Initially, these drugs were thought to slow the progression of the disease. These claims have not been substantiated, and this class is used primarily as adjuncts to levodopa/carbidopa. The adverse effects of the MAO-B inhibitors include insomnia, hallucinations, and orthostatic hypotension.

Amantadine. A randomized, double-blind trial of amantadine in patients with Parkinson disease and dyskinesia showed a 45% reduction in dyskinesia with amantadine compared with placebo. However, the benefit lasted for less than 8 months, and withdrawal of amantadine caused a 10% to 20% rebound increase in the presence of dyskinesias (Thomas et al., 2004). In addition, amantadine is often not well tolerated, limiting its usefulness. The recommended dose is 100 mg twice daily.

Anticholinergics. Anticholinergic drugs appear to improve motor function in Parkinson disease, but effects on individual outcomes are inconsistent across studies (Holloway & Frank, 2004). The primary symptom that anticholinergic drugs appear to affect is tremor. Patients with tremor-predominant Parkinson disease who wish to delay the initiation of L-dopa would be reasonable individuals to try anticholinergics. The side effects include dry mouth, somnolence, and delirium.

Deep Brain Stimulation. Neurosurgical interventions such as deep brain stimulation (DBS) have essentially replaced all other previous forms of surgery, including pallidotomy. The procedure involves placing an electrode in the subthalamic nucleus bilaterally. The electrode is set to provide stimulation aimed at improvements in motor function. While the mechanism of action is not fully known, DBS is thought to result in functional blockade of the site implanted. Patients who have undergone DBS often have more "on" time and fewer dyskinesias. Although there are many instances where DBS has resulted in remarkable and long-lasting improvements, there is considerable cost as well as potential morbidity associated with this procedure. Therefore, selecting the ideal candidate is the key to getting the best results. Patients with cognitive deficits, dementia, atypical Parkinson disease, or significant psychiatric problems are poor candidates for this procedure. Younger age, shorter disease duration, and good preoperative response to levodopa are good predictors of favorable outcomes (Pahwa et al., 2006).

Stem Cell Therapy

Genetic therapies like stem cell therapy hold out hope in diseases like Parkinson disease that have a genetic and cellular basis. There is great hope that such therapies might result in true disease-modifying or curative options for the future.

Alternative Therapies

Ayurvedic medicine—Parkinson disease symptoms are mentioned in an ancient text under the name Kampavata. Ayurvedic medicine is a comprehensive system placing equal emphasis on diet, exercise, meditation, massage, and herbal remedies. One such herb, *Mucuna pruriens*, is gaining attention in conventional circles as its effects mimic synthetic L-dopa, with fewer side effects.

Broad beans—Australian researchers discovered that broad beans are also an extremely effective natural source of levodopa. The highest concentration of levodopa is found in the pod, so they are most effective when consumed whole.

St. John's Wort—Dopamine influences positive feelings in the brain, and since dopamine levels are low in patients with Parkinson disease, depression is often a symptom. St. John's Wort is a herb that has been used in Europe for many years. It has been proven to be effective in alleviating depression and insomnia, but should be used with caution in patients on SSRIs (Selective serotonin reuptake inhibitor).

Botulinum toxin A—This is a bacterium that causes food poisoning (botulism), but has proven to be effective in reducing hand, head, and voice tremors when used in a weak solution (Trosch & Pullman, 1994).

Coenzyme Q10 (CoQ10)—This has been shown to have an effect on the symptoms of Parkinson disease; however, it is unclear whether it actually slows the disease or simply temporarily alleviates symptoms. The drawback is the massive dose required. The effective dose is approximately 1,200 mg/day, well above the 60 to 90 mg recommended by many alternative therapy advocates (Suchowersky et al., 2006).

Acupuncture—Used for centuries in China to correct energy disturbances in the body, acupuncture has become a popular method of treatment for Parkinson sufferers in other parts of the world. So far, there are no placebo-controlled studies that show acupuncture can treat the motor control symptoms of the disease, but there is some evidence that it can assist with sleep disturbances. There is much anecdotal evidence to suggest that it may be effective in increasing feelings of well-being and relaxation.

Massage—While not treating the symptoms directly, it can help reduce some of the discomfort associated with muscle stiffness that is commonly experienced by patients.

Although there may be no cure, there are several Parkinson disease drugs that will improve the quality of life. These drugs do not work to cure the disease, but rather to alleviate symptoms. A lot of research is still underway, in the hope of developing more helpful drugs, and better yet, maybe a cure.

Additional Treatment Strategies

The first step in the clinical management of Parkinson disease is a full discussion of the diagnosis with the patient and family. They should be informed that Parkinson disease is a progressive disease and that most people with this disease have near-normal life expectancy. Patients should be encouraged to participate in physical therapy, have a home exercise program, and engage in a multidisciplinary team approach to the maintenance of functional independence.

When functional status and symptom severity worsen to the point where treatment is indicated, the clinician should consider drug therapy. The efficacy and side effect profile of the drugs along with the patient's age, cognitive status, and degree of motor disability as well as the drug cost should be taken into account.

The clinical trial literature on this subject suggests that levodopa treatment in early Parkinson disease results in greater motor improvement and performance, but also more motor fluctuations and dyskinesias, whereas initial treatment with a dopamine receptor agonist results in less symptom relief, but with a lower incidence of fluctuations and dyskinesias. The practice parameter from the American Academy of Neurology (AAN) considers either levodopa or a dopamine receptor agonist to be a reasonable choice for patients with Parkinson disease who require the initiation of dopaminergic treatment (Miyasaki et al., 2002). In either case, it is best to start with low doses to gauge the effect of the drug and the patient's ability to tolerate the drug. In certain subsets of patients, other therapies may be considered first line. For instance, in the patient with tremor-predominant disease who can tolerate the anticholinergic side effects, these drugs may be helpful.

Pharmacologic Management of Motor Complications in Advanced Disease

Frequently, whether treated with levodopa/carbidopa alone or in combination with a COMT inhibitor, motor complications such as dyskinesias develop. COMT inhibitors often result in reductions in "off" time in patients and are therefore often the first adjunct therapies to be used.

Oral or transdermal dopamine agonists may be considered for the management of motor complications in patients with advanced Parkinson disease. Nonergot agonists (ropinirole, pramipexole, and rotigotine) are preferable to the ergot agonists. In addition, MOA-B inhibitors may be considered for the treatment of motor complications in patients with advanced Parkinson disease.

Management of Nonmotor Symptoms

Neurobehavioral Problems

Dementia is common in patients with Parkinson disease. As these patients are living longer, it is clear that there is cognitive decline that occurs late in the illness. After ruling out drug-associated and secondary causes, it is reasonable to try cholinesterase inhibitors, although the improvements will likely be modest.

Depression is very common in patients with Parkinson disease, and should be treated as in individuals without Parkinson disease.

Psychosis is a common and frightening side effect to many of the medications employed. The standard antipsychotic to be used in patients with Parkinson disease is low-dose clozapine with weekly monitoring for blood counts. Alternatively, the use of quetiapine has been shown helpful. Respiradol and olanzapine are not considered good choices in patients with Parkinson disease (Friedman & Ott, 1998).

Other Symptoms

Constipation is a common occurrence in Parkinson disease as the large bowel muscle activity becomes sluggish. Patients should be encouraged to increase liquid intake and physical activity, to use stool softeners and laxatives, and to discontinue constipating medications such as anticholinergics.

Dysphagia can usually be controlled with simple modifications during meals. Occasionally, referral to a speech therapist might be necessary.

Orthostatic hypotension is a side effect of many of the medications used to treat Parkinson disease. When this becomes symptomatic, consider discontinuing antihypertensives, elevating the head of the bed, and teaching patients how to allow for equilibration with changes in position. Occasionally, the use of fludrocortisone or midodrine becomes necessary. If orthostatic hypotension is particularly profound, consider the diagnosis of Shy–Drager syndrome.

Sleep disturbances are very common and require strict attention to sleep hygiene. Medications, such as dopamine agonists, should be discontinued when sleep disturbance creates a greater burden than the benefit of the medication. Sometimes nighttime awakenings are due to bradykinesia; when this is the case, consider a bedtime dose of the long-acting L-dopa/carbidopa, adjuvant entacapone, or a dopamine agonist. Finally, clonazepam may be necessary when there is a REM sleep behavior disorder.

Urinary urgency should prompt the clinician to recommend a reduction in the evening fluid intake and consideration of tolterodine or oxybutynin.

Sialorrhea occurs occasionally, and clinical trials show that clonidine appears to be beneficial, but blood pressure should be monitored (Serrano-Dueñas, 2003). Glycopyrrolate has been shown to be helpful to decrease moderate to severe sialorrhea (Arbouw et al., 2010). Injection of botulinum toxin type A has been shown to be helpful to decrease hypersalivation (Santamato et al., 2008).

Future Research

Parkinson disease research has improved our knowledge and ability to use gene therapy to alleviate symptoms. Glial-derived neurotrophic factor (GDNF) has been found to protect dopamine-releasing neurons. Trials in humans have been limited, but trials in primates showed that GDNF stimulates the body to produce GDNF naturally (Gill et al., 2002; Grondin et al., 2002). Researchers have also been working with introducing vectors that carry the GDNF gene in monkeys. They have found that substantia nigra (dopamine-producing) cell death decreases. In other research, gene therapy, using stem cells, was found to reduce some cardinal Parkinson disease symptoms, mainly dyskinesias (the abnormal involuntary movements).

Stem cells have the capability of transforming into any other cell in the body. Researchers believe that transplanting embryonic stem cells into target cells in patients with Parkinson disease may allow regeneration of dopamine-producing cells.

Mortality

"Deaths: Preliminary Data for 2010" highlights facts about Parkinson disease. In particular, the report states that age-adjusted death rates for Parkinson disease increased by 4.6%. This could be interpreted secondary to improved treatment and survival of cardiovascular disease and cancer (Parkinson's Disease Foundation, 2013).

Cultural Considerations and Prognosis (Parkinson's Disease Foundation, 2012)

To identify demographic, geographic, and clinical factors that may influence survival of people with Parkinson disease, Allison Willis, MD, and her colleagues at the Washington University School of Medicine examined the health records of over 29 million Medicare beneficiaries with Parkinson disease. They identified 138,000 individuals who were diagnosed with Parkinson disease in 2002 and followed their medical charts through 2008. Dr. Willis and her coworkers gleaned data such as demographics, health service use, and survival from Medicare Beneficiary Annual Summary Files. Then they compared 6-year survival rates among different groups of people with Parkinson disease. Sixty-four percent of people with Parkinson disease died during the 6-year study.

Sex and race significantly predicted survival. Women with Parkinson disease had a 26% lower adjusted risk of death than men. African Americans had the highest crude death rate (66.4%), followed by whites (64.6%), Hispanics (55.4%), and Asians (50.8%).

About 69.9% of the people with Parkinson disease developed dementia by the end of the 6-year study. People with dementia had a higher death rate (71.9%) than those without dementia (46.1%).

Survival rates were similar across the United States—across states, regions of the country, and rural/urban classifications. However, people with Parkinson disease living in urban areas where high levels of manganese were released into the environment had a modestly increased death risk.

After adjusting the data for age, race, and sex, people with Parkinson disease had a nearly four times greater risk of death than people with no disease, and nearly double the risk of death as for those living with other common diseases such as colorectal cancer, stroke, and ischemic heart disease. People with Parkinson disease had nearly the same risk of death as those who had experienced a heart attack or suffered a hip fracture (Willis et al., 2012).

Prevention

There have been suggestions but no good data on strategies to be implemented toward the prevention of Parkinson disease. There are suggestions that avoiding environmental pathogens such as heavy metal exposure and pesticides might prevent the disease. Maintaining an active lifestyle and consuming organic foods are recommended. There has been no known drug proven to prevent Parkinson disease.

REFERENCES

Adams, H. P., Jr., Bendixen, B. H., Kappelle, L. J., Biller, J., Love, B. B., Gordon, D. L., & Marsh, E. E., III. (1993). Classification of subtype of acute ischemic stroke. Definitions for use in a multicenter clinical trial. *Stroke, 24*(1), 35–41.

Adams, H. P., Jr., del Zoppo, G., Alberts, M. J., Bhatt, D. L., Brass L., Furlan A., . . . Wijkicks, E. F. (2007). Guidelines for the early management of adults with ischemic stroke: A guideline from the American Heart Association/American Stroke Association Stroke Council, Clinical Cardiology Council, Cardiovascular Radiology and Intervention Council, and the Atherosclerotic Peripheral Vascular Disease and Quality of Care Outcomes in Research Interdisciplinary Working Groups: The American Academy of Neurology affirms the value of this guideline as an educational tool for neurologists. *Circulation, 115*(20), e478–e534.

Anderson, C. S., Huang Y., Wang, J. G., Arima H., Neal B., Peng B., . . . Chalmers J. (2008). Intensive blood pressure reduction in acute cerebral haemorrhage trial (INTERACT): A randomized pilot trial. *Lancet Neurology, 7*(5), 373–466.

Arbouw, M. E., Movig, K. L., Koopman M., Poels, P. J., Guchelaar, H. J., Egberts, T. C., . . . van Vugt, J. P. (2010). Glycopyrrolate for sialorrhea in Parkinson disease: A randomized, double-blind, crossover trial. *Neurology, 74*(15), 1203–1207.

Barnett, H. J., Taylor, D. W., Eliasziw M., Fox, A. J., Ferguson, G. G., Haynes, R. B., & Spence, J. D. (1998). Benefit of carotid endarterectomy in patients with symptomatic moderate or severe stenosis. *New England Journal of Medicine, 139*, 1415–1425.

Bederson, J. B., Connolly, E. S., Jr., Batjer, H. H., Dacey, R. G., Dion, J. E., Diringer, M. N., . . . Rosenwasser, R. H. (2009). Guidelines for the management of aneurysmal subarachnoid hemorrhage: A statement for healthcare professionals from a special writing group of the Stroke Council, American Heart Association. *Stroke, 40*(3), 994–1025.

Bernheisel, C. R., Schlaudecker, J. D., & Leopold K. (2011). Subacute management of ischemic stroke. *American Family Physician, 84*(12), 1383–1388.

Bower, J. H., Maraganore, D. M., Peterson, B. J., McDonnell, S. K., Ahlskog, J. E., & Rocca, W. A. (2003). Head trauma preceding Parkinson's disease: A case-control study. *Neurology, 60*(10), 1610–1615.

Broderick, J., Connolly, S., Feldmann, E., Hanley D., Kase, C., Krieger, D., . . . Zuccarello, M. (2007). Guidelines for the management of spontaneous intracerebral hemorrhage in adults. *Stroke, 38*(6), 2001–2023.

Checkoway, H., Powers, K., Smith-Weller, T., Franklin, G. M., Longstreth, W. T., Jr., & Swanson, P. D. (2002). Parkinson's disease risks associated with cigarette smoking, alcohol consumption, and caffeine intake. *American Journal of Epidemiology, 155*(8), 732–738.

Chimowitz, M. I., Lynn, M. J., Derdeyn, C. P., Turan, T. N., Fiorella D., Lane, B. F., . . . Cloft, H. J. (2011). Stenting versus aggressive medical therapy for intracranial arterial stenosis. *New England Journal of Medicine, 365*(11), 993–1003.

Chollet, F., Tardy, J., Albucher, J. F., Thalamas, C., Berard, E., Lamy C., . . . Loubinous, I. (2011). Fluoxetine for motor recovery after acute ischaemic stroke (FLAME): A randomised placebo-controlled trial. *Lancet Neurology, 10*(2), 123–130.

Coull, B. M., Williams, L. S., Goldstein, L. B., Meschia, J. F., Heitzman D., Chaturvedi S., . . . Saver, J. L. (2002). Anticoagulants and antiplatelet agents in acute ischemic stroke. Report of the Joint Stroke Guideline Development Committee of the American Academy of Neurology and the American Stroke Association (a division of the American Heart Association). *Stroke, 33*(7), 1934–1942.

de Abreu, T. T., Mateus, S., Carreteiro, C., & Correia, J. (2008). Therapeutic implications of transesophageal echocardiography after transthoracic echocardiography on acute stroke patients. *Vascular Health and Risk Management, 4*(1), 167–172.

DePippo, K. L., Holas, M. A., & Reding, M. J. (1992). Validation of the 3-oz water swallow test for aspiration following stroke. *Archives of Neurology, 49*(12), 1259–1261.

Dick, F. D., De Palma, G., & Ahmadi, A. (2007). Environmental risk factors for Parkinson's disease and Parkinsonism: The geoparkinson study. *Occupational and Environmental Medicine, 64*(10), 666–672.

Doder, M., Johanshahi, M., Turjanski, N., Moseley, I., F., & Lees, A. J. (1999). Parkinson's syndrome after closed head injury: A single case report. *Journal of Neurology, Neurosurgery, and Psychiatry, 66*(3), 380–385.

Driver, J. A., Kurth, T., Buring, J. E., Gaziano, J. M., & Logroscino, G. (2008). Parkinson disease and risk of mortality: A prospective comorbidity-matched cohort study. *Neurology, 70*(16 Pt. 2), 1423–1430.

Driver, J. A., Logroscino, G., Lu, L., Gaziano, J. M., & Kurth, T. (2011). Use of non-steroidal anti-inflammatory drugs and risk of Parkinson's disease: Nested case-control study. *British Medical Journal, 342*, d198.

European Carotid Surgery Trialists' Collaborative Group. (1998). Randomised trial of endarterectomy for recently symptomatic carotid stenosis: Final results of the MRC European Carotid Surgery Trial (ECST). *Lancet, 351*, 1379–1387.

Fang, J., Shaw, K. M., George, M. G., Division for Heart Disease and Stroke Prevention, National Center for Chronic Disease Prevention and Health Promotion, Centres for Disease Control and Prevention. (2012). Prevalence of stroke—United States, *2006–2010. MMWR. Morbidity and Mortality Weekly Report, 61*(20), 379–382. Retrieved from http://www.cdc.gov/mmwr/preview/mmwrhtml/mm6120a5.htm

Friedman, J. H., & Ott, B. R. (1998). Should risperidone be used in Parkinson's disease? *Journal of Neuropsychiatry and Clinical Neuroscience, 10*(4), 473–474.

Furie, K., Kasner, S., Adams, R., Albers, G., Bush, R., Fagan, S., & Wentworth, D. (2011). Guidelines for the prevention of stroke in patients with stroke or transient ischemic attack: A guideline for healthcare professionals from the American Heart Association/American Stroke Association. *Stroke, 42*, 227–276.

Gale, C., & Martyn, C. (2003). Tobacco, coffee, and Parkinson's disease. *British Medical Journal, 326*(7389), 561–562.

Gill, S. S., Patel, N. K., O'Sullivan, K., Brooks, D. J., Hotton, G. R., . . . Svendsen, C. D. (2002). Intraparenchymal putaminal administration of glial-derived neurotrophic factor in the treatment of advanced Parkinson's disease. *Neurology, 58*(Suppl. 3), A241.

Go, A. S., Mozaffarian, D., Roger, V. L., Benjamin, E. J., Berry, J. D., Borden, W. B., . . . Turner, M. B. (2013). Heart disease and stroke statistics–2013 update: A report from the American Heart Association. *Circulation, 127*(1), e6–e245.

Gomes, C. A., Lustosa, S. A., Matos, D., Andriolo, R. B., Waisberg, D. R., & Waisberg J. (2010). Percutaneous endoscopic gastrostomy versus nasogastric tube feeding for adults with swallowing disturbances. *Cochrane Database of Systematic Reviews*, (11), CD008096. doi:10.1002/14651858.CD008096

Grondin, R., Zhang, Z., Yi, A., Cass, W. A., Maswood, N., Anderson, A. H., . . . Gash, D. M. (2002). Chronic, controlled GDNF infusion promotes structural and functional recovery in advanced parkinsonian monkeys. *Brain, 125*(Pt. 10), 2191–2201.

Herzig, S. J., Howell, M. D., Ngo, L. H., & Marcantonio, E. R. (2009). Acid-suppressive medication use and the risk for hospital-acquired pneumonia. *Journal of American Medical Association, 301*(20), 2120–2128.

Hillbom, M., Erila, T., Sotaniemi, K., Tatlisumak, T., Sarna, S., & Kaste M. (2002). Enoxaparin vs heparin for prevention of deep-vein thrombosis in acute ischaemic stroke: A randomized, double-blind study. *Acta Neurologica Scandinavica, 106*(2), 84–92.

Holloway, R., & Frank, S. (2004). Review: Anticholinergic drugs improve motor function and disability in Parkinson disease. *ACP Journal Club, 140*(1), 15.

Hoyert, D. L., Heron, M. P., Murphy, S. L., & Kung, H. C. (2006). *Deaths: Final data for 2003. National Vital Statistics Reports, 54*(13). Retrieved from http://www.cdc.gov/nchs/data/nvsr/nvsr54/nvsr54_13.pdf

Kasner, S. E., & Heather, E. (2010, March). Cerebrovascular disorders. *ACP Medicine Neuro, 1–22.* doi:10.2310/7900.1027

Kissela, B., Schneider, A., Kleindorfer, D., Khoury, J., Miller, R., Alwell, K., . . . Broderick J. (2004). Stroke in a biracial population: The excess burden of stroke among blacks. *Stroke, 35,* 426–431.

Latchaw, R. E., Alberts, M. J., Lev, M. H., Connors, J. J., Harbaugh, R. E., Higashida, R. T., & Walters B. (2009). Recommendations for imaging of acute ischemic stroke: A scientific statement from the American Heart Association. *Stroke, 40,* 3646–3675.

Miyasaki, J. M., Martin, W., Suchowersky, O., Weiner, W. J., & Lang, A. E. (2002). Practice parameter: Initiation of treatment for Parkinson's disease. *Neurology, 58*(1), 11–17.

Molyneux, A. J., Kerr, R. S., Stratton, I., Clarke, M., Shrimpton, J., & Holman R. (2002). International Subarachnoid Aneurysm Trial (ISAT) of neurosurgical clipping versus endovascular coiling in *2143* patients with ruptured intracranial aneurysms: A randomized trial. *Lancet, 360*(9342), 1267–1274.

Molyneux, A. J., Kerr, R. S., Yu L. M., Clarke, M., Sneade, M., Yarnold, J. A., & Sandercock P. (2005). International Subarachnoid Aneurysm Trial (ISAT) of neurosurgical clipping versus endovascular coiling, a randomised comparison of effects on survival, dependency, seizures, rebleeding, subgroups, and aneurysm occlusion. *Lancet, 366*(9488), 809–817.

Nakagawa, T., Sekizawa, K., Arai, H., Kikuchi, R., Manabe, K., & Sasaki, H. (1997). High incidence of pneumonia in elderly patients with basal ganglia infarction. *Archives of Internal Medicine, 157*(3), 321–324.

Ossowska, K. (1994). The role of excitatory amino acids in experimental models of Parkinson's disease. *Journal of Neural Transmission—Parkinson's Disease and Dementia Section, 8*(1–2), 39–71.

Pahwa, R., Factor, S. A., Lyons, K. E., Ondo, W. G., Gronseth, G., Bronte-Stewart, H., . . . Weiner, W. J. (2006). Practice parameter: Treatment of Parkinson disease with motor fluctuations & dyskinesia: Report of the Quality Standards Subcommittee of the American Academy of Neurology. *Neurology, 66*(7), 983–995.

Parkinson's Disease Foundation. (2012) Predicting survival in people with Parkinson's [Newsletter]. Retrieved from http://www.pdf.org/en/science_news/release/pr_1325692019

Parkinson's Disease Foundation. (2013). Statement on *2010* national mortality data. Retrieved from http://www.pdf.org/en/science_news/release/pr_1326314913

Parkinson's Disease Information. (2013a). Retrieved from http://www.parkinsons.org/index.html

Parkinson's Disease Information. (2013b). Parkinson's disease genetic influence. Retrieved from http://www.parkinsons.org/parkinsons-genetics.html

Parkkinen, L., O'Sullivan, S. S., Kuoppamaki, M., Collins, C., Kallis, C., Holton, J. L., & Lees, A. J. (2011). Does levodopa accelerate the pathologic process in Parkinson disease brain? *Neurology, 77*(15), 1420–1426.

Pleis, J. R., & Lethbridge-Cejku, M. (2007). Summary health statistics for U.S. adults: National Health Interview Survey, *2006. Vital Health Statistics, 10*(235), 1–153.

Practice advisory: Thrombolytic therapy for acute ischemic stroke. Report of the Quality of Standards Subcommittee of the American Academy of Neurology. (1996). *Neurology, 47,* 835–839.

Robinson, R. G., Jorge, R. E., Moser, D. J., Acion, L., Solodkin, A., Small, S. L., . . . Arndt, S. (2008). Escitalopram and problem-solving therapy for prevention of poststroke depression: A randomized controlled trial. *JAMA, 299*(20), 2391–2400.

Rothwell, P. M., Eliasziw, M., Gutnikov, S. A., Warlow, C. P., & Barnett, H. J. (2004). Endarterectomy for symptomatic carotid stenosis in relation to clinical subgroups and the timing of surgery. *Lancet, 363*(9413), 915–924.

Sacco, R. L., Adams, R., Albers, G., & Alberts, M. J. (2006). Guidelines for prevention of stroke in patients with ischemic stroke or transient ischemic attack. *Stroke, 2,* 577–617.

Sacco, R. L., Boden-Albala, B., Gan, R., Chen, X., Kargman, D. E., Shea, S., . . . Hauser, W. A. (1998). Stroke incidence among white, black, and Hispanic residents of an urban community: The Northern Manhattan Stroke Study. *American Journal of Epidemiology, 147*(3), 259–268.

Santamato, A., Ianieri, G., Ranieri, M., Megna, M., Panza, F., Fiore, P., & Megna, G. (2008). Botulinum toxin type A in the treatment of sialorrhea in Parkinson's disease. *Journal of American Geriatrics Society, 56*(4), 765–767.

Serrano-Dueñas, M. (2003). Treatment of sialorrhea in Parkinson's disease patients with clonidine. Double-blind, comparative study with placebo. *Neurologia, 18*(1), 2–6.

Suchowersky, O., Gronseth, G., Perlmutter, J., Reich, S., Zesiewica, T., & Weiner, W. J. (2006). Practice parameter: Neuroprotective strategies & alternative therapies for Parkinson disease. American Academy of Neurology. *Neurology*, *66*(7), 976–982.

Thomas, A., Iacono, D., Luciano, A. L., Armellino, K., Di Iori, A., & Onofri, M. (2004). Duration of amantadine benefit on dyskinesia of severe Parkinson's disease. *Journal of Neurology, Neurosurgery, and Psychiatry*, *75*(1), 141–143.

Thomas, R. J. (1995). Excitatory amino acids in health and disease. *Journal of American Geriatrics Society*, *43* (11), 1279.

Trosch, R. M., & Pullman, S. L. (1994). Botulinum toxin A injections for the treatment of hand tremors. *Movement Disorder*, *9*, 601–609.

Wahner, A. D., Bronstein, J. M., Brodelon, Y. M., & Ritz, B. (2008). Statin use and the risk of Parkinson disease. *Neurology*, *70*, 1418–1422.

Wardlaw, J. M. (2004). Diagnosis of stroke on neuroimaging. *BMJ*, *328*(7441), 655–656.

Waters, C. (2000). Catechol-O-methyltransferase (COMT) inhibitors in Parkinson's disease. *Journal of American Geriatrics Society*, *48*(6), 692–698.

Wiebers, D. O., Whisnant, J. P., Huston, J., III, Meissner, I., Brown, R. D., Jr., Piepgras, D. G., . . . Torner, J. C. (2003). Unruptured intracranial aneurysms: Natural history, clinical outcome, and risks of surgical and endovascular treatment. International Study of Unruptured Intracranial Aneurysms Investigators. *Lancet*, *362*(9378), 103–110.

Willis, A. W., Schootman, M., Kung, N., Evanoff, B. A., Perlmutter, J. S., & Racette, B. A. (2012). Predictors of survival in patients with Parkinson disease. *Archives of Neurology*, *69*(5), 601–607.

CHAPTER 7: IT RESOURCES

Websites

American Academy of Neurology
http://www.aan.com/
Parkinson's Disease Foundation
http://www.pdf.org/
National Parkinson's Foundation
http://www.parkinson.org/
American Parkinson's Disease Foundation
http://www.apdaparkinson.org/
5 Things You Need to Know About Neurological Disorders in the Elderly
http://www.livestrong.com/article/9224-need-neurological-disorders-elderly/
Neurological Conditions
http://www.movementforhope.org/what-is-a-neurological-disease/
The Internet Stroke Center
http://www.strokecenter.org/professionals/stroke-diagnosis/stroke-assessment-scales/
Stroke Risk Screening Tools
http://www.neurotexasinstitute.com/clinical-programs/cerebrovascular-stroke-program/resources/stroke-risk-screening-tools.aspx
Stroke Symptoms, Recovery, Types, Signs, Treatments, Causes
http://www.emedicinehealth.com/stroke/article_em.htm
Gait and Balance Disorders in Older Adults
http://www.aafp.org/afp/2010/0701/p61.html
Psychotherapy and Older Adults Resource Guide
http://www.apa.org/pi/aging/resources/guides/psychotherapy.aspx
Stroke Prevention and Management in Older Adults
http://www.nursingcenter.com/pdf.asp?AID=668070

A "Purpose in Life" Lowers Risk of Stroke for Older Adults
http://home.isr.umich.edu/releases/a-purpose-in-life-lowers-risk-of-stroke-for-older-adults/
Gender Differences in Stroke Among Older Adults
http://www.medscape.com/viewarticle/564629
Strokes in People Over 65
http://www.dwp.gov.uk/publications/specialist-guides/
medical-conditions/a-z-of-medical-conditions/stroke/over-65/
"Silent" Strokes Common in Older People
http://www.webmd.com/stroke/news/20071031/silent-strokes-common-in-older-people
Rehabilitation Needs for Older Adults with Stroke Living at Home: Perceptions of Four
Populations
http://www.biomedcentral.com/1471-2318/7/20
Types of Strokes: Hemorrhagic and Ischemic
http://www.everydayhealth.com/stroke/stroke-types-ischemic-and-hemorrhagic.aspx
Transient Ischemic Attack (TIA)
http://www.aplaceformom.com/senior-care-resources/articles/transient-ischemic-attack
Causes of a Transient Ischaemic Attack
http://www.nhs.uk/Conditions/Transient-ischaemic-attack/Pages/Causes.aspx
Subarachnoid Hemorrhage
http://www.nlm.nih.gov/medlineplus/ency/article/000701.htm
Hemorrhagic Stroke—Merck Manual
http://www.merckmanuals.com/home/brain_spinal_cord_and_nerve_disorders/stroke_cva/
hemorrhagic_stroke.html
Subarachnoid Hemorrhage
http://emedicine.medscape.com/article/1164341-overview
Parkinson's Disease in the Elderly
http://www.aplaceformom.com/articles/parkinsons-disease-in-the-elderly
Parkinson's Disease—Complications
http://www.umm.edu/patiented/articles/how_serious_parkinsons_disease_000051_4.htm
Parkinson's Disease and Caregiving
http://www.caregiver.org/caregiver/jsp/content_node.jsp?nodeid=577
Parkinson's Disease Information added to NIHSeniorHealth Web Site
http://www.nih.gov/news/health/sep2008/nia-29.htm
Parkinson's Disease Dementia
http://www.alz.org/dementia/parkinsons-disease-symptoms.asp
Michael J. Fox Foundation for Parkinson's Research
https://www.michaeljfox.org/foundation/publications.html?category=5

PDF Documents

Neurological Disorders: A Public Health Approach
http://www.who.int/mental_health/neurology/chapter_3_a_neuro_disorders_public_h_
challenges.pdf
Neurological Assessment and the Older Adult: A Guide for Nurses: AAN Clinical Practice
Guideline Series
http://www.aann.org/pdf/cpg/aannneuroassessmentolderadult.pdf

Subaracnoid Hemorrhage Non-Traumatic
http://forensicmd.files.wordpress.com/2009/12/subaracnoid-hemorrhage-nontraumadoc.pdf
American Red Cross Scientific Advisory Council—Stroke Assessment Tools
http://www.instructorscorner.org/media/resources/SAC/SAC%20Advisory%20Stroke%20
Assessment%20Tools%20Final%20for%20Posting%2003_2012.pdf

Videos

Rehabilitation for the Parkinson's Disease Patient (2013)
Body in Balance addresses the needs of their Parkinson's Disease patients using the Biodex
Balance System SD, BioStep Elliptical and Gait Trainer 3. Using "Big Step" technique on the
Gait Trainer mitigates the standard shuffle. Patient claims "the more I exercise, the less I
shake." (4:25 minutes)
http://youtu.be/a8tab8Wt55s
Colleen, Person with Parkinson's, UK (2009)
Lundbeck and Teva today announce the launch of www.myPDinfo.com to provide answers
to common questions following a diagnosis of Parkinson's disease. Designed for people with
Parkinson's, their families and carers, the new site provides information on the disease itself,
as well as many aspects of treatment and practical disease management such as medication,
surgery, diet, exercise/physiotherapy, and emotional support. (1:39 minutes)
http://www.youtube.com/watch?v=OJQV8xWnAJU&feature=share&list=PL8E16C944A96
86EF3
Early Diagnosis and Treatment of Parkinson's Disease (2009) (5:04 minutes)
http://youtu.be/T8lXjNUMaWA
Nursing Education for Parkinson's Disease Patients (2012)
This video discusses the role of nurses in improving the transitional care process for patients
with Parkinson's disease. (3:27 minutes)
http://youtu.be/eDWSUsJVWm4

Images

Google images for Neurological Disorders
http://www.google.com/search?q=neurological+disorders+and+older+adults
&source=lnms&tbm=isch&sa=X&ei=gUqjUYSFOenD0AHph4C4Cg&ved=0C
AcQ_AUoAQ&biw=1011&bih=220
Google images for Parkinson's Disease
http://www.google.com/search?q=parkinson's+disease+and+older+adults&source=
lnms&tbm=isch&sa=X&ei=vlijUfbGOuv94AOC_YD4CQ&ved=0CAcQ_AUoAQ&biw=
1011&bih=220

Pulmonary Disease

Joni Goldwasser, RN, DNP, FNP-BC

INTRODUCTION AND BACKGROUND

A 74-year-old man and his wife come to your office reporting, "I get winded walking to the mailbox and never use to; plus my phlegm is harder to get up these days. Is there anything to help get my stamina back?" This example and an array of symptoms usually noting dyspnea, cough, or secretions typically constitute the presentation of breathing concerns by older adults. It is well known that people are living longer and the number of older adults will be significant because of the baby boomer generation. These adults want to live independently and have high expectations for quality health care (Grady, 2011). Pulmonary-related health concerns will be a frequent reason for older adults seeking health care provider visits. Upper respiratory infections (excluding pharyngitis) and chronic obstructive pulmonary disease (COPD) are two of the top-ranked diagnoses attributed to ambulatory care visits according to routinely posted data from the National Ambulatory Medical Care Survey (NAMCS) (Ambulatory Health Care Data, n.d.). In addition, other than infants under 1 year of age, multiple health care data repositories report that ambulatory care office visits overall are highest for persons 75 years old and over. Data from the 2006 NAMCS and National Hospital Ambulatory Medical Care Survey (NHAMCS) were combined to produce annual estimates of ambulatory medical care utilization (Hall et al., 2010). Patients in the United States make an estimated 1.1 billion visits to physician offices and hospital Outpatient Departments and Emergency Departments annually (Centers for Disease Control and Prevention, 2013, n.d.). These reports indicate that nearly one half of ambulatory medical care visits (46.8%) were made to primary care office–based practices. According to the Centers for Disease Control (CDC), National Health Interview Survey, 2011, more than 240,000 office visits were related to respiratory conditions, not including pneumonia and influenza. COPD ranks as one of the top diagnoses needing evaluation with reporting trends that remain steady. The CDC reports lung disease as the third leading cause of death, with 400,000 deaths annually in the United

States, citing final 2010 data (Hall et al., 2010). According to the American Lung Association 2010 Health Disparities report, 35 million Americans are living with lung disease (American Lung Association [ALA], n.d.). The staggering statistics provide evidence that pulmonary problems are not only a significant health concern but also one of the chief complaints for office visits with health care providers.

The older adult with a known history of pulmonary conditions may schedule a visit because of an acute onset of a new health problem, exacerbation of a current condition, or for routine care of chronic disease and multisystem health concerns. Pulmonary concerns include a wide range of complaints frequently characterized as "nagging cough, out of breath, pain, fatigue, or breathlessness" associated with chronic lung disease or an acute upper respiratory infection. Breathing problems may occur with rest or activity or may overlap incapacitating multisystem problems for the older adult. Other medical conditions or medications can cause breathing problems or increased demand on the pulmonary system. Primary care providers will see varying situations involving pulmonary problems in the older adult and must have a comfort level for evaluation and evidence-based treatment. This chapter presents information focusing on health care for the older adult specifically with chronic obstructive lung disease, influenza, and pneumonia, supporting current evaluation and treatment guidelines.

PULMONARY PATHOPHYSIOLOGY

Overall pulmonary structure and function remains relatively unchanged in the healthy older adult, especially in an individual who has never smoked. Several physiologic changes occurring with older age need to be recognized, in order to differentiate normal aging changes from disease pathology. It is important to consider how these aging changes also affect disease pathology and prognosis. According to Bhatt and Wood (2008), the progressive decline in normal lung function with aging is associated with changes in the lung parenchyma, chest wall compliance, and respiratory muscle strength. Pulmonary system alterations occurring with aging include (1) decreasing elastic recoil of lung tissue and reduction in alveolar surface area shifting lung pressure flow volume curves; (2) stiffening of the chest wall related to changes in intercostal muscles, rib–vertebral joint calcification, and age-related osteoporosis all combining to increase kyphosis and chest wall diameter; (3) decreased respiratory and diaphragm muscle strength plus reduced airway diameter increases flow resistance, which results in diminished ventilatory reserve; and (4) alterations in gas exchange because of chemoreceptors that become less sensitive to gas partial pressures with age (Bhatt & Wood, 2008). Anatomically, the diaphragm flattens with aging and the chest wall becomes more rigid (Brashers, 2002). Without adequate conditioning and routine exercise, progressive decline in lung volumes and weakening respiratory muscles occur with aging. Table 8.1 outlines the age-related changes.

The older adult, especially around the eighth decade of life, may experience a decreased compensatory response to hypercapnia and hypoxemia. The combined decreased oxygenation and diminished ventilatory reserve produces much of the exercise intolerance experienced with aging (Brashers, 2002). The dynamic nature of lung volumes is an important area of understanding for providers. Total lung capacity (TLC) is the volume of air within the lungs from a maximal inspiratory effort and depends on chest wall muscle strength and elastic recoil within the lung parenchyma (Enright, 2009). A decrease in TLC represents restriction within the lung parenchyma.

TABLE 8.1 • Pulmonary System Age-Related Changes
1. Increased chest wall stiffness
2. Decreased lung elastic recoil
3. Decreased respiratory muscle strength
4. Decreased airway diameter
5. Decreased alveolar surface area
6. Decreased sensitivity of chemoreceptors altering gas exchange

Residual volume (RV) is the volume of air remaining in the lungs after maximum exhalation and has been shown to increase with aging. The third static lung volume is vital capacity (VC) and is measured after a maximal inhalation and slow, complete exhalation (Brashers, 2002). These three lung volumes are commonly known among health care providers and contribute to further decision making and management of pulmonary health problems.

SCREENING

Spirometry testing is one of the common screening tools used for evaluation of lung function after pulmonary symptoms occur to establish a baseline or changes within lung function. Chronically low oxygen levels associated with aging and poor conditioning can predispose the older adult to respiratory infections or exacerbate existing problems (Enright, 2009). Additional factors can include decreased functional ability to exercise, tobacco use, sleep-related problems, as well as other chronic medical conditions. Certain medications add to the increased risk of respiratory depression and require careful review and reconciliation by the provider. Avoiding smoking is one of the most important ways to minimize the effects of aging on the lungs. An individual who has never used tobacco products and maintained normal lungs may not exhibit changes in breathing throughout the aging process. The older adult who has used tobacco products, had repeated exposure to environmental and/or occupational pathogens, and does not maintain adequate conditioning becomes increasingly symptomatic with aging (Enright, 2009). This older adult is particularly at increased risk for developing various pulmonary problems, either acutely or chronically.

Pulmonary function testing (PFT) is widely used to quantify lung function, evaluate treatment regimen effectiveness, diagnose lung disease, and determine disability (Downs, 2011). Components of PFTs include lung volumes evaluated by spirometry, lung volume response to bronchodilators, gas diffusion, and blood gas analysis. Commonly cited standards for PFT interpretation have been established by the American Thoracic Society (ATS) and the European Respiratory Society (ERS). PFTs are an objective measurement used for differential diagnosis assessment, supporting evaluation of findings and guiding treatment goals for the older adult with pulmonary complaints. All health care providers need to be knowledgeable concerning PFT interpretation because of the increasing volume of individuals with pulmonary problems. Upon presentation of specific pulmonary patient complaints, the provider at that point in time obtains PFTs. Symptoms or spirometry responses may determine additional testing components needed. PFT results categorize problems as obstructive, restrictive, or mixed with other pathology, along with stratification of disease pathophysiology. The spirometry results quantify the percentage of lung function. These data are necessary for determining management strategies and continuity of care. When the PFT report data are received, there may or may not be a summary evaluation and treatment recommendations. Therefore, it is essential for providers to have a basic understanding when reviewing results or to use available PFT interpretation tools (Hyatt et al., 2003).

The provider should initially review the flow–volume curve on the spirometry report. Exhaling from full lung capacity is known as forced vital capacity (FVC). FVC and forced expiratory volume in the first second (FEV_1) are lung capacities tested. Normal values are usually greater than 80%. It has been reported that adults normally experience a loss in FEV_1 about 1 L per decade (Enright, 2009). The FVC also declines with age, but not as great. If there is no loss of area seen on the flow–volume spirometry curve and the FVC is normal, the test is most likely normal. If the FVC is reduced, an obstructive, restrictive problem or mixed problem may be the cause. When the curve is scooped out with a reduced flow–volume slope, an obstructive problem is most likely. If the FVC is reduced and the flow–volume curve shows no loss of area, including the ratio of FVC to FEV_1, a restrictive or nonspecific abnormality may be present (Hyatt et al., 2003). The FEV_1 is an important value to understand. A normal FEV_1 value usually indicates no obstructive or restrictive pulmonary pathology. TLC is needed for further evaluation to determine the specific breathing problem. Further, the individual is assessed for respiratory muscle weakness. If the FEV_1 is reduced more than 15% to 20%, it is generally because of airway obstruction, and the TLC needs to be evaluated. An increased TLC is associated with obstructive disease, whereas a reduced TLC is seen with restrictive disease.

What is the FEV_1/FVC ratio? If the ratio is normal, FEV_1 is more than 80% predicted, FEV_1/FVC is more than 70%, an obstructive problem is excluded. If the ratio is decreased to 65% to 70%, an obstructive process is present. In the older adult, the lower limit of normal (LLN) is about 65% (Hyatt et al., 2003). Response to bronchodilators is usually evaluated. These are important findings and results that identify risk of a rapid decrease in lung function or an increased risk of mortality (Gooneratne et al., 2010). A normal or increased ratio is seen with restrictive problems. Patients with a reduced FVC, reduced FEV_1, normal-to-increased FEV_1/FVC ratio, and normal response to bronchodilators usually have a restrictive process. The TLC should also be decreased. If tested, the noninvasive pulmonary diffusion of carbon monoxide (D_{LCO}) is reviewed. This test reflects the amount of carbon monoxide absorbed into the blood when holding the breath for 10 seconds and supports differentiating airway obstruction and restriction of lung volumes (Brashers, 2002; Enright, 2009). A normal D_{LCO} result is consistent with normal lungs. A reduced finding is characteristic of restrictive disorders, whereas an increased result is seen in conditions that produce pulmonary vascular engorgement (Hyatt et al., 2003). The D_{LCO} is easier than spirometry, reflecting the ability of the lungs to receive oxygen from the environment and deliver it to red blood cells (Enright, 2009).

PFTs and spirometry are recommended as screening tools once symptoms or pulmonary problems have been assessed. Baseline PFTs are obtained only when the older adult is symptomatic with dyspnea or wheezing and periodically with progressive condition worsening, typically every 1 to 2 years. Consultation with specialists dedicated to pulmonary medicine enhances collaborative care planning and supports continuity of care. An overview of spirometry findings is summarized in Table 8.2. The Cleveland Clinic offers a website for PFT interpretation at www.ccjm.org/content/70/866.pdf.

TABLE 8.2 · Generalized Spirometry Findings (Not Including Mixed Disorders, Tumors)

Spirometry	Normal Lung Function	Restrictive Disorder	Obstructive Disorder
Flow–volume curve	No loss of area	Normal or increased slope	Scooped out or decreased slope
FVC	Normal	Normal or decreased	Decreased
FEV_1 (>80%)	Normal	Decreased	Decreased 15%–20%
FEV_1/FVC ratio	Normal	Normal or increased	Decreased to 75% or less; in the Elderly lower limits of normal (LLN) 65%
TLC	Normal	Decreased	Normal or increased
Bronchodilator response (large positive response may indicate- rapid decrease in lung function- severe exacerbations- increased risk for rapid decline and death	Normal (0%–10% $\uparrow FEV_1$)	Normal or positive (FEV_1>12% and 200 ml)	Normal or positive (FEV_1>12% and 200 ml)
DL_{CO}	Normal	Decreased	Decreased

An additional diagnostic tool considered is monitored exercise testing. Exercise testing should be evaluated in individuals with a less than 50% to 60% reduction in predicted diffusing capacity and who are not hypoxemic at rest, especially if supplemental oxygen is being considered to improve exercise capacity (Petrache & Georas, 2007). The distance a patient can walk in 6 minutes is commonly known as the *6-minute walk test,* and results support pulmonary functional ability. Measuring exercise capacity is useful in identifying patients who may benefit from pulmonary rehabilitation, supplemental oxygen, or surgical intervention to improve pulmonary status.

Providers may also include alpha-1 antitrypsin deficiency in the differential diagnoses when evaluating individuals with unexplained airflow obstruction symptoms or unexplained liver disease. Low incidence of the genetic alpha-1 antitrypsin deficiency, identified through genotyping, is an additional finding to consider with suspected but confusing presentation of pulmonary health problems. These individuals produce enzymes that destroy lung connective tissue that results in COPD in about 1% of COPD patients (Yende et al., 2009).

PRESENTATION OF ACUTE AND CHRONIC PULMONARY HEALTH PROBLEMS

Older adults with pulmonary problems can present with acute problems or for routine evaluation of active chronic conditions. Whether acute or chronic health conditions, keen observation beginning with a visual assessment of the older adult's work of breathing, color, and mobility contributes to early diagnosis and recognition of change in functional status. Baseline history common with pulmonary problems includes description of current dyspnea, cough, sputum, hemoptysis, pain, and sleep changes; social history regarding tobacco use, pets/hobbies; occupational or environmental exposures; and family history and medication use. The value of a thorough history and clinical examination is highly contributory to the differential diagnosis and is a key recommendation from multiple professional organizations. This equates to having adequate time or strategies for collecting information needed. Evidence-based studies have shown that patient history, current symptoms, and physical findings combined are most often accurate predictors for pulmonary health problems. The guideline is the official statement of the American College of Physicians (ACP), American College of Chest Physicians (ACCP), ATS, and the ERS and is intended for those providers managing pulmonary disease (Qaseem et al., 2011).

Health assessment of the older adult with pulmonary problems is directed toward obtaining objective data for the differential diagnosis, estimating acuity of the problem and other related conditions. It is not uncommon for older patients to have symptoms related to both restrictive and obstructive lung disease. In addition, health care providers may easily underdiagnose or overdiagnose conditions without a combination of detailed and accurate information (Brashers, 2002).

At each initial observation, the provider can easily evaluate bluish tinge color of the mucus membranes and lips, which may indicate severe airflow limitations, along with the same discoloration noted in the fingers or toes. Later examination may also produce a coolness to touch in these areas. Knowledge of vital signs, room air oxygen saturation (SpO_2), and complete blood count (CBC) complement the assessment of color. During inspection of peripheral color, clubbing of the nail beds can be detected, as well as nicotine staining of the fingers and any presence of fine tremors. Clinical examination of the ears, nose, oral pharynx, and trachea and presence of palpable lymphadenopathy contribute to diagnoses of acute or progressing pulmonary problems. Deformities of the chest wall are seen with thorough inspection and include barrel chest because of hyperinflation, kyphosis, scoliosis, and surgical or traumatic scars. Rate, depth, and regularity of breathing patterns are key influencing assessment findings for both acute and chronic conditions. Hyperventilation or hypoventilation can indicate severe lung pathology. Prolonged expiration and pursed-lip breathing help to maintain higher airway pressures and keep open distal airway supporting assessment of dyspnea. Structural expansion of the lungs helps to confirm shallow breathing depth, pain limitations, and diaphragm weakness common in the older adult or the use of the abdominal muscles for expiration. Asking the patient to take deep breaths through the mouth may assist those older adults with shallow breathing and provide relaxation with acute exacerbations. A brief demonstration of what you expect aids the patient. Breath sounds are produced in the large airways, and clear vesicular breath sounds throughout the posterior and anterior lung fields are considered normal. The presence of additional sounds such as crackles, wheezes, or pleural friction rubs or the absence of sound transmission contributes to confirming the diagnosis. Chronic airflow limitation seen in asthma and obstructive lung disease can produce overlapping findings in the older patient, including hyperinflation of the chest, pursed-lip breathing, and use of accessory muscles to support inspiration. Data helping to predict pulmonary problems are summarized in Table 8.3.

TABLE 8.3 · Predictors of Pulmonary Health Problems	
History	Tobacco use Exposures: environmental, occupational, pets, hobbies Medication use or changes
Current symptoms	Dyspnea or changes Cough frequency or worsening Increasing sputum or phlegm
Physical findings	Changes in functional status Color Chest wall Clubbing Fever Respiratory rate, depth, expansion, SpO_2 Lung sounds

FUNCTIONAL STATUS

Subjective information from the older adult or family regarding participation in everyday activities is needed to support determining patient's conditioning, pulmonary diagnosis, and current management of health. These functional activities include personal hygiene, bathing, dressing, toileting, feeding, transferring bed to chair, and walking. Activities allowing an older adult to have more functional independence include using the telephone, preparing meals, and regular housework, including laundry, managing finances, and transportation needs. These essential data can be elicited during routine conversation and history taking concerning the nature of the visit. The details also need to be routinely updated, in order to have awareness of changing conditions requiring a change in treatment plan. Avoid questionnaires, if possible, to promote a more patient-centered care focus. Use of quick activity of daily living (ADL) tools can be reviewed at initial and routine health maintenance visits to determine functional status as it affects pulmonary health problems in the older adult. For example, the Katz Index of Independence in Activities of Daily Living commonly referred to as the Katz ADL can be accessed online at http://therapeuticresource.ca/CVS/Katzindeptest.pdf. A variety of specific topic ADL tools can also be accessed at http://endoflifecare.tripod.com/embeddedlinks/id17.html. These tools allow for easily obtained, objective data-supplementing assessment findings, individualized care, and continuity of care. Normal aging, acute illness, and chronic pulmonary conditions can affect ADLs. One goal of every health care visit with an older adult should be focused on optimizing function and preserving independence. Documentation describing function and independence with ADLs is essential for monitoring and continuity of care. The plan of care should note pulmonary health problems as stable or unstable; controlled or uncontrolled; and functional status independent or dependent. This specific evaluation also affects billing criteria and reimbursement. Health care providers need to evaluate whether initial impressions are consistent with the individual's story and level of distress. Observing clues such as using mobility assistive devices (walker, wheelchair, etc.), ability to carry on a conversation without respiratory distress, conditioning, body weight, positioning, and use of oxygen delivery systems allows the provider to position the patient and completes a more efficient, comfortable examination with either acute or chronic conditions. In summarizing overall presentation, a thorough health assessment, clinical examination, functional determination, and diagnostic testing together are needed for predicting the presence and acuity of pulmonary problems in the older adult. The history, functional assessment (updated at least annually), routine clinical examinations, and spirometry (or complete PFTs) provide essential data to monitor and manage these health problems. An additional area for providers to explore may include review of echocardiogram results supporting right ventricular hypertrophy and echocardiogram, if completed. Attention to valvular abnormalities and pulmonary artery pressure may provide additional information needed for treatment guidelines. Baseline chest X-ray or comparison with previously obtained chest X-ray provides information for diagnosis and necessary ongoing evaluation. Arterial blood gases are not routinely obtained. A complete health assessment and clinical examination determines specific pulmonary problems and frequency of evaluation needed and supports the differential diagnosis. An encounter example is provided in Table 8.4. Presentation of disease in older adults related specifically to COPD, influenza, and pneumonia is discussed.

TABLE 8.4 • Office Visit–Focused Assessment with Plan of Care

HPI: Joseph D. is a 66-year-old, thin, white male retired factory worker appearing older than stated age. Face is tense and anxious, showing mild distress complaining of increasing difficulty breathing at rest and limiting his activity. He is sitting in a wheelchair accompanied by his wife.

Over the last 2–4 weeks, he has been feeling worse and unable to walk to his mailbox (100′ [30.4 m]) or climb one floor of stairs in his house without stopping to rest, so he scheduled an appointment for evaluation and assistance. Productive cough is present with white-yellow tinged sputum unchanged in amount and consistency, greater in the morning and intermittently throughout the day, using two pillows or the recliner chair for sleep and increasing difficulty showering and getting dressed due to becoming "winded." Fatigue and shortness of breath have been worsening over the last 6–9 months. He denies fever, chest pain, hemoptysis, night sweats, or injury and reports no allergies, hospitalizations, or medication changes. Joseph D. smokes cigarettes 1.5 packs per day × 50 years and drinks one 6-pack beer mostly over the weekends and occasionally two to three beers in the evening if watching television. No routine exercise.

Objective: Transfers from wheelchair using hands to raise self and able to take three to four steps pivoting to exam table without increased work of breathing. Weight 220 lb (99.8 kg) with body mass index calculated 32, heart rate 96, resting, respiratory rate 24/min, shallow with prolonged expiration, increased AP diameter of chest wall and audible expiratory wheezing with loose cough. Clubbing noted all upper extremity digits with brown staining to right thumb and index finger. Oral mucosa pale and dry. Head, eyes, ears, and nose unremarkable with nontender cervical lymphadenopathy. Breath sounds are diminished in the bases posteriorly with coarse expiratory wheezing throughout. No crackles, friction rub, or carotid bruits auscultated. Current with influenza vaccination and pneumovax immunization.

Assessment/Plan: Chronic and increasing dyspnea stable most likely obstructive lung disease related to tobacco abuse, overweight, and deconditioning.

- Baseline ECG, chest X-ray, CBC, chemistry, urinalysis, hepatic panel, B_{12}, vitamin D today and staff to schedule PFTs through pulmonary clinic.
- Albuterol 90 mcg per spray, MDI 2 puffs inhaled every 4–6 hr as needed, no more than 12 puffs per day for bronchospasm/wheezing.
- Complete baseline functional assessment of ADLs—Nurse Case Manager visit 2–4 weeks.
- Dietician consult for meal planning, weight loss plan 2–4 weeks.
- Physical therapy referral for evaluation, strengthening, and conditioning.
- Declines available smoking cessation support and aware of resources available, including 1-800-QUIT NOW.
- Schedule follow-up 1 month and to the Emergency Department/911 with chest pain, unable to breathe or other emergent concerns.
- Advanced Directives discussion next visit.

COPD Presentation

COPD includes chronic bronchitis, emphysema bronchiectasis, and chronic airway obstruction. These diseases are commonly characterized by progressive, irreversible airflow affecting limitation morbidity and mortality. COPD has become a major public health concern and is estimated to become the third most frequent cause of death worldwide by 2020 (Stanley et al., 2013). In 1995, it ranked as the fourth leading cause of death in the United States, accounting for over 100,000 deaths, doubling in 15 years. In 1994, an estimated 16 million individuals in the United States had the diagnosis of COPD. About 80% to 90% of COPD cases are attributable to cigarette smoking. The etiology of COPD is multifactorial. Additional risk factors include occupational exposures, air pollution, respiratory infection, and genetic factors. The relationship of COPD to workplace exposure is well documented for exposure to agents such as coal mine dust, cotton dust, and grain dust (Kim, 1998).

COPD is a slowly progressive disease involving the airways or pulmonary parenchyma that results in partially reversible or nonreversible airflow obstruction (Qaseem et al., 2011). COPD can present as chronic bronchitis or emphysema (or both). Symptoms of COPD may include dyspnea, chronic cough, sputum production, limited exercise capacity, wheezing, right heart failure, or respiratory failure. Spirometry is used to confirm the diagnosis. Chronic conditions with similar symptoms should be carefully evaluated to avoid overdiagnosis or misdiagnosis, which is considered a health care deficit. The National Heart, Lung, and Blood Institute (NHLBI) currently reports COPD as the 3rd leading cause of death in the United States and the 12th leading cause of disability (National Institutes of Health [NIH], National Heart, Lung, and Blood Institute [NHLBI], 2011; Stanley et al., 2013). Medical care for COPD patients is estimated at $29.5 billion annually with an economic burden of almost $50 billion in 2010 (NIH/NHLBI, 2011). Multiple professional organizations contribute to establishing guidelines for diagnosis and management of COPD once the problem has been confirmed. The guidelines reflect cumulative, current data, and research reviewed by the ACP, ACCP, ATS, and the ERS. The World Health Organization (WHO) and the NHLBI formed what is commonly known as the Global Initiative for Chronic Obstructive Lung Disease (GOLD) to increase awareness of growing problems associated with the smoking epidemic and to present guidelines for COPD prevention and treatment. Now age-specific spirometry using the LLNs with FEV_1/FVC ratio below 65% to support the COPD diagnosis is pertinent to correctly identifying breathing problems in the older adult. Structural changes causing narrowing of the airways include mucus hyperplasia, bronchiole edema, smooth muscle hypertrophy, and peribronchiolar fibrosis (Yende et al., 2009). The limited expiratory flow produces the decreased FEV_1/FVC ratio and reduced lung volumes. Most patients with COPD have features of both chronic bronchitis and emphysema, and some patients have been characterized by either chronic bronchitis or emphysema (Corbridge et al., 2012). The patient with chronic bronchitis has decreased alveolar ventilation, pulmonary vasoconstriction, and pulmonary hypertension and presents with symptoms related to hypoxia from the airflow obstruction (Wise and Liu, 2007). This patient may also show right heart strain and peripheral edema. Ventilation is maintained with emphysema mostly because of loss of airway elasticity, resulting in airway collapse on exhalation. This is typically the purse-lipped breather who has loss of muscle mass (Stanley et al., 2013). The provider may see the patient with COPD, presenting with malnourishment, depression, and anxiety, or having concomitant cardiovascular disease (Corbridge et al., 2012; Stanley et al., 2013). The GOLD guidelines for establishing diagnosis and treatment with COPD can be accessed at http://www.goldcopd.org/Guidelines/guidelines-resources.html.

Influenza and Pneumonia Presentation

Congestion, fever, malaise, and achiness are the key features when patients present complaining of influenza. Influenza is known as a global health threat, with older adults being vulnerable during peak seasonal periods October to March. In older adults, influenza infection may progress to one of the most common diseases in this population, which is pneumonia (Cohen et al., 2010). The National Center for Health Statistics reports that infectious pneumonia and influenza together represent the sixth leading cause of death in the United States. Influenza causes between 3,000 and 49,000 deaths annually, depending on the severity of the flu season. Ninety percent of the deaths are with adults 65 years and older. Hospitalizations due to influenza are 26,000 annually. Deaths attributed to pneumonia average 40,000 per year (Aldrich & Keyser, 2008). Influenza can lead to pneumonia, so often these conditions are grouped together. Nearly all deaths result from infectious pneumonia. The common pathogen causing community-acquired pneumonia (CAP) is *Streptococcus pneumoniae*, also referred to as pneumococcus. Safe, available, effective vaccines are not being given to many adults 65 years and older, especially African Americans and Hispanics (Aldrich & Keyser, 2008). This population and these ethnic backgrounds are known to have increased risk and high rates of chronic disease. Knowledge about pneumonia and influenza, and individual attitudes and beliefs are factors requiring counseling during health care visits. Trusting relationships focusing the individual's personal health goals decrease these missed opportunities.

Infectious diseases account for about half of the hospitalizations, and slightly less than half of these were the result of lower respiratory tract infections. The infectious agent involves the terminal bronchioles and alveoli causing an inflammatory response in the body. Typical pneumonia presents with an abrupt onset, high fever, chills, productive cough, and pleuritic chest pain. In the older adult, an increased respiratory rate is a sensitive sign. Typical pneumonias are caused from extracellular bacteria and include *S. pneumonia*, *Streptococcus pyogenes*, and *Haemophilus influenzae*. Globally, *S. pneumonia* is the most common cause of CAP, accounting for 50% of all cases (Marrie, 2009). Pneumonia resulting from viruses has a similar presentation. Atypical pneumonias may have more of a progressive onset, dry cough, headache, myalgias, and diffuse crackles. Positive radiographic finding is the gold standard for diagnosis. Many diagnoses, however, are made on the basis of clinical findings and presentation.

Screening and Risk Factors

Chronic Obstructive Pulmonary Disease. Risk factors for COPD include tobacco abuse, exposure to secondhand smoke, occupational dusts and chemicals, environmental pollutants, childhood illnesses, genetic factors, and low socioeconomic status (Stanley et al., 2013). COPD should be considered in current as well as ex-tobacco users. Screening is based on pertinent history and presentation of symptoms.

Influenza and Pneumonia. Pneumonia is a major health care problem with high morbidity and mortality. Age is a risk factor for pneumonia with every year over age 65 having increasing risk (Marrie, 2009). Additional considerations should include male gender, tobacco use, suspected aspiration, swallowing disorders, low serum albumin, and bedfast state. Pneumonia is high among nursing home residents (1.2 episodes per 1,000 resident days) and is the leading reason for transferring patients to the hospital (Corbridge et al., 2012; Marrie, 2009). Consideration for screening is given to those at high risk, not previously vaccinated, and with presentation of symptoms.

Treatment

COPD Treatment. Once the diagnosis is established, goals for the patient with COPD include (1) slowing disease progression affected strongly by smoking cessation; (2) improving dyspnea, exercise capacity, and other symptoms; and (3) preventing exacerbations and reducing mortality. The provider encounters the patient at various points in the health care continuum. The encounters range from the initial meeting to establish care, routine care, and episodic acute care. The patient may or may not have been diagnosed with COPD; they may present with respiratory distress and no prior management. Where the provider meets the patient on the health care continuum dictates point of care management and planning. In addition, the patient's ability cognitively and physically affects completion of diagnostic testing. Therefore, spirometry alone cannot be used to diagnose COPD in the older adult. The well-established GOLD guidelines identify four stages of COPD severity based on patient symptoms and spirometry. The provider uses these evidence-based guidelines to identify the COPD stage, enact ACP evidence-based clinical treatment recommendations, and reduce risk factors (Marrie, 2009). Realistic treatment goals will depend on the severity of the condition, patient's motivation and confidence for management, and comorbidities. The goals vary among patients because of individualized care and desired quality of life. Planned care includes ongoing education, medication adherence, smoking cessation, if applicable, and routine visits. According to the GOLD guidelines (2013), planned care not only improves quality of life for the COPD patients and caregivers but can also reduce the economic burden by hospitalizations and emergency visits (GOLD, 2013). The detailed GOLD guidelines can be found at http://www.goldcopd.com/guidelines. Additional management strategies are supported with seven evidence-based recommendations from the ACP for diagnosis and management of stable COPD published in 2011 (Qaseem et al., 2011). The ACP Clinical Guidelines can be accessed online at http://www.acponline.org/clinical_information/guidelines/guidelines, and an adapted format is provided in Table 8.5. These collaborative clinical guidelines support the goals of COPD treatment to slow

---

TABLE 8.5 · Diagnosis and Management of COPD

1. Respiratory symptoms must be present prior to obtaining spirometry to screen for airflow obstruction in individuals.
2. EV_1 between 60% and 80% predicted: treatment with inhaled bronchodilators may be used for stable COPD patients with respiratory symptoms.
3. $FEV_1 < 60\%$ predicted treat stable COPD patients with respiratory symptoms using bronchodilators.
4. Monotherapy using either a long-acting inhaled anticholinergics or a long-acting inhaled β-agonists for symptomatic patients with COPD and $FEV_1 < 60\%$ predicted can be used. However, clinicians should base the choice of monotherapy on patient preference, cost, and adverse effect profile.
5. Symptomatic patients with stable COPD and $FEV_1 < 60\%$ predicted may require clinicians to administer combination of inhaled therapies (long-acting inhaled anticholinergics, long-acting inhaled β-agonists, or IHSs).
6. Pulmonary rehabilitation for symptomatic patients with an $FEV_1 < 50\%$ predicted should be prescribed by clinicians. Clinicians may consider pulmonary rehabilitation for symptomatic or exercise-limited patients with an $FEV_1 > 50\%$ predicted.
7. Continuous oxygen therapy in patients with COPD who have severe resting hypoxemia ($PaO_2 \leq 55$ mm Hg or $SpO_2 \leq 88\%$) should be prescribed.

Information from Qaseem, A., Wilt, T. J., Weinberger, S. E., Hanania, N. A., Criner, G., van der Molen, T., . . . Shekelle, P. (2011). Diagnosis and management of stable chronic obstructive pulmonary disease: A clinical practice guideline update from the American College of Physicians, American College of Chest Physicians, American Thoracic Society, and European Respiratory Society. *Annals of Internal Medicine, 155*(3), 179–191.

lung function decline, prevent exacerbations, minimize hospitalizations, reduce mortality, lessen difficulty breathing, and improve exercise capacity and quality of life. The health care provider may benefit from using disease severity tools to enhance the GOLD guidelines and ACP Clinical Practice Guidelines data specific to individualized care. The Modified Medical Research Council (MMRC) Dyspnea Scale and the age, dyspnea, and obstruction (ADO) index have been validated in older adults to identify mortality and provide a more complete clinical picture (Yende et al., 2009).

The progressive nature of COPD indicates a chronic condition that is not curable. Reducing risk factors, managing symptoms, increasing exercise capacity, and maintaining quality of life are desired outcomes. Smoking cessation, oxygen therapy, and lung volume reduction surgical procedures have shown improved survival. The older adult continues to benefit from smoking cessation. Counseling and treatment should be a part of every visit for the older adult with tobacco use. The importance of current immunizations is also a part of COPD management. Studies have supported lower rates of hospitalizations for influenza and pneumonia after the annual influenza vaccine was given to COPD patients, and the pneumococcal polysaccharide vaccine was given to those aged 65 or older. Nutrition, hydration, daily activity, maintaining conditioning, and pulmonary rehabilitation are part of individualized management. Medications reduce symptoms and exacerbations in all patients with COPD. The foundation for pharmacologic treatment is with bronchodilators, beta-2 agonists, and anticholinergic medications. Short-acting beta-2 agonists are recommended for acute rescue therapy relaxing the smooth muscle in the airways. Long-acting beta-2 agonists are effective, have equivalent safety profiles, and are well tolerated in older adults. Individual patients' responses vary, and some may benefit from medications offering a quick onset of action, whereas others benefit from medications with a longer duration of action. Tachypnea, hypokalemia, tremors, tolerance, and existing cardiac conditions influence monitoring. The once daily dry powder, inhaled, long-acting anticholinergics improve dyspnea, FEV_1, and quality of life and decrease exacerbations. Because systemic absorption is limited, side effects such as dry mouth, cough, constipation, and urinary retention are few. In addition, inhaled corticosteroids (ICSs) can be used in patients with moderate to severe airflow limitation and frequent exacerbations (Gelberg & McIvor, 2010; Kim, 1998). Long-term ICS effects include bone density loss, which can be detrimental in an older adult with a history of falls, cataracts, glaucoma, thrush, and skin bruising. Anticholinergic and beta-2 agonist combination therapy is important to consider depending on the staging and classification for COPD in the older adult. Supplemental oxygen therapy, comprehensive outpatient pulmonary rehabilitation, and surgical intervention are necessary aspects of treatment requiring collaboration with pulmonary specialists.

Periodic education programs focusing on self-management and scheduled telephone follow-up are additional management strategies affecting hospital admissions, emergency department visits, and unscheduled office visits (Fromer & Cooper, 2008). COPD exacerbations can occur from related infections, medication nonadherence, metabolic and behavioral factors. When increased dyspnea and increased sputum volume or purulence are present with exacerbations, antibiotic therapy can be effective. Recent publications discuss long-term antibiotic coverage with lower doses to prevent exacerbations in severe end-stage disease. This should be individually evaluated with long-term adverse effects of medication use risk versus benefit openly discussed. When using antibiotics, *Pseudomonas* coverage should be considered when the patient has had prior hospitalizations and frequent antibiotic use from moderate to severe COPD

(Gelberg & McIvor, 2010; Kim, 1998). Brief oral corticosteroid therapy is an additional option to treat COPD exacerbations. Decreased renal function and polypharmacy need ongoing review with the older adult.

Additional long-term treatment by the health care provider for older adults with COPD includes monitoring for cardiovascular disease, osteoporosis, insomnia, weight loss, and behavioral health changes including depression. Two studies conducted in 1995 and 2003 showed decreased anxiety for COPD patients started on Sertraline (Advisor Forum, 2011). There are no respiratory cautions or adverse effects associated with Sertraline in the literature. Depression is seen in up to 40% of the COPD population. Because of the progressive nature of COPD, it is valuable for the provider to have candid discussions with the patient and family concerning advanced directives and end-of-life care. Limited mechanical ventilation trials, cardiopulmonary resuscitation, and palliative care using benzodiazepines and opiates are specific topics to cover during these discussions. Stratification of disease severity and prognostic information should be understood by the patient at every encounter.

Pneumonia and Influenza Treatment. Antibiotic resistance is an emerging problem requiring careful local evaluation when treating the older adult with pneumonia. Suggested treatment for CAP is a macrolide antibiotic (Marrie, 2009). When resistance is common in the community or the patient has multiple comorbidities, a respiratory quinolone can be used. Combination therapy with a beta-lactam antibiotic plus a macrolide can be considered with these increased risk patients. Adequate hydration is a key nonpharmacologic management and can help prevent exacerbation of a change in mental status. Tobacco cessation and the pneumococcal vaccine are two important interventions to prevent pneumonia. The pneumococcal vaccine is recommended to be given at age 65. If given prior to age 65 because of multiple chronic conditions, a booster dose is given 5 years after the initial dose. Patients can receive the pneumococcal and influenza vaccine at the same time.

A recent 2011 study showed a distinct pattern involving winter migration of older adults presenting for health care with pneumonia or influenza (Chui et al., 2011). Influenza is contagious, and presentations may be mild or severe. Symptoms include fever, chills, body aches, cough, sore throat, and headache. However, fever and cough have been the best predictors in the general population. The older adult may present with a more subtle cough and change in baseline temperature. Being aware of local influenza outbreak activity contributes to the differential diagnosis of influenza. Typically, recovery may take about 1 week or so. People aged 65 and older are the most severely affected and have the highest mortality from influenza or influenza-associated pneumonia coinfection. The older adult is one of the most mobile population groups with seasonal migrations (Chui et al., 2011). Consideration for migration patterns is important for prevention in this older adult population. Vaccines for the older adult at increased risk for complications from pneumonia and influenza are a major public health strategy in the United States. Currently, both pneumococcal and influenza vaccination levels among adults 65 years and older remain below the Healthy People 2010/2020 objective for 90% national coverage (Aldrich & Keyser, 2008). Antiviral medications are approved for treating influenza to reduce disease severity and must be given within 48 hours of symptom onset (Loeb, 2009). The antiviral medications have few adverse effects. However, most patients present for treatment later than 48 hours after symptom onset.

ADVANCED DIRECTIVES, END-OF-LIFE CONSIDERATIONS

Increasing age, functional decline, disability resulting in loss of independence, end-stage chronic disease, or severe difficulty breathing produces major distress for the patient and caregiver. Individuals often express opinions wanting to decrease suffering at the end of life and preserve dignity. Advanced Directives, end-of-life planning, and open discussions with the health care providers alleviate a large portion of this distress. Hospice care or inpatient palliative care to relieve suffering often involves sufficient medications, appropriately titrated to produce comfort. The unintended effect of hastening death is morally acceptable, but requires honest communication prior to developing severe disease, as well as ongoing respect for the patient's wishes.

REFERENCES

Advisor Forum. (2011). Sertraline in patients with pulmonary disease. *The Clinical Advisor*, 82.

Aldrich, N., & Keyser, C. M. (2008). CDC says immunizations reduce deaths from influenza and pneumococcal disease among older adults. Retrieved from www.cdc.gov/vaccines/news/media.htm#Reporters

American Lung Association. (n.d.). Lung disease. Retrieved from http://www.lung.org/lung-disease

Bhatt, N. Y., & Wood, K. L. (2008). What defines abnormal lung function in older adults with chronic obstructive pulmonary disease? *Drugs & Aging*, *25*(9), 717–728.

Brashers, V. L. (2002). *Pathophysiology: Structure and function of the pulmonary system*. St. Louis, MO: McCance & Huether, S. E.

Centers for Disease Control and Prevention. (2013). FastStats—Leading causes of death. Retrieved from http://www.cdc.gov/nchs/fastats/lcod.htm

Centers for Disease Control and Prevention. (n.d.). NAMCS/NHAMCS—Ambulatory health care data [Homepage]. Retrieved from http://www.cdc.gov/nchs/ahcd.htm

Chui, K. K., Cohen, S. A., & Naumova E. (2011). Snowbirds and infection—New phenomena in pneumonia and influenza hospitalizations from winter migration of older adults: A spatiotemporal analysis. *BMC Public Health*, *11*, 444.

Cohen, S. A., Klassen, A. C., Ahmed S., Agree, E. M., Louis, T. A., & Naumova, E. N. (2010). Trends for influenza and pneumonia hospitalization in the older population: Age, period, and cohort effects. *Epidemiology and Infection*, *138*(8), 1135–1145.

Corbridge, S., Wilken, L., Kapella, M. C., & Gronkiewcz C. (2012). An evidence-based approach to COPD: Part 1. *American Journal of Nursing*, *112*(3), 46–59.

Downs, C. A. (2011). Functional assessment of chronic obstructive pulmonary disease. *Journal of the American Academy of Nurse Practitioners*, *23*, 161–167.

Enright, P. L. (2009). Aging of the respiratory system. In *Hazzard's geriatric medicine and gerontology* (6th ed., Chap. 82). New York, NY: McGraw Hill Medical.

Fromer, L., & Cooper, C. B. (2008). A review of the GOLD guidelines for the diagnosis and treatment of patients with COPD. Retrieved from http://www.medscape.com/viewprogram/17618_pnt

Gelberg, J., & McIvor, R. A. (2010). Overcoming gaps in the management of chronic obstructive pulmonary disease in older patients: New insights. *Drugs & Aging*, *27*(5), 367–375.

Global Initiative for Chronic Obstructive Lung Disease. (2013). At-a-glance outpatient management reference for chronic obstructive pulmonary disease. Retrieved from http://www.goldcopd.org/uploads/users/files/GOLD_AtAGlance_2013_Feb20.pdf

Gooneratne, N. S., Patel, N. P., & Corcoran A. (2010). Chronic obstructive pulmonary disease and management in older adults. *Journal of the American Geriatric Society*, *58*(6), 1153–1162.

Grady, P. A. (2011). Advancing the health of our aging population: A lead role for nursing science. *Nursing Outlook*, *59*, 207–209.

Hall, M. J., DeFrances, C. J., Williams, S. N., Golosinskiy A., & Schwartzman A. (2010). National hospital discharge survey: 2007 summary. Retrieved from http://www.cdc.gov/nchs/data/nhsr/nhsr029.pdf

Hyatt, R. E., Scanlon, P. D., & Nakamura, M. (2003). *Interpretation of pulmonary tests* (2nd ed.). Philadelphia, PA: Lippincott Williams & Wilkins.

Kim, J. H. (1998). *Atlas of respiratory disease and mortality, United States: 1982–1993* (Publication No. 98–157). Cincinnati, OH: National Institute for Occupational Safety and Health U. S. Department of Health and Human Services. Retrieved from http://www.cdc.gov/niosh/docs/98-157/pdfs/98-157.pdf

Loeb, M. B. (2009). Influenza and respiratory syncytial virus. In *Hazzard's geriatric medicine and gerontology*. New York, NY: McGraw Hill Medical.

Marrie, T. J. (2009). Pneumonia. In *Hazzard's geriatric medicine and gerontology*. New York, NY: McGraw Hill Medical.

National Institutes of Health, National Heart, Lung, and Blood Institute. (2011). COPD. Retrieved from http://www.nhlbi.nih.gov/news/spotlight/success/copd.html

Petrache, I., & Georas S. (2007). Common pulmonary problems: Cough, hemoptysis, dyspnea, chest pain, and abnormal chest x-ray. In *Barker, Burton and Zieve's principles of ambulatory medicine*. Philadelphia, PA:Lippincott Williams & Wilkins.

Qaseem, A., Wilt, T. J., Weinberger, S. E., Hanania, N. A., Criner G., van der Molen T., . . . Shekelle P. (2011). Diagnosis and management of stable chronic obstructive pulmonary disease: A clinical practice guideline update from the American College of Physicians, American College of Chest Physicians, American Thoracic Society, and European Respiratory Society. *Annals of Internal Medicine, 155*(3), 179–191.

Stanley, T., Gordon, J. S., & Pilson, B. A. (2013). Patient and provider attributes associated with Chronic Obstructive Pulmonary Disease exacerbations. *Journal for Nurse Practitioners, 9*(1), 34–39.

Wise, R. A., & Liu, M. C. (2007). Obstructive airway diseases: Asthma and chronic obstructive pulmonary disease. In *Barker, Burton and Zieve's principles of ambulatory medicine* (7th ed., Chap. 60). Philadelphia, PA:Lippincott Williams & Wilkins.

Yende, S., Newman, A. B., & Sin D. (2009). Chronic obstructive pulmonary disease. In *Hazzard's geriatric medicine and gerontology* (6th ed., Chap. 83). New York, NY: McGraw Hill Medical.

CHAPTER 8: IT RESOURCES

Websites

Agingcare.com—Connecting people caring for elderly parents
http://www.agingcare.com/Lung-Disease

American Lung Association
http://www.lung.org/

American College of Chest Physicians
http://www.chestnet.org/accp/

American Thoracic Society
http://www.thoracic.org/

European Respiratory Society
http://www.ersnet.org/

Global Initiative for Chronic Obstructive Lung Disease (GOLD)
http://www.goldcopd.org/

PubMed Health—Chronic Obstructive Pulmonary Disease
http://www.ncbi.nlm.nih.gov/pubmedhealth/PMH0001153/

Consultgerin
http://consultgerin.org/uploads/file/trythis/try_this_2.pdf

Lippincott's Nursing Center
http://www.nursingcenter.com

National Health Statistics Reports: National Hospital Discharge Survey:
2007 Summary
http://www.cdc.gov/nchs/data/nhsr/nhsr029.pdf

Pneumonia—Mayo Clinic
http://www.mayoclinic.com/health/pneumonia/DS00135
Chronic Obstructive Pulmonary Disease (COPD)—Mayo Clinic
http://www.mayoclinic.com/health/copd/DS00916
Influenza—Mayo Clinic
http://www.mayoclinic.com/health/influenza/DS00081
Aging Changes in the Lungs—Medline Plus
http://www.nlm.nih.gov/medlineplus/ency/article/004011.htm
Chronic Obstructive Pulmonary Disease—Medline Plus
http://www.nlm.nih.gov/medlineplus/copdchronicobstructivepulmonarydisease.html
Pulmonary Function Testing—Medline Plus
http://www.nlm.nih.gov/medlineplus/ency/article/003853.htm
Women's Health.gov—A project of the U.S. Department of Health and Human Services Office
on Women's Health
http://womenshealth.gov/publications/our-publications/fact-sheet/lung-disease.cfm
Lung Function Tests
www.webmd.com/lung/lung-function-tests
Lung Disease fact sheet
http://womenshealth.gov/publications/our-publications/fact-sheet/lung-disease.pdf

Videos

Nursing Review Compilation of **Lung Disorder** Part 1 of 2 (2009) (9:29 minutes)
http://www.learningace.com/doc/6152473/e8a1e0e9f2aa912d04f2945a8519ba87/
nursing-review-compilation-of-lung-disorder-part-1-of-2
How COPD develops (2009) (2:32 minutes)
http://youtu.be/2wF1csksp-Q
How Pneumonia occurs (2009) (1:20 minutes)
http://youtu.be/fCFw-eS69i4
How Pneumonia affects the Lungs (2009) (1:33 minutes)
www.youtube.com/watch?v=1rjN2_hDXEY

Images

Google images of Lung Disease
http://www.google.com/search?q=lung+disease&source=lnms&tbm=isch&sa=X&ei=W5
mnUYnKF-jC0AHjiIGIDQ&sqi=2&ved=0CAcQ_AUoAQ&biw=1024&bih=564
Google images of Pneumonia
http://www.google.com/search?q=pneumonia&source=lnms&tbm=isch&sa=X&ei=Jpmn
UcGoOIXO0QHjoYCoDA&sqi=2&ved=0CAcQ_AUoAQ&biw=1024&bih=564
Google images of COPD
http://www.google.com/search?q=copd&source=lnms&tbm=isch&sa=X&ei=f5mnUazZF
pS70AGWsIGwDg&sqi=2&ved=0CAcQ_AUoAQ&biw=1024&bih=564

Diabetes

Carey A. Cole, RN, FNP-BC, DNP

INTRODUCTION

Diabetes mellitus, if not identified early and controlled well, can have a detrimental impact on the health of the older adult. This chapter explores the care and individualized treatment and ways to encourage individuals to optimize their health in the presence of this disease. Diabetes is the seventh leading cause of death among Americans and is estimated to cost $174 billion annually in direct and indirect costs. Direct medical costs are those that include treatments of the disease as well as treatments of complications from the disease. Indirect costs include disability, loss of work hours, and premature death (American Diabetes Association [ADA], 2012; Centers for Disease Control and Prevention [CDC], 2012; Hogan et al., 2003). According to the Centers for Disease Control, it is estimated that there are 11 million Americans over the age of 65 that have the diagnosis of diabetes and approximately 2 million who are undiagnosed. This equates to 27% of this population. The group with the highest prevalence of newly diagnosed diabetes is those aged 45 to 64 (CDC, 2012). These are the older adults of tomorrow whom health providers will care for in their practice settings.

Diabetes in the older adult is frequently underreported as a cause of death because of the plethora of complications that accompany the disease (National Diabetes Education Program, 2012). The actual cause of death may often be a diabetic-related complication. Common complications related to diabetes in the older adult include kidney disease, ophthalmic disorders, peripheral vascular disease, cardiovascular disease, depression, poor wound healing, and cognitive and functional decline. The underlying cause of these complications is poor glycemic control. In a hyperglycemic state with lack of insulin, tissue is unable to uptake proper oxygenation and the nutrients essential to maintain proper function, which causes poor tissue perfusion, resulting in microvascular and macrovascular complications. Microvascular complications of diabetes include nephropathy, neuropathy, and retinopathy. Diabetic nephropathy is the leading cause of renal failure in the older adult necessitating hemodialysis (Mooradian et al., 1999). Retinopathy is the leading cause of blindness in this population, and cataracts occur more commonly and at a younger age in individuals with diabetes. Peripheral neuropathy can be a devastating complication in the older adult causing increased pain, loss of sensation, and gait abnormalities. These complications can increase the risk of falls, foot ulcers, wounds from unintentional injury, and polypharmacy. Macrovascular complications include cardiovascular, cerebrovascular, and peripheral vascular disease. Macrovascular complications increase incidence of myocardial infarction, stroke, decreased cognition, dementia, and leg ulcers. Poor wound healing is also a result of hyperglycemia. The risk of amputations is increased in the diabetic patient from both microvascular and macrovascular complications.

Cognitive and functional declines are also at greater rates in the older adult with diabetes not only because of physiologic changes resulting from diabetic complications, but also because of an increased incidence in depression or emotional changes related to chronic disease. Depression in the older adult is multifactorial and can lead to poor adherence to prescribed treatments as well as marked functional decline. Functional decline and cognitive decline are interrelated. It is difficult to delineate which comes first; the functional decline may cause the cognitive decline or vice versa. All of these conditions can increase the risk of morbidity and mortality in the older adult (Geiss et al., 2006; Mooradian et al., 1999).

PATHOPHYSIOLOGY

Glucose Regulation

Glucose homeostasis is regulated by a negative feedback system in the absence of disease. When there is an increase or decrease in one component or type of hormone, not regulated by a negative feedback, it can cause the system to malfunction and result in a disease state. Diabetes is a disorder that originates in the pancreas. The pancreas is the key organ for the regulation of glucose in the body. Other important organs include the gut, the liver, and the musculoskeletal system. These systems have insulin receptor cells that facilitate the utilization and processing of glucose. In the pancreas, there are three types of cells that are present in the portion known as the islets of Langerhans; these are alpha cells, beta cells (the two most important), and delta cells. Alpha cells are glucagon-secreting cells. Glucagon is released when blood glucose levels drop too low as a compensatory mechanism that prevents hypoglycemia. The beta cells are the cells responsible for insulin secretion. Once food is consumed, blood glucose levels rise, and then the beta cells respond by producing insulin to keep fasting blood glucose levels in a normal range of 60 to 100 mg/dl and to keep postprandial blood glucose level less than 145 mg/dl. There have been two stages identified with glucose regulation and insulin secretion. The first stage occurs within the first 10 minutes of an oral glucose load. The second stage is longer and occurs in direct response to the amount of the glucose stimulus. There are a few key hormones in the gut that have been found to play a role in diabetes and glucose regulation; these incretins are glucose-dependent insulinotropic polypeptide (GIP), glucagon-like peptide 1 (GLP-1), and dipeptidyl peptidase 4 (DPP4). GIP and GLP-1 are secreted in the gut in response to an oral glucose load known as the incretin effect. They are responsible for activating the release of insulin. It has been found that these hormones show a significant decrease during a hyperglycemic state. DPP4 is liable for the degradation of the incretins GLP-1 and GIP, which in turn decreases the stimuli to release insulin (McCance & Huether, 2005).

The liver is responsible for producing endogenous glucose during the fasting state through the hormone glucose-6-phosphatase, which stimulates gluconeogenesis and results in the release of glucose into circulation. The kidneys also secrete glucose-6-phosphatase, but not at the same degree that the liver does and only in extreme fasting states. During normal glucose homeostasis, the liver absorbs the majority of the oral glucose load. Excess glucose is converted into glycogen and stored in the liver as well as in musculoskeletal tissue (McCance & Huether, 2005).

Musculoskeletal tissue, including adipose tissue, is a consumer of glucose but, at the same time, responsible for some of the hormones that cause glucose resistance and affect glucose homeostasis known as adipokines. Adipokines such as leptin, adiponectin, and resistin are believed to play a role in insulin resistance. These hormones are secreted by adipocytes and regulate a multitude of functions. Leptin is responsible for satiety and regulation of eating behavior through the hypothalamus, and assists in insulin sensitization. Adiponectin assists in insulin sensitization and has anti-inflammatory and antiatherogenic properties. The last, resistin, promotes insulin resistance, increases blood glucose levels, as well as inhibits adipocyte differentiation and promotes adipogenesis (McCance & Huether, 2005).

Cytokines, including tumor necrosis factor alpha (TNF-α), interleukin 6 (IL-6), and C-reactive protein (CRP), are also involved in the pathogenesis of diabetes. The exact relationship is unclear, but there is a positive correlation of increased levels of cytokines and obesity. Cytokines increase inflammation, and it is believed that inflammation decreases insulin sensitivity (McCance & Huether, 2005).

C-peptide is created in the pancreas along with insulin in equimolar amounts. This is known as proinsulin and plays a role in transporting insulin into cells. Thus, the measurement of C-peptide levels in the blood is used to help determine how much insulin is being produced by the pancreas. Previously, it was once believed to be a byproduct of insulin and not to have any other beneficial uses, but recent studies have found that it may have protective functions that include protection of renal and vascular tissue. Further studies are underway to determine the efficacy of replacing C-peptide as well as insulin in deficient individuals (Clinical Geriatrics, n.d.; Mooradian et al., 1999).

Type 1 versus Type 2 Diabetes Mellitus

Diabetes mellitus is broken down into two basic groups, type 1 and type 2. Type 1 diabetes develops from the complete destruction of beta cells of the pancreas because of an autoimmune response as evidenced by islet cell antibodies. Type 1 diabetics require insulin replacement as the body does not make its own insulin; hence, it is often called "Insulin-Dependent Diabetes Mellitus (IDDM)." Type 1 diabetes is also known as juvenile diabetes because it commonly occurs before the age of 30, whereas type 2 diabetes is the most common type of diabetes in adults. Type 2 diabetes is primarily caused by insulin resistance (i.e., lack of sensitivity of target cells to insulin) as a result of obesity, and thus it is also known as "Non-Insulin-Dependent Diabetes Mellitus (NIDDM)." In type 2 diabetes, beta cells were not destroyed, but their function is decreased. In type 2 diabetes, the malfunction of beta cells is associated with insulin resistance, but the actual cause is multifactorial, and the specific cause is not always clearly defined (McCance & Huether, 2005).

Age-Related Changes Contributing to Diabetes Mellitus

In the older adults, there is an increased risk of developing diabetes, most commonly type 2, because of both common age-related changes and environmental factors. After age 30, fasting blood glucose levels rise from 1 to 2 mg/dl every decade, and postprandial blood glucose levels rise 15 mg/dl per decade. Central obesity increases with age, which in turn increases visceral fat. Intramuscular fat also increases with age, whereas lean muscle decreases. Besides, the adipokinin hormones in muscle become out of balance with age, affecting the impairment of glucose regulation (Mooradian et al., 1999).

A decrease in mitochondrial function is believed to be a normal age-related change, which may contribute to an increase in insulin resistance and decrease in insulin sensitivity (Gambert & Pinkstaff, 2006). Carbohydrate metabolism changes with age and increases the risk of diabetes twofold; these include reduced insulin sensitivity in muscle tissue, the liver, and adipose tissue as well as decreased insulin production from the beta cells. Recently, there has been an increased awareness of type 2 diabetic patients who are found to have islet cell antibodies. This indicates an autoimmune response that destroys beta cells and is responsible for type 1 diabetes occurring in type 2 diabetic patients and creates an insulin-dependent type 2 diabetic (Gambert & Pinkstaff, 2006).

Multiple studies have noted that there is a marked difference in pathophysiology of the lean older adult with diabetes and the obese older adult with diabetes. In the lean older adult diabetics, there is decreased insulin secretion but good insulin sensitivity. Conversely, in the obese older adult diabetics, there is likely adequate insulin secretion but impairment of glucose usage and poor insulin sensitivity, or a combination thereof (Chau & Edelman, 2001). This information should be taken into consideration when treating these individuals (Clinical Geriatrics, n.d.; Mooradian et al., 1999).

Environmental factors have also been found to increase the incidence of diabetes in older adults. They include decreased activity and dietary choices. Often, a diet high in simple sugars, saturated fats, and low complex carbohydrates becomes the staple of the older adult diet, in part because of convenience. Age-related changes to taste such as loss of taste bud can increase the consumption of sweet foods. Prepackaged meals frequently used for the food to be served as meals for older adults by programs tend to have increased additives.

Concomitant disease processes and multiple medications may also influence the development and treatment of diabetes in the older adult. Common comorbidities that are present in individuals with diabetes include hypertension and hyperlipidemia. Multiple medications can affect glucose metabolism as well as the effectiveness of diabetes medications. Furthermore, pharmacokinetic changes with age can greatly affect the treatment of diabetes in the older adult. Renal function and hepatic function decrease with age, which decreases metabolism and elimination of medications from the body. The provider must have performed a comprehensive assessment when providing care for older adults with diabetes management in older adults (Clinical Geriatrics, n.d.; Mooradian et al., 1999).

PRESENTATION OF DIABETES

The older adult may present to the clinician during any one of the various stages of diabetes. Both acute and chronic presentations are commonly seen, and diabetes or hyperglycemia should also be included in the differential diagnosis. Diabetes becomes more prevalent with age because of the decrease in the function of beta cells and reduced insulin production. An individual who presents in a chronic state of diabetes may be asymptomatic or have a variety of vague complaints. The most common complaints of hyperglycemia include burning, numbness and tingling of extremities, excessive thirst, excessive urination, fatigue, irritability, weight loss, poor wound healing, blurred vision or vision changes, and frequent or unusual infections. The older adult will often not have the common presentation of excessive thirst or urination because of the decreased thirst perception that often occurs with aging (Mooradian et al., 1999). Instead, they may present with dehydration. Unfortunately, by the time these symptoms occur in diabetes, irreversible tissue damage may have already occurred. Moreover, many of these symptoms can be indicative of other disease states. This emphasizes the importance of a complete health history. Early diagnosis and good glycemic control can help reduce further complications and resolve some symptoms.

The acute presentation of diabetes and diabetic-related complications can be catastrophic to the older adult. Unfortunately, it is at these times that diabetes is first diagnosed. The most life-threatening complications of these include diabetic ketoacidosis (DKA), hyperosmolar nonketotic coma (HNC), and lactic acidosis. DKA is the most common complication of diabetes and is the result of total insulin deficiency. This is predominantly found in younger type 1 diabetics, but can present in the older adult with type 2 diabetes. Symptoms associated with DKA include polyuria, polydipsia, polyphagia, weight loss, vomiting, abdominal pain, weakness, and dehydration. DKA can progress rather quickly over a short time frame of usually less than 24 hours. Diagnostic criteria for DKA include hyperketonemia evidenced by a ketone serum level greater than a 1:4 ratio and acidosis—a pH less than 7.3 (Mooradian et al., 1999). HNC is precipitated by hyperglycemia and glucose spilling into the urine. When glucose is present in urine, the kidney is not able to concentrate urine properly, resulting in fluid and electrolyte loss. If proper treatment and rehydration are not begun promptly, hypovolemia occurs along with intracellular and extracellular dehydration, resulting in hyperosmolarity. Symptoms common in HNC include visual disturbances, leg cramps, weakness, and weight loss. On examination, one finds signs of dehydration, dry mucous membranes, poor skin turgor, and a rapid thready pulse. Both DKA and HNC are medical emergencies, and if not recognized and treated promptly, coma and death are likely to occur. Hypoglycemia may also be life threatening and is often the result of diabetic treatment. Red flags that should raise concern about diabetes in the older adult is the new onset of incontinence, cognitive changes, and frequent falls as these could be precursors to more serious life-threatening states (Mooradian et al., 1999).

Associated conditions that may be caused or exacerbated by diabetes in the older adult include dementia, most commonly vascular dementia, but diabetics also have a higher incidence of Alzheimer's disease, stroke, and depression. Many studies have looked at the correlation between diabetes and these comorbidities. It is well known that diabetes affects the vasculature. When blood glucose levels are high, the body is not getting the oxygenation and nutrients delivered to tissue that are required for normal function. This would likely increase the risk of stroke, dementia, and depression.

Numerous studies have indicated that there is an increased incidence of dementia-related conditions in the presence of diabetes; however, there is a lack of sufficient evidence that suggests that diabetes is the cause of these conditions. It is also unclear how diabetic control influences dementia, vascular dementia, and Alzheimer's disease. Future studies are needed for further knowledge of the link between dementia and diabetes (Ahtiluoto et al., 2010; Biessels et al., 2006; Strachan et al., 2008).

Individuals with diabetes are at increased risk of cardiovascular disease, which includes coronary heart disease and stroke. Studies have indicated that there is a two to four times increased risk of those with diabetes having a cardiovascular event. It is estimated that about 20% of deaths in individuals with diabetes are related to cerebrovascular disease and strokes. Studies also suggest that stress hyperglycemia, as well as chronic hyperglycemia, portends a poor outcome in individuals who suffer from a cerebrovascular accident (CVA). These individuals are at an increased risk of having sequential CVAs. Diabetic retinopathy has been studied to determine whether it is an indicator of stroke risk. A direct correlation has not been identified, but studies have suggested that increased retinal venular caliber may be linked to increased stroke incidence. Further studies are needed to predict cardiovascular events and outcomes in older adults with diabetes (Cigolle et al., 2009; Giorda et al., 2007; Sander et al., 2008).

Depression among older adults with diabetes can be devastating. The older adult is already at risk for depression in the absence of chronic diseases due to the aging process and loss. Depression along with diabetes can lead to poor outcomes. The presence of depression is three- to fourfold higher in adults with diabetes. Many studies have indicated poor glycemic control among individuals with depression as comorbidity. There seems to be a direct relationship between mood and treatment adherence. Treating the older adult for underlying depression has improved glycemic control, in turn, decreasing microvascular and macrovascular complications. There is some suspicion that diabetes may cause depression, but studies to date have not been able to indicate this causality other than the correlation of diabetes with depression as one of chronic illnesses (Kilbourne, 2005; Lustman & Clouse, 2005; Lustman et al., 1997; Munshi, 2006). This further stresses the need for a comprehensive assessment, including mental health.

SCREENING

Routine screening for diabetes should be completed for all older adults. The ADA recommends that all adults over the age of 45 be screened for diabetes every 3 years. The most common routine screening test is fasting blood glucose. Two elevated blood glucose levels greater than 126 can confirm the diagnosis of diabetes; however, levels greater than 100 need to be followed up by additional testing. The gold standard laboratory test for diabetes is the elevated fasting glucose followed by a 2-hour glucose tolerance test. Within the last couple of years, the ADA has come out with recommendations for screening with hemoglobin A1C (HbA1C) levels. This gives a broader picture of blood sugar control over a period of up to 3 months. This test can also be performed without fasting, which will increase the opportunity for screening individuals. The ADA included the HbA1C as a screening test in an effort to enhance the ability to diagnose more individuals. The threshold level that would indicate a person has diabetes would be a level greater than 6.5%. A result of 5.7 to 6.4 would indicate an individual with prediabetes. A urinalysis is also useful in the screening of diabetes to detect any glucose present in the urine. Typically, glucose does not spill over into the urine (glycosuria) until prolonged hyperglycemia occurs (Clinical Geriatrics, n.d.; Mooradian et al., 1999).

The older adult should also be screened during any acute presentation that could be associated with the presence of diabetes. This would include falls, acute onset of incontinence, mental status change, or any of the typical signs or symptoms of diabetes, including polydipsia, polyuria, polyphagia, weight loss, weight gain, dizziness, change in cognition, and depression. These symptoms are not exclusive to diabetes. It is important to obtain a thorough history, which can help develop differential diagnoses. Patient history should include the following:

- *Family history* includes individuals in both the mother's and father's immediate family, including parents, grandparents, aunts, and uncles, and collects all disease processes including cause of death.
- *Previous health history* includes current medications, previous surgeries, and past major illnesses.
- *Employment and recreational history* determines risk of prolonged hazardous exposure to any harmful chemicals; there have been links to pesticides as well as Agent Orange with diabetes. (There is a huge disparity in research related to possible links of environmental and chemical exposures to chronic illnesses.)
- *Nutritional history* includes food choices, eating patterns, vitamins and supplements, alcoholic intake, caloric intake, hydration (what and how much the individual drinks throughout the day), and budget for food.
- *Activity history* includes types of exercise/activity and amount of daily exercise.
- *Psychosocial history* includes living arrangements, family members/dynamics, stressors, and brief financial status. (Divulging their complete financial status is not necessary, but having an idea of affordability of treatment is important.)

A thorough history can be beneficial in diagnosing as well as developing a treatment plan (Mooradian et al., 1997, 1999; Norris et al., 2008).

RISK FACTORS

There are many risk factors associated with diabetes. As with all disease processes, there are two types of risk factors, modifiable and nonmodifiable. The majority of the focus should be on modifiable risk factors since these are the things that the patient has control over. These include obesity and sedentary lifestyle. Risk factors that are not modifiable include age, genetics, history of gestational diabetes, and race. African Americans, Hispanic/Latino Americans, Asian Americans, and Alaskan Americans/Pacific Islanders all have an increased risk of developing diabetes compared with Caucasians. Although these risks are not modifiable, there have been studies that suggest that individuals with nonmodifiable risk factors can reduce their risk of developing diabetes by maintaining a healthy weight; eating a diet that is low in simple sugars, low saturated fat, and high complex carbohydrates; and exercising regularly (Durso, 2006; Joslin Diabetes Center, n.d.).

TREATMENT

Treatment of diabetes in older adults should be individualized depending on the patient and their progression of disease. Hypoglycemia can have a detrimental effect on the older adult as does hyperglycemia. Care must be taken in treatment not to cause rapid drops in blood glucose levels. There are several options in treating diabetes: from oral agents to insulin replacement. We will discuss the benefits and disadvantages of all treatments and diabetic agents of the following classes: insulin therapy, sulfonylureas, meglitinides, biguanides, thiazolidinediones, alpha gluco-sidase inhibitor, GLP-1 agonists, DPP4 inhibitors, and a few miscellaneous medications. Dietary considerations as well as exercise and routine examination need to be included in the treatment plan of the older adult. Research of causes and treatments in diabetes is ongoing; today's cutting-edge findings and treatments can be tomorrow's old news. It is important to stay abreast of this information as it changes rapidly.

Lifestyle Modification

Counseling of diet and exercise is most important in treating diabetes in any individual. Diet is instrumental to good glycemic control. There are many tools and rules that studies have shown to help control diabetes through diet. These include carbohydrate counting, the plate method, and eating by the glycemic index (GI). Knowledge of the three types of carbohydrates is important in dietary management—fiber, sugar, and starch. Carbohydrates are what create the largest glucose response. Educating patients in reading labels is key to success. Even good consumers can be fooled by labels or advertising. A good example of this is products that contain "whole grains." Many food labels will report having whole grains, and when comparing nutritional labels, these are not any more nutritionally sound than similar products that do not have "whole grains."

Teaching patients to identify products with the most fiber will be the best choice possible. This will assist in carbohydrate counting for meals. Carbohydrate counting is one of the ways to help patients keep their diabetes under control through diet. It is recommended that they con-sume between 45 and 60 g of carbohydrates with each meal and a 15-g snack. The typical rule of carbohydrates is that a serving is 15 g. Although this method of carbohydrate counting is an effective method of glucose control, a better method to evaluate the individual's glucose response is through monitoring postprandial glucose levels and adjusting the recommendations of carbo-hydrate consumption accordingly (DiabetesCare.net, n.d.).

Another method is the plate method. This method may be an easier concept for patients since it is not as complex as carbohydrate counting. The plate method is simply visualizing the plate and dividing it in half, then half in a half again (one fourth). Half of the plate is filled with veg-etables, a fourth with meat or protein, and the other fourth with starch (DiabetesCare.net, n.d.).

GI is a bit more complicated when teaching patients about appropriate carbohydrate control in the diet, but can be very useful as it measures the glucose response created from individual foods. By consuming carbohydrates with the lowest GI, individuals will have better glycemic control and, in turn, decrease potential complications of their disease. The aforementioned methods of carbohydrate counting and the plate method can be used in conjunction with GI. Unfortunately, there are some disadvantages to the use of the GI in diabetes management. There are factors that may influence the GI of foods, which include how they are cooked and whether they are prepared in combination with other foods. GI does not take into consideration the other nutritional fac-tors of food such as fat, sugar, and calories. When using the GI, proper patient education should include these factors. For a complete list of the GI of foods, there are many books available, or use the website www.glycemicindex.ca/glycemicindexfoods.pdf (Sahyoun et al., 2008).

Exercise is an important adjunct to help tissues optimally utilize insulin. It is recommended that individuals exercise a total of 150 minutes/week or 30 minutes/day most days. Exercise is cumulative, so patients who cannot tolerate exercise or who have been inactive may benefit from breaking up activity, initially, to 10 to 15 minutes two to three times per day. The goal would be to work up to 30 minutes of continuous activity that gets the heart rate up to 50% to 70% of the target heart rate. Starting slow, 5 to 10 minutes/day, and increasing by 5 minutes every week are good goals to set with patients that have been inactive (Sigal, 2006).

Pharmacologic Therapy

Metformin (Glucophage) is the gold standard of diabetic treatment and is typically used as the first line of the drug to treat diabetes. This medication belongs to a group known as the biguanides; they work by decreasing glucose production in the liver. Because of their mechanism of action, hypoglycemia is not a concern with this class when used as monotherapy. It is often combined with medications from other drug classes to give the benefit of two mechanisms of action in the same pill. Another benefit of Metformin is weight loss, which is beneficial in a population that tends to be overweight or obese. The dosing is once to twice a day, so compliance is usually good. Some of the downfalls of this class include common gastrointestinal side effects such as nausea, diarrhea, and flatulence, and it cannot be used in individuals with renal impairment. Metformin can increase the risk of vitamin B_{12} deficiency, which is more common in the older adult and should be monitored while using this medication. A renal function test should be obtained prior to initiation to determine the appropriateness for this medication. The use of Metformin should be discontinued or avoided if serum creatinine level is higher than 1.5 in men and 1.4 in women. This medication should be discontinued prior to undergoing any procedure using intravenous (IV) contrast dye. When Metformin is concurrently used with IV contrast dye, both are metabolized through the kidney and an unsafe buildup could occur (Durso, 2006; Herman et al., 2005; Joslin Diabetes Center, n.d.).

Sulfonylureas are a drug class that stimulates the pancreas to produce more insulin. This group of medications has been around for a long time and is effective at lowering blood glucose. Medications include Glimepiride (Amaryl), Glyburide (DiaBeta), and Glipizide (Glucotrol). Dosing of this medication is typically once to twice daily, which helps with good compliance. Disadvantages of the sulfonylurea drug class include hypoglycemia and a faster decline of beta cell function. Hypoglycemia in the older adult is hazardous when using this class of medications. It is advised to start at a low dose with frequent monitoring of blood glucose levels. Beta cell function decreases because of hyperstimulation of the drug to produce more insulin, eventually causing the cells to wear out, resulting in beta cell death (Durso, 2006; Joslin Diabetes Center, n.d.).

The newest drug class used in the treatment of diabetes is the incretin mimetics. These include GLP-1 agonists and DPP4 inhibitors. The incretin mimetics work in the gut to increase the effect of GLP-1 and GIP in glucoregulation. The GLP-1 agonists are a noninsulin injectable class of drugs. These can be used first line or in combination with the other drug classes. The GLP-1 agonists were discovered when scientists noted that the Gila monster can go without eating for long period. They found that a substance in their saliva delayed gastric emptying. This substance is similar to the hormone that is released in the human gut—GLP-1, which is broken down by DPP4. GLP-1 agonist decreases glucose release from the liver and slows gastric emptying. The same mechanism of action is the premise of another group of medications that are now on the market to treat diabetes, the DPP4 inhibitors. These medications work by blocking DPP4 in the breakdown of GLP-1, in turn increasing the amount of GLP-1 circulating in the gut (Durso, 2006; Joslin Diabetes Center, n.d.).

Meglitinides are another drug group that stimulates increased insulin production in the pancreas. Unlike the sulfonylureas, this drug group does not bind to the insulin receptor cell. Instead, they work on the cell surface through the potassium-based channels. This class of medications is very fast acting and is given prior to meals three times per day. The medications of this class include repaglinide (Prandin) and nateglinide (Starlix). Frequent dosing may decrease compliance. Meglitinides are metabolized through the liver and should not be used in individuals with moderate to severe hepatic impairment, but are safe to use in those with renal impairment. Similar to sulfonylureas, beta cell function is imperative and has been linked to increased beta cell death. In the older adult, it is important to educate and monitor the possibility of hypoglycemia with this drug class. It is recommended to start with a low dose and increase the dose slowly as needed (Durso, 2006; Joslin Diabetes Center, n.d.).

Acarbose (precose) is the medication approved in the alpha glucosidase inhibitors group. It works by delaying the absorption of carbohydrates to decrease or spread out the glucose load. Precose is taken with meals so is dosed three times daily, this can lead to poor compliance. It is not recommended as monotherapy as it does not have good glycemic control when used alone. It does, however, enhance glycemic control when used in conjunction with other antidiabetic agents. Precose has some undesirable side effects that include abdominal cramping, diarrhea, and nausea. These tend to decrease with time and are dose driven, so starting with a low dose, then increasing slowly will help to lessen side effects (Durso, 2006; Joslin Diabetes Center, n.d.; National Diabetes Information Clearinghouse [NDIC], n.d.).

This next class of medications has undergone scrutiny within the treatment modalities of diabetes, but is important to discuss as there are still many individuals taking these medicines and can still be a valuable tool in the treatment of diabetes. The thiazolidinediones work by increasing sensitivity of cells (muscle and fat) to insulin. The two medications in this class are rosiglitazone (Avandia) and pioglitazone (Actos). Benefits of this class include a once daily dosing schedule and a decent decrease in blood glucose levels; this may take up to 12 weeks to reach the maximum effectiveness. There has also been an advantage identified in regard to cholesterol. Actos appears to increase high-density lipoprotein (HDL) and lower triglycerides. However, a 2010 report on drug trials with Avandia indicated a link to an increased risk of heart attack and stroke. Currently, Avandia is no longer being prescribed. If a thiazolidinedione is desired, Actos would be a more appropriate option. In June of 2011, the Food and Drug Administration (FDA) announced a warning of the increased risk of bladder cancer with the use of Actos. Along with these life-threatening side effects, this class of medications is contraindicated in anyone with impaired hepatic function or heart failure. Fluid retention and weight gain have also been associated with these medicines. Weight gain is typically about 12 lb (5.4 kg) to 15 lb (6.8 kg). Although, once thought of as a first-line medication option, these medications need to be used with caution in patients who are not responding to other agents before considering their use (Durso, 2006; Joslin Diabetes Center, n.d.).

Table 9.1 summarizes the major hypoglycemic agents in each drug classification.

The use of insulin therapy should not be viewed as a punishment or used as a threat to increase compliance in patients. Rather, upon diagnosing and educating patients about diabetes, the inevitable need for insulin therapy should be discussed. The majority of patients with type 2 diabetes will eventually require insulin use as their disease progresses. Insulin has delivery options that include injectable and inhaled, but the most commonly used is injectable. Alternatives to injectable insulin include pens, pumps, and the traditional syringe/vial. Insulin options available include rapid-acting, short-acting, intermediate-acting, long-acting, and premixed or combination insulins, which are listed in Table 9.2 (Durso, 2006; Joslin Diabetes Center, n.d.; National Guidelines Clearinghouse, n.d.).

TABLE 9.1 · Oral/Noninsulin Injectable Dosing Chart

Class	Medication	Dosing	Common Side Effect/ Considerations
Sulfonylurea	Glimepiride—Amaryl Glyburide—Diabeta Glipizide—Glucotrol	1–4 mg q.d. Max 8 mg/day 1.25–20 mg q.d. Max 20 mg q.d. 5–10 mg q.d. Max 40 mg q.d.	Hypoglycemia, monitor blood glucose levels
Meglitinides	Repaglinide—Prandin Nateglinide—Starlix	0.5–4 mg t.i.d.–q.i.d. with meals 60–120 mg t.i.d. with meals	Monitor liver and kidney functions
Biguanides	Glucophage— Metformin	500 mg b.i.d. to t.i.d. Max 2,500 mg/day	Nausea, diarrhea, bloating, usually decrease with time
Thiazolidinediones	Rosiglitazone—Actos Pioglitazone—Avandia	2–8 mg b.i.d. or q.d. Max 8 mg q.d. 15–45 mg q.d. Max 45 mg q.d.	Edema, fluid retention, CHF, weight gain, Actos increases risk of bladder cancer
Alpha glucosidase inhibitor	Acarbose—Precose	25 mg t.i.d. with meals max 50–100 mg t.i.d.	Abdominal pain, flatulence, and diarrhea most common
DPP4 inhibitors	Sitagliptin—Januvia Saxagliptin—Onglyza Linagliptin—Tradjenta	50–100 mg q.d. 2.5–5mg q.d. 5 mg q.d.	Dose adjustment needed for creatinine clearance <50 (except with Tradjenta) Risk of pancreatitis
GLP-1 agonists	Byetta Victoza	5–10 mcg b.i.d. 60 min prior to meal 0.6–1.8 mg	Nausea, vomiting, diarrhea—these diminish with time May contribute to medullary thyroid carcinoma

There are many formulas for the initiation of insulin therapy and when and how to add insulin therapy for individuals who are not at their goal. The recent trend is to initiate insulin sooner than later as second- or third-line therapy and typically beginning with basal insulin. The initiation of basal insulin should begin with the formula of either 10 units or 0.1 to 0.25 unit/kg, and then add 1 unit/day until acceptable fasting plasma (blood) glucose (FPG) level is achieved, or if FPG is more than 180 add 6 units, 141 to 180 add 4 units, and 121 to 140 add 2 units. A good rule of thumb for the appropriate dose is when FPG is around 100 or they have reached 100 units of insulin. If HbA1C goal is not achieved with basal insulin, then it is necessary to add a bolus dose. This can be done through two options. The most common is adding fast acting insulin to the largest meal of the day. Start by adding 5 units and adding 2 units every 2 days to reach postprandial goal (see Table 9.3) or by counting carbohydrates for that meal and using the formula of 1 unit for each 50 mg/dl over the 2-hour postprandial goal in addition to 1 unit/15 g of carbohydrates consumed for that meal. Titrate by adding 1 unit/50 mg/dl over the postprandial goal every 2 days. If HbA1C levels are still not at goal, then adding a bolus to the next largest meal would be appropriate. Another option is to initiate premix insulin, which is 70/30 or 75/25. A formula for using a premix is 0.3 to 0.5 unit/kg/day divided into either two or three doses.

TABLE 9.2 · Insulin Chart

Types of Insulin	Onset/Peak/Duration	Usage

Rapid-acting insulins
  Apidra—insulin glulisine
  Humalog—insulin aspart
  NovoLog—insulin lispro
	15 min/30 min—1 hr/3–5 hr
	15 min/30 min—1 hr/4–5 hr
	5–10 min/1–3 hr/3–5 hr
		Bolus/mealtime insulin

Short-acting insulins
  Humulin R—regular insulin
  Novolin R—regular insulin
	30 min–1 hr/2–4 hr/5–7 hr
	30 min–1 hr/2–4 hr/5–7 hr
		Bolus/mealtime insulin

Intermediate-acting insulins
  Humulin N—NPH
  Novolin N—NPH
	1–2 hr/6–14 hr/18–24 hr	Basal/shorter duration

Long-acting insulins
  Lantus—insulin detemir
  Levemir—insulin glargine
	1 hr/peakless/up to 24 hr
	1 hr/peakless/up to 24 hr
		Basal

Premixed insulins
  NovoLog 70/30
  Humalog 75/25
  Humulin 70/30
  Novolin 70/30
	10–20 min/1–3 hr/up to 24 hr
	15–30 min/2–3 hr/14–24 hr
	30–60 min/2–5 hr/14–24 hr
	30–60 min/2–6 hr/14–24 hr
		Basal/bolus combined

If two doses are desired, give two thirds in the morning and one third in the evening, three doses are divided equally (Rodbard & Jellinger, 2010; Texas Diabetes Council—Algorithms & Guidelines, 2012).

There are two formulas to use for intense insulin therapy as follows:

- Basal and basal bolus: Start with 0.5 unit/kg/day for total dose and give 70% as basal and 30% as the bolus. The bolus can be given at the largest meal or divided up between all three meals.
- 80%–80% rule: Using the 0.5 unit/kg/day formula, use 80% of the dose for basal insulin, then 80% of that dose as fast acting or rapid insulin divided into three doses for each meal (Rodbard & Jellinger, 2010; Texas Diabetes Council—Algorithms & Guidelines, 2012).

TABLE 9.3 · Correlation of Blood Glucose Levels with HbA1C

HbA1C	Fasting Blood Glucose	2-Hr Postprandial
6	<110	<130
7	<120	<150
8	<140	<180

An example of the common methods used is demonstrated in the following scenario. A 65-year-old male whose weight is 340 lbs (154.5 kg) is currently taking Metformin and Onglyza, and HbA1C is 9.2, up from his previous reading of 8.6, FPGs are running around 220, and you want to add insulin therapy. You decide to add basal insulin and use the formula of 0.25 unit/kg (he weighs 155 kg) and start with 38 units and instruct him to increase by using the formula of FPG. After therapy initiation, his FPGs are running 160s, so he is to add 4 units and continue adding until he is at 100 units. Three months later he is back. At this time, he is taking 62 units/day because he stopped titrating. His FPGs are running around 200s and his HbA1C time is 8.9. You decide it is time to add a bolus insulin to dinner time using the following formula: He needs to take 1 unit/15 g of carbohydrates and 1 unit/50 mg/dl over the postprandial goal. His current blood glucose log shows that his postprandial blood sugars are running 200s after breakfast, 250s after lunch, and 300s after dinner. He typically eats 60 g of carbohydrates for dinner, which requires 4 units, and with a postprandial of 300 at dinner, you would add 2 to 3 units to get to the goal of less than 180, which is calculated into a total of 7 units as bolus insulin at dinner time as a starting dose and can then be titrated by adding 1 unit for every 50 mg/dl over the postprandial goal of less than 180 every 2 days.

Surgical Therapy

Currently, there are two surgical interventions that are available for the treatment of diabetes. The first is gastric bypass surgery, which has demonstrated some promising results with near instantaneous reversal of hyperglycemia. Like all treatments, this should be used with caution; there are risks of postoperative complications that can be lifelong. Obese individuals who are considered for this option should undergo a preoperative evaluation that includes meeting with a psychiatrist, nutritionist, surgeon, and their primary care physician. Weight loss during this period is encouraged to ensure the motivation of the candidate. Lifestyle changes are imperative along with surgery to prevent future regaining of the weight after surgery. Surgical intervention may be able to offer the older adult many benefits, most importantly weight loss in the obese, a decrease in cardiovascular risks, and decrease or reverse diabetes. This option should be weighed against other treatment options, particularly in the presence of comorbidities that eliminate the individual from being a surgical candidate (Hamza et al., 2010; Morinigo et al., 2007). The other surgical intervention is pancreas transplant. Most commonly, this therapy is indicated for patients with type 1 diabetes mellitus, with 90% being combined pancreas–renal transplants. The success rate has been encouraging, but there have been few such transplants in older adults to date. This option has risks; the usual risk of surgical complications and the risks associated with lifelong immunosuppressant needed.

Complementary Therapy

In addition to medications, there are many complementary and alternative options in the treatment of diabetes. Supplements and over the counter medications should be used with caution. Herbs can contain unknown complex components. Many times, consumers believe that because herbs and dietary supplements are natural, they are safe to use even at higher than recommended doses. Some supplements can affect liver or kidney function. Additionally, these supplements are not regulated like medications by the FDA, so different brands/types may have different concentrations. Thus, it is important to educate patients about possible complications and drug–herb/supplement interactions with the use of supplements, to teach them to read labels carefully, and to know the amount of active ingredient in the product they are taking. It may be beneficial to get a consultation with a reliable complementary physician or use a reliable resource, and when starting medications, start with the smallest effective dose to identify allergic reaction. Common dietary supplements include cinnamon, grapefruit, garlic, onion, almonds, fenugreek, apple cider vinegar, coffee, and turmeric. Many of these supplements have been studied in lab animals and lack sufficient evidence of efficacy in humans, but some studies suggest that they may be beneficial. It is believed that these dietary supplements can increase insulin sensitivity, stimulate insulin production, and inadvertently lower blood sugar (National Center for Complementary and Alternative Medicine [NCCAM], n.d.; NDIC, n.d.; Schoenberg et al., 2004).

Omega 3 fatty acids have been shown to be effective in lowering blood glucose levels, as well as in helping prevent and treat diabetic peripheral neuropathy. They also play a role in improving cholesterol by increasing HDL and decreasing triglycerides. These include flax seed, alpha lipoic acid, and fish oil. Omega 3 fatty acids are high in antioxidants and theoretically these bind to or attack free radicals that are known to cause tissue damage. In addition, they also display anti-inflammatory properties. Chromium and polyphenols' effects have been studied to determine their role in the treatment of diabetes. They both display similar results that suggest they are highly effective in lab animals, but human trials have mixed results. Again, it is imperative to assess all medications and supplements your patients are taking for possible interactions and side effects, and to become familiar with possible hepatic or renal manifestations these supplements may have (NCCAM, n.d.; NDIC, n.d.; Schoenberg et al., 2004).

Monitoring and Managing of Diabetes

Management of chronic disease such as diabetes requires continuous monitoring along with medical treatment. This includes routine lab work and examination to monitor the effectiveness of therapy and development of side effects and prevent diabetes-related complications. Monitoring begins with checking blood glucose levels at home and keeping a log of these values. It is recommended that routine follow-up occur every 3 to 4 months for routine blood work and physical exam. During the exam, important assessment points include vision exam; foot exam; and assess for decreased sensation, numbness, or tingling. Blood work that is monitored during routine exams includes an HbA1C, complete metabolic panel, a lipid profile every 3 months, and a microalbumin yearly. Patients are encouraged to have a yearly comprehensive eye exam to evaluate for retinopathy and a comprehensive foot exam to evaluate for any potential problems, including wounds, decreased circulation, decreased sensation, and diabetic neuropathy. Additional routine care includes dental exam every 6 months and maintaining current immunizations, including pneumonia vaccine and yearly flu immunizations to prevent illness. The following chart displays the recommended tests and timeframes. Creating or providing a log for your patients to use in order to document and follow their progress is a good way to promote self-care in your patients (Table 9.4) (Durso, 2006; Joslin Diabetes Center, n.d.).

Cultural Considerations

Cultural factors should be taken into consideration for the treatment plan of all patients as well as those with diabetes. A comprehensive dietary evaluation must be completed in order to identify problem areas and develop a dietary plan that will work within the realms of the individual's

TABLE 9.4 · Routine Testing and Recommendations

Test	Recommended Frequency
HbA1C	Every 3–6 months
Microalbumin	Yearly
Cholesterol panel—including total cholesterol, HDL, LDL, and triglycerides	Every 3–6 months
Comprehensive foot exam	Yearly
Brief foot exam	Every visit
Diabetic eye exam	Yearly
Blood glucose self-monitoring	Daily—how many times depends on disease progression
Dental exam	Every 6 months
Flu vaccine	Yearly
Pneumonia vaccine	Every 5 years unless using Prevnar 13, which is currently a one-time dose for individuals over age 50

normal diet. An evaluation of the types of activities the individual enjoys is important in order to encourage exercise. Adjusting the treatment plan according to identified cultural beliefs in regard to medications will increase adherence. Acculturation should be assessed as well to determine how much mainstream culture plays a role in a person's health care (Mooradian et al., 1999).

During the review of Healthy People 2020, there were enormous health care disparities and poor health outcomes related to diabetes among ethnic groups. These include African, Asian, Hispanic, and Native Americans. Overall, health care providers have done a poor job of addressing the needs of these ethnic groups and the barriers that prevent them from quality health care compared with their Caucasian counterpart. In order to deliver culturally competent care, the barriers that prevent ethnic groups from obtaining health care need to be identified and understood by the provider. These include spiritual/religious beliefs, cultural beliefs regarding health care, literacy level, language barriers, family dynamics, financial situation, daily activities, and current living situation (Mooradian et al., 1999).

Western medicine tends to be ethnocentric. Providers have been doing a good job of educating patients but a poor job of assessing their unique needs. There is always a reason for a patient to be "noncompliant"; the inquisitive provider can overcome the obstacles that may cause noncompliance. Occasionally, noncompliance is as simple as an individual's decision not to agree with the prescribed treatment because of the conflict of cultural belief. Some common cultural considerations among the following ethnicities when developing a plan for the treatment of diabetes in the older adult are as follows:

- **African Americans:** Diets tend to be high in fat with fried foods and corn. Incorporating traditional foods with modified recipes may be beneficial. Patients may distrust traditional medicine, are leery of treatments, have decreased access to health care, feel that they have no control over health, and have a greater tendency to leave their health in the "hands of the lord" or their faith.

- **Asian Americans:** The risk of diabetes occurs at a lower body mass index (BMI) than other ethnicities (BMI, 23 vs. 25). There is often a tendency to put family obligations before self. There is an increased incidence of renal disease in this population. Again, there may be distrust in western medicine, which might play into the willingness to take traditional and/or complementary therapy over western medicine.
- **Hispanic/Latino Americans:** The traditional diet is low in fat and high in fiber, but has been modified over recent years. There is a respect for hierarchy and placing family needs and priorities first. There is a tendency to believe in good/evil spirits affecting well-being. There are higher rates of nephropathy, retinopathy, and peripheral vascular complications. Hispanic individuals place high value on herbal remedies and other natural treatments, often believing that emotional health and physical health are entwined with each other. There is decreased access to providers.
- **Native Americans/Alaskan Americans:** Traditionally, healing of illness and disease are carried out by a healer with ceremonies and rituals performed as part of healing. As a result of historical events, older adults often mistrust the health care system. There is a focus on recreating traditional dietary fare, which includes fruits, vegetables, lamb, venison, and buffalo, soups and stews. One-on-one demonstration is often more effective than printed materials for disease education (Mooradian et al., 1999).

Individuals from all cultures should receive individualized care. Having knowledge of different cultures is important in treating patients of different ethnicities and culture, and it should not be assumed that all individuals, or a particular ethnicity, have the same beliefs. All cultures are heterogeneous, and the provider will find that some individuals hold on to traditional beliefs and others are more acculturated. The importance of a thorough assessment cannot be overemphasized in developing a treatment plan (Mooradian et al., 1999).

PATIENT EDUCATION

Patient education is important in keeping patients informed of their disease process and one of the best ways to control diabetes and delay progression. There are many resources available to provide patients with information, but first an assessment of their knowledge and willingness to learn is important.

Monitoring blood glucose is important in diabetes self-management. How often patients check their blood sugar is going to depend on the degree to which their disease has advanced. Individuals who are stable might be able to monitor their blood sugar no more than once daily. As insulin is introduced or the patient is hospitalized, monitoring may need to occur up to four times per day. Assessing patients' needs is important when choosing a monitor appropriate for them. Many older adults have decreased vision and hearing, choosing a monitor with large print or even one that verbally announces the reading may be a better choice. Once a monitor has been chosen, patients should be advised when and how often to check their blood glucose level is important. Do not assume that when they are told to check it daily, they will check at an appropriate time. It is wise to suggest to the patient that they should check the blood sugar at various times, rotating from fasting to before meals, 2 hours postprandial and before bedtime. This will provide a better overview of blood glucose levels throughout the day. It is very important for them to log their blood sugars along with the time of day. Patients should be encouraged to bring their log with them during each provider visit. Most monitors also have a function to store a log of blood glucose levels, and thus bringing their monitor to each visit may be an alternative solution to keeping written logs. Free log books from drug companies that promote diabetic products are available to give to patients (BD Diabetes Education Center, n.d.; Haas & Burke, 2010; Kocurek, 2009; Pham, 2005; Sigal, 2006).

Teaching insulin administration can be daunting and time consuming, but proper technique and a patient's comfort level will increase compliance with insulin therapy. Starting insulin in the office allows the patient to ask questions and become comfortable with the process. Insulin pens have made this transition easier as patients can count the clicks to dial up the units to be given. For those patients who are not able to obtain pens because of lack of insurance, using the syringe/vial method may be necessary. Make sure these patients are aware of the importance of getting rid of any bubbles present in the syringe as these may displace part of the prescribed dose. The proper disposal of needles is necessary to address in order to reduce possible injuries to caregivers or public waste workers. All syringes, needles, or lancets should be placed in a heavy-duty plastic container, such as laundry detergent bottle or bleach bottle. It is important that patients use a container that needles would not be able to penetrate. Disposal instructions should be obtained from the local waste facility in the patient's area as instructions vary from facility to facility.

Diabetes management in the older adult includes lifestyle modification: a diet low in fat, low in simple sugars, and high in fiber, as well as daily exercise. Patient education on lifestyle modification is essential to bring optimal patient adherence and achieve optimal diabetes control. This sounds simple, but in the older adult, there are often factors that might make exercise more difficult. In addition to the potential for challenges with access to gyms, older adults often have comorbid musculoskeletal conditions, which make exercise difficult. Increasing activity is important for the older adult; however, providers should consider the above challenges in older adults against physical activities. Increasing activity should be planned with a gradual process starting with 5 to 10 minutes/day, then increasing by small increments but at least 5 minutes/week until they are at the goal of 30 minutes/day. This can be 30 minutes of any activity that increases heart rate. Assessing for types of activity is important; no one is going to do an activity that is not enjoyable to them for any length of time. A gym membership is not necessary to increase activity. Heart rate can be elevated by doing exercises in a chair for those who have limited mobility. There are DVDs or computer-based programs to assist with chair exercises. As a provider, you can recommend some easy exercises that can be done without a DVD or exercise tape. These may include leg lifts, marching in place, using some light weights for bicep curls, triceps exercises, and overhead presses. Walking is one of the best activities to get the heart rate up and has many other health benefits, including decreasing risk of osteoporosis. Another helpful activity is water aerobics; this is particularly beneficial for the older adult with joint pain as being in the water can relieve the pressure on joints.

Compliance with diet can be difficult as older adults may not have as much choice in meal preparation or consistency. Meals are commonly prepared by caregivers, community service organizations, or restaurants. It takes some creative solutions to overcome identified barriers. Dietary obstacles may be harder to overcome, but some recommendations to make are lean proteins such as eggs, chicken, turkey, fish, and lean cuts of beef and pork. Nuts are a good snack as they have many health benefits such as improving cholesterol, and they are high in protein. If fresh fruits and vegetables are not obtainable, advise frozen varieties as an alternative. Frozen vegetables can be prepared quickly and easily and do not spoil as quickly as fresh fruits and vegetables do. Processed foods should be avoided if possible (BD Diabetes Education Center, n.d.; Haas & Burke, 2010; Kocurek, 2009; Pham, 2005; Sigal, 2006).

Resources available for patients regarding their diabetes are bountiful; some of these programs/resources are listed below. There are multiple programs that address routine care, meal planning, carb counting, medications, questions, and answers.

REFERENCES

Ahtiluoto, S., Polvikoski, T., Peltonen, M., Solomon, A., Tuomilehto, J., Winblad, B., & Kivipelto, M. (2010). Diabetes, Alzheimer disease, and vascular dementia: A population-based neuropathologic study. *Neurology, 75*(13), 1195–1202.

American Diabetes Association. (2012). Retrieved from http://www.diabetes.org/

BD Diabetes Education Center. (n.d.). Diabetes Learning Center. Retrieved from http://bd.com/us/diabetes/page .aspx?cat=7001

Biessels, G., Staekenborg, S., Brunner, E., Brayne, C., & Scheltens, P. (2006). Risk of dementia in diabetes mellitus: A systematic review. *Lancet Neurology, 5*(1), 64–74.

Centers for Disease Control and Prevention. (2012, January 10). 2011 National diabetes fact sheet. Retrieved from http://www.cdc.gov/diabetes/pubs/factsheet11.htm

Chau, D., & Edelman, S. (2001). Clinical management of diabetes in the elderly. *Clinical Diabetes, 19*(4), 172–175.

Cigolle, C. T., Blaum, C. S., & Halter, J. B. (2009). Diabetes and cardiovascular disease prevention in older adults. *Clinics in Geriatric Medicine, 25*(4), 607–641.

Clinical Geriatrics. (n.d.). Pathophysiology of diabetes in the elderly. Retrieved from http://www.clinicalgeriatrics.com/ articles/Pathophysiology-Diabetes-Elderly

DiabetesCare.net. (n.d.). Diabetes resource for patients and providers. Retrieved from http://www.diabetescare.net/ index_provider.asp?ut=providers

Durso, S. C. (2006). Using clinical guidelines designed for older adults with diabetes mellitus and complex health status. *JAMA: The Journal of the American Medical Association, 295*(16), 1935–1940.

Gambert, S., & Pinkstaff, S. (2006). Emerging epidemic: Diabetes in older adults—Demography, economic impact and pathophysiology. *Diabetes Spectrum, 19*(4), 121–128.

Geiss, L., Pan, L., Cadwell, B., Gregg, E., Benjamin, S., & Engelgau, M. (2006). Changes in incidence of diabetes in U.S. adults, 1997–2003. *American Journal of Preventive Medicine, 30*(5), 371–377.

Giorda, C. B., Avogaro, A., Maggini, M., Lombardo, F., Mannucci, E., Turco, S., … Ferrannini, E. (2007). Incidence and risk factors for stroke in type 2 diabetic patients: The DAI study. *Stroke, 38*(4), 1154–1160.

Haas, L., & Burke, S. (2010). Diabetes prevention 101: Small and simple changes prevent type 2 diabetes. *Journal on Active Aging, 9*(3), 57–62.

Hamza, N., Abbas, M., Darwish, A., Shafeek, Z., New, J., & Ammori, B. (2010). Predictors of remission of type 2 diabetes mellitus after laparoscopic gastric banding and bypass. *Surgery for Obesity and Related Diseases, 6*(2), 228.

Herman, W. H., Hoerger, T. J., Brandle, M., Hicks, K., Sorensen, S., Zhang, P., … Ratner, R. E. (2005). The cost effectiveness of lifestyle modification or metformin in preventing type 2 diabetes in adults with impaired glucose tolerance. *Annals of Internal Medicine, 142*(5), 323–332. Retrieved from NIH Public Access.

Hogan, P., Dall, T., & Nikolov, P. (2003). Economic costs of diabetes in the U.S. in 2002. *Diabetes Care, 26*(3), 917–932.

Joslin Diabetes Center. (n.d.). *Joslin clinical guidelines.* Retrieved from http://www.joslin.org/joslin_clinical_ guidelines.html

Kilbourne, A. M. (2005). How does depression influence diabetes medication adherence in older patients? *American Journal of Geriatric Psychiatry, 13*(3), 202–210.

Kocurek, B. (2009). Promoting medication adherence in older adults . . . and the rest of us. *Diabetes Spectrum, 22*(2), 80–84.

Lustman, P., & Clouse, R. (2005). Depression in diabetic patients: The relationship between mood and glycemic control. *Journal of Diabetes and Its Complications, 19*(2), 113–122.

Lustman, P. J., Griffith, L. S., Freedland, K. E., & Clouse, R. E. (1997). The course of major depression in diabetes. *General Hospital Psychiatry, 19*(2), 138–143.

McCance, K. L., & Huether, S. E. (2005). *Pathophysiology: The biologic basis for disease in adults & children.* St. Louis, MO: Elsevier Mosby.

Mooradian, A. D., McLaughlin, S., Boyer, C. C., & Winter, J. (1999). Diabetes care for older adults. *Diabetes Spectrum, 12*(2), 70–77. Retrieved from http://journal.diabetes.org/diabetesspectrum/99v12n2/pg70.htm

Morinigo, R., Casamitjana, R., Delgado, S., Lacy, A., Deulofeu, R., Conget, I., … Vidal, J. (2007). Insulin resistance, inflammation, and the metabolic syndrome following Roux-en-Y gastric bypass surgery in severely obese subjects. *Diabetes Care, 30*(7), 1906–1908.

Munshi, M. (2006). Cognitive dysfunction is associated with poor diabetes control in older adults. *Diabetes Care, 29*(8), 1794–1799.

National Center for Complementary and Alternative Medicine. (n.d.). Diabetes and CAM: A focus on dietary supplements [Home page]. Retrieved from http://nccam.nih.gov/health/diabetes/CAM-and-diabetes.htm

National Diabetes Education Program. (2012). NDEP translates the latest science and spreads the word that diabetes is serious, common, and costly, yet controllable and, for type 2, preventable. Retrieved from http://www.ndep.nih.gov/

National Diabetes Information Clearinghouse. (n.d.). Complementary and alternative medical therapies for diabetes. Retrieved from http://diabetes.niddk.nih.gov/dm/pubs/alternativetherapies/

Norris, S. L., Kansagara, D., Bougatsos, C., & Fu, R. (2008). Screening adults for type 2 diabetes: A review of the evidence for the U.S. Preventive Services Task Force. *Annals of Internal Medicine, 148*(11), 855–868.

Pham, H. H. (2005). Delivery of preventive services to older adults by primary care physicians. *JAMA: The Journal of the American Medical Association, 294*(4), 473–481.

Rodbard, H. W., & Jellinger, P. S. (2010). The American Association of Clinical Endocrinologists/American College of Endocrinology (AACE/ACE) algorithm for managing glycaemia in patients with type 2 diabetes mellitus: Comparison with the ADA/EASD algorithm. *Diabetologia, 53*(11), 2458–2460.

Sahyoun, N. R., Anderson, A. L., Tylavsky, F. A., Lee, J. S., Sellmeyer, D. E., & Harris, T. B. (2008). Dietary glycemic index and glycemic load and the risk of type 2 diabetes in older adults. *American Journal of Clinical Nutrition, 87*, 126–131.

Sander, D., Sander, K., & Poppert, H. (2008). Review: Stroke in type 2 diabetes. *British Journal of Diabetes & Vascular Disease, 8*(5), 222–229.

Schoenberg, N. E., Stoller, E. P., Kart, C. S., Perzynski, A., & Chapleski, E. E. (2004). Complementary and alternative medicine use among a multiethnic sample of older adults with diabetes. *Journal of Alternative and Complementary Medicine, 10*(6), 1061–1066.

Sigal, R. J. (2006). Physical activity/exercise and type 2 diabetes: A consensus statement from the American Diabetes Association. *Diabetes Care, 29*(6), 1433–1438.

Strachan, M. J., Reynolds, R. M., Frier, B. M., Mitchell, R. J., & Price, J. F. (2008). The relationship between type 2 diabetes and dementia. *British Medical Bulletin, 88*(1), 131–146.

Texas Diabetes Council—Algorithms & Guidelines. (2012). Retrieved from http://www.tdctoolkit.org/algorithms_and_guidelines.asp

CHAPTER 9: IT RESOURCES

Websites

American Diabetes Association
  www.diabetes.org
Center for Disease Control's Division of Diabetes Translation
  www.cdc.gov/diabetes

The Physicians Committee for Responsible Medicine (PRCM) provides online access to diabetes resources including Nutrition and Cooking Classes; Food for Life TV Webcasts; Diabetes Success Stories; Patient Help; Fact Sheets and Recipes; Scientific Support; Frequently Asked Questions
    www.pcrm.org/health/diabetes-resources/
National Diabetes Education Program
    http://ndep.nih.gov/resources/
National Diabetes Education Initiative
    http://www.ndei.org/
National Diabetes Information Clearinghouse
    http://diabetes.niddk.nih.gov/dm/pubs/statistics/
Drug Company sponsored programs
Merck—Journey for Control
    http://www.journeyforcontrol.com
Novo Nordisk—Cornerstones4Care
    www.cornerstones4care.com
Astra Zeneca and Bristol Myers Squibb—Type2talk
    www.thetype2talk.com/home/aboutus
Sanofi Aventis—A1c Champion Program
    http://www.a1cchampions.com/
Glaxo Smith Kline
    www.diabetes.com
Sharps disposal
    www.epa.gov/epaoswer/other/medical
Screening Adults for Type 2 Diabetes: A Review of the Evidence for the U.S. Preventive Services Task Force
    http://www.uspreventiveservicestaskforce.org/uspstf08/type2/type2art.htm
The following items are available on the PCRM website:
    Diet and Diabetes: Recipes for Success (patient)
    http://www.pcrm.org/search/?cid=129
A fact sheet from Physicians Committee for Responsible Medicine that covers: Diabetes Basics, Dietary Approaches to Diabetes and The New Dietary Approach to Diabetes which includes a four step process: (1) Begin a Vegan Diet: Avoid Animal Products; (2) Avoid Added Vegetable Oils and Other High-Fat Foods; (3) Favor Foods with a Low Glycemic Index; (4) Go High Fiber.
Help Your Patients: Diabetes Resources for Health Care Professionals (patient)
    http://www.pcrm.org/search/?cid=181
Provides printable Patient Education Fact Sheets including: Recipes for Success in English and Spanish; Patient Education Booklets of Vegetarian Starter Kits in English and Spanish; Continuing Education information and book resources

Videos

Tackling Diabetes Part 1 (2011) (14:22 minutes)
    http://youtu.be/oCqCls72amQ

Tackling Diabetes Part 2 (2011) (14:37 minutes)
  http://youtu.be/gFrIDYEEslY
Tackling the Diabetes Epidemic (9:21 minutes)
  http://youtu.be/gFrIDYEEslY
Type 1 Diabetes (2009)
  Dr. Barnard discusses the causes of type 2 diabetes and the current diabetes epidemic. He also
  outlines a healthy plant-based menu that will help you prevent and reverse type 2 diabetes.
  (7:25 minutes)
  http://youtu.be/1nFigsE3Wbk
A New Approach to Type 2 Diabetes (2010)
  Dr. Barnard gives an overview of how insulin is made. He also explains that type 1 diabetes is
  caused when the body produces no insulin. Dr. Barnard also outlines how people already diagnosed with type 1 diabetes can cut down on diabetes complications by eating foods that are
  vegan, low in fat, and have a low glycemic index. (9:48 minutes)
  http://youtu.be/q9UVufDQw-k
The Glycemic Index Lowdown (2010)
  Dr. Barnard explains the glycemic index—a handy tool that lets you know which are the best
  carbohydrate-containing foods. It shows what foods cause blood sugar to rise rapidly compared to those that cause it to rise gently. It's a useful tool for managing diabetes and boosting
  your energy with low-glycemic index foods that cause your blood sugars to rise gently.
  (6:10 minutes)
  http://youtu.be/-AxazN-Vgag

Podcasts (Audio Only)

Preventing Type 2 Diabetes (2010)
  This podcast discusses CDC's work to prevent type 2 diabetes and to reduce complications
  of diabetes. It also focuses on establishing lifestyle intervention programs for overweight or
  obese people at high risk of developing diabetes. Created by: National Center for Chronic
  Disease and Health Promotion (NCCDPHP), Division of Diabetes Translation (DDT)
  (2:12 minutes)
  http://www2c.cdc.gov/podcasts/player.asp?f=6052565
Diabetes Awareness (2009)
  Diabetes is one of the most debilitating diseases in the U.S., affecting nearly 24 million people.
  If it isn't well managed, diabetes can lead to a number of complications, including blindness,
  kidney failure, loss of limbs through amputation, and even death. In this podcast Nilka Rios
  Burrows discuss ways to prevent and control diabetes. Created by: MMWR; Series Name: A
  Cup of Health with CDC (4:49 minutes)
  http://www2c.cdc.gov/podcasts/player.asp?f=359263
Depression and Diabetes in Older Women (2009)
  This women's health podcast focuses on the association between diabetes and depression in
  older women and the importance of getting help when feeling depressed. Created by: Office
  of Women's Health (OWH) and National Center for Chronic Disease Prevention and Health
  Promotion (NCCDPHP) (4:09 minutes)
  http://www2c.cdc.gov/podcasts/player.asp?f=11419

Preventing Vision Loss in Diabetes—Summary (2008)

This podcast is for a professional audience and briefly discusses how to prevent vision loss in people with diabetes. Created by: National Center for Chronic Disease Prevention and Health Promotion (NCCDPHP), Division of Diabetes Translation (DDT), National Diabetes Education Program (NDEP) (1:29 minutes)

http://www2c.cdc.gov/podcasts/player.asp?f=9408

Healthy Feet are Happy Feet (2007)

This podcast offers tips for people with diabetes on foot care to prevent complications, such as foot ulcers and amputation. Created by: National Center for Chronic Disease Prevention and Health Promotion (NCCDPHP), Division of Diabetes Translation (DDT) (2:23 minutes)

http://www2c.cdc.gov/podcasts/player.asp?f=7240

It's Never too Late to Prevent Diabetes (2007)

http://www2c.cdc.gov/podcasts/player.asp?f=7185

This podcast delivers a diabetes prevention message tailored for older adults. Created by: National Center for Chronic Disease Prevention and Health Promotion (NCCDPHP), Division of Diabetes Translation (DDT) (1:20 minutes)

Tips for Helping a Person with Diabetes (2007)

http://www2c.cdc.gov/podcasts/player.asp?f=6915

This podcast gives suggestions for helping a person with diabetes manage the disease. Created by: National Center for Chronic Disease Prevention and Health Promotion (NCCDPHP), Division of Diabetes Translation (DDT) (3:01 minutes)

Nutrition

Nancy Munoz, DCN, MHA, RD, LDN
Melissa Bernstein, PhD, RD, LD

INTRODUCTION

Nutritional well-being has a significant impact on physiological aging and health-related quality of life as a person ages. Eating a nutritious diet, maintaining a healthy body weight and a physically active lifestyle are key factors in helping individuals to lead a healthy life as they age. Five out of the eight most common causes of death in adults 65 years of age and older have a known nutritional influence (Centers for Disease Control and Prevention [CDC], n.d.-e). Eating is an essential part of everyday life and an important pleasure and social element at every age. As the number of older adults grows, and those reaching old age live longer, preventative health and nutrition becomes increasingly important for keeping individuals healthy, independent, and community dwelling.

PHYSIOLOGICAL CHANGES WITH AGE THAT AFFECT NUTRITION

Physiological age-related changes affect our nutritional needs and nutrient status. Nutrient status and nutritional intake, on the other hand, affect biologic aging. Therefore, as a person ages it becomes especially important to eat nutrient-dense, wholesome foods that contribute to health, quality of life, and well-being. There are many aspects of our lifestyle that contribute to a healthier old age that are modifiable. Food, exercise, smoking, and alcohol choices for example, affect not only our risk for chronic disease but also the rate at which we age. Nutrition is a key factor in promoting health and ability to function at advanced ages, as well as through its role in medical nutrition therapy for disease management (Position of the Academy of Nutrition and Dietetics, 2012). This chapter provides an overview of some of the biological and physiological changes and the nutritional implication of these changes that occurs with advancing age (Table 10.1).

TABLE 10.1 • Age-Related Changes and Nutrient Needs

Change in Body Composition or Physiologic Function	Impact on Nutrient Requirement
Decreased muscle mass	Decreased need for energy Increased need for high-quality protein
Decreased bone density	Increased need for calcium, vitamin D
Decreased immune function	Increased need for vitamin B_6, antioxidants, vitamin E, zinc, and high-quality protein
Increased gastric pH	Increased need for vitamin B_{12}, folic acid, calcium, iron, zinc
Decreased skin capacity for cholecalciferol synthesis	Increased need for vitamin D
Decreased skin recoil, thickness of the skin, and size of the rete ridges, vascularity and number of capillaries.	Increased protein with adequate calorie and fluid needs
Increased dry skin due to atrophy of sweat glands	Adequate amount of essential fatty acids
Decreased kidney ability to concentrate urine, constipation, and reduced thirst sensation	Increased fluid needs
Increased oxidative stress, cognitive impairment, cataracts and age-related macular degeneration	Increased need for antioxidants such as beta-carotene, vitamin C, vitamin E
Slowed gastric motility	Increased need for fiber

Changes in Body Weight and Body Composition

Body weight generally increases until the sixth decade of life (Bernstein & Luggen, 2010). Changes in body weight and composition, increases in body fat, and loss of lean muscle are significant health consequences for adults of all ages, and older adults in particular. The growing prevalence of overweight and obese older adults has resulted from poor food choices, consumption of a low quality diet with too many calories, and an inactive lifestyle (Federal Interagency Forum on Aging Related Statistics, 2010). Overweight older adults or those who gain weight with age have an increased risk of chronic diseases such as heart disease, diabetes, metabolic syndrome, and cancer (Bernstein & Luggen, 2010). Increases in body fat and loss of muscle mass lead to declining physical functioning, worsening health, and increased frailty, and interfere with the ability of the older adults to maintain independence in their normal daily activities. Voluntary weight loss in obese older adults has been shown to provide benefits to health, quality of life, and physical function (Zamboni et al., 2005). In contrast, thinness alone is not always a health advantage. Older adults may lose weight due to illness or depression. Unintentional weight loss and low body mass index (BMI) in old age often indicates underlying disease and is associated with poor health outcomes and is a marker for deterioration in well-being (Miller & Wolfe, 2008). Medical, pharmaceutical, social, economic, and environmental causes can contribute to unintentional weight loss in older adults.

Sarcopenia, the loss of skeletal muscle mass and strength, is a widespread problem that affects 8% to 40% of older adults over the age of 60 years and approximately 50% in those over 75 years old (Kim et al., 2010). Sarcopenia is a complex condition with many interrelated causes, often part of a vicious cycle that includes worsening of disease burden and illness, nutritional inadequacy, and increased disability, and functional dependence (Wernette et al., 2011). Interventions including optimizing nutritional intake, specifically adequate high-quality protein and antioxidants, along with progressive resistance strength training have been determined to be the most effective means to prevent and reverse sarcopenia (Boire, 2009; Chaput et al., 2007; Paddon-Jones et al., 2008).

The increasing prevalence of overweight and obesity in older adults mimics the trends seen in younger adults. Thirty-two percent of adults aged 65 years and older are classified as obese resulting from dietary excesses and poor food choices in combination with physical inactivity (Federal Interagency Forum on Aging Related Statistics, 2010). The growing number of older adults and longer life expectancy underscore the burden of ill health resulting from excess body weight and body fat and is likely to continue to increase in the older adult population. Obesity is a complex problem in older adults that contributes to increased morbidity and reduced quality of life. The combination of sarcopenia and obesity together is termed sarcopenic obesity.

Sarcopenic obesity results from the deterioration of muscle composition and quality in combination with increased fat mass (Rolland et al., 2009). A number of causes have been implicated in the etiology and pathophysiology of sarcopenic obesity, for example, excess energy intake, physical inactivity, low-grade inflammation, insulin resistance, and changes in hormonal environment, as well as peptides produced by adipose tissue (Houston et al., 2009; Rolland et al., 2009). Sarcopenic obesity worsens disability and is detrimental to physical functioning and health of older adults (Houston et al., 2009). In an effort to implement effective treatment and minimize the clinical impact of this condition, identification of older adults with sarcopenic obesity is clinically relevant and should become more widespread.

Should older adults be encouraged to lose weight? Adults who have medical conditions or functional impairments and would benefit from reduced body weight should be identified. Evidence suggests, however, that intentional weight loss in older adults results in loss of muscle even when excess fat mass is targeted. Loss of lean muscle mass correlates negatively with functional capacity for independent living (Berger & Doherty, 2010). Healthcare professionals must give careful consideration to whether the benefits of weight loss outweigh the risks (Stenholm et al., 2008). A comprehensive nutritional assessment, completed by a registered dietitian that takes into consideration existing comorbidities, weight history, and potential adverse health effects of excess body weight should be completed before beginning a weight loss program with an older adult (Vincent et al., 2010). Obese older adults for whom weight loss can be advantageous must be identified so that effective, supportive nutritional care, that promotes health and well-being can be provided (Position of the Academy of Nutrition and Dietetics, 2012). Goals of weight-loss treatment in older adults are to minimize adverse effects on nutritional status, preserve muscle and bone mass and reduce body weight and body fat under qualified medical supervision.

Olfactory Changes

In older adults, the taste threshold, the minimum amount of flavor needed for a person to detect taste, increases with age. Along with taste, the sense of smell diminishes, affecting how we choose and prepare foods. To make matters worse, older adults often use multiple medications that can alter taste, flavor perception, and appetite. Poor oral health, dentition, and problems with chewing and swallowing can impair the ability to eat a nutritious diet. Meats, fresh fruits, and fresh vegetables may be avoided because they are difficult to chew and swallow.

Gastrointestinal Changes

Gastrointestinal changes occurring along the length of the GI tract affect older adults. Beginning in the mouth, the production of saliva declines with age and can be a side effect from medication. Reduced digestive secretions lower the amount of nutrients older adults absorb from the foods. Reductions in the stomach secretions of hydrochloric acid and pepsin can alter the ability of the stomach to adequately digest foods. This can contribute to the development of atrophic gastritis, interfering with normal absorption of vitamin B_{12}, leading to a deficiency of this vitamin. While a reduction of lactase production is associated with aging, intolerance to milk and dairy products is less common than older adults.

Slowing of gastrointestinal motility with age, along with a diet low in fiber, and low fluid intake contribute to constipation (discussed later on in this chapter), one of the most common gastrointestinal conditions of older adults. Myths and misinformation about the gastrointestinal effects of various foods, among older adults and even among the medical community, may lead to unnecessary dietary restrictions and to inadequate nutrient intake.

Cardiovascular Changes

Anatomical changes include decrease in heart size, decrease in the size of the cavity in the left ventricle, and increase in the size of the left atrium. Heart valves become more rigid and thick as collagen deposits increase. Calcification in the aortic valves also takes place. The heart of an older adult has a decreased ability to utilize oxygen and does not tolerate physical stress such as increased blood pressure, fever, and strenuous exercise as well as a the younger counterpart (Larsen, 2008). In a healthy older adult, cardiac output can be adequate to meet the body's needs and allow continued physical activity as part of their lifestyle (Beers & Berkow, 2000). However, with aging, the heart rate decreases and end-diastolic as well as end-systolic volumes increase. Older adults are vulnerable to the development of heart failure (Larsen, 2008). Overweight and obesity as well as modifiable lifestyle choices such as poor diet as well as poor diet and physical inactivity place older adults at increased risk for heart disease. Physical activity is valuable for older adults, even those with difficulties executing activities of daily living like ascending stairs or walking (CDC, 2011b). Physical activity coupled with consuming a nutrient-dense diet is key in the prevention of cardiovascular disease.

Respiratory Changes

Lung function weakens with age. Decreased alveolar surface and progressive loss of elastic recoil in the lung tissue lessen the proficiency of gas exchange and make it arduous for older adults to exercise. Optimum breathing power and voluntary ventilation of the lungs also declines as part of the aging process (Larsen, 2008). As a result of these changes, an older adult has reduced ability to fully expire all the air that was inhaled, causing more residual air in the lungs at expiration, leading to a higher residual lung volume. In addition, maximum breathing capacity declines with age. Older adults, particularly those who are frail or malnourished, are more susceptible to pulmonary infections such as pneumonia, bronchitis, and tuberculosis as well as aspiration pneumonia (Bernstein & Luggen, 2010).

Integumentary System

Covering the entire body, the skin is the largest organ. Aside from serving as a protective buffer against heat, light, injury, and infection, the skin regulates body temperature, stores water and fat, and serves as a sensory organ (Baranoski & Ayello, 2012). The skin goes through textural changes as we age. The dermis thins and becomes more susceptible to skin tears. Thinning subcutaneous fatty layers accentuate bony prominences and increase the risk of pressure ulcers (PUs) in these areas. Skin loses elasticity as collagen decreases, and elastin loses its ability to recoil. The size of the rete ridges decreases as we age, allowing for easier separation of the epidermis from the dermis. With a reduction of sweat glands, we see drier skin that has much slower epidermal regeneration (Baranoski & Ayello, 2012).

Immune System Changes

After the age of 50, the functions carried out by the immune system begin to deteriorate. Changes in the immune system may cause the body to lose the ability to combat viruses, bacteria, and other foreign bodies. The clinical consequence of these changes translates into increased susceptibility to upper respiratory tract infections such as influenza, pneumonia, urinary tract infections, pressure sores, and foodborne illnesses. Physical barriers to infectious agents, foreign bodies, and chemicals such as the skin, the acid environment in the stomach, and swallowing and coughing reflexes decline as well.

Nutrition plays an important role in immune response. Inadequate consumption of macronutrients, vitamins, minerals, and some antioxidants can contribute to the age-related immune system dysregulation often seen in older adults. Decreased appetite, difficulty chewing, financial limitations, and potential for food allergies such as lactose intolerance contribute to reduced intake of meat, dairy products, and fresh fruits and vegetables, making it difficult for older adults to get all the calories, protein, and other important nutrients needed. Decreased nutrient intake can lead to impaired immunity, sarcopenia, reduced ability for wound healing, and osteoporosis.

Nervous System Changes

As we age, the brain and the nervous system go through natural variations. The number of nerve cells and the total weight of the brain and the spinal cord are reduced. Time for message processing may take a little longer (Health Central, n.d.). Changes in the nervous system can affect the senses and contribute to reduced or loss reflexes that can impact mobility and overall safety. Falls are a primary reason for fractures in older adults. Low vitamin D levels have been linked to increased risk of falling. The relationship between vitamin D and falls has not been fully defined. Falls can occur as a result of debilitated bones prone to spontaneous fractures or from other consequence of vitamin D on brain function, nerve health, or muscle strength (HealthinAging.org, n.d.).

Endocrine System Changes

The aging process is characterized by widespread reduction in hormone production and activity. The reduction in different hormone levels touches most metabolic functions of the body. These changes can cause alterations in water, mineral, electrolyte, carbohydrate, protein, lipid, and vitamin metabolism. Insulin resistance and development of glucose intolerance are common conditions in older adults, with important health consequences. Hyperinsulinemia may contribute to the incidence of vascular disease in older adults (Medline Plus, 2012).

With aging, thyroid hormone and estrogen hormone levels decrease. The reduction in estrogen level can impact bone metabolism and, in the presence of other risk factors, the development of osteoporosis (Medline Plus, 2012). Osteoporosis increases the risk of falls and injury in older adults.

Urinary System Changes

Changes commonly seen in the aging genitourinary system include decrease bladder capacity, enlarged prostate gland, alterations in pelvic support and diminished vaginal and cervical secretions. As a result of these changes, older adults can suffer from urinary incontinence, urethral obstruction, and pruritus (Beers & Berkow, 2000). Fluid intake can be affected, thus contributing to the risk of dehydration in older adults. The reduced ability of the kidneys to concentrate urine can also be an important factor contributing to dehydration in older adults.

Like other organs, the aging process affects both the structure and the function of the kidneys. As we age, the glomerular rate begins to decline by as much as 7% per decade, starting with the third decade of life. It is estimated that by the age of 60, the average person has lost approximately 25% of his or her kidney function. With aging, the blood vessels that transport blood to the kidney can become hardened, thus reducing the rate at which the kidneys filter blood (Weinstein & Anderson, 2010).

Kidneys are affected not only by the aging process, but also by illness, medications, and other conditions. Kidney changes in an older adult can impact the older adult's ability to concentrate water and maintain fluid balance. With age, older adults are at increased risk for acute and chronic kidney failure, bladder control issues and infections, and urinary system cancers such as prostate cancer (Weinstein & Anderson, 2010).

DIETARY GUIDELINES AND NUTRIENT REQUIREMENTS

Dietary Guidelines for Americans, 2010 provide recommendations for Americans aged 2 and older, including healthy older adults and those that are at increased risk for chronic diseases. The guidelines encourage Americans to emphasize the consumption of a healthy diet to obtain or maintain a healthy weight, promote health, and minimize disease risks. The guidelines reflect the latest research and scientific knowledge outlining the relationship between diet, health promotion, and disease prevention (United States Department of Agriculture [USDA] & U.S. Department of Health and Human Services [HHS], 2010).

Modifiable lifestyle choices such as poor diet and lack of physical activity are significant factors contributing to the obesity epidemic affecting older adults in similar patterns as younger individuals. Older adults are commonly affected and at higher risk of developing degenerative conditions associated with morbidity and mortality. The Dietary Guidelines for Americans encourage Americans at every age to balance caloric intake with physical activity to control weight. Selecting a healthier diet rich in vegetables, fruits, whole grains, fat-free and low-fat dairy products, and seafood poses additional challenges for older adults owing to social, economic, medical, and functional limitations. Choosing foods that are lower in sodium, saturated and trans fats, added sugars, and refined grains as well as increasing daily physical activity are additional guidelines that are underscored advancing age when choosing a nutrient-dense diet to meet nutritional requirements without too many calories becomes increasingly difficult. Good nutrition is essential to promoting health and well-being at any age, and therefore in effort to help Americans implement the Dietary Guidelines for Americans, the MyPlate eating pattern is intended to support individuals in making healthier food selections http://www.choosemyplate.gov.

MyPlate delivers the key messages from the *Dietary Guidelines for Americans, 2010* using a plate, a familiar everyday icon. Modifications to MyPlate to highlight the specific nutritional needs of older adults can be seen in the Modified MyPlate for Older adults (Fig. 10.1). The Tufts University version of MyPlate emphasizes the nutritional concerns of the older population, including various beverage choices to promote adequate hydration, socialization, physical activity and easy-to-prepare wholesome foods.

The *Dietary Guidelines for Americans* and MyPlate offer dietary guidance of whole foods and food groups rather than individual nutrient values; after all, foods are what we think about in planning our daily meals and shopping lists. A healthful diet is healthful, because of the balance

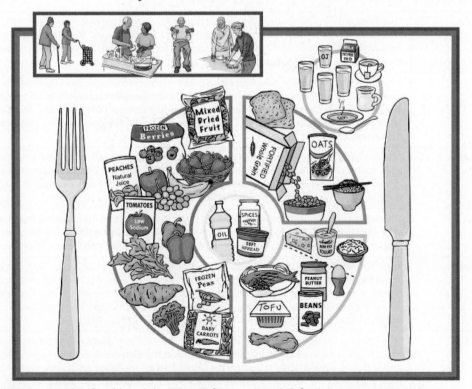

MyPlate for Older Adults

FIGURE 10.1. MyPlate for older adults. (From Tufts Now. [2011]. Tufts University nutrition scientists unveil MyPlate for older adults. Retrieved from http://now.tufts.edu/news-releases/tufts-university-nutrition-scientists-unveil-, with permission.)

of *nutrients* it contains. Dietary standards define healthful diets in terms of specific amounts of the nutrients. To assess nutritional adequacy, diet planners can compare the nutrient composition of their food plans to recommended intake values. The Dietary Reference Intakes, the DRIs, reflect intake levels for dietary adequacy and also for optimal nutrition recommended for healthy people. The DRIs are the dietary standards for the United States and Canada and serve as reference values for nutrient intakes to be used in assessing and planning diets, help the governments set nutrition policy and can also be used as a guide in the planning and evaluation of diets for groups and individuals. The DRIs include four basic groups (see Table 10.2): Estimated Average Requirement (EAR), Recommended Dietary Allowance (RDA), Adequate Intake (AI), and Tolerable Upper Intake Level (UL). In the DRI report on macronutrients, two other concepts were introduced: the Estimated Energy Requirement (EER) and the Acceptable Macronutrient Distribution Ranges (AMDRs) (Institute of Medicine [IOM], Food & Nutrition Board [FNB], 2005a). When dietary standards are used as comparison values for individual diets, this information should be interpreted with caution to ensure that the dietary intake data provide an accurate

TABLE 10.2 · Dietary Reference Intakes

DRI Value	Key Features
RDA	"The average daily dietary nutrient intake that is sufficient to meet the nutrient requirements of nearly all (97% to 98%) healthy individuals in a particular life stage and [sex] group" (IOM, FNB, 2006). People with consumption that meets the RDA most often have suitable intake. The RDA exceeds the requirements of most individuals (American Dietetic Association, 2011).
AI	"The recommended average daily intake level based on observed or experimentally determined approximations or estimates of nutrient intake by a group (or groups) of apparently healthy people that are assumed to be adequate; used when an RDA cannot be determined" (IOM, FNB, 2006). The RDA could not be defined for some nutrients due to the limited research on the nutrient individuals (American Dietetic Association, 2011).
EAR	"The average daily nutrient intake that is estimated to meet the requirement of half the healthy individuals in a particular life stage and [sex] group" (IOM, FNB, 2006). Very often, the desired level is based on consumption desired for an appropriate level of function instead of the amount required to avoid deficit and disease (American Dietetic Association, 2011).
UL	"The highest average daily nutrient intake level that is likely to pose no risk of adverse health effects to almost all individuals in the general population. As intake increases above the UL, the risk of adverse effects may increase" (IOM, FNB, 2006). The UL should not be surpassed (American Dietetic Association, 2011).
AMDR	The AMDR represents "a range of intakes for a particular energy source that is associated with reduced risk of chronic disease while providing adequate intakes of essential nutrients" (IOM, FNB, 2005a). AMDRs calculated as a percentage of total energy consumed have been defined for carbohydrate, protein, and total fat, n-3 and n6-6 polyunsaturated fatty acids. The goal is for both individuals and population to consume nutrients between the ranges defined (American Dietetic Association, 2011).
EER	"The EER is the average dietary energy intake that is predicted to maintain energy balance in healthy adults of defined age, weight, height, and level of physical activity consistent with good health. In children and pregnant and lactating women, the EER is taken to include the needs associated with the deposition of tissues or the secretion of milk at rates consistent with good health" (IOM, FNB, 2006). This is an initial step in planning appropriate energy intake. Body weight is a more suitable assessment parameter when determining energy intake (American Dietetic Association, 2011).

representation of the usual diet (dietary assessment is discussed below). An intake that is less than the RDA/AI doesn't necessarily mean deficiency; the individual requirement for a nutrient may be less than the RDA/AI value. You can use the RDA/AI values as targets for dietary intake, while avoiding nutrient intake that exceeds the UL; this is especially true when evaluating the diets of older adults.

POSITION OF THE ACADEMY OF NUTRITION AND DIETETICS: FOOD AND NUTRITION FOR OLDER ADULTS: PROMOTING HEALTH AND WELLNESS

It is the position of the Academy of Nutrition and Dietetics that all Americans aged 60 years and older receive appropriate nutrition care; have access to coordinated, comprehensive food and nutrition services; and receive the benefits of ongoing research to identify the most effective food and nutrition programs, interventions, and therapies. (Position of the Academy of Nutrition and Dietetics, 2012)

NUTRIENT NEEDS CHANGE WITH AGE

The aging process has an impact on the nutrient requirements of older adults. Changes in body composition and decrease in cardiac and respiratory function coupled with a limited ability for prolonged exercise may affect nutrient requirements. Understanding of the nutritional needs of older adults is increasing; however, research to define the specific needs of older adults is an area of significant investigation. Dietary recommendations for calories and some essential nutrients and food components, such as dietary fiber, have been identified in the DRIs (USDA, Food and Nutrition Information Center, 2010). The DRIs include the age groups of 51 to 70 years and over 70 years. The precise nutrient needs of an older adult at any age are multifactorial due to the diversity of this population group. The MyPlate for Older Adults icon shows the recommendations of the 2010 Dietary Guidelines for Americans and MyPlate primarily personalized for older adults by emphasizing subjects such as consuming adequate fluids, securing convenient, affordable and readily available foods and physical activity (Tufts Now, 2011).

A decrease in food intake in an older adult can have many undesirable effects. Older adults often have numerous medical conditions that require a change in nutrient intake as well as the use of various prescriptions and over-the-counter medications that can decrease food intake or modify digestion, absorption, metabolism, and excretion. Efforts to consume a healthy diet can be negatively impacted by social factors, economic hardships, functional limitations while shopping for or preparing foods, decreased mental ability, as well as alterations in taste perception, decreased olfactory ability, difficulty chewing and swallowing, and changes in digestion and absorption (Bernstein & Luggen, 2010). These factors may occur naturally with aging or as a result of illness or as a side effect of medication use. Changes in body composition or physiological function that occur with age may also influence nutritional requirements. Declines in muscle mass, bone density, immune function, and nutrient absorption and metabolism may interfere with the capability of older adults to meet nutritional needs especially when calorie needs are reduced. Nutrients of particular concern for older adults are reviewed in Table 10.3.

TABLE 10.3 · Nutrients of Particular Concern for Older Adults (51–70 years old)

Nutrient	DRI Value[a]	Key Functions[a]	Considerations for Older Adult[a]
Water	M: 3.7 L/day F: 2.7 L/day	Sustains homeostasis in the body and aids in moving nutrients to cells and elimination of waste products of metabolism.[a]	Sufficient fluids must be provided in efforts to prevent dehydration and its comorbidities.[a]
Fiber	M: 30 g/day F: 21 g/day	Improves laxation, decreases chance for coronary heart disease, supports maintaining glucose levels.[a]	Consuming too much fiber can cause gastrointestinal distress.[a]
Calcium	1,200 mg/day	With vitamin D, calcium is essential in promoting bone health.[a] It also plays an important role in blood clotting, muscle contraction, nerve transmission, and tooth formation.[a]	Consuming too much calcium from dietary sources can contribute to the development of kidney stones.[a]
Vitamin D	10 µg/day	With calcium, vitamin D is essential in promoting bone health.[a]	Excessive consumption of vitamin D can contribute to hypercalcemia, thus leading to diminished renal function and hypercalciuria, kidney failure, cardiovascular system failure, and calcification of soft tissues.[a] Deficiency can contribute to chronic conditions like osteoporosis.
Zinc	8 mg/day	Zinc is a constituent of many enzymes and proteins. It is involved in the regulation of gene expression.[a]	Zinc deficiency can contribute to loss of appetite, hair loss, delayed wound healing, skin abnormalities, impaired taste, and depression.[b]
Folate	400 µg/day	Folate is a coenzyme in the breakdown and absorption of nucleic acid. Avoids megaloblastic anemia.[a]	High consumption of folic acid can contribute to vitamin B_{12} deficiency.
Vitamin B_6	M: 1.7 mg/day F: 1.5 mg/day	Vitamin B_6 is a coenzyme in the metabolism and absorption of amino acids, glycogen, and sphingoid bases.[a]	Sensory neuropathy has occurred from high intake of B_6 in supplement form.[a] Deficiency can contribute to high homocysteine, depression, and impaired immune function.
Vitamin B_{12}	2.4 µg/day	Vitamin B_{12} is a coenzyme in nucleic acid metabolism. Prevents megaloblastic anemia.[a]	It is estimated that 10%–30% of older adults may suffer from B_{12} malabsorption from food-bound sources. Older adults should consume foods fortified with vitamin B_{12} or a vitamin supplement.[a] B_{12} deficiency can lead to peripheral neuropathy, balance disturbances, and high homocysteine.
Iron	8 mg/day	It is a constituent of hemoglobin and various enzymes. Averts microcytic hypochromic anemia.[a]	Anemia related to iron deficiency is the most common form of anemia in older adults. Blood loss, poor nutrition intake, medication side effects, cancer treatment, and malabsorption contribute to iron deficiency.[c]

[a]Institute of Medicine, Food and Nutrition Board. (2006). *Dietary reference intake: The essential guide to nutrient requirement.* Washington, DC: National Academy Press.

[b]Sallit, J. (2012, January). Rationale for zinc supplementation in older adults with wounds. *Annals of Long-Term Care, 20*(1), 39–41.

[c]Center for Disease Control and Prevention. (n.d.-d). Iron and iron deficiency. http://www.cdc.gov/nutrition/everyone/basics/vitamins/iron.html

Energy

The estimated energy requirement (EER) equations are the same for both older and younger adults. Individual energy needs depend on activity, lean body mass, and the existence of illness. A person who is bed- or chair-ridden, for example, usually needs fewer calories than an ambulatory person. Decreased energy needs signify a challenging nutritional situation for the older adult since vitamin and mineral requirements often stay constant or may even rise for several nutrients. Eating a diet that meets nutritional needs without surpassing energy needs adds an extra challenge for older adults and would necessitate close monitoring of the intake of discretionary calories. Current data on dietary trends are alarming. Everyday consumption for a sizeable percentage of older adults aged 51 to 70 years and those 71 years and older was lower than recommended for the nutrient-rich food groups. Greater than 90% of persons aged 51 to 70 years and over 80% of persons aged 71 years and older consume empty calories above the discretionary calorie allowances (Krebs-Smith et al., 2010). This disproportion between calorie needs and calories consumed produces a nutritionally challenging situation, as food and dining practices significantly add to the quality of life and general well-being of older adults. It is important to work with older adults to balance nutrient requirements and intake to promote health.

Reduced physical activity and the decrease in lean body mass that accompanies the aging process contribute to the decreased energy requirements seen in older adults. For instance, a 60-year-old man will need to increase his physical activity and/or reduce his caloric intake to support his weight as he ages. This generates a challenge for older adults who adopt a more sedentary lifestyle, thus contributing further to reduced caloric requirements. To maintain a healthy body weight and avoid increases in body weight, older adults should choose a nutrient-dense diet that includes all nutrients needed for optimum health without consuming too many calories. Physical activity raises energy needs while also delaying the loss in lean mass, thus permitting us to eat more without adding weight and increase the probability that the diets of older adults will be adequate in indispensable nutrients.

Water

Water is vital to all body functions; if consumption is insufficient, cellular metabolism becomes arduous, if not impossible. Decreased thirst response coupled with reduced kidney function increases the risk of dehydration in older adults (IOM, FNB, 2004). Diuretic prescriptions and alcohol intensify fluid elimination and can contribute to dehydration. Fluid references are the same for young and older adults: 3,700 ml/day for men and 2,700 ml/day for women (IOM, FNB, 2004). Fluid needs are met by consuming both beverages and foods.

The daily water requirement from food and fluids is set at a level projected to replenish usual daily losses and avert the consequences of dehydration; however, the recommended level is often not met by many older adults (IOM, FNB, 2004). Dehydration, a form of malnutrition, is a major problem in older adults, especially persons over 85 years and institutionalized older adults. Fear of incontinence and arthritic pain related to frequent trips to the toilet may hinder opportunity to consume adequate amounts of fluids. Dehydration can contribute to constipation, fecal impaction, cognitive impairment, functional decline, and even death.

Protein

For healthy older adults, the RDA for protein is 0.8 g/kg of body weight, which, on average, translates into 46 g/kg BW for women and 56 g/kg BW for men. Protein requirements (as grams per kilogram of body weight [g/kg BW]) may be more difficult for older adults to meet as the overall energy needs decrease, ability to chew and swallow becomes more difficult, taste changes, and the cost of nutrient-dense foods may be out of reach. With decreased caloric needs and protein needs remaining constant, a suitable diet must contain comparatively more protein. There is some debate about total protein requirements for older adults to maintain nitrogen equilibrium. Recent research supports providing older adults with 1.0 g of protein/ kg of body weight with additional amount needed to heal skin injury (Houston et al., 2008). The precise role of dietary protein in the prevention of sarcopenia remains unclear, however, a protein intake slightly above 1.0 g/kg may be beneficial to enhance muscle protein anabolism and reduce progressive loss of muscle mass with age (Millward, 2008; Paddon-Jones et al., 2008). Some experts suggest that a protein intake of 1.0 to 1.6 g/kg daily is safe and adequate to meet the needs of healthy older adults (American Dietetic Association Standards of Practice, 2009; Houston et al., 2008). To meet protein requirements and augment muscle protein synthesis, older adults should strive to consume 25 to 30 g of high-quality protein with every meal (Paddon-Jones & Rasmussen, 2009).

Consuming sufficient protein can be challenging for older adults (Chernoff, 2004). Selecting food items with high-quality protein throughout the day is advocated by MyPlate as an effective approach to help improve protein intake (Position of the Academy of Nutrition and Dietetics, 2012). Trauma, stress, and infection may also increase protein needs. However, there are risks associated with high protein intake, including dehydration, nitrogen overload, and possible adverse effects on the kidneys. Although protein undernutrition has been found to contribute to both sarcopenia and morbidity, aging does not appear to cause impaired ability to synthesize muscle protein when high quality protein is consumed (Symons et al., 2007, 2011). Consuming too few animal products as part of a dietary regime can contribute to reduced dietary protein intake and deficiency of vitamins and minerals such as calcium, iron, zinc, vitamin D and vitamin B_{12}.

Carbohydrates and Fiber

Carbohydrates should contribute 45% to 65% of the calories in the diet. Carbohydrate selection should consist of complex carbohydrates, including whole grains and breads and pastas that are unrefined. Fiber, a complex carbohydrate, has numerous health benefits, and along with adequate water is of primary importance in efforts to help an older adult avoid constipation and maintain bowel health. Additionally, fiber is important in helping to support a healthy body weight and helpful in managing blood glucose. Older adults normally do not consume sufficient dietary fiber. Foods with decreased fiber content have a tendency to replace more nutritious foods vital to maintain health and weight management goals of older adults. Since the AI for fiber is based on caloric intake (14 g/1,000 kcal/day), and energy requirement is reduced with age, the AI for fiber is 21 and 30 g/day for women and men over age 50 respectively. Fiber may help to decrease blood cholesterol levels, making these recommendations particularly significant for those who are at risk for heart disease. Five or more servings of fruits and vegetables daily, in addition to whole-grain breads or cereals high in bran, will provide the recommended amount while at the same time providing vitamins, minerals, and phytochemicals required by older adults. To prevent abdominal distress that can result as a side effect of increasing fiber in the diet, increase dietary fiber consumption slowly. When increasing dietary fiber consumption, it is important to ensure sufficient fluids—preferably water—to avoid dehydration and constipation.

Fat

Consuming too much dietary fat at any age can contribute to obesity, which in turn can contribute to the possibility of developing diabetes, heart disease, and some types of cancer. While younger people should limit their dietary cholesterol and fat intake, it is important to note that severe restrictions in older adults may be of little benefit and could contribute to inadequate calorie and nutrient intake and essential fatty acids.

Healthy individuals of any age should strive to obtain 20% to 35% of their daily caloric allowance from fat, while also limiting saturated fat intake to 8% to 10% of this amount. Total cholesterol intake should be limited to no more than 300 mg/day. Individuals at high risk for heart disease may need to limit saturated fat and cholesterol even further, as per their physicians' recommendation. As a rule, to help maintain a healthy body weight, older adults should limit excess dietary fat.

Micronutrients

Micronutrient needs and availability of nutrients changes as we age. In many instances, age-related decreases in absorption, use, or activation of nutrients contributes to higher dietary vitamin and mineral requirements. In some instances, our vitamin requirements stay unchanged, as our energy needs decrease. Vitamins D and B_{12} are examples of vitamins that are affected by physiological changes that occur with age. This makes the need for older adults to consume nutrient-dense foods particularly important. To maintain a healthy body weight or avert unhealthy increases in weight, older adults must consume a nutrient-dense diet for optimum health without overdoing calories, while still ensuring that the diet contains all necessary nutrients.

The B Vitamins

The B vitamins are of special concern in older adults. Research supports that inadequate folate, vitamin B_6, and vitamin B_{12} can contribute to elevated levels of plasma homocysteine, which is linked with an increased risk of cardiovascular disease and mortality (Dangour et al., 2008). High levels of homocysteine have also been defined as an independent risk factor for cognitive impairment and dementia (Green, 2009; Haan et al., 2007).

With age, the occurrence of vitamin B_{12} deficiency increases. It is estimated that 6% of adults aged 60 or older are vitamin B_{12} deficient, and approximately 20% have negligible levels (Allen, 2009). While the intake of most adults shows sufficient intake of vitamin B_{12}, 10% to 30% of older adults fail to absorb protein-bound vitamin B_{12} from foods due to pernicious anemia, lack of intrinsic factor, and atrophic gastritis. Consumption of folic acid, in excess of recommended levels, may conceal vitamin B_{12} deficiency and interfere with diagnosis (Position of the Academy of Nutrition and Dietetics, 2012). Neurological symptoms like variations in mental status should prompt further assessment in older adults and should not be credited to "old age." A daily consumption of 2.4 mg of vitamin B_{12} is suggested for all adults 51 years and older. Since it is easier to absorb synthetic B_{12} than food-bound B_{12}, it is frequently recommended that adults older than 50 use fortified foods or supplements that contain B_{12} to help meet their vitamin B_{12} needs.

Vitamin D and Calcium

Vitamin D is an important component of bone health and the prevention of osteoporosis. Insufficient intake of dietary vitamin D can contribute to frail bones that are predisposed to fractures. Vitamin D has been studied for its possible role in the prevention and treatment of cancer, types 1 and 2 diabetes mellitus, hypertension, glucose metabolism, heart disease, arthritis and multiple sclerosis (National Institutes of Health [NIH], Office of Dietary Supplements [ODS], n.d.-d). The current DRIs are based on the evidence that supports the role of vitamin D and calcium in supporting bone health. The Institute of Medicine forewarns consumers of all ages that some research shows that too much of these nutrients may be harmful. Low levels of vitamin D are common in older adults (IOM, FNB, 2011). As we age, tissues are less efficient in processing serum vitamin D; also, the aging skin is less effective in manufacturing vitamin D when exposed to sunlight. Older adults have a tendency to spend more time indoors, thus limiting exposure to sunlight. While the use of sunscreens is a good strategy in the skin cancer prevention effort, it also reduces vitamin D synthesis. Older adults with lactose intolerance add a particular challenge as avoidance of dairy products further compromises vitamin D status. The RDA for vitamin D for young adults as well as adults aged 51 through 70 is 600/day. For adults 70 years and older, the RDA is 800 IU/day (IOM, FNB, 2011).

Calcium absorption decreases with age, partly because of a loss of vitamin D receptors in the gut. Stomach inflammation and increase in fiber consumption also decrease calcium absorption. As with vitamin D intake, real or perceived lactose intolerance promotes reduced consumption of dairy products and consequently of calcium. As a result of these factors, adequate intake of calcium is essential to reduce the rate of age-related bone loss as well as the incidence of fractures, particularly of the hip (IOM, FNB, 2011). For women aged 51 to 70 years, the RDA for calcium has been established at 1,200 mg/day. The RDA for men in this age group is 1,000 mg/day. For older adults over the age of 70, the RDA for calcium is 1,200 mg/day, regardless of the sex (IOM, FNB, 2011).

Low fat dairy products are good sources of calcium, vitamin D and protein while being low in calories and fat, making them a good food choice for older adults. It is difficult to consume the recommended amount of calcium and vitamin D from food alone, especially for older adults. Ensuring adequacy of other nutrients involved in bone health such as protein, vitamins A and K, magnesium, and phytoestrogens is also imperative when working with older adults.

Minerals

Iron is an important nutrient during the life cycle. For postmenopausal women, the RDA for iron is the same as the RDA for men, 8 mg/day. Reduced meat consumption associated with taste changes, economics, and poor dentition can contribute to iron deficiency. Iron depletion may result from prolonged malabsorption, restricted dietary intake or intestinal bleeding. As a rule, most iron is absorbed in the small intestine. Gastrointestinal ailments that result in inflammation of the small intestine can contribute to diarrhea, poor absorption of dietary iron, and iron depletion (CDC, n.d.-f). Chronic GI bleeding and blood loss can contribute to anemia and symptoms such as decreased energy, episodes of syncope, pale skin, irregular heartbeat, cold extremities, and headaches. Once the cause of the bleeding has been identified, iron supplementation can be considered appropriate (Anemia.org, 2009).

Although clinical zinc insufficiency is rare, the average zinc intake for older adults tends to be below the RDA. Stress, particularly in hospitalized older adults, seems to raise the risk of zinc deficit and impaired immune function. Research supports that zinc supplementation can contribute to wound healing, but only in those who are zinc deficient. Since excess zinc may affect immune function and the absorption of other minerals and may work to lower HDL cholesterol, people of all ages should avoid unnecessary and incessant zinc supplementation.

Magnesium is involved in 100s of enzyme reactions. Energy metabolism, protein and fatty acid synthesis, and glucose metabolism occur in the presence of magnesium. It is also needed for muscle contraction (Vaquero, 2002). Older adults are less likely to consume adequate amounts of magnesium than younger adults; therefore, they must be encouraged to consume magnesium-rich foods such as green leafy vegetables, whole grains, and nuts. The RDA for magnesium is 420 mg/day for men 51 years and older, and 320 mg/day for women in the same age group. Magnesium deficiency is rare, and high intake of dietary magnesium has not been linked to adverse effects. Hypomagnesaemia can occur in individuals with compromised renal function (NIH, ODS, n.d.-a).

Antioxidants

Dietary antioxidant intake is associated with lower prevalence of degenerative diseases and maintenance of physiological functions in older adults. This is thought to be due to the role of antioxidant nutrients and phytochemicals in reducing oxidative stress that contributes to aging and disease pathogenesis. Antioxidants such as those naturally occurring in fruits and vegetables are vital to prevent the damage caused by oxidative stress and progressive diseases frequently seen in older adults. Antioxidants may have a protective effect against the impairment to the brain that may result in Alzheimer's disease and other deteriorations in cognition that are common in aging (Devore et al., 2010).

Vitamin E is vital in maintaining cell integrity by preventing lipid peroxidation. It also plays a role in immune function and the blood clotting process (NIH, ODS, n.d.-e). The RDI for vitamin E is 15 mg/day for both men and women over the age of 51. Older adults seem to have overall inadequate vitamin E. Good sources of vitamin E include vegetable oil, nuts, seeds, whole grains, and dark green leafy vegetables (NIH, ODS, n.d.-e).

Vitamin C is an antioxidant that plays a vital role in collagen synthesis and wound healing, immune function and facilitates iron absorption. Fruits and vegetables are the best sources of vitamin C (NIH, ODS, n.d.-c).

Two forms of vitamin A are available in dietary form, preformed and provitamin. Provitamin A includes Carotenoids. Carotenoids have antioxidant qualities, thus protecting against cellular peroxidation and cellular DNA damage. While the main dietary carotenoids include alpha carotene, beta-carotene, beta cryptoxanthin, lycopene, lutein, and zeaxanthin, over 700 carotenoids have been identified (NIH, ODS, n.d.-b). Carotenoids are found in red, yellow, and orange fruits and vegetables such as carrots, pumpkin, spinach, tomatoes, and watermelon. Vitamin A deficiency is rare in the United States. People with cystic fibrosis are at increased risk for developing vitamin A deficiency owing to difficulty absorbing fat (NIH, ODS, n.d.-b).

ACTUAL DIETARY INTAKE

Older adults along with many Americans are not compliant with national dietary guidance. Many Americans, older adults included, eat foods that are high in fats and added sugars, sacrificing the intake of recommended more nutrient-dense food groups (Bachman et al., 2008). The significance of the aggregate outcome of a lifespan of poor nutritional selections has a strong influence on one's well-being and quality of life. Older adults who follow a dietetic pattern consisting of high-fat dairy foods and high sugar content foods and desserts have a greater risk of mortality than older adults that sustained a healthy eating pattern (Anderson et al., 2011). Both the quantity of food and energy intake may decrease with age, thereby emphasizing the critical importance of a nutrient-dense diet for older adults. The decreased energy needs contribute to reduced micronutrient intakes, particularly calcium, zinc, iron, and B vitamins. Older adults run the risk of not meeting the RDA or AI values for calcium; vitamins D, E, and K; potassium; and fiber, while potentially consuming too much folate and sodium in their diets (Lichtenstein et al., 2008).

A number of barriers make it difficult for older adults to consume sufficient fruits and vegetables. Financial limitations, functional disability, and the physical demands of shopping and preparing foods, oral cavity dysfunction such as reduced number of teeth, inflamed gums, and ill-fitting dentures could all be hindrances making observance of fruit and vegetable recommendations difficult for the older adult. Education and counseling, whether face to face, web based, or via telephone, have produced positive results in improving the intake of fruit and vegetables in this population (Pomerleau et al., 2005).

Adults 51 years and older are recommended to decrease sodium in their diets to 1,500 mg/day in efforts to reduce the risk of high blood pressure and associated comorbidities (USDA & HHS, 2010). Working towards consuming a low-sodium diet has unique challenges for older adults. Functional and physical disability can make food preparation demanding. As a result, older adults often turn to processed, preprepared, and ready-to-eat meals that can be higher in sodium. Changes in the ability to perceive taste due to illness or medication side effect can lead to excessive salt use.

Nutritional Supplementation

Many older adults use vitamin supplements. There are two main reasons that older adults take nutritional supplements: first, to delay age-related chronic diseases, and second, for the potential health-promoting effects of these nutrients (Buhr & Bales, 2010). Nutritional supplements can affect the absorption of other nutrients or interfere with the absorption and metabolism of prescription medications, contribute to polypharmacy, and, in large amounts, can have toxic or other negative effects on health.

A great number of adults aged 51 and older do not meet the recommended amounts of many nutrients from foods alone (Sebastian et al., 2007). When dietary variety is limited, nutrient supplementation with low-dose multivitamin and mineral supplements can assist older adults in meeting recommended intake levels. Nutrients consistently found to be deficient in the diet of older adults such as antioxidants, calcium, vitamin D, and those for which the digestion, absorption, or metabolism declines with age such as vitamin B_{12} should be considered for supplementation. Healthcare professionals should inquire of older adults about the use of dietary supplements such as phytochemical and herbal products during the nutrition assessment process.

HEALTH CONDITIONS THAT AFFECT NUTRITIONAL STATUS AND FOOD INTAKE

Many people reach old age with the cumulative effects of a lifetime of suboptimal health habits, including poor nutrition and physical inactivity, putting them at risk for many chronic degenerative conditions. Older adults may be required to make numerous dietary changes to manage symptoms or treat illness. Many conditions can alter the nutritional requirements of older adults.

Arthritis

Arthritis pain may impair food intake and make it hard to prepare meals. Some arthritis medications may inhibit nutrient absorption. There is no proven cure for arthritis, and treatment is aimed at reducing symptoms. Weight management plays a role in treating arthritis because excess body weight adds stress to the hips and knees. Therefore, for those that are overweight or obese, weight loss may reduce the risk of developing osteoarthritis, particularly of the knee (National Institute of Arthritis and Musculoskeletal and Skin Diseases, 2010).

Adding foods that are high in unsaturated fatty acids, particularly the omega-3 fatty acids in flaxseed and cold-water fish, may benefit older adults who have rheumatoid arthritis by decreasing inflammation and thereby reducing discomfort (Patterson et al., 2012). Dietary antioxidants may provide protection against arthritis; however, high coffee consumption, alcohol intake (especially among smokers) as well as obesity tend to increase the risk of rheumatoid arthritis (Lahiri et al., 2012).

Cardiovascular Disease

Despite increased survival and reduced mortality rates, cardiovascular disease is one of the leading causes of morbidity and mortality in older adults. CVD affects many adults as they advance through their later years of life. Veins become tauter, collagen collects, smooth muscle cells move, vasomotor role deteriorates, and the biology of the circulatory system is altered (Larsen, 2008). Implementation of healthy lifestyles is essential for the deterrence of CVD. Chief lifestyle changes effective in the management of CVD include achieving and maintaining a healthy weight, implementing the Dietary Approaches to Stop Hypertension (DASH) eating plan, which is rich in potassium and calcium as well as low in dietary sodium, regular physical activity, and consuming alcohol in moderation. Lifestyle modifications can help to decrease blood pressure, improve antihypertensive drug effectiveness, and lessen cardiovascular risk (CDC, 2011a).

Diabetes

Individuals whose body does not produce sufficient insulin, or the insulin produced is ineffective, are diagnosed with type-2 diabetes. Approximately 25.6% of adults over the age of 65 have diabetes (American Diabetes Association [ADA], n.d.). Risk factors for the development of diabetes include genetic predisposition, history of excessive caloric intake, being overweight and obese, and hyperlipidemia. Common complications of diabetes in older adults include depression, falls and fractures, urinary incontinence, forgetfulness and other mental problems, chronic pain, as well as the traditionally recognized cardiovascular problems (ADA, n.d.).

Care goals for the diabetic older adult include weight reduction to improve glucose tolerance, control of hyperlipidemia, secure positive metabolic outcomes such as glycated hemoglobin (A1C), and maintaining blood sugar within an acceptable range. Type 2 diabetes in the older adult can often be controlled with diet alone. Consuming a diet with adequate calories, a low-fat diet with appropriate amounts of fruits, vegetables, and whole grains coupled with 30 minutes of exercise most days of the week are adequate to promote weight loss and maintenance and delay comorbidities associated with the disease. Diet should include 45% to 65% of calories from carbohydrate, 15% to 20% of calories from protein, less than 30% of calories from fat and adequate fiber (5 to 50 g/day) (ADA, n.d.).

Cancer

Cancer is a multifactorial illness that grows from an interface between family history and the environment. Avoiding tobacco items, maintaining a healthy weight, maintaining an active lifestyle, and consuming a healthy diet may significantly decrease an individual's risk of developing cancer. These factors can also contribute to a decreased risk of developing heart disease and diabetes (American Cancer Society [ACS], n.d.). Older adults who suffer from cancer frequently have altered medical needs. They develop comorbidities like heart failure, arthritis, impaired glucose tolerance, or high blood pressure. At times, treatment must be deferred until chronic conditions are effectively managed (CDC, n.d.-b). The goals of nutrition management include promoting adequate intake, identifying individualized interventions for each person, preventing or reversing nutrient deficits, maintaining lean body mass, enabling the patient to tolerate treatments, and reducing side effects and complications (Academy of Nutrition and Dietetics [AND.], Evidence Analysis Library [EAL], n.d.-b). Changes in diet texture or supplementary diet controls such as consistent carbohydrate or limitations in sodium can help ease some of the symptoms.

Anorexia is often a comorbidity associated with cancer diagnosis. In many instances, the treatment will cause GI distress including nausea, vomiting and loss of appetite. Chemotherapy can contribute to an augmented sensitivity to scents and a distorted perception of smells (CDC, n.d.-b). The ability to taste food may also change throughout the time the older adult receives chemotherapy treatments. Foods may taste metallic, old, bitter, or freezer burned. For these older adults, finding the comfort food that will entice them to eat and providing the food item at a time that the older adult will accept is an important component of the care provided.

The American Cancer Society Nutrition Guidelines recommends consumption of a diet with emphasis on plant sources, including five or more servings of fruits and vegetables per day, whole grains, three cups of low-fat milk or equivalent, limiting salt, and choosing foods that help to maintain a healthy weight (ACS, n.d.).

Obesity

The importance of maintaining a healthy body weight is underscored in older adults where both overweight and underweight have a significant impact on health and well-being. Obesity in older adults can contribute to reduced independence by interfering with health and normal physical function and increased difficulty accomplishing daily tasks. Additional weight gain is discouraged for overweight and obese older adults (USDA & HHS, 2010). The presence of nutritional deficiencies in overweight and obese older adults can result from long-term intake of a high-calorie, poor-nutrient diet and a physically inactive lifestyle (Anderson et al. 2011).

Weight loss in older adults is not straightforward, and careful consideration should be given to identify older adults for whom medically supervised weight loss is appropriate. Voluntary weight loss has been shown to be beneficial to the health, quality of life, and physical functioning of older adults; however, even when targeting fat mass, weight loss accelerates muscle loss (Miller &

Wolfe, 2008). For older adults following a hypocaloric diet for weight loss, careful attention should be given to protein, fluid, fiber, vitamins B_{12} and D, calcium and discretionary energy intake. Unintentional weight loss, on the other hand, can be detrimental to health and often signifies underlying disease.

Changes in Mental Status: Alzheimer Disease, Depression and Dementia

In later life, changes in mental functioning and cognition as well as depression can lead to anorexia (loss of appetite) or overeating and contribute to malnutrition. Individuals with Alzheimer disease and dementia often lose the ability to obtain, prepare, and consume an optimal diet. Antioxidants may offer some protection from the disease; however, supplemental antioxidants have not been conclusively shown to be beneficial and may lead to undesirable side effects (Devore et al., 2010). Antioxidants from food should therefore be encouraged for older adults to reduce the risk of Alzheimer disease (AND, EAL, 2012). Wandering, a common consequence of Alzheimer disease, can affect the person's ability to maintain weight. Overactivity can drain nutritional reserve and increase calorie needs. Diets must be carefully planned to meet psychological and physical needs.

Depression can influence health by causing changes in appetite. An increase in appetite can result in weight gain and resulting health threats such as hypertension, diabetes, and cardiovascular disease. A decrease in appetite can contribute to weight loss and the comorbidities associated with consuming inadequate calories, vitamins, minerals, and fiber. Decreased intake may cause the person to feel sluggish, moody, and fatigued. Some nutrient deficiencies, such as B complex, can contribute to signs and symptoms of depression (CDC, n.d.-c).

Osteoporosis

Lifelong diet and physical activity habits are among the preventable risk factors for development of osteoporosis. Good nutrition and regular weight-bearing exercise throughout life play a significant role in the development and progression of osteoporosis. Following a diet that is rich in calcium and vitamin D and engaging in regular physical activity, in particular weight-bearing exercises, such as walking, reduces osteoporosis risks.

Osteoporosis contributes to an increase in the possibility of bone fractures commonly seen in the wrist, hip, and spine as well as falls in older adults. Calcium is an essential mineral needed for healthy bones, teeth, as well as proper heart function, muscles, and nerves. Calcium is not produced for the body. The calcium needed to sustain a healthy body must be obtained for foods. Dairy products such as low-fat or non-fat milk, yogurt, cheese and calcium fortified foods such as breakfast cereal and orange juice, and nuts such as almonds are good sources of calcium (NIH Osteoporosis and Related Bone Diseases National Resource Center, 2013).

Vitamin D plays a significant role in calcium absorption and bone health. Food sources of vitamin D include egg yolks, saltwater fish, and liver. While most adults obtain sufficient vitamin D via sun exposure, studies support that vitamin D production declines in older adults, people that are confined to their homes or live in institutions, and the population at large during the winter months (unless you live in a tropical zone all year round) (NIH Osteoporosis and Related Bone Diseases National Resource Center, 2013).

Exercise is a vital component of an osteoporosis prevention and treatment regime. Exercise helps to improve bone health, increase muscle strength, coordination, and balance. Older adults should consult with their physician before starting an exercise program (NIH Osteoporosis and Related Bone Diseases National Resource Center, 2013).

Constipation

Constipation is one of the most common health complaints among older adults. Age-related decreases in intestinal motility and transit time, accompanied by poor food intake, may exacerbate gastrointestinal problems such as constipation. Excessive laxative use leading to decreased transit time may prevent the adequate absorption of nutrients and contribute to nutritional deficiencies and dehydration. Fiber intake of older adults consistently falls below recommended levels. Increasing dietary fiber and fluid is one of the most effective treatments for constipation. To help reduce constipation, older adults should gradually adopt a high-fiber diet. Care should be taken to ensure sufficient fluid intake and that dietary fiber does not lead to excess satiety and limit food intake.

Vision: Cataracts and Age-Related Macular Degeneration

Preventing or slowing progression of cataracts and age-related macular degeneration could potentially save the vision of many people. The National Eye Institute's Age-Related Eye Disease Study (AREDS) found that taking a specific high-dose formulation of antioxidants and zinc (beta-carotene; vitamins A, C, and E; copper; and zinc) significantly reduces the risk of advanced age-related macular degeneration and its associated vision loss (National Eye Institute, n.d.). Foods that contain the carotenoids lutein and zeaxanthin are widely investigated for their ability to reduce the risk of macular degeneration by preventing free radical damage in the eye and blood vessels (Academy of Nutrition and Dietetics, n.d.-a; Carpentier et al., 2009).

Alcoholism

Disproportionate alcohol consumption can lead to the added possibility of health complications such as injuries, violence, and liver diseases (CDC, n.d.-a). Older adults have a unique set of challenges associated with alcohol consumption. Physiological changes associated with aging, the presence of chronic conditions, and medications taken to manage chronic ailments can make alcohol consumption a problem for older adults (NIH Senior Health, 2013). People who consume excessive amounts of alcohol often have poor diets that are low in numerous essential nutrients. Socially isolated or depressed older adults may be at risk for alcoholism. Chronic alcohol consumption is linked with deficits in vitamins and minerals as a result of decreased food consumption. Vitamins A, C, D, E, K, and the B vitamins can be affected by increased alcohol intake (National Institute on Alcohol Abuse and Alcoholism, 2013).

Older adults can develop sensitivity to alcohol effects. The slower rate of alcohol metabolism seen in older adults allows the alcohol to stay longer in their bodies. As a result, older adults have a higher percentage of alcohol in their blood than their younger counterparts after consuming the same amount of alcohol. Aging decreases the body's ability to tolerate alcohol. Side effects such as slurred speech and lack of coordination are readily observed (NIH Senior Health, 2013). Over time, alcohol consumption can contribute to liver damage, heart disease, and brain damage as well as increasing the risk of cancer and immune system disorders. Chronic conditions such as diabetes, hypertension, congestive heart failure, and memory deficits can intensify in the presence of alcohol use (NIH Senior Health, 2013).

Interaction between medications and alcohol consumption can contribute to greater challenges in the health management of older adults. Older adults consuming aspirin or arthritis medications are at increased risk for gastrointestinal bleeding. Pain medications taken in the presence of alcohol can contribute to liver damage. Alcohol can intensify the effects of some medications such as antihistamines, sleep aids, or medications taken for depression and anxiety. Symptoms such as drowsiness, sleepiness, poor coordination, and in extreme cases difficulty breathing can be present (NIH Senior Health, 2013).

Pressure Ulcers

Maintaining adequate parameters of nutrition is considered a best practice in both the prevention and treatment of PUs. Older adults with PUs or who are at risk for developing PUs should strive to achieve or maintain adequate nutrition parameters.

Sufficient macronutrients (carbohydrates, protein, fats, and water) and micronutrients (vitamins and minerals) are vital for the body to support tissue integrity and prevent breakdown. Weight loss and difficulties with eating can increase the incidence of PUs (Horn et al., 2004). Other nutrition-related risk factors that can contribute to PU development include a change in appetite, compromised dental health, gastrointestinal and elimination disturbances, decreased self-feeding abilities, drug–nutrient interactions, and alcohol and substance abuse (American Dietetic Association, n.d.; AND, n.d.-b; Center for Medicare and Medicaid Services, 2011; Stechmiller et al., 2008).

Restrictive diets can contribute to a decreased intake of nutrients (Position of the American Dietetic Association, 2010). A diet too low in protein will lack the amino acids needed for protein synthesis. Additional nutrients imperative for skin integrity include essential fatty acids, adequate carbohydrates, water, vitamin A, vitamin C, and zinc. Table 10.4 provides a list of nutrients involved in the treatment and prevention of wounds as well as the role these nutrients play.

Aside from the role of vitamins and minerals, the role of individual amino acids in wound healing has been explored. Arginine stimulates growth factors and boosts the immune system. Current research does not support the use of arginine to promote PU healing (AND, n.d.-b; Dorner et al., 2009). Glutamine is a conditionally-essential amino acid that serves as a fuel source for fibroblasts and epithelial cells in the healing process. Further research is needed to determine the effectiveness of glutamine and arginine supplementation on wound healing (AND, n.d.-b).

Malnutrition

Malnutrition in older adults can have many interrelated etiologies and great significance. Consuming a poor-quality diet can contribute to insufficient energy and essential nutrient consumption, which can contribute to malnutrition, deteriorating health conditions, frailty, and disability. Loss of appetite is considered an important predictor of malnutrition in older adults. Decreased appetite is a contributing factor in the undernutrition often assessed in older adults in community dwelling and institutionalized settings. Other factors linked with increased risk or incidence of malnutrition in older adults include weight loss, functional dependence, cognitive impairment, loneliness, living without a partner, history of lung or heart disease, and acute vomiting (Jurschik et al., 2010). When conducting a nutrition assessment, healthcare professionals need to pay attention to this type of malnutrition, its sources, and consequences. Aside from the malnutrition normally identified in frail, infirm older adults, a shift in paradigm of growing concern is the manifestation of malnutrition in overweight and obese older adults. Long-term intake of a high-calorie, decreased-nutrient diet along with age-related reduction in physical activity can increase the number of older adults that are overweight, obese, have reduced muscle mass, functional limitations, and many nutrient deficits.

Frequently labeled as "anorexia of aging," physiological, psychosocial, social, and cultural elements all combine to contribute to the decreased food consumption and appetite often seen in

TABLE 10.4 · Nutrients Involved in Treatment and Prevention of Wounds

Nutrient	Role in Wound Healing
Protein	Plays a major role in the production of enzymes involved in wound healing, cell multiplication, and collagen and connective-tissue manufacture. Caloric needs must be met in order for protein to be spared for buildup and repair (Baranoski & Ayello, 2012). Although the amount of protein needed by patients with PUs is debatable, protein levels higher than the adult recommendation of 0.8 g/kg of body weight/day are generally accepted and recommended. The National Pressure Ulcer Advisory Panel (NPUAP) recommends 1.2–1.5 g of protein/kg of body weight/day and 30–35 kcal/kg of body weight/day for wound healing (Dorner et al., 2009).
Fatty acids	Essential to maintain the lipid barrier.
Carbohydrates	Essential for the cells to carry out basic functions of metabolism and prevent gluconeogenesis from protein stores (Baranoski & Ayello, 2012).
Water	Plays a role in wound-site hydration and oxygen perfusion, is a solvent for nutrients and other small molecules to diffuse into and out of cells, and removes waste from cells. Dehydration is a risk factor for wound development. Patients with draining wounds need additional fluids to replace losses.
Vitamin A	Fuels cellular differentiation in fibroblasts and is involved in collagen development. Research supports vitamin A's role in reversing the adverse effects caused by corticosteroids in terms of wound healing (MacKay & Miller, 2003).
Vitamin C	Vital for collagen production. Vitamin C has been associated with prolonged wound healing time, decreased wound strength, and decreased immune function (Baranoski & Ayello, 2012). It is important to note that mega-doses of vitamin C have not been linked to an increased wound-healing rate (Dorner et al., 2009). While not appropriate for all patients, vitamin and mineral supplementation is most beneficial for patients with poor vitamin C intake, since they are likely to have limited nutrient stores, and for patients with a diagnosed vitamin C deficiency (Baranoski & Ayello, 2012.)
Zinc	Associated with collagen formation, protein metabolism, vitamin A transport, and immune function (Baranoski & Ayello, 2012; Dorner et al., 2009). Zinc deficiency can emerge as a result of severe wound drainage or GI losses, corticosteroid use, or a long-term decreased dietary intake (Baranoski & Ayello, 2012). The amount of zinc in a multivitamin and mineral supplement is generally adequate. Supplementing to no more than the upper tolerable limit of the DRI (40 mg of elemental zinc) until the deficiency is corrected can be recommended (Dorner et al., 2009).

older adults. Anorexia of aging, defined as poor food intake that accompanies age, can result in significant undernutrition in older adults (Chapman, 2007). Malnutrition, in turn, can contribute to the worsening of many ailments, including immune insufficiencies, anemia, falls, and cognitive degeneration. It can be challenging to identify treatment approaches for anorexia in older adults. Loss of appetite can result from medical, pharmacological, social and psychological issues. Identifying the cause of anorexia is important because managing even one component of the problem can offer at least provisional improvement.

DIET INDIVIDUALIZATION

Eating a varied diet has been at the forefront of nutrition recommendations for many years. Individuals, including older adults who eat a more diverse diet, are rewarded with improved health and overall well-being (Bernstein et al., 2003; Hollis & Henry, 2007). Dietary constraints linked with chronic illnesses and therapeutic diets can further compromise nutritional status among older adults (Shatenstein, 2008). A diet that is too limiting can be undesirable to the older adult, thus promoting poor food or fluid intake that can cause undernutrition and decreased quality of life and adverse health consequences (Position of the American Dietetic Association, 2010). The risks and benefits coupled with therapeutic diets for older adults should be weighed prior to implementing dietary restrictions. Research supports that less restrictive diets contribute to improved quality of life and improved nutritional status in older adults (Position of the American Dietetic Association, 2010). Care goals for older adults should focus on promoting health and presenting quality of life. Allowing older adults to participate in making meal and dining choices can help them to maintain a sense of control and dignity (Position of the American Dietetic Association, 2010).

DRUG–NUTRIENT INTERACTIONS

Foods and nutrients can enhance or interfere with the effects of drugs. Grapefruit juice, for example, contains a compound that increases the absorption of some drugs and can enhance their effects. Medication can alter food intake and the way the body uses nutrients. Many older adults take multiple medications that can lead to increased nutritional risk.

Use of nutritional supplements, including vitamins, minerals, or herbal preparations, should be evaluated by healthcare professionals for their interactions with prescription and over-the-counter medications. Older adults may neglect to list nutritional supplements along with medications, and therefore healthcare providers should routinely inquire about their use when obtaining a medication list so that possible interactions can be avoided (Tables 10.5 and 10.6).

TABLE 10.5 · Examples of Food/Drug Interactions

Drug Class	Food That Interacts	Effect of the Food	What to Do
Antihistamine diphenhydramine (Benadryl), chlorpheniramine (Chlor-Trimeton)	Alcohol	Increased drowsiness	Avoid alcohol
Antihyperlipemic lovastatin (Mevacor)	Food	Enhances drug absorption	Take with food
Antihypertensive felodipine (Plendil), nifedipine	Grapefruit juice	Increases drug absorption	Consult your physician or pharmacist before changing diet
Anti-inflammatory naproxen (Naprosyn), ibuprofen (Motrin)	Food or milk Alcohol	Decreases GI irritation Increases risk for liverDamage or stomach bleeding	Take with food or milk Avoid alcohol
Diuretic spironolactone (Aldactone)	Food	Decreases GI irritation	Take with food
Psychotherapeutic MAO inhibitors: isocarboxazid (Marplan), tranylcypromine (Parnate), phenelzine (Nardil)	Foods high in tyramine: aged cheeses, Chianti wine, pickled herring, Brewer's yeast, fava beans	Risk for hypertensive crisis	Avoid foods high in tyramine

TABLE 10.6 • Examples of Drug/Nutrient Interactions

Drug Class	Nutrient That Interacts	Effect of the Nutrient	What to Do
Acid Blocker ranitidine (Zantac), cimetidine (Tagamet), famotidine (Pepcid), nizatidine (Axid)	Vitamin B_{12}	Decrease vitamin absorption	Consult your physician regarding B_{12} supplementation
Antihyperlipemic cholestyramine (Questran), colestipol (Colestid)	Fat soluble vitamins (A, D, E, K)	Decreases vitamin absorption	Include rich sources of these vitamins in the diet
Antineoplastic methotrexate	Folic acid, vitamin B_{12}	Decreases vitamin absorption	Consult your physician regarding supplementation
Diuretic furosemide (Lasix), hydrochlorothiazide (HCTZ)	Many minerals	Increases mineral loss in urine	Include fresh fruits and vegetables in the diet
Laxative fibercon, Mitrolan	Vitamins and minerals	Decreases nutrient absorption	Consult your physician regarding supplementation

From Bobroff, L. B., Lentz, A., & Turner, R. E. (2009). *Food/drug and drug/nutrient interactions: What you should know about your medications*. Gainesville, FL: University of Florida. Publication FCS 8092 in a series of the Department of Family, Youth and Community Sciences, Florida Cooperative Extension Service, Institute of Food and Agricultural Sciences. Retrieved from http://edis.ifas.ufl.edu/pdffiles/HE/HE77600.pdf, with permission.

NUTRITIONAL ASSESSMENT

Nutritional health can be simply defined as the process of securing all nutrients in the quantities needed to sustain body processes. Nutritional health can be measured in many ways. Taken together, the data collected can give you a better understanding of the current and long-term well-being of an individual older adult. The procedures used to measure nutritional health are normally defined as a nutrition assessment.

Nutrition assessment can serve a number of purposes. The completion of a nutrition assessment in all care settings helps to evaluate nutrition-related risks that could threaten the health and well-being of older adults. In a medical setting, nutrition assessment helps to identify risks as well as determine the efficacy of medical nutrition therapy and dietary interventions. Completing a nutrition assessment is a component of the care provided to all hospitalized patients. In this care setting, the nutrition evaluation helps identify risks and also quantify the efficacy of treatments. In public health, nutrition evaluations assist in identifying people in need of nutrition-related interventions and in monitoring the efficacy of intervention programs. At times, assessments can assist in determining the nutritional health of an entire population, detecting health risks shared in a population, for example, so that specific policy measures can be established for prevention or treatment.

There are a number of measures that help us determine the nutritional health of a person. Nutrition assessment involves the gathering of different forms of data—anthropometric measurements, biochemical values, clinical assessment, and dietary consumption—for a comprehensive depiction of one's nutritional well-being. The data obtained are compared with conventional standards to identify nutritional deficits, detect dietary deficiencies, or measure changes resulting from the implementation of dietary changes. The measures of nutritional status examine many factors by using a variety of assessment tools often referred to as the ABCDs of nutrition assessment: anthropometric measurements, biochemical tests, clinical observations, and dietary intake (see Table 10.7).

Anthropometric Measurements

Anthropometric measurements include physical dimensions of the body, such as height and weight, waist circumference, girth measurement, or skinfold measurement.

Height and Weight

To allow the clinician to make an accurate assessment, height and weight must be precisely measured. Older adults lose some height due to bone compression and curvature of the spine; therefore, it is vital to obtain an actual *measurement of* height rather than relying on remembered value reported by the patient. An accurate weight is an important component in a nutrition assessment. This measurement is used to predict energy expenditure and protein needs and to calculate body mass index (BMI).

Body Mass Index

Body Mass Index (BMI) is an assessment parameter calculated using a person's height and weight. BMI is considered a dependable indicator of body fat measurement for most people. This assessment calculation is used to screen for weight categories that may lead to chronic diseases. Centered on benchmarks issued by the NIH and embraced by the Dietary Guidelines for Americans, body weight status is classified as underweight, healthy weight, overweight, and obese (Bernstein & Luggen, 2010).

Waist Circumference

While waist circumference and BMI measurements are interrelated, waist circumference offers an independent prediction of risk for patients classified as normal or overweight on the BMI scale (Guidelines on Overweight and Obesity: Electronic Textbook). Once the BMI measurement is greater than 35, the waist circumference measurement loses its predictive value (Guidelines on Overweight and Obesity: Electronic Textbook). Waist circumference is a good indicator of abdominal fat and risk of chronic diseases in adults (Nelms & Habash, 2011).

Skinfold Measure

Skinfold measurement serves to determine the subcutaneous fat layer thickness. Skinfold measurement is used for a number of purposes, the most common of which is to estimate the percentage of body fat so that it can be compared with percentile tables for specific sex and age categories. This measurement can be useful in evaluating the physical fitness of an athlete or to predict the risk of obesity-related syndrome. Skinfold measurements are also helpful dimensions in cases of illness; the maintenance of fat stores in a patient's body may be an important marker of dietary adequacy.

TABLE 10.7 · Nutritional Assessment of the Older Adult

Tool	Key Features	Special Considerations in Older Adults
Anthropometric Data(height, weight, BMI, circumference, and skinfold)	■ Determine and monitor changes in body weight, height, body composition, and body fat distribution. ■ Establish energy and protein reserves ■ Assess changes that can reflect risk for acute or chronic conditions ■ Monitor effectiveness of nutritional intervention and MNT	■ Physiologic changes in body size and composition may influence measurements ■ Comparison with reference standards based on age can lead to misclassification of nutritional status ■ Lack of appropriate standards for older adults ■ Hydration status can influence measurements ■ Physical impairments can limit ability to obtain accurate measures
Biochemical Data(serum protein—albumin, prealbumin, transferrin, retinol binding capacity C-Reactive Protein Total Lymphocyte Count Serum Cholesterol)	■ Provides objective evaluation of nutrient intake and nutritional status ■ Determine stored and functional levels of nutrients ■ Determine risk and monitor changes for nutrition-related conditions ■ Evaluating the effectiveness of nutritional intervention programs	■ Age-related changes in biochemical parameters must be considered when interpreting biochemical values ■ Lack of appropriate normative values for older adults ■ Polypharmacy may influence measures and interfere with assays ■ Multiple medical conditions may influence interpretation of results ■ Sample collection may be challenging in older adults
Clinical Data(medical history, social history, cognition, physical function, medication food and drug interaction)	■ Useful to obtain a complete medical, personal, social and nutritional history ■ Includes measures of cognition, physical function, functional status, oral status ■ Determine the presence of signs and symptoms related to a nutritional deficiency and malnutrition ■ Evaluation of medication use and food, nutrient, drug interactions	■ Evaluation of MNT and dietary restrictions should be considered on an individual basis to ensure that dietary restrictions do not limit intake and contribute to under/malnutrition ■ Polypharmacy and multiple dietary supplement use must be considered ■ Malnutrition can coexist with obesity, and risk factors should not be overlooked
Dietary Data(food and fluid intake, food security, supplementation, cultural preferences and beliefs, food preferences)	■ Obtain and monitor food and beverage consumption to determine overall diet quality ■ Identify and evaluate dietary patterns ■ Assessment of ability to obtain, prepare, and consume a nutritious diet ■ Evaluate food security ■ Evaluation of nutritional supplement usage, food-related behaviors, food preferences, cultural and ethnic food practices and beliefs, access to and use of food assistance programs	■ Evaluation of social setting, support, and access for food and nutrition programs is important for determining food security ■ Diet liberalization may be important to improve food intake ■ Memory, mental status, and cognition can affect recall and reporting of food intake ■ Access to caregiver involved in food preparation and feeding ■ Participation in federal feeding programs improves intake

Adapted from Bernstein MA, Luggen AS. *Nutrition for the Older Adult.* Sudbury, MA: Jones and Bartlett; 2010.

Biochemical Examination

Biochemical indicators are useful when assessing the adequacy of dietary intake. Biochemical evaluation may include determining the amount of a nutrient metabolite, a storage or transport compound, an enzyme that relies on a vitamin or mineral, or another indicator of the body's performance in comparison with a specific nutrient. The concentration of albumin, an important transport protein in the blood, for example, it is important in regulating blood volume by maintaining the oncotic pressure of the blood compartment. The amount of nutrients lost in the urine or feces also provides important information when assessing the nutrient status of older adults. Values, however, should be interpreted with consideration of the overall health status and medication use of the individual.

Clinical Examination

Clinical observations—The physical examination component of a nutrition assessment is crucial to the determination of the overall nutritional health. As part of conducting a nutrition-focused nutrition assessment, the clinician examines the hair, nails, skin, eyes, lips, mouth, bones, muscles, and joints of the patient. Observations like cheilosis (indicative of riboflavin, vitamin B_6, or niacin insufficiency) or petechiae (small, pinpoint hemorrhages on the skin indicative of vitamin C insufficiency) need further assessment. Obtaining a health history (past medical history) is an important component of completing a nutrition assessment. Information about previous medical illnesses and existing health conditions, life stage, family history, and social, environmental, and economic conditions may affect dietary needs and should be discussed as part of a medical interview. The information collected via the physical examination and interview should be integrated with the information collected from other assessment parameters when creating and evaluating medical and plans of care for individuals.

In addition to collecting information about the older adult's physiology, obtaining information about the older adult's environment and social conditions is fundamental for determining appropriate nutrition interventions in older adults. Older adults may also lack knowledge of what is adequate nutrition. Factors such as economic resources and social isolation can play a role in the older adult's ability to consume a nutritious diet. Those that live on a fixed income, for example, may have to choose between purchasing foods versus securing medications. Social isolation, lack of reliable transportation, and living in a food desert are examples of factors that can impact the older adult's ability to consume an adequate diet. Loneliness and depression diminish the pleasure associated with preparing and consuming meals.

Dietary Assessment

Information on dietary intake is an important component in describing the nutritional status of an older adult. Information from dietary intake can validate the absence or surplus of a dietary component identified by anthropometric, biochemical, or clinical assessments. There are different ways to obtain dietary intake data. It is important to note that the quality of the dietary intake information obtained from patients often relies on people's ability to remember the food items and quantity consumed, as well as their honesty in sharing those recollections. For example, can you remember everything you ate for lunch yesterday and the exact amounts and methods of preparation? Common methods for assessing nutritional intake include a diet history, food

TABLE 10.8 · Dietary Assessment and Key Features

Dietary Assessment Method	Key Features
Diet history	The most comprehensive form of obtaining dietary intake information is the diet history. Using this technique, a trained interviewer probes the client to find out what the client has been eating recently and also the client's long-term food intake practice.
Food records or diaries	Can provide meticulous information about day-to-day eating behavior. Usually, a person records all foods and beverages consumed during a specific period, normally 3–7 successive days.
Food Frequency Questionnaire (FFQ)	Records how often the person consumes certain foods or groups of foods, rather than specific foods consumed on a daily basis. These data are used to calculate that person's average daily intake.
24-Hour dietary recall	The easiest form of dietary intake data retrieval. In a 24-hr recall, the examiner walks the client through a recent 24-hr period (usually midnight to midnight) to define what foods and beverages the client consumed.

record, food frequency questionnaire, and 24-hour diet recall (Table 10.8). The value of these methods depends on the information desired and the skill of the interviewer collecting the information. In older adults, memory and cognitive status as well as the attention of a caregiver to food intake are important factors in the accuracy of the information.

Comparison with Dietary Standards

Once dietary data are gathered, the next step is to define the nutrient composition of the diet and assess that data in terms of dietary standards or other benchmark. This is usually done using nutrient analysis software. It is possible to compare data collected from nutrient intake reports with dietary standards such as the RDA or AI values. While this will give a quantitative idea of dietary adequacy, it should not be considered an absolute assessment of a person's diet as we do not know the person's individual nutrient needs.

The MyPlate system, for example, has many online tools for evaluating dietary intake. Individuals and assessors can use the Analyze My Diet function on the ChooseMyPlate Web site to compare a typical day's food intake with the MyPlate groups and *Dietary Guidelines*. The use of these tools can assist in providing a general idea of whether the person's diet is adequate in saturated fat, or whether the person is consuming sufficient fruits, vegetables, and whole grains.

Outcomes of Nutrition Assessment

Assessment parameters such as anthropometric measures, biochemical tests, clinical exams, and dietary evaluation, along with the individual's family history, socioeconomic situation, and other factors, can assist in depicting a comprehensive picture of nutritional health. A complete nutritional assessment can provide the information needed to make alterations in nutrition interventions to generate a change in diet to promote weight loss or blood cholesterol, the addition of a vitamin or mineral supplement to address a deficiency, or just the attestation that dietary intake is adequate for current nutrition needs.

FOOD AND NUTRITION ASSISTANCE

Countless older adults are at nutritional risk due to financial situation, social isolation, limited mobility, inability to shop for and/or cook meals, and medical ailments. Currently, there are many ways that older adults can maintain their independence and have access to a suitable diet. Independent and assisted-living facilities allow older adults to live carefree and independent lives. Senior citizen apartment buildings and retirement villages provide an assortment of amenities, including nutritious meals. Government-sponsored programs such as Meals on Wheels and the Older Americans Act Nutrition Program deliver meals to community-dwelling older adults that are homebound, as well as those in congregate meal settings. Programs offer meals at least five times per week. The Supplemental Nutrition Assistance Program (SNAP) is another program that offers low-income older adults the resources to secure food. The SNAP conveys a "welfare" stigma; as a result, some older adults are unwilling to participate. Additionally, not all older adults that need assistance with purchasing food meet the eligibility criteria. Research supports that the older adults that participate in the Older Americans Act Nutrition Program have higher nutrient levels than nonparticipants. Program participants also have a higher number of regular social contacts, another important factor in promoting adequate nutrition intake (Academy of Nutrition and Dietetics, Evidence Analysis Library, n.d.-c).

FACTORS THAT AFFECT FOOD CHOICES

Food is a vital element of daily life. Meals contribute to a sense of security, meaning, and structure to an older adult's day, affording older adults with feelings of freedom and control and a sense of mastery over their environment (Amarantos et al., 2001). Food practices of older adults are influenced by a lifetime of inclinations and physiological changes as well as elements such as living arrangements, finances, transportation, and disability. The positive psychological and social features of eating are significant pleasures of life. When determining the care of older adults, clinicians must recognize that food habits make a substantial influence to well-being.

Lifetime eating habits, spiritual and religious principles, sociocultural effects, infirmities, caregivers, and living arrangements can have a substantial influence on the food consumption of older adults. By understanding and accepting the short- and long-term issues that impact the food and lifestyle preferences of older adults, clinicians can better support their well-being.

Disability is normally defined by limited ability in conducting activities of daily living (ADL) and/or instrumental activities of daily living (IADL). Challenges with physical performance are more common as we age. A number of health conditions augment the risk of functional restrictions; for instance, approximately 20% of stroke survivors, 11% of older adults with diabetes, and 10% of older adults with ischemic heart disease need assistance conducting ADLs (Pfizer Facts, 2007). Sarcopenic obesity is independently linked with IADL disability in the community-dwelling older adult (Baumgartner et al., 2004).

Living arrangements and the presence of a caregiver can influence diet quality. Almost 29.3% of noninstitutionalized older adults, 8.1 million women, and 3.2 million men live alone (Administration on Aging [AOA], n.d.-b). This results in a demand for a variety of housing choices to meet the unique needs of each older adult. Caregivers and families can play an important role by encouraging good nutrition and by assisting in activities such as shopping, meal preparation, and, as needed, administration of home enteral nutrition. Healthcare providers must recognize that care givers may lack the knowledge and skill required to adjust the diet to meet recommendations for diet therapy, or, for example, to change diet consistency if needed.

The ability to prepare and obtain food, including transportation to/from the store, and economic resources such as limited income can have profound effects on the food intake and nutritional status of older adults. Shopping for food and preparing meals can become an everyday challenge. Physical limitations, such as muscle weakness, loss of strength and flexibility and poor balance, resulting from chronic conditions, can make the simple task of meal preparation overwhelming. Being alone can impact the older adult's appetite, resulting in decreased meal intake. In 2010, 72% of men between the ages of 65 and 74 lived with their partners, versus 42% of women in the same age group (Federal Interagency Forum on Aging-Related Statistics, 2012). Participation in USDA and OAA programs can improve food and nutrient intake, increase food and vegetable intake, and serve to stimulate the desire to consume healthy foods (AND, EAL, n.d.-a). For many elders, physical limitations, illness, depression, and isolation are common factors that can reduce the willingness to cook and eat meals. For community-dwelling adults, dependency on transportation resources can impact their ability to procure fresh, wholesome foods. In addition, financial constraints and a limited income are significant contributors to food insecurity for this age group. In 2010, 9% of the older adult population lived in poverty, and 26% of the older population was in the low-income group (Federal Interagency Forum on Aging-Related Statistics, 2012).

FEDERAL PROGRAMS

Adequate nutrition and food security are essential factors in promoting healthy aging. A large system of federally funded programs offers food to millions of older adults on a yearly basis (Position of the American Dietetic Association, American Society for Nutrition, and Society for Nutrition Education, 2010). Participation in food assistance programs can have nutritional and nonnutritional benefits. These programs allow older adults to obtain nutrient-dense foods and nutritionally balanced meals. They also contribute to improved nutritional status and support health, independence with ADLs, and quality of life via directed nutrition screening, assessment, nutrition education, and counseling. Preventing and/or reducing the undesirable nutritional consequences linked with food insecurity are some of the benefits associated with participation in food assistance programs (Kirang & Frongillo, 2007).

OLDER AMERICANS ACT PROGRAMS

Publicly funded programs, by the US Administration on Aging and the US Department of Agriculture (USDA), provide food and nutrition services for older adults. Participation in the OAA programs facilitates access to nutritious foods. Consumption of nutrient dense foods gives older adults an edge in their pursuit of wellness and health as well as quality of life. However, universal access across all communities is limited in part to availability of programs in all localities, eligibility requirements for participants, perceived social stigma, and limited funding.

Older Americans Act

This is perhaps the earliest and most comprehensive program to provide a variety of services and support to help older adults aged 60 years and older to remain independent in home and in community settings (AOA, n.d.-a). The OAA targets those persons who are poor, members of minority groups, and those living in rural areas with limited access to services. The OAA is unique in that it sets parameters and general requirements to support a bottom-up, community-based planning and service delivery system. Decisions are made at the individual community level concerning local area plans, specific programs, and services to be provided and their delivery mechanism, and methods to monitor effectiveness and quality (AOA, n.d.-a).

The OAA is administered by the US Administration on Aging through the National Aging Services Network (OAA Network), consisting of 244 Tribal or Native organizations or 56 State Units on Aging in collaboration with 629 local Area Agencies on Aging, 20,000 service providers, and 2 Native Hawaiian organizations representing 400 tribes (HHS, 2010). Title III of the OAA authorizes a broad array of community-based nutrition, health, and supportive services (AOA, n.d.-a). These services may include information, referral, transportation, adult day care, senior center activities, pension counseling, and health and physical activity programs. In-home care may include home maintenance assistance, home-health and personal care. Caregiver support can include respite services, nutrition advice, and assistance with care coordination (AOA, n.d.-a). The OAA provides meals to older adults in a variety of settings, including senior centers, or home delivery to older adults that are homebound due to illness, disability, or geographic isolation. Services are targeted at those with social and economic need with special attention to low-income elders, minorities, people in rural communities, those with limited English proficiency as well as elders at risk for institutional care. One key objective of the Nutrition Services Programs is to help older individuals to remain independent and in their communities by providing nutritious food to qualified participants (AOA, n.d.-a).

USDA Food and Nutrition Assistance Programs

The USDA administers community-based food and nutrition assistance programs, including the Supplemental Nutrition Assistance Program (SNAP), the Senior Farmers Market Nutrition Program, the Child and Adult Care Food Program, the Emergency Food Assistance Program, and the Commodity Supplemental Food Program to provide Americans, including older adults, with access to food, a healthful diet, and nutrition education (USDA, 2013; USDA, Food and Nutrition Services [FNS], 2010). Every single program functions as a discrete unit, regarding income and asset eligibility requirements. Each state may select different populations based on their demographics targeting vulnerable populations such as children, needy families, and older adults. Thus, these important USDA programs differ from the more comprehensive coordinated nutrition, health, and supportive services provided under the OAA. USDA programs, particularly the SNAP and the Senior Farmers Market Nutrition Program, promote primary prevention through better access to food and a more healthful diet by way of its food assistance programs and comprehensive nutrition education efforts. Collaboration among dietetics professionals, extension, and other community resources help increase referrals across programs (USDA, FNS, 2010).

Supplemental Nutrition Assistance Program (SNAP)

The SNAP, available to all eligible persons meeting need and asset requirements, provides older adults with access to nutrient-dense foods to improve quality and variety of dietary intake.

Senior Farmers Market Nutrition Program

Grants are used to provide low-income seniors with coupons to be used for eligible foods at farmers' markets, roadside stands, and community-supported agriculture programs. Eligible foods are defined as fresh, nutritious, unprepared, locally grown fruits, vegetables, herbs, and honey (USDA, FNS, 2013). Although there is variation in program administration, there is evidence that the Senior Farmers Market Nutrition Program is successful in increasing fruit and vegetable consumption, stimulating interest in healthy foods, and improving quality of life (Academy of Nutrition and Dietetics, Evidence Analysis Library, n.d.-c).

COMMUNITY RESOURCES

An older person's requirement for community services can change as they age. At times, defining the community services needed by an older adult can be multifactorial, and financial concerns may add limitations to the access to services that can help older adults in their homes.

CULTURAL SENSITIVITY

As the older population continues to flourish, it becomes more diverse, imitating the demographic transformations of the US population in the last 20 to 30 years. Cultural patterns influence and help to develop eating patterns and behaviors. By 2050, programs and amenities for older adults will necessitate more flexibility to accommodate the needs of a much more diverse population (Federal Interagency Forum on Aging-Related Statistics, 2012). Our culture determines how foods are prepared and how meals are served. Providing nutrition services to a diverse population requires for healthcare providers to become familiar with other cultures and possibly learn basic communication on other languages.

PHYSICAL ACTIVITY

Physical activity cannot stop biological aging; regular exercise can, however, minimize the physiological effects of a sedentary lifestyle and limit the progression of disabling conditions and chronic diseases (Salem et al., 2009). The U.S. Department of Health and Human Services' 2008 *Physical Activity Guidelines for Americans* states, "regular physical activity is essential for healthy aging" and recommends that all adults should avoid inactivity; recommendations that are echoed in the *Dietary Guidelines for Americans 2010*. Despite these recommendations, however, fewer than 5% of adults participate in 30 minutes of physical activity each day, and participation in physical activity declines with age (USDA & HHS, 2010). Lack of physical activity contributes to sarcopenia, functional decline, and frailty that commonly accompany aging (Fiatarone-Singh & Bernstein, 2010). Advanced age and degenerative conditions should not automatically prevent older adults from participating in physical activity with qualified supervision. In fact, they may instead provide good reason for appropriate exercises for the older adult (Position of the American Dietetic Association, 2010).

The health benefits of a professionally designed and individualized exercise prescription to increase physical activity that includes aerobic activities, flexibility exercises, and progressive resistance strength training are interconnected and far reaching, especially in older adults. Illness, medication use, and nutritional deficiencies, and notably dehydration, may lead to impaired motor function; therefore, older adults should be evaluated by their physician prior to beginning a new exercise program.

FOOD SAFETY

While food safety is important for everyone, it is particularly important for older adults. The physiological changes associated with aging make older adults more susceptible to foodborne illness. The chronic conditions from which older adults suffer or the side effect of one of the many medications they take on a daily basis can weaken the immune system, causing the older adult to be more prone to foodborne illness. Older adults need to prepare, store, and handle foods following HACCP guidelines. When preparing foods, work surfaces and hands should be washed often with hot soapy water. All foods must be cooked to a safe temperature, raw foods must be kept away from cooked foods, and all foods must be refrigerated per manufacturer recommendations.

ROLE OF THE REGISTERED DIETITIAN AND DIET TECHNICIAN, REGISTERED

In many care settings, the registered dietitian (RD) will partner with a dietetic technician registered (DTR) to collect data, complete nutrition assessments and deliver nutrition care. The DTR along with the RD both can provide patient education, while the RD completes the actual in-depth assessment and provides education counseling to the patient. All members of the interdisciplinary team play a crucial part in guaranteeing that older adults with specific dietary requirements, food beliefs, and disabilities are provided with optimum nutrition. The healthcare team works together to develop and implement a plan of care that addresses health promotion and independence, acute and chronic disease management, and quality of life for older adults.

REFERENCES

Academy of Nutrition and Dietetics. (n.d.-a). *Food and nutrition for older adults: promoting health and wellness evidence analysis project*. Retrieved from Academy of Nutrition and Dietetics Evidence Analysis Library Web site: http://www.andevidenceanalysislibrary.com/topic.cfm?cat=3987

Academy of Nutrition and Dietetics. (n.d.-b). *Nutrition care manual products*. Retrieved from http://nutritioncaremanual.org/auth.cfm?p=%2Findex%2Ecfm%3F&err=NotLoggedIn

Academy of Nutrition and Dietetics, Evidence Analysis Library. (2012). *Nutrition across the spectrum of aging. Evidence Analysis project. Aging programs*. Retrieved from http://www.adaevidencelibrary.com/topic.cfm?cat=4072

Academy of Nutrition and Dietetics, Evidence Analysis Library. (n.d.-a). *Encourage participation in USDA and OAA programs*. Retrieved from http://andevidencelibrary.com/default.cfm?auth=1

Academy of Nutrition and Dietetics, Evidence Analysis Library. (n.d.-b). Retrieved from http://andevidencelibrary.com/default.cfm?auth=1

Academy of Nutrition and Dietetics, Evidence Analysis Library. (n.d.-c). *Aging programs—Evidence based practice guidelines*. Retrieved from http://www.ada.portalxm.com/eal/topic.cfm?cat=4552

Administration on Aging. (n.d.-a). *Older Americans Act*. Retrieved from http://www.aoa.gov/AoARoot/AoA_Programs/OAA/index.aspx

Administration on Aging. (n.d.-b). *Profile of older Americans 2011*. Retrieved from http://www.aoa.gov/AoARoot/Aging_Statistics/Profile/index.aspx

Allen, L. H. (2009). How common is vitamin B-12 deficiency? *American Journal of Clinical Nutrition, 89*(2), 693S–696S.

Amarantos, E., Martinez, A., & Dwyer, J. (2001). Nutrition and quality of life in older adults. *Journals of Gerontology. Series A, Biological Sciences and Medical Sciences, 56A*, 54–64.

American Cancer Society. (n.d.). *ACS guidelines on nutrition and physical activity for cancer prevention*. Retrieved from http://www.cancer.org/healthy/eathealthygetactive/acsguidelinesonnutritionphysicalactivityforcancerprevention/acs-guidelines-on-nutrition-and-physical-activity-for-cancer-prevention-intro

American Diabetes Association. (n.d.). *Diabetes statistics*. Retrieved from http://www.diabetes.org/diabetes-basics/diabetes-statistics/?loc=DropDownDB-stats

American Dietetic Association. (2011). Practice paper of the American Dietetic Association: Using the Dietary Reference Intakes. *Journal of the American Dietetic Association, 111*(5), 762–770.

American Dietetic Association. (n.d.). *ADA nutrition care manual*. Retrieved from http://www.nutritioncaremanual.org/

American Dietetic Association standards of practice and standards of professional performance for registered dietitians (generalist, specialty, advanced) in sports dietetics (2009). *Journal of the American Dietetic Association, 109*(3), 544–552. e530.

Anderson, A. L., Harris, T. B., Tylavsky, F. A., Perry, S. E., Houston, D. K., Hue, T. F., … Sahyoun, N. R. (2011). Dietary patterns and survival of older adults. The Health ABC Study. *Journal of the American Dietetic Association, 111*(1), 84–91.

Anemia.org. (2009, June 17). Recognizing concomitant anemia secondary to digestive disease. Retrieved from http://anemia.org/professionals/feature-articles/content.php?contentid=395&sectionid=15

Bachman, J., Reedy, J., Subar, A., & Krebs-Smith, S. (2008). Sources of food group intakes among the US population, 2001–2002. *Journal of the American Dietetic Association, 108*(5), 804–814.

Baranoski, S., & Ayello, E. A. (Eds.). (2012). *Wound care essentials: Practice principles* (3rd ed.). Ambler, PA: Wolter Kluwer/Lippincott Williams & Wilkins.

Baumgartner, R., Wayne, S., Walters, D., Janssen, I., Gallagher, D., & Morley, J. (2004). Sarcopenic obesity predicts instrumental activities of daily living disability in the elderly. *Obesity Research, 12*(12), 1995–2004.

Beers, M. H., & Berkow, R. (2000). *The Merck manual of geriatrics* (3rd ed.). West Point, PA: Merck Research Laboratories. Retrieved from http://www.merckmanuals.com/professional/geriatrics.html

Berger, M., & Doherty, T. (2010). Sarcopenia: Prevalence, mechanisms and functional consequences. *Interdisciplinary Topics in Gerontology, 37*, 94–114.

Bernstein, M., Tucker, K., Ryan, N., et al. (2003). Higher dietary variety is associated with better nutritional status in frail elderly people. *Journal of the American Dietetic Association, 102*(8), 1096–1104.

Bernstein, M. A., & Luggen, A. S. (2010). *Nutrition for the older adult*. Sudbury, MA: Jones and Bartlett.

Boire, Y. (2009). Physiopathological mechanisms of sarcopenia. *Journal of Nutrition, Health & Aging, 13*(8), 717–723.

Buhr, G., & Bales, C. W. (2010). Nutritional supplements for older adults: Review and recommendations-part II. *Journal of Nutrition for the Elderly, 29*(1), 42–71.

Carpentier, S., Knaus, M., & Suh, M. (2009). Associations between lutein, zeaxanthin, and age-related macular degeneration: An overview. *Critical Reviews in Food Science and Nutrition, 49*(4), 313–326.

Centers for Disease Control and Prevention. (2011a). Heart disease: Guidelines and recommendations. Retrieved from http://www.cdc.gov/HeartDisease/guidelines_recommendations.htm.

Centers for Disease Control and Prevention. (2011b, November). Make physical activity a part of an older adult's life. Retrieved from http://www.cdc.gov/physicalactivity/everyone/getactive/olderadults.html

Centers for Disease Control and Prevention. (n.d.-a). Cancer. Retrieved from http://www.cdc.gov/alcohol/index.htm

Centers for Disease Control and Prevention. (n.d.-b). Cancer prevention and treatment. Retrieved from http://www.cdc.gov/cancer/

Centers for Disease Control and Prevention. (n.d.-c). Depression. Retrieved from http://www.cdc.gov/Features/Depression/

Centers for Disease Control and Prevention. (n.d.-d). Dietary supplements—Nutrition for everyone. Retrieved from http://www.cdc.gov/nutrition/everyone/basics/vitamins/iron.html

Centers for Disease Control and Prevention. (n.d.-e). 10 Leading causes of death by age group, United States—2009. Retrieved from National Vital Statistics System, National Center for Health Statistics, Centers for Disease Control and Prevention Web site: http://www.cdc.gov/Injury/wisqars/pdf/10LCD-Age-Grp-US-2009-a.pdf

Centers for Disease Control and Prevention. (n.d.-f). Nutrition for everyone: Iron and iron deficiency. Retrieved from http://www.cdc.gov/nutrition/everyone/basics/vitamins/iron.html

Centers for Medicare and Medicaid Services. (2011). *State operations manual appendix PP—Guidance to surveyors for long term care facilities.* Baltimore, MD: Author. Retrieved from http://www.cms.gov/Regulations-and-Guidance/Guidance/Manuals/downloads/som107ap_pp_guidelines_ltcf.pdf

Chapman, I. M. (2007). The anorexia of aging. *Clinics in Geriatric Medicine, 23*(4), 735–756.

Chaput, J., Lord, C., Coutier, M., et al. (2007). Relationship between antioxidant intakes and class l sarcopenia in elderly men and women. *Journal of Nutrition, Health & Aging, 11*(4), 363–369.

Chernoff, R. (2004). Protein and older adults. *Journal of the American College of Nutrition, 23*(6 Suppl.), 627S–630S.

Dangour, A. D., Breeze, E., Clarke, R., et al. (2008). Plasma homocysteine, but not folate or vitamin B12, predicts mortality in older adults in the United Kingdom. *Journal of Nutrition, 138*, 1121–1128.

Devore, E., Kang, J., Stampfer, M., & Grodstein, F. (2010). Total antioxidant capacity of diet in relation to cognitive function. *American Journal of Clinical Nutrition, 92*, 1157–1164.

Dorner, B., Posthauer, M. E., & Thomas, D., National Pressure Ulcer Advisory Panel. (2009). *The role of nutrition in pressure ulcer prevention and treatment: National pressure ulcer advisory panel White Paper.* Washington, DC: National Pressure Ulcer Advisory Panel.

Federal Interagency Forum on Aging Related Statistics. (2010). *Older Americans 2010: Key indicators of well-being.* Retrieved from http://www.agingstats.gov/agingstatsdotnet/Main_Site/Data/2010_Documents/Docs/OA_2010.pdf

Federal Interagency Forum on Aging-Related Statistics. (2012). *Older Americans 2012: Key indicators of well-being.* Retrieved from http://www.agingstats.gov/agingstatsdotnet/Main_Site/Data/2012_Documents/Docs/EntireChartbook.pdf.

Fiatarone-Singh, M. A., & Bernstein, M. A. (2010). Exercise for the older adult: nutritional implications. In: M. S. Bernstein & A. S. Luggen (Eds.), *Nutrition for the older adult.* Sudbury, MA: Jones & Bartlett.

Green, R. (2009). Is it time for vitamin B-12 fortification? What are the questions? *American Journal of Clinical Nutrition, 89*(2), 712S–716S

Haan, M. N., Miller, J. W., Aiello, A. E., et al. (2007). Homocysteine, B vitamins, and the incidence of dementia and cognitive impairment: results from the Sacramento Area Latino Study on Aging. *American Journal of Clinical Nutrition, 85*(2), 511–517.

Health Central. (n.d.). Retrieved from http://www.healthcentral.com/alzheimers/stages-8783-108.html?ic=506019

HealthinAging.org. (n.d.). Retrieved from http://www.healthinaging.org/aging-and-health-a-to-z/topic:nutrition/info:unique-to-older-adults/

Hollis, J., & Henry, C. (2007). Dietary variety and its effect on food intake of elder adults. *Journal of Human Nutrition and Dietetics: The Official Journal of the British Dietetic Association, 20*(4), 345–351.

Horn, S. D., Bender, S. A., Ferguson, M. L., et al. (2004). The National Pressure Ulcer Long Term Care Study: Pressure ulcer development in long-term care residents. *Journal of the American Geriatrics Society, 52*, 359–367.

Houston, D. K., Nicklas, B. J., Ding, J., Harris, T. B., Tylavsky, F. A., Newman, A. B., … Kritchevsky, S. B. (2008). Dietary protein intake is associated with lean mass change in older, community-dwelling adults: The Health, Aging, and Body Composition (Health ABC) Study. *American Journal of Clinical Nutrition, 87*(1), 150–155.

Houston, D. K., Nicklas, B. J., & Zizza, C. A. (2009). Weighty concerns: The growing prevalence of obesity among older adults. *Journal of the American Dietetic Association, 109*(11), 1886–1895.

Institute of Medicine, Food and Nutrition Board. (2004). *Dietary Reference Intakes for water, potassium, sodium, chloride, and sulfate.* Washington, DC: National Academies Press.

Institute of Medicine, Food and Nutrition Board. (2005a). *Dietary Reference Intakes for energy, carbohydrate, fiber, fat, fatty acids, cholesterol, protein, and amino acids (Macronutrients).* Washington, DC: National Academy Press.

Institute of Medicine, Food and Nutrition Board, Standing Committee on the Scientific Evaluation of Dietary Reference Intakes, Panel on Dietary Reference Intakes for Electrolytes and Water. (2005b). *Dietary Reference Intakes for water, potassium, sodium, chloride, and sulfate.* Washington, DC: National Academies Press. Retrieved from http://www.nap.edu/catalog.php?record_id=10925

Institute of Medicine, Food and Nutrition Board. (2006). *Dietary Reference Intake: The essential guide to nutrient requirement.* Washington, DC. National Academy Press.

Institute of Medicine, Food and Nutrition Board. (2011). *Dietary Reference Intakes for calcium and vitamin D.* Washington, DC: National Academies Press. 2011. Retrieved from http://books.nap.edu/openbook.php?record_id=13050.

Jurschik, P., Torres, J., Sola, R., Nuin, C., Botigue, T., & Lavedan, A. (2010). High rates of malnutrition in older adults receiving different levels of health care in Lleida, Catalonia: An assessment of contributory factors. *Journal of Nutrition for the Elderly, 29*(4), 410–422.

Kim, J., Wilson, J., & Lee, S. (2010). Dietary implications on mechanisms of sarcopenia: Roles of protein, amino acids and antioxidants. *Journal of Nutritional Biochemistry, 21*(1), 1–13.

Kirang, K., & Frongillo, E. (2007). Participation in food assistance programs modifies the relation of food insecurity with weight and depression in elders. *Journal of Nutrition, 137*(4), 1005–1010.

Krebs-Smith, S. M., Guenther, P. M., Subar, A., Kirkpatrick, S. I., & Dodd, K. W. (2010). Americans do not meet federal dietary recommendations. *Journal of Nutrition, 140*(10), 1832–1838.

Lahiri, M., Morgan, C., Symmons, D. P., & Bruce, I. N. (2012). Modifiable risk factors for RA: Prevention, better than a cure? *Rheumatology (Oxford), 51*(3), 499–512.

Larsen, P. (December 2008–January 2009). A review of cardiovascular changes in the older adult. *Gerontology.* Retrieved from http://www.rehabnurse.org/pdf/GeriatricsCV.pdf

Lichtenstein, A. H., Rasmussen, H., Winifred, Y., Epstein, S., & Russell, R. (2008). Modified MyPyramid for older adults. *Journal of Nutrition, 138*(1), 5–11.

MacKay, D., & Miller, A. (2003). Nutritional support for wound healing. *Alternative Medicine Review: A Journal of Clinical Therapeutic, 8,* 359–377.

Medline Plus. (2012, September 2). Aging changes in hormone production. Retrieved from http://www.nlm.nih.gov/medlineplus/ency/article/004000.htm

Miller, S. L., & Wolfe, R. R. (2008). The danger of weight loss in the elderly. *Journal of Nutrition, Health & Aging, 12*(7), 487–491.

Millward, D. J. (2008). Sufficient protein for our elders? *American Journal of Clinical Nutrition, 88*(5), 1187–1188.

National Eye Institute. (2012). The AREDS formulation and age-related macular degeneration. Are these high levels of antioxidants and zinc right for you? Retrieved from http://www.nei.nih.gov/amd/summary.asp

National Institute of Arthritis and Musculoskeletal and Skin Diseases. (2010, July). Handout on health: osteoarthritis (Revised). Retrieved from http://www.niams.nih.gov/Health_Info/Osteoarthritis

National Institutes of Health, Office of Dietary Supplements. (n.d.-a). Dietary supplement fact sheet: Magnesium. Retrieved from http://ods.od.nih.gov/factsheets/Magnesium-HealthProfessional/

National Institutes of Health, Office of Dietary Supplements. (n.d.-b). Dietary supplement fact sheet: Vitamin A. Retrieved from http://ods.od.nih.gov/factsheets/VitaminA-HealthProfessional/

National Institutes of Health, Office of Dietary Supplements. (n.d.-c). Dietary supplement fact sheet: Vitamin C. Retrieved from http://ods.od.nih.gov/factsheets/VitaminC-HealthProfessional/#h5

National Institutes of Health, Office of Dietary Supplements. (n.d.-d). Dietary supplement fact sheet: Vitamin D. Retrieved from http://ods.od.nih.gov/factsheets/vitamind/#en61

National Institutes of Health, Office of Dietary Supplements. (n.d.-e). Dietary supplement fact sheet: Vitamin E. Retrieved from http://ods.od.nih.gov/factsheets/VitaminE-QuickFacts/

National Institute on Alcohol Abuse and Alcoholism. (2013). Retrieved from http://pubs.niaaa.nih.gov/publications/aa22.htm

Nelms, M., & Habash, D. (2011). Nutrition assessment: Foundations of the nutrition care process. In M. Nelms, K. P. Sucher, K. Lacy, & S. Long Roth (Eds.), *Nutrition therapy and pathophysiology* (2nd ed.). Belmont, CA: Wadsworth Cengage.

NIH Osteoporosis and Related Bone Diseases National Resource Center. (2013). Osteoporosis overview. Retrieved from http://www.niams.nih.gov/Health_Info/Bone/Osteoporosis/overview.asp#g

NIH Senior Health. (2013). Alcohol and aging. Retrieved from http://nihseniorhealth.gov/alcoholuse/alcoholandaging/01.html

Paddon-Jones, D., & Rasmussen, B. B. (2009). Dietary protein recommendations and the prevention of sarcopenia. *Current Opinion in Clinical Nutrition and Metabolic Care, 12*(1), 86–90.

Paddon-Jones, D., Short, K. R., Campbell, W. W., et al. (2008). The role of dietary protein in sarcopenia and aging. *American Journal of Clinical Nutrition, 87*(Suppl.), 1562s–1566s.

Patterson, E., Wall, R., Fitzgerald, G. F., Ross, R. P., & Stanton, C. (2012). Health implications of high dietary omega-6 polyunsaturated fatty acids. *Journal of Nutrition and Metabolism, 2012,* 539426. Published online 2012 April 5. doi:10.1155/2012/539426

Pfizer Facts. (2007). *Health status of older adults. Findings from the National Health and Nutrition Examination Survey (NHANES) 1999–2004, the National Health Interview Survey (NHIS) 2005, and the Compressed Mortality File (CMF) 2003.* Retrieved from http://www.pfizer.com/files/products/The_Health_Status_of_Older_Adults_2007.pdf

Pomerleau, J., Lock, K., Knai, C., & McKee, M. (2005). Interventions designed to increase fruit and vegetable intake can be effective: A systematic review of the literature. *Journal of Nutrition, 135*(10), 2486–2495.

Position of the Academy of Nutrition and Dietetics: Food and nutrition for older adults: Promoting health and wellness. (2012). *Journal of the Academy of Nutrition and Dietetics, 112*(8), 1255–1277.

Position of the American Dietetic Association: Individualized nutrition approaches for older adults in health care communities. (2010). *Journal of the American Dietetic Association, 110*(10), 1549–1553.

Position of the American Dietetic Association, American Society for Nutrition, and Society for Nutrition Education: Food and nutrition programs for community-residing older adults. (2010). *Journal of Nutrition Education and Behavior, 42*(2), 72–82.

Rolland, Y., Lauwers-Cances, V., Cristini, C., et al. (2009). Difficulties with physical function associated with obesity, sarcopenia, and sarcopenic-obesity in community-dwelling elderly women: The EPIDOS (EPIDemiologie de l'OSteoporose) Study. *American Journal of Clinical Nutrition, 89*(6), 1895–1900.

Salem, G. J., Skinner, J. S., Chodzko-Zajko, W. J., et al. (2009). Exercise and physical activity for older adults. *Medicine and Science in Sports and Exercise, 41*(7), 1510–1530.

Sebastian, R., Cleveland, L., Goldman, J., & Moshfegh, A. (2007). Older adults who use vitamin/mineral supplements differ from nonusers in nutrient intake adequacy and dietary attitudes. *Journal of the American Dietetic Association, 107*(8), 1322–1332.

Shatenstein, B. (2008). Impact of health conditions on food intakes among older adults. *Journal of Nutrition for the Elderly, 27*(3–4), 333–361.

Stechmiller, J. K., Cowan, L., Whitney, J. D., et al. (2008). Guidelines for the prevention of pressure ulcers. *Wound Repair and Regeneration, 16*, 151–168.

Stenholm, S., Harris, T., Rantanen, T., Visser, M., Kritchevsky, S., & Ferrucci L. (2008). Sarcopenic obesity definition, etiology and consequences. *Current Opinion in Clinical Nutrition and Metabolic Care, 11*(6), 693–700.

Symons, T., Schutzler, S., Cocke, T., Chinkes, D., Wolfe, R., & Paddon-Jones, D. (2007). Aging does not impair the anabolic response to a protein-rich meal. *American Journal of Clinical Nutrition, 86*(2), 451–456.

Symons, T. B., Sheffield-Moore, M., Mamerow, M. M., Wolfe, R. R., & Paddon-Jones, D. (2011). The anabolic response to resistance exercise and a protein-rich meal is not diminished by age. *Journal of Nutrition, Health & Aging, 15*(5), 376–381.

Tufts Now. (2011). Tufts University nutrition scientists unveil MyPlate for older adults. Retrieved from http://now.tufts.edu/news-releases/tufts-university-nutrition-scientists-unveil-

United States Department of Agriculture. (2013). *USDA Senior's Farmers Market Nutrition Program Fact Sheet*. Retrieved from http://www.fns.usda.gov/wic/SFMNP-Fact-Sheet.pdf

United States Department of Agriculture, Food and Nutrition Information Center. (2010). Dietary guidance DRI tables. Retrieved from http://fnic.nal.usda.gov/nal_display/index.php?info_center=4&tax_level=2&tax_subject=256&topic_id=1342

United States Department of Agriculture, Food and Nutrition Services. (2010). *USDA Food and Nutrition Services—Nutrition Assistance programs*. Retrieved from http://www.fns.usda.gov/fns

United States Department of Agriculture, Food and Nutrition Services. (2013). *Seniors Farmers Market Nutrition Program*. Retrieved from http://www.fns.usda.gov/wic/seniorfmnp/sfmnpmenu.htm

United States Department of Agriculture & U.S. Department of Health and Human Services. (2010, December). *Dietary guidelines for Americans*, 2010 (7th ed.). Washington, DC: U.S. Government Printing Office. Retrieved from http://www.cnpp.usda.gov/Publications/DietaryGuidelines/2010/PolicyDoc/PolicyDoc.pdf

U.S. Department of Health and Human Services. (2008). Active older adults. In: *2008 Physical activity guidelines for Americans*. Rockville, MD: Author.

U.S. Department of Health and Human Services. (2010, August 27). Older Americans Act. Retrieved from http://www.hhs.gov/asl/testify/2010/08/t20100827a.html

Vaquero, M. P. (2002). Magnesium and trace elements in the elderly: Intake, status, and recommendations. *Journal of Nutrition, Health & Aging, 6*(2), 147–153.

Vincent, H., Vincent, K., & Lamb, K. (2010). Obesity and mobility disability in the older adult. *Obesity Reviews: An Official Journal of the International Association for the Study of Obesity, 11*(8), 568–579.

Weinstein, J. R., & Anderson, S. (2010). The aging kidney: Physiological changes. *Advances in Chronic Kidney Disease, 17*(4), 302–307. Retrieved from http://www.ncbi.nlm.nih.gov/pmc/articles/PMC2901622/

Wernette, C. M., White, B. D., & Zizza, C. A. (2011). Signaling proteins that influence energy intake may affect unintentional weight loss in elderly persons. *Journal of the American Dietetic Association, 111*(6), 864–873.

Zamboni, M., Mazzali, G., Zoico, E., Harris, T. B., Meigs, J. B., Di Francesco, V., … Bosello, O. (2005). Health consequences of obesity in the elderly: A review of four unresolved questions. *International Journal of Obesity, 29*(9), 1011–1029.

CHAPTER 10: IT RESOURCES

Websites

Academy of Nutrition and Dietetics (formerly the American Dietetic Association)
http://www.eatright.org/

Centers for Disease Control and Prevention—Nutrition
http://www.cdc.gov/nutrition/

Food and Nutrition Board—Institute of Medicine
http://www.iom.edu/About-IOM/Leadership-Staff/Boards/Food-and-Nutrition-Board.aspx

National Institute of Health—Nutrition
http://health.nih.gov/topic/Nutrition

United States Department of Agriculture—Nutrition for Older Adults: SNAP-Ed Connection
http://snap.nal.usda.gov/professional-development-tools/hot-topics-z/nutrition-older-adults

United States Department of Agriculture—National Agriculture Library—Aging
http://fnic.nal.usda.gov/lifecycle-nutrition/aging

Older Adults: 9 Nutrients You May Be Missing
http://www.webmd.com/healthy-aging/nutrition-world-2/missing-nutrients

Special Nutrient Needs of Older Adults
http://www.eatright.org/Public/content.aspx?id=6839

Using the Nutrition Facts Label: A How-To Guide for Older Adults
http://www.fda.gov/Food/ResourcesForYou/Consumers/ucm267499.htm

Dietary Reference Intakes (DRIs)/Recommended Dietary Allowances (RDAs) for Older Adults
http://www2.fiu.edu/~nutreldr/SubjectList/D/DRI_RDA.htm

Academy of Nutrition and Dietetics—Academy Position and Practice Papers
http://www.eatright.org/positions/

ChooseMyPlate.gov
http://www.choosemyplate.gov/

Estimated Energy Requirement Calculator
http://moritzcycling.com/eer.cgi

Assessment and Management of Nutrition in Older People and its Importance to Health
http://www.ncbi.nlm.nih.gov/pmc/articles/PMC2920201/

Nutrition in Older Adults: Intervention and Assessment Can Help Curb the Growing Threat of Malnutrition
http://journals.lww.com/ajnonline/Fulltext/2005/03000/Nutrition_in_Older_Adults__Intervention_and.20.aspx

Tufts University—The Top Nutrition Guide
http://enews.tufts.edu/stories/777/2003/11/10/TopNutritionGuide

Nutrition Services (Older Americans Act Title IIIC)
http://www.aoa.gov/AoA_programs/HCLTC/Nutrition_Services/index.aspx

Supplemental Nutrition Assistance Program (SNAP)
http://www.fns.usda.gov/snap

Senior Farmers' Market Nutrition Program (SFMNP)
http://www.fns.usda.gov/sfmnp

PDF Documents

Try This Issue 9—Assessing Nutrition in Older Adults
   http://consultgerirn.org/uploads/File/trythis/try_this_9.pdf
Current Dietary Reference Intakes for Older Adults
   http://www.lifeclinic.com/focus/seniorcare/DRI.pdf
Dietary Guidelines for Americans 2010
   http://www.cnpp.usda.gov/Publications/DietaryGuidelines/2010/PolicyDoc/PolicyDoc.pdf
Calculating BMI and Estimated Energy Requirements (EER)
   http://faculty.mccneb.edu/CVanRiper/Unit%201/Calculating%20BMI%20and%20EER.pdf
The Mini Nutritional Assessment—This tool can identify malnutrition in older adults before
   changes in biochemistry or weight are evident.
   http://www.tuftshealthplans.com/providers/pdf/assessing_nutrition.pdf
The Health Status of Older Adults—Pfizer Facts
   http://www.pfizer.com/files/products/The_Health_Status_of_Older_Adults_2007.pdf

Videos

Choose My Plate Videos
   http://www.choosemyplate.gov/videos.html
Nutrition for the Older Adult (2009) (2:16 minutes)
   http://youtu.be/kgbOEs8BINE
Diets for Older Adults (2011)
   Our body's need for good nutrition doesn't diminish as we age. Though their needs are very
   different from those of younger people, there are some crucial nutritional considerations to
   keep in mind for older adults. (3:35 minutes)
   http://youtu.be/YhGsssLHFcI
Nutrition for the Aging Population (2012)
   This free course teaches the importance of nutrition in aging population (old people, retired
   people, adults). This is a free presentation that is being produced by United States University
   for the benefit of the public. http://www.usuniversity.edu (23:18 minutes)
   http://youtu.be/tviaPuZg_XQ
MNA Mini Nutritional Assessment (2009)
   MNA Video demonstrates step-by-step directions for using the MNA in clinical practice
   to identify malnutrition in the elderly. More information on www.mna-elderly.com
   (10:59 minutes)
   http://youtu.be/9oT7pF_Gck8

Images

Google images for Nutrition and the Older Adult
   http://www.google.com/search?q=nutrition+and+the+older+adult&source=lnms&tbm=isch
   &sa=X&ei=-MaiUYnyCIXe4AOlyICgDw&ved=0CAcQ_AUoAQ&biw=1011&bih=220

Exercise

Margaret B. Sproule, PhD, CHES

INTRODUCTION AND BACKGROUND

Walter Bortz, a physician and expert on aging, commented, "An unused engine rusts; a still stream stagnates; an untended garden tangles—much of what we pass as 'age' is disuse" (Bortz, 2007). The underlying message in this for the aging population is to move, to use the body, and to be physically active.

For a majority of the US population, increasing age after maturation is accompanied by a concomitant decline in physical activity and exercise behaviors. This decrease occurs for a variety of reasons, both lifestyle-related and health-related. This phenomenon has been presented as the Exercise and Aging Cycle (Canadian Centre for Activity and Aging, 2000). This cycle is a downward spiral, with the decline in physical activity leading to changes in fitness level, which in turn lead successively to decreased ability to be active, to lowered self-esteem, and, ultimately, to changes in health status. This cycle can be ended with regular, consistent physical activity.

Physical activity is a global term that describes any movement of the skeletal muscles. Among older adults, the goal of physical activity is to use the large muscle groups to expend energy (e.g., raking leaves or walking). The Physical Activity Guidelines for Americans recommend that older adults be as active as their abilities allow (U.S. Department of Health & Human Services [HHS], 2008). At a basic level, older adults should strive for 2½ hours of moderate-intensity activity or 1¼ hours of vigorous activity or a combination of moderate and vigorous activities each week.

Exercise is a specific type of physical activity. Exercise is planned and structured and uses the large muscle groups in repetitive ways to improve fitness. Fitness or physical fitness refers to the body's ability to be active. Having a certain level of fitness allows an individual to meet the demands of daily life, to successfully complete activities of daily living, and to ensure a good quality of life. The components of fitness for an older adult include cardiorespiratory endurance, muscular strength and endurance, flexibility, balance, and body composition. The national recommendations for physical activity encompass exercise and fitness, encouraging older adults to engage in muscle strengthening and balance exercises, in addition to the moderate- and vigorous-intensity cardiorespiratory activities.

Physical activity, incorporated as part of the lifestyle, and exercise, even when begun late in life, can provide both health and fitness benefits to the older adult. It is recommended that older adults be as active as possible within the context of their own lives and abilities.

PATHOPHYSIOLOGY AND HEALTHY ALTERNATIVES

Physical inactivity is a risk factor for a plethora of health conditions, and there are multiple mechanisms by which it causes physical impairment. On the flip side, there is ample evidence that shows that *physical activity*, particularly exercise, plays a preventative role in certain diseases and health conditions. For the older adult, exercise is strongly associated with a lower risk of heart disease, stroke, hypertension, hypercholesterolemia, metabolic syndrome, type 2 diabetes, and cancers of the colon and breast. Exercise is also strongly associated with weight loss and prevention of weight gain; with improved cardiovascular, respiratory, and muscular fitness; with fall prevention; and with improved cognitive function and decreased rates of depression (HHS, 2000). Exercise is also associated with increased bone density, lower risk of hip fracture, improved sleep quality, and improved functional health among older adults. Following is a brief discussion of the role of exercise in select health conditions. For further information on these diseases, refer to previous chapters.

Cardiovascular diseases (including hypertension, atherosclerosis, coronary heart disease, and stroke) remain the primary cause of morbidity, mortality, and disability in the United States and the world (Hoyert & Xu, 2012; World Health Organization [WHO], 2012). The American Heart Association estimates that roughly 84 million Americans have some form of cardiovascular disease. Furthermore, 42 million of these individuals are over 60 years of age (American Heart Association [AHA], 2013). Cardiovascular disease adversely affects not only these individuals but society as a whole in terms of financial, care-taking, and treatment burdens. Physical inactivity is strongly linked to the incidence of myocardial infarction, angina, and stroke, and is considered one of the leading modifiable risk factors for cardiovascular diseases. Inactivity impairs cardiac function through multiple mechanisms, including changes to such markers as high-density lipoprotein (HDL) cholesterol, apolipoprotein A, hemoglobin A, and vitamin D (Chomistek et al., 2011). The benefits of regular activity have long been recognized to offset cardiovascular disease, not only as a preventive measure but as a treatment option (Thompson et al., 2003).

Obesity, type 2 diabetes, and metabolic syndrome are unfortunate buzz words in the current culture and are coexisting conditions for many Americans. Metabolic syndrome, which has garnered attention in recent years, is a multifaceted condition whose diagnosis is based on clinical measures, including elevated waist circumference (abdominal obesity), elevated triglycerides, decreased HDL, elevated blood pressure, and elevated fasting glucose levels. Together, these risk factors promote the development of atherosclerotic heart disease and type 2 diabetes (Leutholtz & Ripoll, 2011; Rikli & Jones, 2001; Taylor & Johnson, 2008). Physical inactivity is implicated as a risk factor for metabolic syndrome, and it is indicated for both prevention and treatment (Boule et al., 2001; Ivy et al., 1999). Obesity, now considered an epidemic in the United

States, has increased to 27% among older adults aged 60 years and older (Schiller et al., 2012). Obesity is a risk factor for a number of chronic health conditions, including type 2 diabetes, cardiovascular disease, and arthritis. Again, physical inactivity is a major contributor to obesity. Type 2 diabetes is a chronic disease, with typical onset occurring after age 40, whose hallmarks are insulin resistance and ineffective insulin secretion.

Although type 2 diabetes is multifactorial, obesity is a significant contributor to insulin resistance, and it is estimated that the majority of people with new-onset type 2 diabetes are obese (Schiller et al., 2012). Once more, physical inactivity greatly impacts both prevention and treatment.

Cancer, or the uncontrolled growth of cells, can occur in any cell line, organ, or system in the body and can metastasize to other sites. It is generally believed that physical inactivity plays a role in the development of various cancers, and there is strong evidence showing a relationship between physical inactivity and colon cancers and breast cancers. Specifically, there is a demonstrated inverse relationship showing the greater the exercise level, the lower the risk of cancer of the colon or breast (International Agency on Research for Cancer, 2002; Slattery, 2004). In addition to research indicating the preventive benefits of physical activity and exercise, there is evidence to support the role of physical activity in effective cancer treatment (Holmes et al., 2005; Meyerhardt et al., 2006a, 2006b).

Musculoskeletal disorders, such as sarcopenia, osteoporosis, and arthritis, may not be immediately life-threatening, but they cause pain, immobility, and weakness and can certainly contribute to decreased functional ability and loss of independence in an older adult. Sarcopenia, a decline in skeletal muscle mass, size, and strength, is relatively common in the older adult. Although sarcopenia is attributed to the aging process, it is unclear whether the loss is due to that or to an increase in inactivity. Regardless of the cause, however, the changes in muscle tissue are not inevitable and may be offset with exercise (Hughes et al., 2001; Iannuzzi-Sucich et al., 2002). Osteoporosis and its precursor, osteopenia, both describe bone loss after maturation and affect approximately 28 million Americans (Durstine & Moore, 2003). The primary concern with osteoporosis is fracture of the back and/or hips, which can result in pain, vertebral deformities (which in turn could lead to respiratory problems), and loss of independence. Although some bone loss is inevitable with advancing age, the extent and rate of the loss may vary depending on the accompanying risk factors, one of which is a lack of physical activity. To prevent osteoporosis, there should be a focus with young- to middle-aged adults on attaining peak bone mass through good health behaviors, including weight-bearing exercise. Weight-bearing exercise may also be beneficial as part of the treatment regimen for older adults with diagnosed osteoporosis. Arthritis and other rheumatologic diseases are a common cause of pain and functional limitation among older adults (Dunlop et al., 2005). Osteoarthritis (a degenerative disease of specific joints) and rheumatoid arthritis (a disease of the immune system that affects multiple joints and systems) are two of the most common forms of arthritis. The pain, stiffness, and inflammation that accompany these forms of arthritis often start a cycle of reduced activity. Regular activity and exercise can improve the fitness, health, and flexibility of older adults with both osteoarthritis and rheumatoid arthritis. Furthermore, appropriate exercise is associated with decreased joint swelling and pain and increased ability to engage in activities of daily living (Durstine & Moore, 2003).

Mental disorders, conditions that affect an individual's emotions, thoughts, mood, or behavior, are commonly diagnosed, affecting approximately 26% of American adults (Kessler et al., 2005). Older adults may suffer from mental disorders such as depression, dementias (including Alzheimer disease), substance use, sleep disorders, and anxiety. These disorders may be exacerbated by changes to an elder's social support network, by poor coping mechanisms, and by the presence of comorbid health conditions. Physical activity can positively impact the older adults' mental health by improving self-concept, improving mood state, decreasing anxiety, lessening depression, and improving sleep (American Psychiatric Association [APA], 1994; Durstine & Moore, 2003; Singh et al., 2001).

PRESENTATION OF PHYSICAL INACTIVITY

There is a wide range of physical activity patterns and exercise behaviors among older adults. In the community-dwelling adult population, approximately 16% of adults aged 65 to 74 and 12% of adults over age 75 report being active at the recommended levels. Among this same population, 28% to 34% of adults aged 65 to 74 years and 35% to 44% of those 75 years and older are inactive. As evidenced by these values, physical inactivity increases with advancing age—by 75 years of age one in three men and one in two women engage in no physical activity (Centers for Disease Control and Prevention [CDC], 1996, 2000; HHS, 2000).

Among residents of long-term care institutions, physical activity levels decrease more markedly. Ruuskanen and Parkatti (1994) noted that more than 30% of new admissions to a long-term care facility reported reductions in daily physical activity. Historically, these institutions were designed to provide medical and nursing care for the sick and infirm. Despite recent restructuring to accommodate younger rehabilitative clients, such care facilities still predominately provide medical care for the sick and frail. Because of the medical focus on acute needs, there is often little emphasis placed on long-term preventive health for these seniors. As a result, residents lead a sedentary lifestyle (Ruuskanen & Parkatti, 1994).

The presence of physical inactivity in the older adult population overall is a result of real and perceived "barriers" to exercise and activity. As much as 87% of older adults report at least one barrier to being active (Chen, 2010; O'Neill & Reid, 1991). Inactivity among older adults may be due to underlying disease states or health conditions (discussed previously) and poor health status. Physical activity is further limited because of decreased functional capacity and frailty, particularly among residents in long-term care environments. Inactivity may also be due to lifestyle factors or self-selection. Independent older adults may opt out of physical activity because they feel "too old" to be active or because they perceive other barriers to leading an active lifestyle, such as lack of motivation, time constraints, and fear of injury. Social issues, such as lack of an exercise partner, also affect activity. Another limiting factor to physical activity among older adults is lack of information and advice from health care providers (Cherry et al., 2003; Lees et al., 2005; Schutzer & Graves, 2004).

There is a large body of evidence describing the benefits of physical activity and exercise, and many older adults know that physical activity is an important part of their lifestyle. Simply having this awareness of the importance of physical activity, however, is not enough to make someone become more active. In the United States, the general practitioner is often the main source of health information for older adults. This is not surprising given that older adults average over three office visits per year to their physician (Lees et al., 2005). What is surprising, however, is that the percentage of adults receiving advice from their health care provider to initiate or continue some form of physical activity declines with advancing age. Twenty-nine percent of adults aged 65 to 74 years, 22% of adults aged 75 to 84 years, and 14% of adults over age 85 years report physician counseling of activity and/or exercise (Schonberg et al., 2005).

SCREENING AND RISK FACTORS

Physical activity and exercise have multiple benefits for older adults. Although the majority of older adults can safely participate in a low- to moderate-intensity physical activity program, there may be contraindications for specific individuals to engage in vigorous activity. Individuals having recent myocardial infarction, severe aortic stenosis, unstable coronary artery disease or angina, uncontrolled arrhythmias, third-degree atrioventricular block, thrombus/embolus, and/or acute congestive heart failure should refrain from vigorous activity (American College of Sports Medicine [ACSM], 2010; Taylor & Johnson, 2008). Furthermore, individuals with chronic conditions such as chronic obstructive pulmonary disease (COPD), coronary artery disease, diabetes, and arthritis should be evaluated and counseled about appropriate activity and condition-specific risks, and activity should be tailored for these individuals. The medical evaluation should also include a review of medications, paying attention to polypharmacy, to ensure that the older adult is following appropriate treatment and to minimize potential risks with increased physical activity. For example, an older adult taking an antihypertensive may be prone to postural hypotension and should be cautioned to change positions slowly during exercise. It is also advisable for the practitioner to obtain information about musculoskeletal issues (e.g., back pain), sensory impairments (e.g., vision or hearing loss), and history of fall and fracture.

Because of the increasing prevalence of sedentary behaviors among older adults, it is important to screen them and identify those who are inactive. The Rapid Assessment of Physical Activity (RAPA), a questionnaire developed for clinicians to easily assess an older adult's activity during a typical week, may be helpful in determining an individual's activity and exercise behaviors (Fig. 11.1). It may also help the practitioner initiate a conversation about incorporating physical activity into the lifestyle (University of Washington Health Promotion Research Center, 2006). Alternatively, the practitioner could simply ask about activity and exercise behaviors as part of the routine health history interview.

Physical activity and exercise are behaviors, and as such, there are multiple determinants that play a role in an older adult's choice to engage in them. The transtheoretical model (or stages of change) was initially developed to describe individual behavior change in smoking cessation programs but is applicable for exercise and physical activity behaviors. The stages include precontemplation, contemplation, preparation, action, and maintenance, and the central idea is that people cycle through the various stages, often relapsing to a previous stage, when making a behavior change (Marcus et al., 1992).

In the first stage, precontemplation, the individual is not physically active and is not considering pursuing activity within the next 6 months. In the second stage, contemplation, the individual may have realized that he or she needs to become more active and so starts considering becoming more physically active within a 6-month time frame. In the preparation stage, the individual starts making concrete plans to become active. For example, she may decide to walk 3 days a week and may purchase walking shoes. The action stage occurs when the individual is engaged in the physical activity behavior on a regular basis. An individual in the action stage has been pursuing the behavior change for less than 6 months. An individual is considered to be in the maintenance stage when she (or he) has been engaged in the physical activity for longer than 6 months. It is normal and expected that individuals may revert to periods of inactivity, and the goal is to help them return to the physical activity as readily as possible.

How Physically Active Are You?

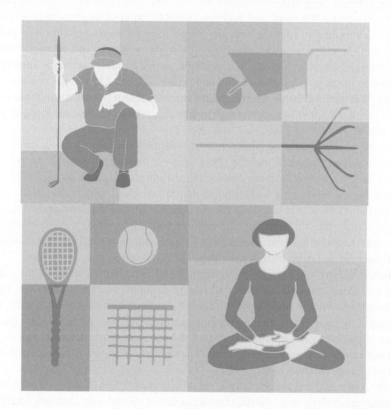

An assessment of level and intensity of physical activity

FIGURE 11.1.   The RAPA Questionnaire. (With permission, University of Washington Health Promotion Research Center, ©2006.)

Rapid Assessment of Physical Activity

Physical Activities are activities where you move and increase your heart rate above its resting rate, whether you do them for pleasure, work, or transportation.

The following questions ask about the amount and intensity of physical activity you usually do. The intensity of the activity is related to the amount of energy you use to do these activities.

Examples of physical activity intensity levels:

Light activities • your heart beats slightly faster than normal • you can talk and sing	Walking Leisurely Stretching Vacuuming or Light Yard Work
Moderate activities • your heart beats faster than normal • you can talk but not sing	Fast Walking Aerobics Class Strength Training Swimming Gently
Vigorous activities • your heart rate increases a lot • you can't talk or your talking is broken up by large breaths	Stair Machine Jogging or Running Tennis, Racquetball, Pickleball or Badminton

FIGURE 11.1. *(Continued).*

How physically active are you? *(Check one answer on each line)*

		Does this accurately describe you?	
		Yes	**No**
1	I rarely or never do any physical activities.	☐	☐
2	I do some **light** or **moderate** physical activities, but not every week.	☐	☐
3	I do some **light** physical activity every week.	☐	☐
4	I do **moderate** physical activities every week, but less than 30 minutes a day or 5 days a week.	☐	☐
5	I do **vigorous** physical activities every week, but less than 20 minutes a day or 3 days a week.	☐	☐
6	I do 30 minutes or more a day of **moderate** physical activities, 5 or more days a week.	☐	☐
7	I do 20 minutes or more a day of **vigorous** physical activities, 3 or more days a week.	☐	☐
1	I do activities to increase muscle **strength**, such as lifting weights or calisthenics, once a week or more.	☐	☐
2	I do activities to improve **flexibility**, such as stretching or yoga, once a week or more.	☐	☐

RAPA 1

RAPA 2
3 = Both 1 & 2

ID # _____

Today's Date _____

FIGURE 11.1. *(Continued).*

Scoring Instructions

RAPA 1: Aerobic

To score, choose the question with the highest score with an affirmative response. Any number less than 6 is suboptimal.

For scoring or summarizing categorically:

Score as sedentary:

1. I rarely or never do any physical activities.

Score as under-active:

2. I do some light or moderate physical activities, but not every week.

Score as under-active regular – light activities:

3. I do some light physical activity every week.

Score as under-active regular:

4. I do moderate physical activities every week, but less than 30 minutes a day or 5 days a week.

5. I do vigorous physical activities every week, but less than 20 minutes a day or 3 days a week.

Score as active:

6. I do 30 minutes or more a day of moderate physical activities, 5 or more days a week.

7. I do 20 minutes or more a day of vigorous physical activities, 3 or more days a week.

RAPA 2: Strength & Flexibility

I do activities to increase muscle strength, such as lifting weights or calisthenics, once a week or more. (1)

I do activities to improve flexibility, such as stretching or yoga, once a week or more. (2)

Both. (3)

None (0)

FIGURE 11.1. *(Continued)*.

"Exercise" is any moderate physical activity you do in your free time (e.g. walking, swimming, bicycling, dancing, active gardening, et cetera). "Regular exercise" is done at least 3 times per week for at least 20 minutes per day.

Directions:
Read the following statements and place an X in the box next to the statement which most closely corresponds with your response.

	AGREE
I have been exercising regularly for more than 6 months	
I have been exercising regularly for less than 6 months	
I am not exercising, but I am planning to start exercising in the next 6 months	
I am not exercising, and I don't plan to start in the next 6 months	

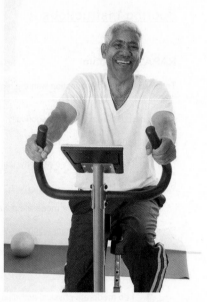

FIGURE 11.2. Exercise stage of Change Questionnaire.

A stage of change questionnaire can help the practitioner identify patterns of inactivity along this continuum and then tailor recommendations for the individual. Various strategies are helpful at each stage to assist an individual advance to the action and maintenance stages (see Fig. 11.2).

In addition to determining the older adult's current activity behavior, it may be helpful to ask about activity history, goals, and interests. Helping the older adult set short-term goals for physical activity is a way to make the activity manageable and concrete while encompassing activities that are important for the individual. Goal-setting also helps to ensure adherence and success. A SMART goal is, in essence, a recipe to create a goal that is *s*pecific, *m*easurable, *a*ction-oriented, *r*ealistic, and that adheres to a *t*ime frame. Often the tendency is to state a vague goal, based on a perception of the ideal. For example, "I want to begin a fitness program." A better goal would be "I will start walking at the mall, 3 days a week, for 15 minutes each time for the next 2 weeks." This goal is specific (walking at the mall), measurable (3 days, 15 minutes), action-oriented (something the individual can do), and realistic (starts gradually with room to grow), with attention to a time frame (2 weeks).

Fitness testing for the older adult, while not a preactivity requirement, may be beneficial and provides additional objective information about fitness level and ability prior to designing the physical activity/exercise program. The goal with any fitness testing should be to guide the exercise/activity prescription rather than to eliminate people or to discourage them from becoming physically active. Any exercise testing should be well planned and individualized to garner the most effective information. The American College of Sports Medicine's "Exercise Management for Persons with Chronic Diseases and Conditions" is an excellent resource for fitness testing with specific populations, providing suggestions and contraindications for testing (Durstine & Moore, 2003).

In lieu of sophisticated laboratory testing, the Senior Fitness Test (SFT) developed by Rikli and Jones (2001) provides objective information about fitness level and may be conducted relatively easily and inexpensively. The SFT includes a battery of tests that assess cardiorespiratory endurance, flexibility, muscular endurance, and dynamic agility. The SFT can be a useful tool in that it provides a baseline for comparison, identifies personal limitations, and provides direction for the activity program. It can also provide external motivation to the active older adult.

Additionally, the health care provider may be able to use information already available from the individual's medical record (e.g., ECG, pulmonary function tests, bone mineral density, lipid panels) to guide the creation of the exercise prescription and tailor it specifically to the individual.

TREATMENT: THE EXERCISE PRESCRIPTION

The basic recommendations for older adults call for 2½ hours of moderate-intensity physical activity, or 1¼ hours of vigorous activity, or a combination of both each week. The older adult can increase the time to 5 hours of activity per week for additional health benefits. While daily lifestyle activity (e.g., housework) certainly counts toward these goals, a specific exercise program may be warranted. Developing an exercise prescription is the process of using information from the health history (including health status, activity history/status, stages of change, SMART goals, and/or fitness testing) to create an individualized exercise program that specifies certain parameters for exercise (ACSM, 2010). This section will address exercise appropriate for a healthy, mobile older adult and functional exercise appropriate for a less healthy, frail, and/or primarily sedentary older adult.

When designing an exercise program for a healthy, mobile older adult, the practitioner should address four components: cardiorespiratory endurance, muscular strength and endurance, flexibility, and balance. There are an additional four variables to consider in each component, collectively referred to as the FITT approach: frequency (F), intensity (I), time (T), and type (T) of exercise. Frequency refers to how often the exercise is conducted, usually expressed as a certain number of days per week. Intensity refers to the difficulty of the exercise session. Time is the duration of exercise, usually expressed in minutes. The type of exercise, sometimes called the mode, is the activity that the individual selects.

Cardiorespiratory Endurance for the Independent Older Adult

The older adult should strive to exercise 3 to 5 days per week to build cardiorespiratory endurance, using moderate- to vigorous-intensity activities that elevate heart rate and increase respiration for approximately 20 to 30 minutes. The selected type, or mode, of exercise may vary, but should be enjoyable for the older adult and should not place any orthopedic stress on the individual or cause pain. Examples of the types of activities include walking (treadmill, track, outdoors), swimming, bicycling (stationery or outdoors), elliptical or stair machines, rowing, and arm ergometry. When selecting the mode for a beginning exerciser, consider ease of movement as well as safety. For example, walking is a much easier activity for a beginning exerciser than is a stair machine.

The key to any exercise prescription should be to progress in gradual increments to the ultimate goal. Initially, the beginning exerciser should be recommended to increase the time to the 20- to 30-minute goal. This progression may need to occur slowly, in small steps. An extremely deconditioned older adult, who is not accustomed to exercise, may be able to walk only for 5 minutes on the first day. She/he should be encouraged to add several minutes each time until the 30-minute goal is a reality. At that point, when the time goal is satisfied, the older exerciser can begin to focus on the intensity of the exercise. Another strategy for the de-conditioned older adult is to perform smaller exercise bouts throughout the day. For example, the elder could walk 10 minutes in the morning, 10 minutes around noon, and 10 minutes in the mid-afternoon.

Intensity, an indicator of how hard an individual is working, is historically based on the heart rate response during exercise. Typically, an individual will exercise within a target heart rate range based on one's maximal heart rate and resting heart rate, referred to as the heart rate reserve (HRR). The target range identified as most effective is between 40% and 80% of the HRR, depending on the individual's starting level of fitness. Exercise at the lower end of the range is considered low- to moderate intensity, while exercise at the upper end of the range is considered moderate- to vigorous intensity. The calculation of this target heart rate range using both the age-predicted maximal rate and the resting rate is called the Karvonen formula, and it is appropriate even for individuals receiving certain pharmacotherapy (i.e., beta blockers). A calculation of the Karvonen formula starts with the theoretical maximum heart rate of 220 beats per minute (bpm). With advancing age, however, that maximum heart rate decreases 1 bpm/year. This age-predicted maximal heart rate may be determined by subtracting the individual's age from 220 bpm. For example, a 70-year-old man has a resting heart rate of 72 bpm. His age-predicted maximal heart rate is 150 bpm (220 bpm − 70 years = 150 bpm). To determine the HRR, subtract the resting heart rate from the age-predicted maximal heart rate (150 bpm − 72 bpm = 78 bpm HRR). Multiply the HRR by the desired target range percentages and add the resting heart rate. An example of this calculation is shown in Table 11.1.

TABLE 11.1 · Example of Karvonen Formula for Determining Heart Rate Training Zone

A 70-year-old man with a resting heart rate of 72 bpm would have a heart rate training zone between 103 and 134 bpm.

Calculation:

220 bpm	Theoretical maximal heart rate
− 70 years of age	
150 bpm	Age-predicted maximal heart rate
− 72 bpm	Resting heart rate (RHR)
78 bpm	HRR

Lower end of zone		Upper end of zone	
HRR	78	HRR	78
	× 0.4		× 0.8
	31.2		62.4
	+ 72 bpm RHR		+ 72 bpm RHR
	103.2 bpm		134.4 bpm

Target heart rate training zone

6	No exertion at all
7	
8	Extremely light
9	Very light
10	
11	Light
12	
13	Somewhat hard
14	
15	Hard (heavy)
16	
17	Very hard
18	
19	Extremely hard
20	Maximal exertion

FIGURE 11.3. Borg scale of "Rating of Perceived Exertion." (With permission, Borg-RPE-skalan, Gunnar Borg, ©1970, 1985, 1994, 1998.)

Ideally, to attain the resting heart rate, the older adult would be asked to monitor one's heart rate upon waking naturally in the morning. Alternatively, the individual may be asked to monitor the pulse after resting quietly for about 10 to 15 minutes. She or he would count the number of beats felt in 60 seconds, beginning the count with "0." The pulse may be taken at the wrist (radial pulse) or the neck (carotid pulse), whichever is easier for the individual to palpate. To monitor this training zone during exercise, the older adult may take a carotid or radial pulse, usually counting the number of beats felt during 6 seconds and multiplying by 10. A pulse, particularly the radial pulse, may be difficult for an untrained person to feel; thus, another option for the older adult is to use a heart rate monitor worn on the body. There are two other recognized methods of assessing intensity, both of which require less work on the part of the exerciser. The first of these is a Rating of Perceived Exertion (RPE) Scale developed by Borg (1998). This scale is a subjective measure of an individual's intensity level while exercising. Participants use a 10-point scale to rate their work or fatigue. A rating from 4 to 6 ("somewhat strong" to "strong") is ideal for submaximal exercise (see Fig. 11.3). The second alternate method is the Talk Test (Persinger et al., 2004). The Talk Test (Table 11.2) is also a subjective rating and is especially appropriate for a novice exerciser. An older adult should be encouraged to exercise at a level that requires him/her to breathe more heavily than at rest but still allows conversation.

Muscular Fitness for the Independent Older Adult

For the older adult, having sufficient muscular fitness (which includes muscular strength, muscular endurance, and power) is key to offsetting the muscular and neural decrements that occur

TABLE 11.2 · "Talk Test" to Determine Exercise Intensity

Too Light	Just Right	Too Hard
The person exercising can talk easily and could even sing a song during activity	The person exercising can talk, somewhat breathily, during activity	The person exercising cannot speak during activity

during the process of sarcopenia. Muscular fitness not only helps spare the muscle tissue loss, but is crucial for the older adult to maintain the capacity to perform both recreational activities and activities of daily living. Resistance training occurs when the muscles work against a resistive force. This resistive force may be in the form of free weights (e.g., dumbbell, barbell), elastic bands, body weight (e.g., push-ups), or machines (e.g., Cybex, Nautilus). In order for the resistance-training program to be most effective for the older adult, the practitioner should consider and apply progressive overload in the exercise prescription. Since the body adapts to training, additional stimuli are required for improvement. This means that a resistance-training program needs to be varied over time. Multiple variables—type of exercises, resistance/weight (also called the load), repetitions (i.e., lifting and lowering the weight), and sets (i.e., groups of repetitions)—can be adjusted to ensure that progressive overload is occurring. It is recommended that resistance-training sessions for the older adult be supervised, at least initially, to ensure proper technique, build confidence, and ascertain adequate intensity (ACSM, 2010; Skinner, 2005).

In terms of frequency of resistance training, the older adult should strive for two, possibly three, sessions per week. The body needs adequate time to recover from the resistive force exercises, and so 24 to 36 hours should be allowed between sessions. A variety of exercises should be selected for each session, and these should target the major muscle groups. Exercises that use larger muscle groups and involve multiple joints are called multijoint exercises, and they mimic the coordinated muscle use inherent in many activities of daily living. Some examples of multijoint exercises include squats, dead lifts, chest press, and lat pulldowns. Exercises that attempt to isolate a muscle group are referred to as single-joint, for example, bicep curls and knee extensions. In order to minimize fatigue, it is preferable to incorporate multijoint exercises early in the workout, alternate upper and lower body exercises, and utilize single-joint exercises toward the end of the session.

For the older adult who is just starting a resistance-training program, one set of 10 to 15 repetitions would be appropriate for each exercise. The older adult should choose a load that allows him/her to complete 10 to 15 repetitions, rating the effort required as 13 to 15 (somewhat hard to hard) on the RPE scale. If the older adult cannot accomplish a minimum of 10 repetitions, the load is too heavy and should be decreased. Conversely, if the older adult is able to accomplish 15 repetitions easily and could do more, the load should be increased. The load should be lifted or pushed smoothly into place in about 4 seconds during each repetition, using a full, pain-free range of motion. There should be a brief pause, and then the load should be returned to its starting position, again taking about 4 seconds and moving smoothly. The older adult should be encouraged to breathe regularly, preferably exhaling as one pushes or lifts and inhaling during the return phase. The rest period between sets is another variable to consider since this affects fatigue. In a basic, low-load resistance-training program, a rest period of 1 to 3 minutes should be adequate between sets, but this may be adjusted. In general, shorter rest periods may enhance muscular endurance, while longer rest periods may allow for greater recovery and greater gains in muscular strength (ACSM, 2010). The total time required to complete a resistance-training session will vary, but in general it would be completed in approximately 30 minutes.

The type of resistance exercises selected depends on personal preference, health/functional status, access, availability, and affordability. To improve compliance and adherence, however, the older adult should be given choices for resistance training: group versus individual setting, home versus gym or clinic, and free weights versus body weight versus machines. In terms of the mode of resistance training, there are advantages and disadvantages to each type. Machines often allow greater isolation of the working muscle group while providing support for other areas of the body. The load on machines is usually changed by moving a pin in a self-contained weight stack, so it is not necessary for the individual to do a lot of preparation for each exercise, and there is little risk of the individual dropping a weight on himself/herself. Usually machines are set up in a circuit format and the exerciser can move from one to another relatively quickly and easily. One drawback to machines is that there are often multiple seat adjustments, which may be confusing initially. Supervision is key in this situation. Free weights, such as dumbbells, barbells, and medicine balls, are beneficial in that they can be used in many different settings. They also provide a more total-body workout because the individual must engage core muscles to stabilize and balance the working muscle groups. Free weights, however, may be intimidating to the older adult. One recommendation for using free weights with the older adult population is to incorporate exercises gradually. Certain free weight exercises done with heavy loads may pose safety issues for a novice exerciser, so supervision and/or the use of a spotter is highly recommended.

Flexibility for the Independent Older Adult

Flexibility, or the range of motion around a joint, is an important component of physical fitness for the older adult. It allows for greater freedom of movement in activities of daily living and potential emergency situations (e.g., a fall). Flexibility is joint specific, so the stretching program should address multiple muscle groups and joints. A good rule of thumb is to stretch what is strengthened. Stretching to improve range of motion should be performed when the muscles are warm, usually at the end of a workout program or as part of the cooldown. Flexibility exercises should be performed a minimum of 2 to 3 days per week. While performing a stretch, the older adult should use slow, static movements to elongate the muscle gently. The end stretch should be held for 10 to 30 seconds. The individual should return to the starting position, allowing the muscle to rest briefly for several seconds, and then repeat the stretch (up to four times total) holding for 10 to 30 seconds each time. This type of static stretching should not be painful for the older adult, and the individual should be cautioned not to push past the normal range of motion. Other recommendations for stretching include having the older adult release any tension in other muscles (e.g., holding tension in the shoulders while performing a sit-and-reach stretch) and focusing on breathing naturally and not holding the breath while stretching.

Balance Training for the Independent Older Adult

Balance, or control of the center of gravity, involves three domains (base of support, center of mass, and sensory pathways), each of which should be included in a balance training program. Improving balance in an older adult can be beneficial for mobility, fall prevention, and fall response and outcome (ACSM, 2010; Skinner, 2005). In terms of frequency, balance training can be performed every day. As discussed in the previous section, resistance training improves balance and mobility; so from a programmatic standpoint, the older adult might prefer to do balance exercises on the days when she or he is not performing resistance training. The intensity of balance training refers to the difficulty of the postures, positions, or movements, and the older adult should strive to practice at a level that is challenging but does not induce a fall. In order to ensure safety, the older adult should have available a bar, chair, countertop, or spotter for support. Each exercise that is selected should be performed initially with the older adult holding onto the support with both hands. As the older adult becomes more proficient, one can use one hand on the support, then progress to fingertip touch, and then progress to hands off but several inches above the support. The time required for balance training is variable and is specific to the balance exercise performed. The mode of balance training should ideally address each of the three domains, but each is progressively more complex and the older adult may need time to build gradually to the final domain. The first domain is narrowing the base of support. The older adult should be instructed to practice standing in progressively more difficult positions, again using support as needed. Some positions to practice include feet apart, feet together, feet together heel to toe, one-legged stand with foot flat, ball-of-foot stand (with both or one foot on ground), and/or heel stand (toes of both feet raised off ground) (ACSM, 2010). The older adult should start with the least difficult position and attempt to hold that pose for 15 seconds. When the individual can hold the position for 15 seconds without support, without moving the feet, or without leaning, she or he can progress to the next position. The second domain involves changing the center of mass. The objective in this domain is to move the body through space without losing balance. Suggestions for exercises in this domain include standing with the feet slightly apart and leaning the torso forward, backward, and sideways; turning in a circle; shifting weight from side to side; or walking in a variety of patterns (crossover, backward, etc.). The third domain involves changing sensory pathways used in balance. This type of training is more sophisticated and should be used with caution, taking safety measures into account. Suggestions for exercises that change the sensory pathways include performing any of the postures with eyes closed or while standing on a variable surface (e.g., pillow, blanket, foam pad).

Exercise for the Frail, Sedentary Older Adult

There is ample evidence which suggests that the frail or sedentary older adult can benefit from exercise (Stuck & Ross, 2006). Consideration should be given to the type of exercise for the frail elder, with attention to medical history, setting, and goals or care plan. In general, walking, pool exercise, and seated exercise are most appropriate for this population, but it is still possible to incorporate resistance training, flexibility training, motor skills coordination, and fall prevention and recovery.

Functional exercise sessions may be especially beneficial to the frail elder. As the name implies, functional exercise is intended to improve function and activities of daily living. Functional exercise ideally should address the cardiorespiratory and musculoskeletal systems, but it will be more adaptive in nature, to account for the limitations of the frail, sedentary elder. Depending on the setting, the frail elder may be able to incorporate exercise into his/her lifestyle, such as walking to the mailbox and back or, in the case of a residential patient, standing from the wheelchair used for transportation to sit in a dining-room chair. The frail elder, even when confined to a sitting position, can still perform resistance training and flexibility exercises (with no load or extremely light load) for the total body. Such exercises include lifting the arms out to the sides, rotating the wrists, reaching overhead, bending side to side gently, marching in place, extending the lower leg, rotating the ankles, and lifting the heels and toes.

The frail elder may also enjoy the use of equipment such as foam balls, scarves, rhythm wands, and elastic bands. This type of equipment is light and easy to hold and manipulate, and it may be used in much the same way as free weights (e.g., bicep curls with a foam ball) or for games (e.g., passing the ball from person to person). Additional benefits of using equipment are that it may encourage larger movements, it can provide social interaction, and it may not seem so much like exercise.

CULTURAL CONSIDERATIONS

When creating the exercise program, it is important to be sensitive to the individual and tailor the prescription whenever possible. There are many variables within the FITT approach, and the exercise prescription should not be one size fits all. At a minimum, the practitioner should be cognizant of the individual's limitations, abilities, interests, and goals. It may also be helpful to be aware of the individual's knowledge of, attitude toward, and beliefs about activity or exercise. These may be linked to upbringing, social norms of the generation, and ethnic or religious background, and they may influence the individual's self-efficacy for exercise. For example, some older women may not feel it is appropriate to break a sweat in mixed company. One way to address this and similar issues is to offer dedicated programs, such as a women-only exercise class or a special senior time in the weight room.

Additional considerations may arise from the physical limitations of the older adult. For those with vision problems, it is important to have good lighting and legible signage and give attention to trip hazards. Individuals who have limited vision may need additional help getting on and off exercise equipment, and they may need to be cautioned to terrain and/or flooring changes. Those with auditory limitations may need visual instruction or loud, clear verbal instruction. They may also benefit from changes to background noise (e.g., a lower volume on the stereo system). Individuals with arthritis may need weights with a special strap or lever so they do not have to grip. They may also benefit from exercise modalities in a warm pool. Many older adults, particularly those who are disengaged in some way, may benefit from group exercise settings. Group exercise allows for social interaction and social support, and it may improve adherence to the activity program. In general, when working with an older adult with a limitation, the practitioner should not automatically discount an exercise or assume that the individual cannot perform certain activities. Instead, the practitioner should communicate with the individual, seek ways to modify the activity, and be prepared to suggest alternatives.

PREVENTION OF PHYSICAL INACTIVITY

The Exercise and Aging Cycle described early in this chapter paints a rather bleak picture of increasing age in the absence of physical activity. The good news, however, is that this cycle can be prevented or broken with regular physical activity. The key to an effective exercise or activity program is consistency. Skinner (2005) comments that for the older adult we should "emphasize that the *process* of being active is more important than the *product* of being fit."

The health care provider certainly has a role in this process, because she or he is on the front lines to reach and engage the older adult. The provider should be prepared to initiate a conversation about the role of an active lifestyle and to give basic advice about appropriate activity. The health care team should also be familiar with local activity/fitness/exercise programs, both traditional and nontraditional, and should be prepared to offer either an exercise prescription or referral to an appropriate fitness professional who works with the older adult population.

PATIENT EDUCATION COMPONENTS FOR PROVIDERS

Exercise behavior, like various health conditions, requires follow-up from the health care team or fitness professional. It is not enough simply to give older adults an exercise prescription and hope the patients will fill it by themselves. The older adult needs instruction, skill development, practice opportunities, and the option of revision. Ideally, a periodized, or phased, program would be developed for the older adult. In this scenario, the elder would be started on an appropriate activity program to follow for 4 to 6 weeks. Toward the end of this time frame, the program would be altered gradually, either by including additional exercises or by changing the frequency, intensity, or time. This amended program would be followed for an additional 4 to 6 weeks at which time the program could again be revised.

Providers who are unaccustomed to developing an exercise prescription for the older adult may benefit from the wealth of resources available and may find that they do not need to reinvent the wheel. The National Institute on Aging (NIA) (2009) has created the Exercise & Physical Activity guide for older adults, which outlines the basics of exercise and lifestyle activity and provides sample exercises along with worksheets and activity logs. The American College of Sports Medicine and the American Medical Association have launched an initiative called Exercise is Medicine to encourage health care providers to discuss physical activity with patients. Their Web site (www.exerciseismedicine.org) provides information not only for providers but also for fitness professionals and the general public. The American Heart Association also offers provider and patient resources such as an interactive Web site (www.startwalkingnow.org), which contains an individualized walking plan builder, an activity tracker, and applications to locate area walking trails via smart phone technology. The Arthritis Foundation, while providing arthritis-specific information, also promotes lifetime physical activity through their program called *Let's Move Together*. *Let's Move Together* offers an online movement tracker for individuals to log their activity and keep track of their daily activity patterns. This site is accessible at www.lmt.arthritis.org. The Administration on Aging (AOA) also provides a variety of health and wellness information for older adults, caregivers, and health care providers. Of particular interest in this case is the AOA's Disease Prevention and Health Promotion Services webpage, which provides a list of evidence-based physical activity and wellness interventions available in many communities. The web address for the AOA is www.aoa.gov.

As the age wave in America continues, there will certainly be a demand for effective preventive health measures and treatment options. Physical activity and exercise will have a role in both. Health care providers should recognize that recommending physical activity is a valuable tool in their medical kits, keeping in mind that, in the words of author Jennie Brand-Miller, "[t]here are really only two requirements when it comes to exercise. One is that you do it. The other is that you continue to do it."

REFERENCES

American College of Sports Medicine. (2010). *Resource manual for guidelines for exercise testing and prescription* (6th ed.). Philadelphia, PA: Wolters Kluwer/Lippincott Williams & Wilkins.

American Heart Association. (2013). Heart disease and stroke statistics—2013 update. *Circulation, 127*, e6–e245.

American Psychiatric Association. (1994). *Diagnostic and statistical manual of mental disorders* (4th ed.). Washington, DC: Author.

Borg, G. (1998). *Borg's perceived exertion and pain scales*. Champaign, IL: Human Kinetics.

Bortz, W. M. (2007). *We live too short and die too long: How to achieve and enjoy your natural 100-year-plus life span*. New York, NY: Select Books.

Boule, N. G., Haddad, E., Kenny, G. P., Wells, G. A., & Sigal, R. J. (2001). Effects of exercise on glycemic control and body mass in type 2 diabetes mellitus: A meta-analysis of controlled clinical trials. *JAMA: The Journal of the American Medical Association, 286*(10), 1218–1227.

Canadian Centre for Activity and Aging. (2000). *Canada's physical activity guide to healthy active living for older adults*.

Centers for Disease Control and Prevention. (1996). *Physical activity and health: A report of the Surgeon General*. Atlanta, GA: U.S. Department of Health and Human Services.

Centers for Disease Control and Prevention. (2000). *Behavioral risk factor surveillance system*.

Chen, Y. M. (2010). Perceived barriers to physical activity among older adults residing in long-term care institutions. *Journal of Clinical Nursing, 19*(3–4), 432–439.

Cherry, D.K., Burt, C. W., and Woodwell, D.A. (2003). National Ambulatory Medical Care Survey: 2001 Summary. Advance Data, 337 (1–44).

Chomistek, A. K., Chiuve, S. E., Jensen, M. K., Cook, N. R., & Rimm, E. B. (2011). Vigorous physical activity, mediating biomarkers, and risk of myocardial infarction. *Medicine and Science in Sports and Exercise, 43*(10), 1884–1890.

Dunlop, D. D., Semanik, P., Song, J., Manheim, L. M., Shih, V., & Chang, R. W. (2005). Risk factors for functional decline in older adults with arthritis. *Arthritis and Rheumatism, 52*(4), 1274–1282.

Durstine, L. G., & Moore, G. E. (2003). *ACSM's exercise management for persons with chronic diseases and disabilities* (2nd ed.). Champaign, IL: Human Kinetics.

Holmes, M. D., Chen, W. Y., Feskanich, D., Kroenke, C. H., & Colditz, G. A. (2005). Physical activity and survival after breast cancer diagnosis. *Journal of the American Medical Association, 293*(20), 2479–2486.

Hoyert, D. L., & Xu, J. Q. (2012). Deaths: Preliminary data for 2011. *National Vital Statistics Reports, 61*(6). Retrieved from http://www.cdc.gov/nchs/data/nvsr/nvsr61/nvsr61_06.pdf

Hughes, V. A., Frontera, W. R., Wood, M., Evans, W. J., Dallal, G. E., Roubenoff, R., & Fiatarone Singh, M. A. (2001). Longitudinal muscle strength changes in older adults: Influence of muscle mass, physical activity, and health. *Journals of Gerontology: Series A, Biological Sciences and Medical Sciences, 56*(5), B209–B217.

Iannuzzi-Sucich, M., Prestwood, K. M., & Kenny, A. M. (2002). Prevalence of sarcopenia and predictors of skeletal muscle mass in healthy, older men and women. *Journals of Gerontology: Series A, Biological Sciences and Medical Sciences, 57*(12), M772–M777.

International Agency on Research for Cancer. (2002). *IARC handbooks of cancer prevention. Weight control and physical activity* (Vol. 6). Lyon, France: Author.

Ivy, J. L., Zderic, T. W., & Fogt, D. L. (1999). Prevention and treatment of non-insulin-dependent diabetes mellitus. *Exercise and Sport Sciences Reviews, 27*, 1–35.

Kessler, R. C., Chiu, W. T., Demler, O., & Walters, E. E. (2005). Prevalence, severity, and comorbidity of twelve-month DSM-IV disorders in the National Comorbidity Survey Replication (NCS-R). *Archives of General Psychiatry, 62*(6), 617–627.

Lees, F. D., Clark, P. G., Nigg, C. R., & Newman, P. (2005). Barriers to exercise behavior among older adults: A focus-group study. *Journal of Aging and Physical Activity, 13*(1), 23–33.

Leutholtz, B. C., & Ripoll, I. (2011). *Exercise and disease management* (2nd ed.). Boca Raton, FL: CRC Press, Taylor & Francis.

Marcus, B. H., Selby, V. C., Niaura, R. S., & Rossi, J. S. (1992). Self-efficacy and the stages of exercise behavior change. *Research Quarterly for Exercise and Sport, 63*, 60–66.

Meyerhardt, J. A., Giovanucci, E. L., Holmes, M. D., Chan, A. T., Chan, J. A., Colditz, G. A., & Fuchs, C. S. (2006a). Physical activity and survival after colorectal cancer diagnosis. *Journal of Clinical Oncology, 24*(22), 3527–3534.

Meyerhardt, J. A., Heseltine, D., Niedzwiecki, D., Hollis, D., Saltz, L. B., Mayer, R. J., … Fuchs, C. S. (2006b). Impact of physical activity on cancer recurrence and survival in patients with stage III colon cancer: Findings from CALGB 89803. *Journal of Clinical Oncology, 24*(22), 3535–3541.

National Institute on Aging. (2009). *Your everyday guide from the NIA: Exercise & physical activity* (Publication No. 09-4258). Retrieved from www.nia.nih.gov

O'Neill, K., & Reid, G. (1991). Perceived barriers to physical activity by older adults. *Canadian Journal of Public Health, 82*, 392–396.

Persinger, R., Foster, C., Gibson, M., Fater, D., & Porcari, J. (2004). Consistency of the talk test for exercise prescription. *Medicine and Science in Sports and Exercise, 36*(9), 1632–1636.

Rikli, R. E., & Jones, J. (2001). *Senior fitness test kit.* Champaign, IL: Human Kinetics.

Ruuskanen, J. M., & Parkatti, T. (1994). Physical activity and related factors among nursing home residents. *Journal of the American Geriatric Society, 42*(9), 987–991.

Schiller, J. S., Lucas, J. W., Ward, B. W., & Peregoy, J. A. (2012). Summary health statistics for U.S. adults: National Health Interview Survey, 2010. *Vital and Health Statistics, 10*(252), 1–80.

Schonberg, M. A., Marcantonio, E. R., & Wee, C. C. (2005). Physician counseling about exercise to older women. *Journal of General Internal Medicine, 20*(Suppl. 1), 295.

Schutzer, K. A., & Graves, B. S. (2004). Barriers and motivations to exercise in older adults. *Preventive Medicine, 39*, 1056–1061.

Singh, N. A., Clements, K. M., & Fiatarone Singh, M. A. (2001). The efficacy of exercise as a long-term antidepressant in elderly subjects: a randomized, controlled trial. *Journal of Gerontology: Medical Sciences, 56*(8), M497–M504.

Skinner, J. S. (2005). *Exercise testing and exercise prescription for special cases: Theoretical basis and clinical application* (3rd ed.). Philadelphia, PA: Lippincott Williams & Wilkins.

Slattery, M. L. (2004). Physical activity and colorectal cancer. *Sports Medicine, 34*(4), 239–252.

Stuck, B. D., & Ross, K. M. (2006). Health promotion in older adults: Prescribing exercise for the frail and home bound. *Geriatrics, 61*(5), 22–27.

Taylor, A. W., & Johnson, M. J. (2008). *Physiology of exercise and healthy aging*. Champaign, IL: Human Kinetics.

Thompson, P., Buchner, D., Pina, I. L., Balady, G. J., Williams, M. A., Marcus, B. H., … Wenger, N. K. (2003). Exercise and physical activity in the prevention and treatment of atherosclerotic cardiovascular disease: A statement from the Council on Clinical Cardiology and the Council on Nutrition, Physical Activity, and Metabolism. *Circulation, 107*, 3109–3116.

University of Washington Health Promotion Research Center. (2006). *Rapid Assessment of Physical Activity* (Funded in part by the Centers for Disease Control. Reproduced with permission). Seattle, WA: Author.

U.S. Department of Health & Human Services. (2000). *Healthy people 2010* (2nd ed.). Washington, DC: Author.

U.S. Department of Health & Human Services. (2008). *2008 Physical activity guidelines for Americans*. Washington, DC: Author.

World Health Organization. (2012, September). Cardiovascular diseases (Fact sheet No. 317). Retrieved from www.who.int/mediacentre

CHAPTER 11: IT RESOURCES

Websites

American College of Sports Medicine
http://www.acsm.org/

Canadian Centre for Aging and Activity
http://www.uwo.ca/actage/

Physical Activities Guidelines for Americans, taken from the President's Council on Fitness, Sports & Nutrition
http://www.fitness.gov/be-active/physical-activity-guidelines-for-americans/

Exercise for the Elderly, taken from Agingcare.com: Connecting People Caring for Elderly Parents
http://www.agingcare.com/Articles/Exercise-benefits-for-the-Elderly-95383.htm

Exercise and Seniors, taken from FamilyDoctor.org
http://familydoctor.org/familydoctor/en/seniors/staying-healthy/exercise-and-seniors.html

Exercise for the Elderly, taken from Livestrong.com
http://www.livestrong.com/exercise-elderly/

The Best Anti-Aging Therapy. You are never too old to start exercising; in fact, exercise only gets more important with advancing age
http://fitness.mercola.com/sites/fitness/archive/2011/09/30/you-are-never-too-old-to-start-exercising.aspx

Promoting and Prescribing Exercise for the Elderly, taken from the American Academy of Family Physicians
http://www.aafp.org/afp/2002/0201/p419.html

Exercise and Cardiovascular Health, taken from the American Heart Association
http://circ.ahajournals.org/content/107/1/e2.full

Heart Disease and Exercise, taken from WebMD
http://www.webmd.com/heart-disease/heart-disease-prevention-exercise

Exercise Helps Your Immune System Protect Against Future Cancers
http://fitness.mercola.com/sites/fitness/archive/2012/11/30/exercise-protects-immune-system.aspx

Exercise for Osteoporosis
http://www.webmd.com/osteoporosis/features/exercise-for-osteoporosis

Osteoporosis Exercise, from WebMD
  http://www.webmd.com/osteoporosis/guide/osteoporosis-exercise
Exercise helps ease arthritis pain and stiffness
  http://www.mayoclinic.com/health/arthritis/AR00009
The Arthritis Foundation Exercise Program
  http://www.arthritis.org/resources/community-programs/excercise/
Alzheimer's Disease and Exercise
  http://physicaltherapy.about.com/od/typesofphysicaltherapy/ss/Alzheimers.htm
Introduction to Alzheimer's Disease and Exercise, taken from National Center on Health,
  Physical Activity, and Disability
  http://www.ncpad.org/116/896/Alzheimer˜s˜Disease˜and˜Exercise
Physical Activity Assessment Tools including the Rapid Assessment of Physical Activity (RAPA)
  questionnaire, and the Telephone Assessment of Physical Activity, taken from the University
  of Washington, Health Promotion Research Center
  http://depts.washington.edu/hprc/rapa
The Transtheoretical model of behavior change
  http://www.umbc.edu/psyc/habits/content/the_model/
The Senior Fitness Test
  http://www.topendsports.com/testing/senior-fitness-test.htm
Karvonen Formula
  http://www.topendsports.com/fitness/karvonen-formula.htm
Perceived Exertion (BORG Rating of Perceived Exertion scale), taken from CDC
  http://www.cdc.gov/physicalactivity/everyone/measuring/exertion.html
The Talk Test
  http://www.unm.edu/˜lkravitz/Article%20folder/talktest.html
The Talk Test Assesses Exercise Intensity
  http://diabeteshealth.com/read/2011/10/08/7312/the-talk-test-assesses-exercise-intensity/
Elderly Balance Exercises For Seniors to Help Prevent Falls
  http://www.eldergym.com/elderly-balance.html
Elderly Flexibility Stretching Exercises for Seniors
  http://www.eldergym.com/elderly-flexibility.html
National Institute on Aging, Exercise for all Older Adults
  http://www.nia.nih.gov/newsroom/features/
  exercise-all-older-adults-nia-guide-shows-and-tells
US Department of Health & Human Services – Staying Fit Together (2013)
  http://www.hhs.gov/news/healthbeat/2013/01/20130129a.html

Books

Reach for It: A Handbook for Health, Exercise and Dance for Older Adults
  http://www.amazon.com/Reach-It-Handbook-Health-Exercise/dp/0945483767

Videos

Pilates Chair Workout (2009)
  Stay seated in front of the TV and exercise your body and mind in a fun and effective way.
  This chair-based workout will help you improve your stamina, flexibility, balance and

confidence in the comfort of your own home. It's one of the secrets to living a healthier and longer life. (2:50 minutes)

http://youtu.be/xuzBm8O19o4

Stronger Seniors Strength (2010)

Senior Exercise Aerobic Video, Elderly Exercise, Chair Exercise. This clip focuses on the lower body. This Chair Exercise program helps seniors and the disabled get a great cardio workout. (8:30 minutes)

http://youtu.be/m7zCDiiTBTk

10 Daily Posture Exercises for Seniors (2011)

This video is derived from the presentation Ms. Burnell gave at the National Council on Aging Annual Convention in 2010. Walking straight and tall, sitting straight and tall, and working with the proper posture will improve your health in so many ways. It will improve your breathing, internal organ function, and energy. Alleviate back pain with better posture. Your overall health will improve noticeably. (5:40 minutes)

http://youtu.be/WJspJaFL_l8

How to Do Balance Exercises for Seniors (2011)

Learning how to do balance exercises for seniors is important for the elderly. This video includes step-by-step instructions for doing balance exercises for seniors. (3:30 minutes)

http://youtu.be/fdW3vHF1828

Images

Google images of exercise and aging cycle

http://www.google.com/search?q=Exercise+and+Aging+Cycle&hl=en&tbm=isch&tbo=u&source=univ&sa=X&ei=-1ZgUfLjMoWi4AO_g4CgBA&ved=0CGEQsAQ&biw=1280&bih=705

Google image of transtheoretical model of behavior change

http://www.google.com/search?q=transtheoretical+model+of+behavior+change&hl=en&tbm=isch&tbo=u&source=univ&sa=X&ei=HGhgUcfEHq3B4APl0ICIDw&sqi=2&ved=0CEsQsAQ&biw=1280&bih=705

Osteoporosis

Karen A. Roberto, PhD
Marya C. McPherson, MS
Deborah T. Gold, PhD

INTRODUCTION

Osteoporosis is a major public health concern. An estimated 10 million people in the United States have osteoporosis (National Osteoporosis Foundation [NOF], 2011a), a metabolic bone disease that leads to reduced bone mineral content and increased risk of nontraumatic fractures of the spine, hip, and wrist. Another 34 million individuals have low bone mass, the clinical precursor of osteoporosis. Although women are at highest risk for osteoporosis, 20% of Americans with osteoporosis are men (Curtis et al., 2009).

TYPES OF FRACTURES

The principal fractures associated with osteoporosis are clinical vertebral fractures (Ettinger et al., 2010); other common fracture sites include the radial shaft and ulna (wrist), proximal humerus (shoulder), proximal femur (hip), and distal radius (pelvis). Once an osteoporotic fracture occurs, an older person's likelihood of experiencing subsequent fractures increases dramatically (Kanis et al., 2004a; Lindsay et al., 2001). Approximately one in two women and one in four men aged 50 or older will have an osteoporosis-related fracture during the remaining years of their lifetime (Bonura, 2009). These osteoporotic fractures, particularly vertebral and hip fractures, result in significant morbidity and mortality for both female and male patients (Cummings & Melton, 2002). If treatment is not initiated soon after a traumatic fracture, the potential for chronic, disabling pain, severe deformity, and reduced quality of life is substantial (Gold, 2003). Compression fractures of the vertebrae may result in chronic pain and physical deformity, including increased kyphosis (dowager's hump), decreased lordosis (flattened curve in lower back), forward head position, and other postural abnormalities (Avioli, 2000; U.S. Department of Health and Human Services, 2004). Hip fractures almost invariably are associated with chronic pain, reduced mobility, disability, and increased dependence (Marks, 2010; Randell et al., 2000). After hip fracture, half of the patients will experience loss of mobility and will never return to prefracture mobility levels; 25% of these patients will require long-term care (Bonura, 2009).

DIRECT AND INDIRECT COSTS

Over 2 million fractures occur in the United States annually, with direct medical costs associated with osteoporosis in 2005 exceeding $19 billion (NOF, 2011a). By 2025, with the aging of the baby boomers, annual fractures and costs are projected to increase by 50% and $25 billion, respectively (Burge et al., 2007). The care necessitated from osteoporosis-related fractures is often complex and prolonged; fractures are not only associated with significant increases in acute inpatient care, but also have marked effects on use of all forms of postacute care, including inpatient facility stays, home health care, and physical and occupational therapy (Becker et al., 2010). Most costs incurred by fracture patients result from inpatient care (57%) and long-term care (30%) as opposed to outpatient treatment (13%) (Burge et al., 2007). The indirect costs of osteoporosis, including caregiver time and the nonmonetary costs of poor health, are also extensive (Becker et al., 2010).

QUALITY OF LIFE

In addition to the financial cost to society, osteoporosis has a substantial impact on quality of life (Papaioannou et al., 2009). Impaired health-related quality of life resulting from functional impairments, psychological distress, and social isolation are possible consequences associated with osteoporosis (Becker et al., 2010; Stone & Lyles, 2006). Because of the physical discomfort of pain, older persons with osteoporosis may develop a range of undesirable consequences, including impaired mobility, reduced productivity, decreased socialization, depression, and sleep disturbances (Bonura, 2009; Morgan, 2007). Furthermore, less obviously, related phenomena may be worsened by pain, such as gait disturbances, falls, malnutrition, slow rehabilitation, and cognitive dysfunction (Williams, 1995). Though each individual living with osteoporosis may experience a common set of symptoms, the impact of the disease depends largely on how profoundly it affects the roles and activities that have previously defined a person's life (Morgan, 2007; Roberto & Reynolds, 2001).

Research on managing osteoporosis and coping with related functional changes (e.g., pain, limited mobility) and psychosocial consequences (e.g., depression, anxiety, low self-esteem, and social dysfunction) is based primarily on investigations of older women, reflecting an overwhelming gender bias in osteoporosis research. Women reported multiple ways of coping with osteoporosis. Some women used physical coping strategies (e.g., exercise), whereas others depended on avoiding pain-inducing activities such as bending, reaching, and carrying heavy objects (Hjalmarson et al., 2007; Roberto, 2004; Roberto & Reynolds, 2001). They also relied on emotional strategies, concentrating on keeping a positive attitude and being grateful for being no worse off. Other psychosocial variables associated with the ways in which women managed their pain included experiencing distress (e.g., depression, anxiety) (Gold & Solimeo, 2006), receiving help from family and friends (Roberto, 1992; Roberto et al., 2004), and engaging with formal community services (Forster-Burke et al., 2010).

BONE PATHOPHYSIOLOGY

Peak bone mass (PBM) for women is reached somewhere in an individual's 20s or 30s and, in the absence of risk factors or other diseases, remains reasonably stable or diminishes slightly until menopause. Throughout the early part of life, more new bone is formed than old bone is lost, ultimately resulting in PBM. Once PBM is reached, the remodeling process—bone resorption (the breakdown and removal of older bone by osteoclasts) and bone formation (the development of new bone by osteoblasts)—is balanced. As age increases and other factors influence bone remodeling, however, bone resorption increases and bone formation decreases so that the net result is a loss of bone mineral density (BMD). The first 5 years post menopause is the time during which bone density loss is most precipitous.

As noted above, age and hypogonadism (low estrogen levels from surgical or biological menopause) can decrease bone density and lead to what has been called postmenopausal osteoporosis (PMO). However, there are also a multitude of other factors that contribute in varying degrees and ways to the degradation of bone. Some potentially influential and modifiable risk factors include mutable weight below 127 lb (57.6 kg), smoking, excessive alcohol intake, deficient calcium and vitamin D intake, and inactivity. Nonmodifiable factors include age, gender, menopausal status, family history, a previous fracture, or having lost more than 1" (2.54 cm) in height.

Among the most potent causal factors related to the onset of bone loss are certain medications. The dose and duration of use of these medications play a role in their impact on bone. The best known of these are the glucocorticoids (i.e., corticosteroids) such as prednisone, cortisone, and dexamethasone. Typically, these medications are necessary to treat chronic conditions and once started, cannot be stopped. There is strong evidence, however, that those women who take at least 7.5 mg of steroids over 3 months or longer are at high risk of experiencing bone loss. Those taking a corticosteroid dose of 5 mg or more daily for 3 or more months are at highest risk of developing glucocorticoid-induced osteoporosis (GIO; Kanis et al., 2004b). In addition to steroids, other medications that cause bone loss include, but are not limited to: chemotherapy, antirejection drugs, proton pump inhibitors, selective serotonin reuptake inhibitors, and excess thyroid replacement. See the NOF Web site for a more complete list of medications associated with increased risk of osteoporosis (http://www.nof.org/aboutosteoporosis/detectingosteoporosis/medicineboneloss).

In addition to medications, there are certain conditions or diseases that can increase the risk of osteoporosis. The risk of osteoporosis can be attributed to prescribed treatments, disease-specific physiologic changes, or a combination of both. Conditions associated with increased risk of osteoporosis include various cancers, endocrine disorders (e.g., diabetes, hyperparathyroidism), autoimmune disorders (e.g., rheumatoid arthritis, lupus), and nervous system conditions (e.g., Parkinson disease, stroke). Women with estrogen-sensitive breast cancer, for instance, are commonly treated with aromatase inhibitors, which lower the amount of estrogen in the body and can lead to bone loss and broken bones. For persons with rheumatoid arthritis, both the disease itself and the steroid medications used to treat it can contribute to bone loss. The increased risk of osteoporosis for individuals suffering from Parkinson or stroke results from limited mobility and subsequent decreased activity and increased fall risk. A more complete list of osteoporosis-associated conditions and the specific risk factors stemming from these conditions is available at the NOF Web site (http://www.nof.org/node/233).

PRESENTATION OF OSTEOPOROSIS IN OLDER ADULTS

Bone density loss is not in itself problematic. Osteoporosis is asymptomatic through its early stages until a fracture occurs. Thus, the fractures are the cause of pain, deformity, reduction in quality of life, depression, and excess morbidity and mortality. The two most common osteoporotic fractures occur in the vertebra and hip.

Vertebral Fracture

Vertebral fractures are often "silent" or asymptomatic fractures that can occur without an individual or health care provider being aware of their existence. Some women can have multiple vertebral fractures and still be unaware until the changed position of the spine (kyphosis) alerts them to the fact that something is wrong. Physical consequences of vertebral fractures include acute and chronic pain, deformity or dowager's hump, and increased morbidity and mortality (Cauley et al., 2001). Thirty years ago, vertebral fractures were not considered severe. Research since that time indicates that they play a critical role in reduced quality of life, depression, social isolation, and ultimately in death (Gold, 2003). Health care professionals should watch for the cardinal signs of vertebral fractures in women with low bone mass or osteoporosis. Height loss of greater than 1 inch (2.54 cm) can often be the first indication that vertebral fractures have occurred. They can be verified by x-ray or vertebral assessment using dual x-ray absorptiometry (DXA). Two surgical procedures, kyphoplasty and vertebroplasty, can be performed to help reduce pain, and in the case of kyphoplasty, restore vertebral height (Boonen et al., 2011). Vertebral fracture prevention with appropriate calcium and vitamin D intake, weight-bearing and strength-training exercise, and appropriate osteoporosis medication is critical following either the first or a subsequent fracture.

Hip Fracture

Hip fracture occurs in older women and men and can often have devastating effects. Some of these are well-known: pain, immobility, loss of independence, and reduced ability to perform activities of daily living (ADLs), increased morbidity, and nursing home placement (Stevens, 2005). Hip fractures have also long been associated with increased mortality. In a recent study, LeBlanc et al. (2011) noted that short-term mortality (in the year after hip fracture) increased twofold in women aged 65 to 79 years and exceptionally healthy women aged 80 and over.

SCREENING AND RISK FACTORS

Screening for Osteoporosis

The best way to avoid osteoporotic fractures is to engage in routine preventive actions, among which screening is exceptionally important. A bone density or bone mass measurement test is the appropriate way to screen for and diagnose osteoporosis. The gold standard of these tests is DXA or central DXA. These tests measure density at the hip and spine and are noninvasive and painless; in most cases, they can be done without undressing. They take only about 15 minutes, yet the physician who interprets them gets a wealth of information about the skeleton. Most important is the T-score, which conveys information on the skeleton's bone density when compared with that of a young normal skeleton. The World Health Organization (World Health Organization [WHO], 1994) developed criteria by which to compare individual T-scores and determine bone health (Table 12.1). Bone density scores are essential in diagnosing osteoporosis. Medicare covers the costs of DXA tests; however, because they are not sensitive to small changes, they are typically done only once every 18 to 24 months.

Other techniques are also used to measure bone mass, but they are far less precise and predictable. They are peripheral tests done on the heel, lower arm, wrist, or finger and are called pDXA (peripheral dual energy x-ray absorptiometry), QUS (quantitative ultrasound), or pQCT (peripheral quantitative computed tomography). These tests should be used only to determine whether a central DXA should also be ordered or if a central DXA is not available. They are not to be used to diagnose osteoporosis or to monitor treatment.

FRAX

Bone density is but one of many factors that can put older women at risk of developing osteoporosis. The WHO, under the leadership of Dr. John Kanis, developed FRAX (http://www.shef .ac.uk/FRAX/), a screening tool that integrates analysis of clinical risk factors and measurement of BMD to determine fracture risk. One of the unique aspects of FRAX is that separate algorithms have been designed for use with women in different countries, each based on data specific to that country. In the United States, FRAX also has different algorithms for men, and for women of Caucasian, Asian, African American, and Hispanic races, again using race-specific data in the formulations.

TABLE 12.1 · Understanding T-Scores

Category	Fracture Risk	Action
Normal: BMD < 1 SD below young adult reference range	Below average	Be watchful for clinical triggers.
Osteopenia: BMD 1–2.5 SD below young adult reference range	Above average	Consider prevention in peri/postmenopausal women, be watchful for clinical triggers, and possibly repeat investigation in 2–3 years.
Osteoporosis: BMD > 2.5 SD below young adult reference range	High	Exclude secondary causes; therapeutic intervention indicated for most patients.
Severe osteoporosis: BMD > 2.5 SD below young adult reference range, plus one or more fragility fractures	Established osteoporosis	Exclude secondary causes; therapeutic intervention indicated for most patients.

FRAX requires the answers to 12 straightforward questions that inquire about age (or date of birth), sex, weight, height, previous fracture, parent fractured hip, current smoking, glucocorticoid use, presence of rheumatoid arthritis, secondary osteoporosis, alcohol use, and femoral neck BMD. Health care professionals should complete these primarily yes/no questions and then submit them for immediate scoring. The scoring provides two percentages: 10-year absolute risk of major osteoporotic fractures and 10-year absolute risk of hip fracture. Unlike T-scores, which provide an estimation of the relative risk of fracture, FRAX provides the absolute risk of osteoporotic fractures for the individual. According to work done by Kanis et al. (2011), if a person has a 20% or greater absolute risk of major osteoporotic fracture or a 3% or greater absolute risk of hip fracture, it is cost-effective to treat that person with prescription osteoporosis medications.

The FRAX approach to assessment of risk factors and fracture risk is also more intuitive in its scoring and application than are T-scores, making it easier for lay people to understand. FRAX is intended for use only in postmenopausal women and men 50 years of age and older who have never been treated with osteoporosis medications. Its results must be combined with clinical expertise to make appropriate treatment decisions.

TREATMENT OF OSTEOPOROSIS

Calcium and Vitamin D

All individuals, regardless of menopausal or fracture status, should be ingesting sufficient calcium and vitamin D so that the medications they take can work. Calcium and vitamin D are to bone strength what bricks and mortar are to a wall. Without vitamin D to enhance the effect of calcium, and without calcium—the primary substance that gives strength to the skeleton—bone-active medications cannot be effective. Although the daily required amounts of calcium and vitamin D differ according to different information sources, the NOF has established gender- and age-specific recommendations for calcium and vitamin D intake (Table 12.2). The importance of calcium and vitamin D for bone health is further discussed in the prevention section of this chapter.

TABLE 12.2 · National Osteoporosis Foundation Total Daily Calcium and Vitamin D Recommendations

	Calcium[a] (mg)	Vitamin D (International Units)
Women		
Under age 50	1,000	400–800
Aged 50+	1,200	800–1,000
Men		
Under age 50	1,000	400–800
Aged 50–70	1,000	800–1,000
Aged 71+	1,200	800–1,000

[a]Note: Calcium recommendations include the total amount the person gets from both food and supplements.

Pharmaceutical Treatments

Currently, there are nine FDA-approved medications designed to prevent and/or treat osteoporosis. Both health care professionals and patients unfamiliar with osteoporosis are often overwhelmed by the many choices. Below, we describe five categories of medications: hormonal treatments, bisphosphonates, selective estrogen receptor modulators (SERMs), parathyroid hormone, and Rank Ligand (RANKL) inhibitors. In this section, we discuss their specific indications and fracture-prevention qualities, note their side effects, and point out black box warnings (i.e., particularly serious side effects or life-threatening risks) imposed by the FDA.

Hormonal Treatments—Estrogen

Beginning in the early 1970s, the FDA noted that estrogen was "probably effective" for selected cases of osteoporosis. By 1990, it became a mainstay of osteoporosis prevention and treatment as well as for the management of menopausal symptoms. Since the release of the estrogen-related results of the Women's Health Initiative (WHI), estrogen's FDA approval changed from treatment of osteoporosis to prevention of osteoporosis only in women with vasomotor symptoms related to menopause. According to the new safety guidelines, estrogen should be prescribed in the smallest possible doses over the shortest period (Wyeth Pharmaceuticals, Inc., 2011). The use of various estrogen preparations reduces the risk of vertebral fractures significantly. The common side effects of estrogen are well-known—headaches, nausea, and vomiting. More serious, and far less prevalent, are breast and uterine cancer, stroke, heart attack, and blood clots (Rossouw et al., 2002). In 2003, the FDA required a black box warning for estrogen products to show that estrogen increases risks of heart disease, myocardial infarction, stroke, and breast cancer for postmenopausal women.

Hormonal Treatments—Calcitonin

The first nonestrogen drug that the FDA approved for the treatment of osteoporosis was calcitonin, approved in injectable form in 1984 and in a nasal spray in 1995 (Miacalcin; Novartis, 2011a). Calcitonin is a synthetic hormone approved for use in women who have osteoporosis (are already undergoing treatment) and who are at least 5 years past menopause. Calcitonin has been shown to reduce the risk of vertebral fractures but has not been effective at other fracture sites. One of the reasons for the popularity of calcitonin was that there were virtually no side effects. A second reason was that, because the nasal spray delivery method was so easy, patients seemed to be more compliant with it than with oral or other drugs (Novartis, 2009). Unfortunately, the bone effects of calcitonin in clinical trials were never strong (Chestnut & Azria, 2010). Calcitonin does not have any black box warning on its prescribing information.

Bisphosphonates

In 1995, the first of a family of drugs called bisphosphonates was approved by the FDA and released for public sale. Alendronate (Merck and Co., Inc., 2012) is approved for the prevention and treatment of osteoporosis in postmenopausal women and the treatment of osteoporosis in men. It is also approved for the treatment of GIO in both women and men who have had extended exposure to steroids. It was initially released in a daily tablet form, but is now available in a once-weekly tablet as well as a weekly tablet that includes vitamin D. Alendronate has been shown to be effective in preventing vertebral, hip, and nonvertebral fractures. In 2000, the FDA approved a second bisphosphonate, risedronate (Actonel; Warner Chilcott, 1998), for the prevention and treatment of PMO, the treatment of osteoporosis in men, and the prevention and treatment of GIO in women and men. Risedronate has been effective in preventing vertebral fractures and a composite set of nonvertebral fractures including hip fractures.

Ibandronate (Boniva) was the third bisphosphonate to be approved by the FDA. Although the pivotal Boniva trial showed it to be effective in preventing vertebral fractures, it did not achieve statistical significance for its ability to prevent hip or other nonvertebral fractures. It has been approved for the prevention and treatment of postmenopausal osteoporosis (Genentech USA, Inc., 2011a, 2011b). Ibandronate, although initially approved as a daily drug, was never marketed in that dose. Instead, it was marketed as a once-monthly drug, something many marketing experts believed would make it the drug of choice for women with compliance and persistence problems. The marketing push around ibandronate was startlingly good; Sally Field was identified as the spokesperson for this medication. However, its lack of nonvertebral efficacy made some women and many physicians reluctant to use it. Ultimately, ibandronate was also available as a quarterly IV medication (Genentech USA, Inc., 2011b).

In 2002, the final bisphosphonate approved by the FDA made its appearance. Zoledronic acid was originally approved (as Zometa) for hypercalcemia, bone metastases, and multiple myeloma. In 2007, zoledronic acid (under the name Reclast; Novartis, 2011b) was approved as the only once-yearly medication for the prevention and treatment of PMO, the treatment of osteoporosis in men, and prevention and treatment of GIO. A health care provider in a setting that has specialized infusion equipment must administer the infusion annually. Zoledronic acid has been shown to be effective in preventing vertebral, hip, and nonvertebral fractures. Not only did this medication have to be taken only once a year, but because it was delivered in an IV infusion, it eliminated some of the class problems with oral bisphosphonates (discussed below).

Class Effects of Bisphosphonates.   Without question, the bisphosphonates are the most widely used and arguably the most effective treatments for osteoporosis. From the beginning, however, oral bisphosphonates presented consumer challenges as the regimen for taking them was complex and essential (first thing in the morning on an empty stomach; only with plain water and must drink 8 oz [236.6 ml] of water; no food or drink for 30 to 60 minutes after administration; cannot lie down or recline for 30 minutes after taking). Even when these rules were followed, only a small proportion of the bisphosphonates were bioavailable (Cremers & Papapoulos, 2011). Thus, patients who deviated from this strict regimen (e.g., took it with orange juice or coffee; ate right after taking it) were unlikely to receive therapeutic benefit from the treatment.

The most common immediate or short-term side effects of the oral bisphosphonates are esophageal irritation and gastric distress or heartburn. Use of IV zoledronic acid eliminates those problems, but this medication has potential side effects of its own: joint pain, fever, headaches, and flu-like symptoms. However, none of these side effects occurs in all persons. Unfortunately, many individuals terminate their oral bisphosphonate use because of side effects, despite the fact that most of the IV bisphosphonate effects are transient, and can be expected to disappear after a few days (Eekman et al., 2009).

Of greater concern to patients is the association between bisphosphonate use and more serious side effects. Three such problems have received substantial media attention: osteonecrosis of the jaw (ONJ) (Sambrook et al., 2006), atrial fibrillation (Rhee et al., 2012) and subtrochanteric fractures (Black et al., 2010). ONJ is most likely to occur in patients having major dental work or oral surgery or in those who have cancer and are receiving the cancer dose of zoledronic acid. The data on these outcomes are equivocal at best. They appear in case reports and anecdotally at scientific meetings, but randomized controlled trial data reexamined for these outcomes show that they are very rare, and that no clear causal links between taking bisphosphonates and experiencing these outcomes exist.

Atrial fibrillation may also be a consequence of bisphosphonate use. After several studies that showed no such relationship, a large study of cancer patients showed an increased risk of this problem (Erichsen et al., 2011). The use of bisphosphonates to prevent and treat osteoporotic fractures is extremely effective, and the likelihood of any of these serious outcomes is minimal (Shane et al., 2010). Despite these potential serious adverse events, no bisphosphonate has a black box warning on its prescribing information.

Selective Estrogen Receptor Modulators

SERMS comprise a class of drugs that work like estrogen in some ways and anti-estrogens in other ways. The only SERM currently approved for the prevention and treatment of PMO is raloxifene (Evista; Eli Lilly and Company, 2011). In addition, raloxifene is approved for the reduction of risk of invasive breast cancer in postmenopausal women with osteoporosis and postmenopausal women with high risk of invasive breast cancer. Needless to say, the compound approval encourages some women to use raloxifene who might not otherwise consider medications for OP, despite the fact that raloxifene has been shown to be effective in reducing only vertebral fractures. This daily medication can be taken any time, with or without food, and has no restrictions such as remaining upright. Side effects are minimal and include leg pain, hot flashes, sweating, and flu-like symptoms. However, raloxifene does have a black box warning on its prescribing information, mandated by the FDA. Consumers and health care providers are warned that very serious adverse events can occur in the following areas: deep vein thrombosis and pulmonary embolism, increased risk of death from stroke in women with heart disease or major risk factors for heart disease.

Parathyroid Hormone

Although parathyroid hormone has been implicated in bone loss and osteoporosis, a new formulation of it, teriparatide (Forteo; Eli Lilly and Company, 2012), was approved by the FDA in 2002 for the treatment of PMO, male osteoporosis, and GIO. Clinical trials have shown teriparatide to be effective in preventing vertebral and nonvertebral fractures. Because there are potential side effects from teriparatide, it should be used only in patients with severe osteoporosis and high risk of fracture.

Teriparatide is a daily self-administered subcutaneous injection. The FDA has approved 24 months as the maximum time any patient should take this medication. It is the only anabolic drug in the osteoporosis group, meaning it actually builds bone rather than just slowing the loss of bone. However, it stops working as soon as a patient stops taking it, so an antiresorptive therapy should be prescribed when teriparatide is stopped to sustain BMD gains. Primary side effects that result from the use of teriparatide are leg cramps and dizziness, occasional headache, and nausea (Neer et al., 2001).

In early studies of teriparatide, researchers found that the medication appeared to cause osteosarcoma in rats (Vahle et al., 2004). Despite the fact that no human patient had manifested osteosarcoma in conjunction with teriparatide, the FDA mandated a black box warning on the prescribing information noting the potential of osteosarcoma as an outcome (Eli Lilly and Company, 2012). Since that time, two human patients have been reported with a teriparatide-related osteosarcoma (Subbiah et al., 2010). It is worth noting that this osteosarcoma prevalence rate in OP patients on teriparatide is the same as would be expected in the general population.

RANK Ligand Inhibitor

The newest FDA-approved medication XGEVA (Amgen, Inc., 2010) for the treatment of osteoporosis is an entirely new approach to maintaining sufficient bone density and strength. Denosumab (Amgen, Inc., 2011) is a fully human monoclonal antibody that has been approved to treat PMO in women, to treat osteoporosis in men receiving androgen deprivation therapy for prostate cancer, and to increase bone mass in women who are receiving adjuvant aromatase inhibitor therapy for breast cancer. By inhibiting the action of RANKL, denosumab reduces the survival and activity of osteoclasts, thereby slowing the rate of bone resorption. Denosumab is dosed once every 6 months via a subcutaneous injection that must be administered by a health care provider. It reduces vertebral, hip, and nonvertebral fractures. Side effects of denosumab include infections (of the urinary and respiratory tracts), constipation, and joint pain. Patients with insufficient calcium and vitamin D levels should not be put on denosumab until calcium levels return to normal. A more serious consequence of denosumab use is ONJ. Although extremely rare, ONJ can occur in patients having major dental work or oral surgery done and/or who have cancer. Denosumab does not have any black box warnings on its prescribing information.

Alternative Treatments

Women frustrated by the cost, side effects, and other negatives associated with pharmacological therapy for osteoporosis have been searching for alternative treatments to help improve bone density and prevent fracture. Few of these alternatives have been studied empirically, so the use of many alternative medications is anecdotal rather than evidence based.

Common examples of alternative approaches to sustaining bone health include the use of omega-3 fatty acids and dietary and herbal therapy. The Agency for Healthcare Research and Quality (AHRQ) published a technical report in 2004 on omega-3 fatty acids and their impact on certain chronic diseases (MacLean et al., 2004). Five studies of the impact of omega-3 fatty acids on BMD were reviewed; no studies with fracture end points were available. Current research suggests no consistent effect of omega-3 fatty acids on BMD or fracture.

Beyond the use of calcium and vitamin D, few dietary and herbal therapies have been appropriately tested to determine whether they play a significant role in bone health and good bone metabolism. Researchers in the United Kingdom (Putnam et al., 2007) have suggested that such therapies can strengthen mineralization and resorption of bone. Recommended substances include common vegetables, including onion, garlic, and parsley; essential oils derived from sage, rosemary, thyme, and other herbs; soya; and cannabinoids. However, the level of proof is very low, and controlled studies with large samples are needed to provide sufficient scientific support for these suggestions.

A recent article on herbal products that help prevent osteoporosis (Leung et al., 2011) described a study of 150 Chinese women at least 1 year since their last menstrual period. The women were randomly assigned to either a treatment group that received a triple herb product, Bo-gu Ling (ELP), or a placebo group. BMD of the spine and secondary end points was measured at baseline,

6 months, and 12 months. The spine BMD scores of the ELP group increased at 12 months, though not significantly, whereas those in the placebo group declined. However, in a subgroup analysis, spinal BMD in the treatment group of women more than 10 years past menopause was significantly higher than BMD for those in the placebo group. Although this intervention does not appear to be equally effective in all women with osteoporosis, the results may be promising for older women at least a decade past menopause.

COMPLIANCE AND PERSISTENCE WITH OSTEOPOROSIS MEDICATIONS

Perhaps the biggest challenge to the prevention and treatment of osteoporosis in postmenopausal and older women, as well as in men, is the lack of compliance and persistence with FDA-approved medications, as well as with calcium and vitamin D supplementation, and weight-bearing and strength-training exercise. Despite the fact that there are nine FDA-approved drugs available in a wide variety of dosing styles and frequencies, nearly 50% of women have stopped their osteoporosis medication within 1 year after they started it (Gold et al., 2007; Yood et al., 2003). In general, medications for all chronic diseases, especially those that are asymptomatic like osteoporosis, have poor compliance and persistence rates. We examine osteoporosis-specific medication compliance and persistence issues below.

The Problem

As noted above, asymptomatic chronic diseases such as osteoporosis do not compromise quality of life or functionality in women until or unless a fracture occurs. Conceptually, it is difficult for people to understand why they should take medication for something they "can't feel" or "can't see." Unlike pain medication or those for symptomatic diseases like diabetes or asthma, osteoporosis medications do not have a discernible impact on the patient. Just as pain medications stop pain, osteoporosis medications stop bone loss; but the latter type of change cannot be detected by the patient. Furthermore, positive medication outcomes (e.g., increased BMD) are difficult to determine over a short period. Typically, patients start antiresorptive medication and return 12 to 24 months later for a follow-up DXA to see if it is working. Thus, it is not surprising that many patients stop taking medication when they receive no feedback for their behaviors (Compston, 2003).

The Evidence

The number of scholarly articles on compliance increases exponentially each year. Most report results from analyses of administrative claims data that both compliance and persistence are poor (Papaioannou et al., 2007). An early article on compliance with hormone replacement therapy showed that only 34% of postmenopausal women still took their hormone replacement 2 years after initiation (Steel et al., 2003). Recent reports indicated that compliance and persistence with all osteoporosis medications remained poor over a decade later (Kothawala et al., 2007).

The Issues

Beginning with the release of alendronate in 1995, the pharmaceutical companies that produced osteoporosis medications (especially bisphosphonates) realized that consumers would dislike the detailed regimens required for maximum absorption of medications, especially when they had to follow these guidelines on a daily basis. As noted above, the daily dose of alendronate was approved by the FDA in 1995; its first competitor, risedronate, had its daily dose approved in 1998. At that point, these two daily administrations of oral bisphosphonates were the only ones available. Many people thought of this as a "drug war" between the two and assumed that alendronate would win out as it was first to market.

Daily and Weekly Dosing Intervals

Changes in dosing intervals were just about to begin, however. Marketers believed that the dosing regimen for bisphosphonates would be much better tolerated for weekly than for daily doses. Alendronate weekly dosing was approved in 2000, only 2 years after its competitor—risedronate—released a daily dose. Not surprisingly, most women preferred a weekly rather than a daily dose (Kendler et al., 2004; Simon et al., 2002). Given the overwhelming evidence that women were far more likely to comply with bisphosphonate challenges weekly rather than daily (Baroutsou et al., 2004; Ettinger et al., 2006), a weekly dose of risedronate was FDA-approved in 2002. With patients having two weekly options to choose from, compliance and persistence with the weekly dosing continued to be better than with daily regimens (Silverman & Gold, 2008). However, Cramer and colleagues (2005) found that while weekly bisphosphonate users had better persistence than daily users, neither group was anywhere near the level of compliance necessary to reduce overall prevalence of osteoporosis. Regardless of the dosing interval, the two oral bisphosphonates required a strict dosing regimen and had side effects that were bothersome. Strong evidence suggested that poor compliance and persistence would, in fact, result in the very fractures medication was designed to prevent (Rabenda et al., 2008; Siris et al., 2006).

Another daily drug, raloxifene (Eli Lilly and Company, 2011), was introduced in 2007. Because it could be taken at any time during the day, with or without food, it did not raise the same controversy or concerns over compliance and persistence as the bisphosphonates. Physicians anticipated they would see improvements in raloxifene use when the FDA released the following indication for raloxifene in 2007: reduction in risk of invasive breast cancer in postmenopausal women at high risk for invasive breast cancer (Eli Lilly and Company, 2011). Few studies have examined compliance and persistence with raloxifene, however, to confirm or refute whether physician beliefs were accurate.

Delivery System

The approval of Teriparatide in 2002 not only brought a different dosing approach and regimen, but also introduced the first and only anabolic therapy to treat bone loss—one that actually built new bone instead of just slowing the rate of bone loss. Teriparatide was, as alendronate and risedronate were originally, a daily medication. However, there were several distinct differences in dosing, with some advantages and some drawbacks. First, teriparatide could be taken at any time of day, an advantage over the "first thing in the morning" problem with bisphosphonates. Next, the delivery system for teriparatide (i.e., daily subcutaneous injections) did not cause the negative gastrointestinal impact of oral bisphosphonates. Finally, the FDA indicated that 24 months was the maximum dosing duration for teriparatide. After accruing bone during that time, women needed to go back on an antiresorptive medication to avoid losing their new gains in bone density.

Given the complexity of subcutaneous dosing and daily timing, health care professionals expressed concerns about compliance and persistence with this drug. An observational study called Direct Assessment of Nonvertebral Fractures in Community Experience (DANCE) was initiated to examine real-world behaviors with regard to this new drug (Miller et al., 2006). Initial analyses of data from this trial suggested that compliance and persistence were higher than might have been expected. Unlike data from bisphosphonate users who reported significant discontinuation, only 7% ($n = 919$) reported early discontinuation of teriparatide and just 10% ($n = 68$) reported late discontinuation (Gold et al., 2011). Perhaps those willing to initiate a daily injection were more committed to beating osteoporosis than those taking a less invasive medication. For whatever reason, teriparatide users appeared to have the best compliance and persistence rates of all anti-osteoporotic medication users.

Monthly Dosing and More

The improvement in compliance and persistence that occurred between daily and weekly bisphosphonates convinced the pharmaceutical industry that the timing of doses was a critical component of osteoporosis medication adherence. In 2005, a new bisphosphonate—ibandronate (Boniva)—was brought to the FDA for approval. Several studies purported to show that compliance and persistence was optimal with monthly dosing, especially in direct competition with weekly bisphosphonates. This interval allowed those who struggled with bisphosphonate-related side effects to deal with them only 12 times a year. The early study on patient preferences for ibandronate was called the *Boniva ALendronate Trial in Osteoporosis* (BALTO) and was a comparison of weekly alendronate and monthly ibandronate (Emkey et al., 2005). In it, patients were randomized to 6 months of either once-weekly alendronate or once-monthly ibandronate. At the end of the 6 months, these groups crossed over and completed another 6-month segment with the other option. Significantly more women preferred ibandronate and its dosing to alendronate and its dosing, with the primary reason being convenience. A second study, named Monthly Oral iBandronate In LadiEs (MOBILE), compared monthly ibandronate with daily ibandronate and found that patients strongly preferred monthly over daily regimens (Reginster et al., 2006). A third study (BALTO II) reinforced the findings from the original BALTO study by comparing once-monthly ibandronate with once-weekly alendronate (Hadji et al., 2008). Because these studies supported intuition (that women would prefer monthly over weekly or daily dosing), they received instant credibility.

Further study of the situation, however, identified a flaw in BALTO that was not identified in previous publications using these data (Keen et al., 2006). Keen and colleagues pointed out that the women in the BALTO sample were led to believe that the two drugs (i.e., ibandronate and alendronate) were equally efficacious when questioned about preferences for weekly versus monthly dosing. As noted previously, this is not true. Alendronate has been shown to have efficacy in preventing fractures at the spine, hip, and wrist; ibandronate has only been shown to be efficacious in the spine. When women were given correct effectiveness information in the Keen et al. study, 82% of the women preferred a weekly dose with proven efficacy at the spine and hip to a monthly medication with only spinal efficacy. Similar findings were shown in a study of weekly risedronate versus monthly ibandronate (Gold et al., 2006).

The final dosing change in bisphosphonates occurred in 2007 when zoledronic acid was approved as a once-yearly IV infusion (Novartis, 2011b). Many believed, despite several complicating factors, that this medication would eliminate problems of compliance and adherence with osteoporosis medications. A health care professional must administer zoledronic acid. It is given in an IV infusion, so patients have to go to infusion centers, often not conveniently located.

The infusion must be given over at least a 15-minute interval; thus, the timing of administration was longer than that for any other drug (Novartis, 2011b). Nevertheless, this was billed as the drug that had to succeed (Ringe, 2010).

Given the short time since zoledronic acid has been approved and the long time lag between doses, few data have been published on its compliance and persistence. Recently, Curtis and colleagues (2012) compared adherence with two osteoporosis drugs: zoledronic acid and ibandronate. They found that adherence for more than 1 year with these two drugs was about the same and slightly better than that of oral bisphosphonates. Yet, more than 33% of IV bisphosphonate users discontinued in the first year (Curtis et al., 2012).

Conclusions about Compliance and Persistence

Space limitations preclude a thorough inventory of the entire literature on compliance and persistence with osteoporosis medications. One compelling conclusion, however, emerges from every study: Patients taking osteoporosis medication, for the most part, are not continuing to take the medication as long as necessary. Although there have been some interventions designed to improve compliance and persistence with these drugs (e.g., Clowes et al., 2004), none has been found to be truly efficacious. Continuing research to further understand why osteoporosis patients are not compliant and what might help them to become so is crucial.

CULTURAL CONSIDERATIONS

White postmenopausal women have predominantly garnered the attention of osteoporosis researchers and health care providers because they are the group at highest risk for fracture and account for about 90% of disease-related costs (Melton & Marquez, 2008). The landscape of osteoporosis management will change, however, with population aging. Although fewer men are diagnosed with osteoporosis, they account for almost 30% of osteoporosis-related hip fractures and experience a higher rate of morbidity and mortality than female osteoporosis patients (Khosla et al., 2008). As the number of older men increases, therefore, sex (biologic) and gender (social/cultural) differences will demand further scrutiny (Dy et al., 2011). Owing to increasing ethnic and racial diversity among older adults in the United States, the greatest increase in future osteoporotic fractures is projected to be in the nonwhite population; yet, the literature on the cultural factors that affect osteoporosis prevention, identification, and treatment among diverse populations is extremely scant (Melton & Marquez, 2008). However, there are some general cultural issues affecting chronic disease management, societal beliefs about osteoporosis and aging, and differences with respect to race, gender, and geographic setting that should be considered.

MANAGING OSTEOPOROSIS

Similar to patterns of other chronic conditions, individuals with the lowest health literacy about osteoporosis prevention and management are likely to carry the greatest disease burden due to lifestyle, diet, and lack of access to health resources (Shaw et al., 2009). Osteoporosis health disparities within and between different socioeconomic, geographic, and minority groups, however, have not been fully explored (Melton & Marquez, 2008). Because of the dearth of information about the unique health needs of different ethnic and social groups, a "personalized" medical approach that integrates patient preferences and values is recommended to overcome hidden cultural, educational, geographic, or financial barriers that might otherwise compromise osteoporosis prevention and treatment (Katz, 2001; Melton & Marquez, 2008). There is always a danger with such an approach, however, that systemic differences across socioeconomic, ethnic, and racial groups regarding the perceived risks and benefits of health interventions may exacerbate, rather than alleviate, health disparities (Katz, 2001). In addition to including patients in decision-making processes, culturally sensitive osteoporosis screening and management must offer active outreach and education to minority populations for improved health literacy and provide translation services to overcome language barriers and navigate different culture-specific explanatory models for disease (Shaw et al., 2009). When there is conflict between the best evidence-based practice for osteoporosis response and a patient's cultural beliefs or customs, health professionals are advised to incorporate cultural practices that are "beneficial or neutral" into the treatment plan, but to provide ample time for discussion and explanation if a cultural custom is deemed potentially harmful (Hulme, 2010). Even such strategies are not enough, however, to guarantee quality patient outcomes. They must be accompanied by the development of broader knowledge systems about the cultural groups being served by a specific health provider and organizational level monitoring of treatment outcomes for different groups (Hulme, 2010).

Racial and Ethnic Differences

Researchers have identified some physiological differences in bone morphology and osteoporosis manifestation patterns along racial and gender lines. These differences do not, however, provide adequate justification for differences in prevention practices or treatment among various groups (racial/ethnic minorities, men) (Neuman et al., 2011). African American and Hispanic children have been shown to demonstrate greater bone strength than Caucasian children from an early age (Wetzsteon et al., 2009); yet, in a national sample, Mexican American adults exhibited lower bone density than non-Hispanic Whites (Looker et al., 2009). Asian Americans on Medicare experience the highest prevalence of osteoporosis and related fractures compared with other ethnic Medicare recipient groups (White, Hispanic, African American). Conversely, non-Hispanic Blacks have the highest BMD of any ethnic group (Looker et al., 2009), and Black women have the lowest hip fracture rate in the United States—almost half that of Whites and Hispanics (Stone & Lyles, 2006). Even when controlling for physiological differences, socioeconomic disparities, and other factors, a dramatic gap between current NOF treatment guidelines and the receipt of prescription medications for osteoporosis exists for African American women and male patients. These groups, even when exhibiting high risk for fracture, are substantially less likely to receive osteoporosis medications than White females (Curtis et al., 2009). This may be due to lack of uniformity in osteoporosis guidelines, inappropriate interpretation of screening results for non-Caucasians and men, or physician failure to identify high-risk African Americans or males since they are aware that these groups are generally at lower risk for osteoporosis. Overall, more than three fourths of White males and more than one half of African American females may be at high enough osteoporosis risk to warrant further evaluation and possible treatment with prescription medications (Curtis et al., 2009).

Gender and Age Differences

Given the complexity of cultural issues and the current lack of specific information regarding the needs of various patient groups, health professionals offering osteoporosis outreach, education, and intervention can begin with an improved understanding of how general patient beliefs—those that are not culture-specific—may influence prevention practices and care decisions. Both older men and women, despite strong beliefs in the severity of osteoporosis and the effectiveness of osteoporosis screening, concurrently have low belief in their own personal susceptibility to osteoporosis (Nayak et al., 2010). Differences in beliefs may exist across age cohorts regarding the perceived seriousness of osteoporosis and importance of prevention practices, but neither older nor younger women are inclined to consider themselves susceptible to the disease (Piehowski et al., 2010). This may be due in part to older adults relying on "worst-case scenarios" as explanatory models for the disease (Reventlow & Bang, 2006). These beliefs, which run counter to adoption of lifelong osteoporosis prevention measures and early diagnosis, should be specifically targeted with patient education to improve prevention practices and increase osteoporosis screening rates (Nayak et al., 2010; Piehowski et al., 2010). Once patients have received osteoporosis diagnosis, other common beliefs may come into conflict with treatment adherence. Specifically, one difference between those who choose to initiate medical treatment and those who do not seek treatment relates to beliefs about osteoporosis medications. Individuals with a distrust of medications and lack of faith in their benefits are least likely to pursue treatment even after diagnosis (Yood et al., 2008). Practitioners and researchers need to explore various approaches to addressing concerns and questions about the pharmaceutical aspects of osteoporosis intervention. It is crucial for health care professionals to tease out whether the broad beliefs guiding health habits and treatment choices among those at risk for or experiencing osteoporosis differ among their patients along the dimensions of gender, race, and ethnicity.

Recent research offers some insight into the gender gap between treatment and outcome patterns of osteoporosis; preliminary findings that can help guide educational outreach and health provider interactions with men. Compared with women, men with an existing diagnosis seem to: (a) dismiss osteoporosis as an immediate or serious threat to their current health (seeing it as a "women's disease"), (b) perceive that medications have little effect, and (c) ignore both the pain signals of osteoporosis and physician guidelines to prevent fracture (Solimeo et al., 2011). Once diagnosed, men collectively suggest they are given inadequate information about interventions, are reluctant to take medications or tolerate side effects, and have a general lack of faith in care management or medication efficacy (Solimeo et al., 2011). These documented beliefs that interfere with effective treatment of males, in conjunction with the higher morbidity and mortality among male osteoporosis patients, illuminate how dramatically prevention efforts with male patients lag behind interventions with female patients (Dy et al., 2011). With the aging of the population and increasing health problem of osteoporosis among men, further research and improved practices with respect to gender and sex differences, across and between different ethnic groups, will be paramount (Khosla et al., 2008).

Geographic Considerations

Finally, geographic setting may impact osteoporosis prevalence, incidence, and the effectiveness of response efforts. It is not clear exactly how the rural–urban divide affects osteoporosis manifestations and response. In general, chronic disease management in rural areas often poses different and greater challenges than in urban settings owing to disparities in preventable chronic diseases and infrastructure or capacity to address health needs (Gamm et al., 2002). The findings of national population studies suggest that older residents of rural areas have a higher age-adjusted rate for most chronic conditions, including musculoskeletal problems and orthopedic impairments, than their urban counterparts (Jones et al., 2009) and limited access to both primary and specialized health care (Gamm et al., 2002). Rural community members exhibit a higher rate of smoking, which may exacerbate susceptibility to osteoporosis, but also experience a higher rate of obesity, and higher body weight is generally associated with higher bone density (Bonura, 2009; Eberhardt & Pamuk, 2004; Looker et al., 2007). There is some evidence that clinical guidelines for improved osteoporosis management may not be embraced as readily in rural versus urban areas, perhaps due to resource or educational barriers (Dagenais et al., 2010). Although the influence of geographic setting on osteoporosis occurrence and outcomes remains unclear, the limited research available suggests that women with osteoporosis living in a rural environment report being socially isolated and often lack access to supportive services; thus the complexity of coping with this disease may be magnified (Roberto, 2004; Roberto & Reynolds, 2001).

OSTEOPOROSIS PREVENTION

Osteoporosis prevention can be divided into three main areas: (a) primary prevention (e.g., education about health habits across the life span that decrease chances of osteoporosis); (b) secondary prevention of disease progression after risk factor identification or early diagnosis (e.g., screenings, supplements, exercise, and medications); and (c) tertiary prevention of further physical deterioration and the specific osteoporosis-related injuries that increase morbidity/mortality and decrease quality of life for individuals living with the disease (e.g., fall prevention, pain management, modified medication, and exercise regimens). Proper nutrition and beneficial exercise practices are crucial components of any osteoporosis prevention efforts, while fall prevention is usually viewed as a disease management strategy. Screening measures and the prescription medications involved in osteoporosis prevention and intervention have been addressed extensively in previous sections of this chapter. In this section, we focus attention primarily on how nutritional choices and exercise habits across the life span impact osteoporosis outcomes, as well as the specific approaches employed to prevent falls and serious injuries in persons with osteoporosis.

HEREDITY AND ENVIRONMENT

Genetic factors play a large role in the development of osteoporosis and BMD, accounting for an estimated 60% to 90% of variation in PBM (Duncan & Brown, 2010). Currently, these genetic factors are not modifiable, but an understanding of the ways in which genetic and environmental factors interact may influence interventions aimed at modifying health behaviors and lifestyle choices of those who are genetically predisposed to developing osteoporosis (Grossman, 2011; Lorentzon et al., 2007). Modifiable environmental factors, such as nutrition and exercise habits, may account for up to 40% of PBM variance (Bonjour et al., 2009). Researchers continue to explore how heredity, hormonal factors (e.g., premature menopause or amenorrhea in women, hypogonadism in men), nutrient intake, and mechanical forces (e.g., physical activity, weight) converge to either undermine or optimize long-term bone health.

IMPORTANCE OF EARLY DEVELOPMENT AND PREVENTION

While osteoporosis is commonly associated with old age, osteoporotic prevention is a lifelong process beginning *in utero* (Grossman, 2011). Owing to the prevalence of bone fractures in older adults, educational efforts and medical interventions have focused mainly on this population.

However, more recent research has revealed that preventative measures may be most effective when implemented early in the life course (Dontas & Yiannakopoulos, 2007).

Evidence has accrued that maximization of PBM and minimization of fracture risk begins with intrauterine life (Cooper et al., 2009). Several studies have demonstrated a strong association between low birth weight, low BMD, and increased risk of hip fracture later in life, suggesting that *in utero* development plays a critical role in the attainment of PBM (Baird et al., 2010; Cooper et al., 2006). Risk factors associated with suboptimal acquisition of PBM *in utero* include vitamin D deficiency, maternal smoking, and maternal lack of exercise (Cooper et al., 2009; Javaid et al., 2006).

Researchers have also suggested that because 90% of adult bone mass will have formed by the end of puberty, prepuberty and adolescence may be critical times to modify both nutritional and exercise factors for maximum impact on long-term BMD and bone strength (Nikander et al., 2010; Stránský & Ryšavá, 2009). Children and adolescents demonstrate markedly better absorption of calcium and more dramatic improvements in bone strength in response to targeted exercise programs than adults who participate in similar interventions (Nikander et al., 2010, Stránský & Ryšavá, 2009). Not only is this a time during which bone health appears most malleable (as compared with the years after puberty has ended), but PBM during a child's early years could be the "single most important factor for prevention of osteoporosis in later life," with a 10% increase in PBM potentially reducing the risk of future fracture in postmenopausal women by 50% (Bonjour et al., 2009, p. S8).

ELEMENTS OF LONG-TERM BONE HEALTH

There are several health choices pivotal to successful osteoporosis prevention. Although many of these factors may have the greatest influence on long-term bone health if addressed in the early years of childhood development, they can still continue to have a significant impact on osteoporosis outcomes in middle and late life. Nutritional elements such as calcium, vitamin D, vitamin K, protein, magnesium and potassium, vitamin C, and phytochemicals from fruits and vegetables; physical activity; excessive alcohol; and tobacco use may all play an important role in lifelong bone health (Grossman, 2011; Tucker, 2009; Tylavsky et al., 2008). Professionals are still struggling, however, to define the optimal guidelines for intake of nutrients and alcohol, or the ideal prescription of exercise for bone health at different life phases (Grossman, 2011; Nikander et al., 2010; Tucker, 2009).

Nutrition

There is general consensus that both calcium and vitamin D are essential elements of bone health and osteoporosis prevention throughout the life cycle (Lanham-New, 2008; Stránský & Ryšavá, 2009). Neither the complexities of calcium uptake (regarding absorption of different forms, interactions with other nutritional elements, or the synergy of calcium and exercise) nor vitamin D interactions with calcium are, however, fully understood (Grossman, 2011; Tucker, 2009). To date, collective research suggests that calcium intake is protective against osteoporosis, but its effectiveness is heavily dependent on how it is utilized in the body. Absorption depends on many nuanced factors, including its chemical form and the presence of other complementary or interfering nutrients in foods. While adequate vitamin D consumption is necessary for calcium absorption, high doses of vitamin D can also increase renal secretion of calcium

(Stránský & Ryšavá, 2009; Tucker, 2009). Age of calcium intake may also create varying outcomes or differential benefits. Studies indicate that calcium intake before pubertal maturation can have the greatest impact on BMD (Bonjour et al., 2009), and suggest that calcium supplements can be effective in reducing bone loss among late postmenopausal women and reducing fracture rates among institutionalized older adults (Lanham-New, 2008). Findings across several studies also suggest a strong calcium and physical activity interaction, with calcium supplementation enhancing the positive impacts of exercise on bone growth and an active lifestyle enhancing the body's absorption of calcium (Bonjour et al., 2009; Stránský & Ryšavá, 2009).

Although calcium and vitamin D have historically been the primary components of osteoporosis nutritional prevention efforts, recent research has highlighted the importance of many other nutrients and food choices for support of bone health (Tucker, 2009). Data suggest, for instance, that vitamin K (available in leafy green vegetables and vegetable oils) plays a key role in maintenance of skeletal integrity over the life course and fracture reduction among osteoporosis patients (Lanham-New, 2008). Higher levels of vitamin K intake have reduced hip fracture rates in some older populations (Tucker, 2009), and combining supplementation of vitamin K with calcium and vitamin D has increased BMD measurements among healthy older women more significantly than calcium and vitamin D alone (Bolton-Smith et al., 2007). There have been conflicting outcomes in studies, however, regarding the impact of vitamin K in different chemical forms. While there is conclusive evidence that vitamin K is important for activation of crucial bone proteins, more research is needed to further understanding of which sources and amounts of this nutrient are optimal for prolonged bone health (Tucker, 2009).

Magnesium and potassium are other nutrients that protect against bone loss by helping maintain an acid–base balance in the body, and their interactions with other nutritional elements, such as protein, calcium, and sodium, are crucial to homeostasis of bone health (Tucker, 2009; Tylavsky et al., 2008). Particularly, these nutrients seem to buffer against the acid-producing effects of high protein intake and related urinary calcium loss. Protein also has a complex relationship with bone health. Although excess protein intake without adequate balance of certain nutrients can contribute to loss of calcium, low protein intake has been associated with increased risk of fracture among older adults. Irrespective of other dietary factors, high levels of protein intake (even several times higher than the current US recommended daily allowance) have consistently resulted in reduced risk of bone and hip fracture among older adult study participants (Misra et al., 2011; Tucker, 2009; Tylavsky et al., 2008).

Other specific dietary elements, including vitamin C, B vitamins, and various phytochemicals from fruits and vegetables, have just begun to draw attention regarding their potential protective effects on bone. The exact roles of these substances require much further exploration before their specific benefits can be confirmed (Tucker, 2009). However, experts tend to agree that: (a) a balanced diet emphasizing high intake of fruits and vegetables and adequate levels of calcium and protein from low-fat dairy products and lean meats is important and (b) healthy diversity in the diet interacts in pivotal ways with calcium and vitamin D supplementation to confer the greatest benefits on long-term bone health (Tucker, 2009; Tylavsky et al., 2008). Though not yet fully illuminated, "the effects of nutrition on the skeleton are powerful and wide-ranging" (Lanham-New, 2008, p. 173).

Exercise

Exercise may act alone or interact with nutritional factors to help maximize bone density and strength. Growing bones, before pubertal maturation, are most responsive to "mechanical loading" through exercise (Bonjour et al., 2009). Analysis of several studies related to osteoporosis prevention and exercise suggested that programs incorporating regular weight-bearing exercises can result in 1% to 8% improvements in bone strength at loaded skeletal sites for children and improvements of 0.5% to 2.5% among postmenopausal women with high exercise compliance (Nikander et al., 2010). Overall gains are significant in children but not adults. This does not negate, however, the protective effects exercise can have against loss of bone in adulthood or the significance of exercise-induced improvements in mobility, muscle strength, and balance that can minimize falls and increase quality of life for osteoporosis patients (Bonura, 2009; Dontas & Yiannakopoulos, 2007).

Evaluating the effectiveness of exercise programs for osteoporosis prevention and management is challenging owing to the heterogeneous nature of prescribed exercise regimens, varied lengths of interventions, and variety of study target groups (Grossman, 2011). Although an ideal exercise plan for use across the life course has not been clearly defined, the most effective exercise interventions with children incorporate a combination of moderate- to high-impact weight-bearing activities that are variable/multidirectional in nature and applied rapidly (e.g., skipping, dancing, jumping, hopping) (Nikander et al., 2010). For middle-aged to older adults, optimal exercise approaches are less definitive, but there is general consensus that low- to moderate-impact weight-bearing exercises in combination with progressive resistance and agility training are probably the most effective for improving BMD and preventing bone loss (Nikander et al., 2010). Exercise programs for individual osteoporosis patients must, of course, be tailored to multifactorial risk assessments by physicians with the goal of maximizing benefits and minimizing vulnerability to falls (Dontas & Yiannakopoulos, 2007). It is also important to note that excessive exercise in any life phase, especially for persons with restricted diets or low body weight, can impair the acquisition and maintenance of bone mass through a combination of hormonal and nutritional deficiencies, creating higher risk for osteoporosis (Bonjour et al., 2009). Professional female dancers, for example, have exhibited high risk for low bone density and early onset of osteoporosis (Hoch et al., 2011).

Lifestyle

Just as poor nutritional and activity practices can increase osteoporosis risk, there are specific, negative lifestyle choices that can interfere with healthy bone development and maintenance of BMD over the life course. For example, studies have found lower bone density among adolescents, females, and postmenopausal women who smoke as compared with nonsmokers in these groups (Bonura, 2009). Meta-analyses by several scholars have also suggested that there is an increased risk of hip fracture among smokers (Grossman, 2011).

Heavy consumption of alcohol (three or more drinks per day) has also been linked to low bone density and increased risk for both falls and fracture (Bonura, 2009; Stránský & Ryšavá, 2009). However, several studies in recent years have indicated that moderate alcohol intake may have a positive effect on BMD (Grossman, 2011; Tucker, 2009). This positive effect appears to be strongest among postmenopausal women and results more from consumption of wine or beer than distilled spirits, but the mechanisms of protection or optimal levels of alcohol intake are not yet clear (Tucker, 2009). Current clinical recommendations are to limit alcohol consumption (Stone & Lyles, 2006) and place knowledge of alcohol's potential protective effects within the context of "well-known harmful effects, including increased risk for falls and greater risk for breast cancer" (Tucker, 2009, p. 115).

An inverse relationship has also been established between consumption of carbonated soft drinks and BMD. In particular, the presence of phosphoric acid in colas has raised concern since it is known to bind with calcium in the body and possibly reduce calcium absorption (Tucker, 2009). In studies of children, lower BMD among soft drink consumers has generally been attributed to displacement of milk in the diet and has been associated with consumption of all types of sodas. Among adult women, those consuming cola daily have exhibited a BMD 4% to 5% lower than women avoiding soft drinks or consuming noncola sodas (Tucker, 2009). In sync with clinical recommendations for a balanced, nutrient-rich diet, limiting consumption of soft drinks and other nutrient-poor drinks or foods may be a prudent component of osteoporosis prevention.

CONTINUED PREVENTION IN ADULTHOOD AND INJURY REDUCTION

PBM is maintained until approximately age 28 to 30 years, at which time age-related bone loss may begin (Lanham-New, 2008; Stránský & Ryšavá, 2009). Throughout middle and late adulthood, therefore, continued healthy choices with respect to lifestyle, diet, and exercise are paramount to maintenance of skeletal integrity (Stone & Lyles, 2006). Bone is a living tissue, and even after PBM is reached in early life, there is a continuous cycle—a turnover process called bone remodeling—through which the body maintains bone density (Lanham-New, 2008; Stone & Lyles, 2006). Because this process requires adequate input of the crucial nutrients for bone health, the NOF (2011b) has higher recommendations for calcium and vitamin D intake after age 50 when bone loss is accelerated (1,200 mg calcium and 800 to 1,000 international units of vitamin D daily). Unfortunately, many older adults do not consume adequate levels of calcium or vitamin D (Stone & Lyles, 2006). The average postmenopausal diet provides only about half of the recommended levels of calcium per day (Bonura, 2009). Older adults living in care facilities and those with low body weight seem to benefit the most from additional calcium and vitamin D supplementation (Stránský & Ryšavá, 2009).

Falls and Fractures

More than one third of US adults aged 65 and older fall each year, and 20% to 30% of these accidents result in moderate-to-severe injuries. Between 90% and 95% of hip fractures—the injuries with the most detrimental impact on osteoporosis patients—result from falls (Dontas & Yiannakopoulos, 2007). Fall and related fracture avoidance is therefore a critical component of tertiary osteoporosis prevention.

Many of the same risk factors for osteoporosis contribute to increased fracture risk due to weakening of bones or increased susceptibility to falls. Basic preventative measures such as regular physical activity, adequate nutrient intake, cessation of smoking, and reduction of alcohol consumption, therefore, remain important components of injury prevention measures. There are a myriad of issues, however, that can influence the various types of falls and resultant injuries, and there are age-related trends that are important to consider (Dontas & Yiannakopoulos, 2007). Falls in older adults are typically low velocity with impact to the hip area, whereas middle-aged adults are more prone to high-velocity falls with the point of impact on the arms, specifically the humerus and distal forearm (Dennison et al., 2005). According to Dontas and Yiannakopoulos (2007, p. 271), there are an extensive range of personal risk factors for falls that should be part of patient assessment for fall and fracture vulnerability. These include: (a) previous falls, (b) lack of physical activity, (c) muscle weakness, (d) gait and balance problems, (e) neuromuscular diseases, (f) disability of the lower extremities, (g) inadequate footwear, (h) functional limitations regarding ADLs, (i) proprioceptive impairment, (j) dizziness, (k) fainting or loss of consciousness, (l) cardiovascular conditions (e.g., arrhythmia, hypertension), (m) visual problems, (n) urinary incontinence, (o) cognitive impairment, and (p) use of certain medications (e.g., antidepressants, sedatives). Other researchers also draw attention to the key roles of exercise and maintenance of good vision and hearing in fall prevention, as well as regular physician review of patient medication regimens to avoid unnecessary use of medications (i.e., those prescribed for hypertension and anxiety) that are known to increase risk of falls (Bonura, 2009; Stone & Lyles, 2006).

Environmental factors are also a central component of fall prevention. Home and residential environments should regularly be inspected for any tripping hazards, such as "throw rugs, slippery surfaces, and dimly lit corridors" (Stone & Lyles, 2006, p. 66). Additionally, environmental assessment should take into account lack of stair railings or bath mats and bars (Dontas & Yiannakopoulos, 2007). The most significant risk factor for fracture is a previous osteoporosis-related fracture (Stone & Lyles, 2006). Simply monitoring and screening (e.g., with yearly risk assessment questions, BMD measurements, FRAX use) individuals at most risk for the disease or with an existing osteoporosis diagnosis can, therefore, have a dramatic impact on the reduction of fractures (Bonura, 2009; Stone & Lyles, 2006).

PATIENT EDUCATION

The information and interpersonal exchanges that characterize disease prevention and management are shaped by overarching physician and health care system philosophies of care. Experts in the United States and many other countries (e.g., Denmark, United Kingdom, Australia), as well the World Health Organization, have embraced patient-centered care (PCC) as a critical component of effective medical response to complex chronic conditions such as osteoporosis (Davis et al., 2005; WHO, 2002), which are "long term, variable, and often degenerative" (Jordan et al., 2008, p. S9).

The WHO, in a report entitled *Innovative Care for Chronic Conditions* (2002, p. 46), described patients and their families as "the most undervalued assets in the healthcare system," and presented a framework for innovative care elevating the role of patients and their families to one of "partners" with communities and health care providers. Although definitions of PCC often differ across sources, frequently identified dimensions of PCC (Davis et al., 2005; Hudon et al., 2011; van Mossel et al., 2011) include:

- Acknowledgment of both the disease and illness experience
- Respect for the patient's values, preferences, and expressed needs
- Treating the whole person (biopsychosocial perspective)
- Emotional support to relieve fear and anxiety
- Incorporation of prevention and health promotion
- Information sharing and education
- Enhancing the patient–doctor relationship (sharing power and responsibility)
- Access to care
- Involvement of family and friends
- Continuity and secure transition between health care settings
- Physical comfort
- Coordination of care

Although PCC has emerged as a core value of US family medical practice, the implementation of PCC guiding principles has proven very challenging (Davis et al. 2005; Hudon et al., 2011; van Mossel et al., 2011). It is not entirely clear what a successful partnership between patient and provider looks like, or how shared decision-making is fully realized.

A recent review of patient-focused post-fracture osteoporosis interventions indicated that these PCC principles, if fully embraced, might operate to greatly strengthen osteoporosis response. Osteoporosis interventions with any potential to generate behavior changes in patients need to consider the patient's perception of "factors such as susceptibility, self-efficacy, subjective norm, barriers to and benefits of behavior change" (Sujic et al., 2011, p. 2217). To date, osteoporosis interventions have lacked grounding in behavior change theories (e.g., Health Belief Model, Social Cognitive Theory, Stages of Change Model). Implementing interventions informed and refined on the basis of tested theories of behavior change can help ensure that patients are fully engaged in their treatment rather than being passive recipients of information from health care providers (Sujic et al., 2011).

International initiatives targeting osteoporosis and incorporating concepts of PCC also recognize the complexity of these ideals, and that systemic change has to proceed before improved patient care can occur. Researchers and practitioners trying to optimize chronic disease self-management in Australia, for example, suggest that health care systems must improve "self-management support" for patients. They assert that osteoporosis and other chronic conditions require a high level of patient self-management that demands expanded resources and efforts to enable patients to improve management of their own health (Jordan et al., 2008). These health and social service systemic supports might include education programs, physical aids and devices, support groups, counseling, awareness and promotion campaigns, and efforts to keep physicians well informed about both disease management advances and the community resources available to patients. Supports can potentially be delivered in individual or group settings, through a variety of mediums such as face-to-face consultation, telephone contact, Internet sites, group-based courses, written handouts, or TV and multimedia sources (Jordan et al., 2008).

Similarly, the Ontario Osteoporosis Strategy exemplifies a broad, integrated approach to improving osteoporosis care through five main components: (1) health promotion through a wide range of media, (2) improved BMD testing, access, and quality, (3) improved postfracture care and secondary fracture prevention, (4) professional education to improve health providers' utilization of clinical practice guidelines, and (5) a research and evaluation work group to evaluate the impact of the strategy on osteoporosis prevention and treatment in Ontario (Jaglal et al., 2010). Components of this population-based strategy hold great potential for applicability in other countries and smaller communities around the world, "with the caveat that it would need to be tailored to the unique needs of each jurisdiction and health care system" (Jaglal et al., 2010, p. 908).

Taken together, the insights from PCC efforts in the United States and early indications of success from population-based osteoporosis interventions in other countries suggest that the most successful osteoporosis initiatives should attempt to simultaneously embrace the micro-level nuances of PCC (e.g., improved patient–physician communication, inclusion of family and friends) and initiate macro-level changes (e.g., coordination of patient and physician education programs for mutual reinforcement, fostering confidence among health professionals regarding effectiveness and sustainability of community education services). Micro- and macro-level changes in osteoporosis care that are synchronized, systematic, and grounded firmly in behavior change theory seem to have the most potential for bringing the patient-centered approach to full fruition (Jaglal et al., 2010; Jordan et al., 2008; Sujic et al., 2011).

Support Groups

Various efforts to improve osteoporosis knowledge and adherence to osteoporosis treatment have met with mixed results, with few interventions proving to have a marked impact on long-term behavior change among patients (Gleeson et al., 2009; Jaglal et al., 2009; Nielsen et al., 2010). There is evidence, however, that follow-up interactions between patients and providers can be beneficial (Gleeson et al., 2009) and that osteoporosis support groups might be an important aspect of self-management support that can enhance patient experiences and outcomes (Jordan et al., 2008). Those who participate in support groups tend to be happier and cope better with the challenges of managing chronic conditions such as osteoporosis (Vann & Jones, 2012). According to the NOF (2011c), the movement toward more PCC means that many patients today take more responsibility for their care and seek out avenues of information and support to help them cope with disease.

Support groups available in communities nationwide through the NOF network "provide a way to learn more about osteoporosis while providing an opportunity to share information, feelings, and goals with others in a similar situation." Benefits of support group participation include: (a) learning more about the disease and treatment choices; (b) receiving free brochures and educational materials; (c) feeling a sense of caring and understanding; (d) not feeling alone in dealing with osteoporosis; (e) improving coping skills by learning how others handle the disease; (f) exchanging information about community resources, including health care providers who treat osteoporosis; (g) improving mental and physical well-being; and (h) finding hope and encouragement (NOF, 2011c). To find out about the nearest NOF-sponsored support group, individuals can complete an online request for information form at http://nof.org/connect/community-groups/support-groups.

For persons who do not live near an active NOF support group, NOF's online health community helps people connect with others who have osteoporosis. This online health community includes blogs, individual Web pages, discussions, message boards, and more. One of the ways members can expand their social network within the community is through a personal profile, so that the NOF can link health community members by gender, the topics in which they are interested, and where they live. This helps people more easily find and connect with others in similar situations (NOF, 2011c).

EDUCATION RESOURCES

A wide variety of valuable resources is available to support individual and systemic improvements in osteoporosis prevention and response. Osteoporosis research implications and practice innovations include:

- **OsteoEd** (http://depts.washington.edu/osteoed): An educational Web site from the University of Washington School of Medicine that provides evidence-based information for students, residents, and primary care providers on the prevention, diagnosis, and treatment of osteoporosis. The site offers a combination of: (a) *case-based learning* to strengthen professional knowledge of prevention measures, screening and evaluation techniques, drug therapy, secondary causes of osteoporosis, and male osteoporosis; (b) answers to *common questions* related to osteoporosis prevention and treatment; and (c) detailed descriptions of *clinical calculators and guidelines* for use in osteoporosis risk assessment and identification.

- **FORE:** The Foundation for Osteoporosis Research and Education (http://www.fore.org)—provides updated information to various stakeholders in osteoporosis care, with different sections of the organization's Web site dedicated to patients, family and friends, health care providers, and scholars. The foundation describes itself as a "non-profit resource center dedicated to preventing osteoporosis through research and education of the public and medical community to increase awareness of risk, detection, prevention, and treatment." Most FORE resources are available nationwide through the organization's Web site, though certain educational events, certification courses for health professionals, and a speakers bureau are available only in the Bay Area near the foundation main office in Oakland, California.

- **Healthy Bones, Build Them for Life Webinar Series** (http://www.nof.org/aboutosteoporosis/moreresources/consumer-webinar-series): A series of free, educational webinars developed by the NOF that allows viewers (patients and physicians alike) access to seminars from the nation's leading bone health experts. Example modules include *Balancing the Benefits and Risks of Osteoporosis Treatment, Update on Osteoporosis Treatment Options,* and *Exercise for Your Bone Health.*

- **United States Department of Agriculture (USDA) National Agricultural Library** has compiled a number of resources about osteoporosis, accessible through their Web site (http://fnic.nal.usda.gov/nal_display/index.php?info_center=4&tax_level=2&tax_subject=278&topic_id=1385). Available information includes osteoporosis fast facts, a report of the Surgeon General on bone health and osteoporosis, descriptions of well-established Extension and Mayo Clinic initiatives for better bone health, and connections to various national and international sites, associations, and foundations offering osteoporosis prevention and care resources.

- **Osteoporosis Canada** (http://www.osteoporosis.ca): It is the only national organization in Canada serving people who have, or are at risk for, osteoporosis. The organization works to educate, empower, and support individuals and communities in the risk reduction and treatment of osteoporosis by providing medically accurate information to patients, health care professionals, and the public. Services include free publications, a bilingual toll-free information line, educational programs, and referrals to self-help groups and community resources, as well as their Web site. They offer a wide range of fact sheets, booklets, and newsletters that can be downloaded for free via the Internet.

As is evident from these examples, there are many starting points that persons with osteoporosis, as well as professionals, can turn to for resources and support to enhance osteoporosis prevention and response. How to optimize uptake of information for lasting behavior change among osteoporosis patients, however, remains an ongoing challenge (Sujic et al., 2011; van Mossel et al., 2011).

REFERENCES

Amgen, Inc. (2010). *Xgeva™ highlights of prescribing medication.* Retrieved from http://pi.amgen.com/united_states/xgeva/xgeva_pi.pdf

Amgen, Inc. (2011). *Prolia® highlights of prescribing information.* Retrieved from http://pi.amgen.com/united_states/prolia/prolia_pi.pdf

Avioli, L. V. (Ed.). (2000). *The osteoporotic syndrome: Detection, prevention and treatment* (4th ed.). San Diego, CA: Academic Press.

Baird, J., et al. (2011). Does birthweight predict bone mass in adulthood? A systematic review and meta-analysis. *Osteoporosis International, 22*(5), 1323–1334.

Baroutsou, B., et al. (2004). Patient compliance and preference of alendronate once weekly administration in comparison with daily regimens for osteoporotic postmenopausal women. *Annals of the Rheumatic Diseases, 63*(1), 455.

Becker, D., Kilgore, M., & Morrisey, M. (2010). The societal burden of osteoporosis. *Current Rheumatology Reports, 12*(3), 186–191.

Black, D. M., et al. (2010). Bisphosphonates and fractures of the subtrochanteric or diaphyseal femur. *New England Journal of Medicine, 362*(19), 1761–1771.

Bolton-Smith, C., et al. (2007). Two-year randomized controlled trial of vitamin K1 (phylloquinone) and vitamin D3 plus calcium on the bone health of older women. *Journal of Bone and Mineral Research, 22*(4), 509–519.

Bonjour, J. P., Chevalley, T., Ferrari, S., & Rizzoli, R. (2009). The importance and relevance of peak bone mass in the prevalence of osteoporosis. *Salud Pública de México, 51*(1), S5–S17.

Bonura, F. (2009). Prevention, screening, and management of osteoporosis: An overview of the current strategies. *Postgraduate Medicine, 121*(4), 5–17.

Boonen, S., et al. (2011). Balloon kyphoplasty and vertebroplasty in the management of vertebral compression fractures. *Osteoporosis International, 22*(12), 2915–2934.

Burge, R., et al. (2007). Incidence and economic burden of osteoporosis-related fractures in the United States, 2005–2025. *Journal of Bone and Mineral Research, 22*(3), 465–475.

Cauley, J. A., et al. (2001). Risk of mortality following clinical fractures. *Osteoporosis International, 11*(7), 556–561.

Chestnut, C. H., & Azria, M. (2010). Salmon calcitonin: An update on its clinical utility in osteoporosis. *Contemporary Endocrinology*, 423–441.

Clowes, J. A., Peel, N. F., & Eastell, R. (2004). The impact of monitoring on adherence and persistence with antiresorptive treatment for postmenopausal osteoporosis: A Randomized Controlled trial. *Journal of Clinical Endocrinology & Metabolism, 89*(3), 1117–1123.

Compston, J. (2003, May). *Do we need to monitor anti-osteoporosis treatment anyway?* Paper presented at the 30th European Symposium on Calcified Tissues, Rome, Italy.

Cooper, C., et al. (2006). Review: Developmental origins of osteoporotic fracture. *Osteoporosis International, 17*(3), 337–347.

Cooper, C., Harvey, N., Cole, Z., Hanson, M., & Dennison, E. (2009). Developmental origins of osteoporosis: The role of maternal nutrition. In K. Berthold et al. (Eds.), *Early nutrition programming and health outcomes in later life* (Advances in experimental medicine and biology, *Vol. 646*, pp. 31–39). Netherlands: Springer.

Cramer, J. A., Amonkar, M. M., Hebborn, A., & Altman, R. (2005). Compliance and persistence with bisphosphonate dosing regimens among women with postmenopausal osteoporosis. *Current Medical Research and Opinion, 21*(9), 1453–1460.

Cremers, S., & Papapoulos, S. (2011). The pharmacology of bisphosphonates. *Bone, 49*(1), 42–49.

Cummings, S. R., & Melton, L. J., Jr. (2002). Epidemiology and outcomes of osteoporotic fractures. *Lancet, 359*(9319), 1761–1767.

Curtis, J., et al. (2009). Population-based fracture risk assessment and osteoporosis treatment disparities by race and gender. *Journal of General Internal Medicine, 24*(8), 956–962.

Curtis, J. R., et al. (2012). Adherence with intravenous zoledronate and intravenous ibandronate in the United States Medicare population. *Arthritis Care & Research, 65*(7), 1054–1060.

Dagenais, P., Vanasse, A., Courteau, J., Orzanco, M. G., & Asghari, S. (2010). Disparities between rural and urban areas for osteoporosis management in the province of Quebec following the Canadian 2002 guidelines publication. *Journal of Evaluation in Clinical Practice, 16*(3), 438–444.

Davis, K., Schoenbaum, S., & Audet, A. M. (2005). A 2020 vision of patient-centered primary care. *Journal of General Internal Medicine, 20*(10), 953–957.

Dennison, E., Cole, Z., & Cooper, C. (2005). Diagnosis and epidemiology of osteoporosis. *Current Opinion in Rheumatology, 17*(4), 456–461.

Dontas, I. A., & Yiannakopoulos, C. K. (2007). Risk factors and prevention of osteoporosis-related fractures. *Journal of Musculoskeletal & Neuronal Interactions, 7*(3), 268.

Duncan, E. L., & Brown, M. A. (2010). Genetic determinants of bone density and fracture risk—State of the art and future directions. *Journal of Clinical Endocrinology & Metabolism, 95*(6), 2576–2587.

Dy, C., LaMont, L. E., Ton, Q. V., & Lane, J. M. (2011). Sex and gender considerations in male patients with osteoporosis. *Clinical Orthopaedics and Related Research, 469*(7), 1906–1912.

Eberhardt, M. S., & Pamuk, E. R. (2004). The importance of place of residence: Examining health in rural and nonrural areas. *Rural Health and Health Care Disparities, 94*(10), 1682–1686.

Eekman, D. A., et al. (2009). Treatment with intravenous pamidronate is a good alternative in case of gastrointestinal side effects or contraindications for oral bisphosphonates. *BMC Musculoskeletal Disorders, 10*(86), 1–5.

Eli Lilly and Company. (2011). *Evista® highlights of prescribing information.* Retrieved from http://pi.lilly.com/us/evista-pi.pdf

Eli Lilly and Company. (2012). *Forteo® highlights of prescribing information.* Retrieved from http://pi.lilly.com/us/forteo-pi.pdf

Emkey, R., et al. (2005). Patient preference for once-monthly ibandronate versus once-weekly alendronate in a randomized, open-label, cross-over trial: The Boniva Alendronate Trial in Osteoporosis (BALTO). *Current Medical Research & Opinion, 21*(12), 1895–1903.

Erichsen, R., Christiansen, C. F., Frøslev, T., Jacobsen, J., & Sørensen, H. J. (2011). Intravenous bisphosphonate therapy and atrial fibrillation/flutter risk in cancer patients: A Nationwide Cohort study. *British Journal of Cancer, 105*(7), 881–883.

Ettinger, B., Black, D. M., Dawson-Hughes, B., Pressman, A. R., & Melton, L. J. (2010). Updated fracture incidence rates for the US version of Frax®. *Osteoporosis International, 21*(1), 25–33.

Ettinger, M. P., Gallagher, R., & MacCosbe, P. E. (2006). Medication persistence with weekly versus daily doses of orally administered bisphosphonates. *Endocrine Practice, 12*(5), 522–528.

Forster-Burke, D., Ritter, L., & Zimmer, S. (2010). Collaboration of a model osteoporosis prevention and management program in a faith community. *Journal of Obstetric, Gynecologic, & Neonatal Nursing, 39*(2), 212–219.

Foundation for Osteoporosis Research and Education. (2011). Retrieved from http://www.fore.org/

Gamm, L., Hutchison, L., Bellamy, G., & Dabney, B. J. (2002). Rural healthy people 2010: Identifying rural health priorities and models for practice. *Journal of Rural Health, 18*(1), 9–14.

Genentech USA, Inc. (2011a). *Boniva® (ibandronate sodium) injection.* Retrieved from http://www.gene.com/gene/products/information/boniva/pdf/pi.pdf

Genentech USA, Inc. (2011b). *Boniva® tablets highlights of prescribing information.* Retrieved from http://www.gene.com/gene/products/information/boniva/pdf/boniva_prescribing_tablets.pdf

Gleeson, T., et al. (2009). Interventions to improve adherence and persistence with osteoporosis medications: A systematic literature review. *Osteoporosis International, 20*(12), 2127–2134.

Gold, D. T. (2003). Osteoporosis and quality of life psychosocial outcomes and interventions for individual patients. *Clinics in Geriatric Medicine, 19*(2), 271–280.

Gold, D. T., et al. (2007). A claims database analysis of persistence with alendronate therapy and fracture risk in postmenopausal women with osteoporosis. *Current Medical Research & Opinion, 23*(3), 585–594.

Gold, D. T., et al. (2011). Factors associated with persistence with teriparatide therapy: Results from the DANCE Observational study. *Journal of Osteoporosis, 2011*, 314970. doi:10.4061/2011/314970

Gold, D. T., Safi, W., & Trinh, H. (2006). Patient preference and adherence: Comparative US studies between two bisphosphonates, weekly risedronate and monthly ibandronate. *Current Medical Research & Opinion, 22*(12), 2383–2391.

Gold, D. T., & Solimeo, S. (2006). Osteoporosis and depression: A historical perspective. *Current Osteoporosis Reports, 4*(4), 134–139.

Grossman, J. M. (2011). Osteoporosis prevention. *Current Opinion in Rheumatology, 23*(2), 203–210.

Hadji, P., et al. (2008). Treatment preference for monthly oral ibandronate and weekly oral alendronate in women with postmenopausal osteoporosis: A Randomized, Crossover study (BALTO II). *Joint, Bone, Spine: Revue du Rhumatisme, 75*(3), 303–310.

Hjalmarson, H. V., Strandmark, M., & Klässbo, M. (2007). Healthy risk awareness motivates fracture prevention behaviour: A Grounded Theory study of women with osteoporosis. *International Journal of Qualitative Studies on Health and Well-Being, 2*(4), 236–245.

Hoch, A. Z., et al. (2011). Association between the female athlete triad and endothelial dysfunction in dancers. *Clinical Journal of Sport Medicine, 21*(2), 119–125.

Hudon, C., et al. (2011). Measuring patients' perceptions of patient-centered care: A systematic review of tools for family medicine. *Annals of Family Medicine, 9*(2), 155–164.

Hulme, P. A. (2010). Cultural considerations in evidence-based practice. *Journal of Transcultural Nursing, 21*(3), 271–280.

Jaglal, S. B., et al (2009). A demonstration project of a multi-component educational intervention to improve integrated post-fracture osteoporosis care in five rural communities in Ontario, Canada. *Osteoporosis International, 20*(2), 265–274.

Jaglal, S. B., et al. (2010). The Ontario osteoporosis strategy: Implementation of a population-based osteoporosis action plan in Canada. *Osteoporosis International, 21*(6), 903–908.

Javaid, M. K., et al. (2006). Maternal vitamin D status during pregnancy and childhood bone mass at age 9 years: A Longitudinal study. *Lancet, 367*(9504), 36–43.

Jones, C. A., Parker, T. S., Ahearn, M., Mishra, A. K., & Variyam, J. N. (2009, August). *Health status and health care access of farm and rural populations.* Retrieved from http://www.ers.usda.gov/ersDownloadHandler.ashx?file=/media/155453/eib57_1_.pdf

Jordan, J. E., Briggs, A. M., Brand, C. A., & Osborne, R. H. (2008). Enhancing patient engagement in chronic disease self-management support initiatives in Australia: The need for an integrated approach. *Medical Journal of Australia, 189*(Suppl. 10), S9–S13.

Kanis, J. A., et al. (2004a). A meta-analysis of previous fracture and subsequent fracture risk. *Bone, 35*(2), 375–382.

Kanis, J. A., et al. (2004b). A meta-analysis of prior corticosteroid use and fracture risk. *Journal of Bone and Mineral Research, 19*(6), 893–899.

Kanis, J. A., et al. (2011). Task force of the FRAX initiative. Interpretation and use of FRAX in clinical practice. *Osteoporosis International, 22*(9), 2395–2411.

Katz, J. N. (2001). Patient preferences and health disparities. *JAMA: The Journal of the American Medical Association, 286*(12), 1506–1509.

Keen, R., et al. (2006). European women's preference for osteoporosis treatment: Influence of clinical effectiveness and dosing frequency. *Current Medical Research & Opinion, 22*(12) 2375–2381.

Kendler, D., et al. (2004). Patients with osteoporosis prefer once weekly to once daily dosing with alendronate. *Maturitas, 48*(3), 243–251.

Khosla, S., Amin, S., & Orwoll, E. (2008). Osteoporosis in men. *Endocrine Reviews, 29*(4), 441–464.

Kothawala, P., Badamgarav, E., Ryu, S., Miller, R. M., & Halbert, R. J. (2007). Systematic review and meta-analysis of real-world adherence to drug therapy for osteoporosis. *Mayo Clinic Proceedings, 82*(12), 1493–1501.

Lanham-New, S. A. (2008). Importance of calcium, vitamin D and vitamin K for osteoporosis prevention and treatment. *Proceedings of the Nutrition Society, 67*(2), 163.

LeBlanc, E. S., et al. (2011). Hip fracture and increased short-term but not long-term mortality in healthy older women. *Archives of Internal Medicine, 171*(20), 1831–1837.

Leung, P.-C., Cheng, K.-F., & Chan, Y.-H. (2011). An innovative herbal product for the prevention of osteoporosis. *Chinese Journal of Integrative Medicine, 17*(10), 744–749.

Lindsay, R., et al. (2001). Risk of new vertebral fracture in the year following a fracture. *JAMA: The Journal of the American Medical Association, 285*(3), 320–323.

Looker, A., et al. (2009). Age, gender, and race/ethnic differences in total body and subregional bone density. *Osteoporosis International, 20*(7), 1141–1149.

Looker, A. C., Flegal, K. M., & Melton, L. J. (2007). Impact of increased overweight on the projected prevalence of osteoporosis in older women. *Osteoporosis International, 18*(3), 307–313.

Lorentzon, M., Eriksson, A. L., Nilsson, S., Mellström, D., & Ohlsson, C. (2007). Association between physical activity and BMD in young men is modulated by catechol-O-methyltransferase (COMT) genotype: The Good study. *Journal of Bone and Mineral Research, 22*(8), 1165–1172.

MacLean, C. H., et al. (2004). *Effects of omega-3 fatty acids on lipids and glycemic control in type II diabetes and the metabolic syndrome and on inflammatory bowel disease, rheumatoid arthritis, renal disease, systemic lupus erythematosus, and osteoporosis* (Evidence Report/Technology Assessment No. 89. Prepared by Southern California/RAND Evidence-based Practice Center, under Contract No. 290-02-0003. AHRQ Publication No. 04-E012-2). Rockville, MD: Agency for Healthcare Research and Quality.

Marks, R. (2010). Hip fracture epidemiological trends, outcomes, and risk factors, 1970–2009. *International Journal of General Medicine, 8*, 1–7.

Melton, L. J., & Marquez, M. A. (2008). Opportunities in population-specific osteoporosis research and management. *Osteoporosis International, 19*(12), 1679–1681.

Merck and Co., Inc. (2012). *Fosamax® highlights of prescribing information.* Retrieved from http://www.merck.com/product/usa/pi_circulars/f/fosamax/fosamax_pi.pdf

Miller, P. D., et al. (2006). Rational, objectives and design of the Direct Analysis of Nonvertebral Fracture in the Community Experience (DANCE) study. *Osteoporosis International, 17*(1), 85–90.

Misra, D., et al. (2011). Does dietary protein reduce hip fracture risk in elders? The Framingham Osteoporosis study. *Osteoporosis International, 22*(1), 345–349.

Morgan, M. J. (2007). Maintaining independence and quality of life. In S. H. Gueldner et al. (Eds.), *Osteoporosis: Clinical guidelines for prevention, diagnosis and management* (pp. 153–165). New York, NY: Springer.

National Osteoporosis Foundation. (2011a). Fast Facts 2011. Retrieved from http://www.nof.org/node/40

National Osteoporosis Foundation. (2011b). Calcium: What you should know. Retrieved from http://www.nof.org/aboutosteoporosis/prevention/calcium

National Osteoporosis Foundation. (2011c). Community groups. Retrieved from http://www.nof.org/node/57

Nayak, S., Roberts, M. S., Chang, C. C., & Greenspan, S. L. (2010). Health beliefs about osteoporosis and osteoporosis screening in older women and men. *Health Education Journal, 69*(3), 267–276.

Neer, R. M., et al. (2001). Effect of parathyroid hormone (1–34) on fractures and bone mineral density in postmenopausal women with osteoporosis. *New England Journal of Medicine, 344*(19), 1434–1441.

Neuman, M. D., Kennelly, A. M., & Tosi, L. L. (2011). Breakout session: Sex/gender and racial/ethnic disparities in the care of osteoporosis and fragility fractures. *Clinical Orthopaedics and Related Research, 469*(7), 1936–1940.

Nielsen, D., et al. (2010). Patient education in groups increases knowledge of osteoporosis and adherence to treatment: A Two-Year Randomized Controlled trial. *Patient Education and Counseling, 81*(2), 155–160.

Nikander, R., et al. (2010). Targeted exercise against osteoporosis: A systematic review and meta-analysis for optimising bone strength throughout life. *BMC Medicine, 8*(1), 47.

Novartis. (2009). *Miacalcin®*. Retrieved from http://www.pharma.us.novartis.com/product/pi/pdf/miacalcin_injection.pdf

Novartis. (2011a). *Miacalcin® (calcitonin-salmon) nasal spray*. Retrieved from http://www.pharma.us.novartis.com/product/pi/pdf/miacalcin_nasal.pdf

Novartis. (2011b). *Reclast® highlights of prescribing information*. Retrieved from http://www.pharma.us.novartis.com/product/pi/pdf/reclast.pdf

OsteoEd. (2012). Osteoed: Osteoporosis Education. M. Laya & H. Powell (Eds.). Retrieved from http://depts.washington.edu/osteoed

Osteoporosis Canada. (2011). Retrieved from http://www.osteoporosis.ca/

Papaioannou, A., Kennedy, C. C., Dolovich, L., Lau, E., & Adachi, J. D. (2007). Patient adherence to osteoporosis medications: Problems, consequences and management strategies. *Drugs Aging, 24*(1), 37–55.

Papaioannou, A., et al. (2009). The impact of incident fractures on health-related quality of life: 5 years of data from the Canadian Multicentre Osteoporosis study. *Osteoporosis International, 20*(5), 703–714.

Piehowski, K. E., Nickols-Richardson, S. M., Clymer, E. K., & Roberto, K. A. (2010). Osteoporosis health beliefs in women differ by menopausal status and across age cohorts. *Family and Consumer Sciences Research Journal, 38*(3), 345–355.

Putnam, S. E., et al. (2007). Natural products as alternative treatments for metabolic bone disorders and for maintenance of bone health. *Phytotherapy Research, 21*(2), 99–112.

Rabenda, V., et al. (2008). Adherence to bisphosphonates therapy and hip fracture risk in osteoporotic women. *Osteoporosis International, 19*(6), 811–818.

Randell, A. G., et al. (2000). Deterioration in quality of life following hip fracture: A Prospective study. *Osteoporosis International, 11*, 460–466.

Reginster, J. Y., et al. (2006). Efficacy and tolerability of once-monthly oral ibandronate in postmenopausal osteoporosis: 2 year results from the MOBILE study. *Annals of the Rheumatic Diseases, 65*(5), 654–661.

Reventlow, S., & Bang, H. (2006). Brittle bones: Ageing or threat of disease—Exploring women's cultural models of osteoporosis. *Scandinavian Journal of Public Health, 34*(3), 320–326.

Rhee, C. W., Lee, J., Oh, S., Choi, N. K., & Park, B. J. (2012). Use of bisphosphonate and risk of atrial fibrillation in older women with osteoporosis. *Osteoporosis International, 23*(1), 247–254.

Ringe, J. D. (2010). Development of clinical utility of zoledronic acid and patient considerations in the treatment of osteoporosis. *Patient Preference and Adherence, 4*, 231–245.

Roberto, K. A. (1992). The role of social support in older women's recovery from hip fractures. *Journal of Applied Gerontology, 11*(3), 314–325.

Roberto, K. A. (2004). Care practices and quality of life of rural old women with osteoporosis. *Journal of the American Medical Women's Association, 59*(4), 295–301.

Roberto, K. A., Gold, D. T., & Yorgason, J. (2004). The influence of osteoporosis on the marital relationship of older couples. *Journal of Applied Gerontology, 23*(4), 443–456.

Roberto, K. A., & Reynolds, S. G. (2001). The meaning of osteoporosis in the lives of rural older women. *Health Care for Women International, 22*(6), 599–611.

Rossouw, J. E., et al. (2002). Risks and benefits of estrogen plus progestin in healthy postmenopausal women: Principal results from the Women's Health Initiative Randomized Controlled trial. *Journal of the American Medical Association, 288*(3), 321–333.

Sambrook, P. N., Olver, I., & Goss, A. N. (2006). Bisphosphonates and osteonecrosis of the jaw. *Australian Family Physician, 35*(10), 801–803.

Shane, E., et al. (2010). Atypical subtrochanteric and diaphyseal femoral fractures: Report of a task force of the American Society for Bone and Mineral Research. *Journal of Bone Mineral Research, 25*(11), 2267–2294.

Shaw, S. J., Huebner, C., Armin, J., Orzech, K., & Vivian, J. (2009). The role of culture in health literacy and chronic disease screening and management. *Journal of Immigrant and Minority Health, 11*(6), 460–467.

Silverman, S. L., & Gold, D. T. (2008). Compliance and persistence with osteoporosis therapies. *Current Rheumatology Reports, 10*(2), 118–122.

Simon, J. A., et al. (2002). Patient preference for once-weekly alendronate 70 mg versus once-daily alendronate 10 mg: A Multicenter, Randomized, Open-Label, Crossover study. *Clinical Therapeutics, 24*(12), 1871–1886.

Siris, E. S., et al. (2006). Adherence to bisphosphonate therapy and fracture rates in osteoporotic women: Relationship to vertebral and nonvertebral fractures from 2 US claims databases. *Mayo Clinical Proceedings, 81*(8), 1013–1022.

Solimeo, S. L., Weber, T. J., & Gold, D. T. (2011). Older men's explanatory model for osteoporosis. *Gerontologist, 51*(4), 530–539.

Steel, S. A., Albertazzi, P., Howarth, E. M., & Purdie, D. W. (2003). Factors affecting long-term adherence to hormone replacement therapy after screening for osteoporosis. *Climacteric, 6*(2), 96–103.

Stevens, J. A. (2005). Falls among older adults - risk factors and prevention strategies. *Journal of Safety Research, 36*(4), 409–411.

Stone, L. M., & Lyles, K. W. (2006). Osteoporosis in later life. *Generations, 30*(3), 65–70.

Stránský, M., & Ryšavá, L. (2009). Nutrition as prevention and treatment of osteoporosis. *Physiological Research, 58*(Suppl. 1), S7.

Subbiah, V., Madsen, V. S., Raymond, A. K., Benjamin, R. S., & Ludwig, J. A. (2010). Of mice and men: Divergent risks of teriparatide-induced osteosarcoma. *Osteoporosis International, 21*(6), 1041–1045.

Sujic, R., Gignac, M. A., Cockerill, R., & Beaton, D. E. (2011). A review of patient-centred post-fracture interventions in the context of theories of health behaviour change. *Osteoporosis International, 22*(8), 2213–2224.

Tucker, K. L. (2009). Osteoporosis prevention and nutrition. *Current Osteoporosis Reports, 7*(4), 111–117.

Tylavsky, F. A., Spence, L. A., & Harkness, L. (2008). The importance of calcium, potassium, and acid-base homeostasis in bone health and osteoporosis prevention. *Journal of Nutrition, 138*(1), 164S–165S.

U.S. Department of Agriculture, National Agricultural Library. (2011). Diet and disease: Osteoporosis. Retrieved from http://fnic.nal.usda.gov/nal_display/index.php?info_center=4&tax_level=2&tax_subject=278&topic_id=1385

U.S. Department of Health and Human Services. (2004). *Bone health and osteoporosis: A report of the Surgeon General.* Washington, DC: Author. Retrieved from http://www.surgeongeneral.gov/library/reports/bonehealth/

Vahle, J. L., et al. (2004). Bone neoplasms in F344 rats given teriparatide [rhPTH(1-34)] are dependent on duration of treatment and dose. *Toxicologic Pathology, 32*(4), 426–438.

van Mossel, C., Alford, M., & Watson, H. (2011). Challenges of patient-centered care: Practice or rhetoric. *Nursing Inquiry, 18*(4), 278–289.

Vann, M., & Jones, N. (2012). *The benefits of joining Osteoporosis Support Groups.* Everyday Health. Retrieved from http://www.everydayhealth.com/osteoporosis/osteoporosis-support-groups.aspx

Warner Chilcott, LLC. (1998). *Actonel® highlights of prescribing information.* Retrieved from http://www.actonel.com/global/prescribing_information.pdf

Wetzsteon, R. J., et al. (2009). Ethnic differences in bone geometry and strength are apparent in childhood. *Bone, 44*(5), 970–975.

Williams, M. E. (1995). *American geriatric society's complete guide to aging and health.* New York, NY: Harmony.

World Health Organization. (1994). *Assessment of fracture risk and its application to screening for postmenopausal osteoporosis* (Technical Report Series). Geneva, Switzerland: Author.

World Health Organization. (2002). Innovations in care: Meeting the challenge of chronic conditions. In *Innovative care for chronic conditions* (Chap. 3). Geneva, Switzerland: World Health Organization.

Wyeth Pharmaceuticals, Inc. (2011). *Premarin®.* Retrieved from http://labeling.pfizer.com/showlabeling.aspx?id=131

Yood, R. A., et al. (2003). Compliance with pharmacologic therapy for osteoporosis. *Osteoporosis International, 14*(12), 965–968.

Yood, R. A., et al. (2008). Patient decision to initiate therapy for osteoporosis: The influence of knowledge and beliefs. *Journal of General Internal Medicine, 23*(11), 1815–1821.

CHAPTER 12: IT RESOURCES

Web sites

National Osteoporosis Foundation
http://www.nof.org/
Agency for Healthcare Research and Quality
http://www.ahrq.gov/
Osteoporosis Health Center: Spine-Health
http://www.spine-health.com/conditions/osteoporosis
Osteoporosis: Causes, Symptoms, Diagnosis, Treatment
http://www.emedicinehealth.com/osteoporosis/article_em.htm
Falls among Older Adults: An Overview
http://www.cdc.gov/HomeandRecreationalSafety/Falls/adultfalls.html/
Ontario Osteoporosis Strategy
http://www.osteostrategy.on.ca/
Osteoporosis Online Health Information
http://www.fletcherallen.org/services/orthopedic_care/specialties/osteoporosis/patient_resources/health_resources_links/health_resources_links.html
The NOF (National Osteoporosis Foundation) Web site provides a list of medications associated with increased risk of osteoporosis.
http://www.nof.org/aboutosteoporosis/detectingosteoporosis/medicineboneloss
The NOF Web site provides a list of osteoporosis-associated conditions and specific risk factors stemming from these conditions.
http://www.nof.org/node/233
The WHO (World Health Organization), under the leadership of Dr. John Kanis, developed FRAX, a screening tool that integrates analysis of clinical risk factors and measurement of bone mineral density to determine fracture risk.
http://www.shef.ac.uk/FRAX/
To find out about the nearest NOF-sponsored support group, individuals can complete an online request for information form at
http://nof.org/connect/community-groups/support-groups

Osteoporosis research implications and practice innovations include:

OsteoEd
http://depts.washington.edu/osteoed
FORE—The Foundation for Osteoporosis Research and Education
http://www.fore.org
Healthy Bones, Build Them for Life Webinar Series
http://www.nof.org/aboutosteoporosis/moreresources/consumer-webinar-series
United States Department of Agriculture (USDA) National Agricultural Library has compiled a number of resources about osteoporosis, accessible through their Web site:
http://fnic.nal.usda.gov/nal_display/index.
php?info_center=4&tax_level=2&tax_subject=278&topic_id=1385
Osteoporosis Canada
http://www.osteoporosis.ca

PDF Documents

Reducing the Risk of Bone Fracture: A Review of Research for Adults with Low Bone Density (2012) Agency for Healthcare Research and Quality Consumer Report
http://www.effectivehealthcare.ahrq.gov/ehc/products/160/1049/lbd_cons_fin_to_post.pdf

Government-approved Drugs for Postmenopausal Osteoporosis in the United States and Canada (2012)
http://www.menopause.org/otcharts.pdf

Osteoporosis in Men (2012)—National Institutes of Health
http://www.niams.nih.gov/Health_Info/Bone/Osteoporosis/men_osteoporosis.pdf

Videos

Postmenopausal Osteoporosis (2012) (2:55 minutes)
http://youtu.be/c5tc01WFYks

What is Osteoporosis? (2012) (2:49 minutes)
http://www.youtube.com/watch?v=LS_0fvI_uxY

Osteoporosis Risk Factors and Symptoms (2012) (3:22 minutes)
http://www.youtube.com/watch?v=eyzwBMH7hws

Osteoporosis Screening and Prevention (2012) (3:31 minutes)
http://www.youtube.com/watch?v=dT95P37jjhc

Treatment for Osteoporosis (2012) (3:17 minutes)
http://www.youtube.com/watch?v=9clDtErR4Y0

True Life Story: Osteoporosis (2012)

Every woman should consider the risk of developing osteoporosis later in life. Janet talks about the lifestyle habits that help keep her bone density at safe levels. (2:15 minutes)
http://www.youtube.com/watch?v=KDHUrbBHYNY

Images

Google images of Osteoporosis
http://www.google.com/search?q=osteoporosis&hl=en&qscrl=1&nord=1&rlz=1T4A DFA_enUS417US433&prmd=imvns&source=lnms&tbm=isch&sa=X&ei=ka4NUITfCo-x 0QG26MHmAw&ved=0CEgQ_AUoAQ&biw=960&bih=414

Google images of Osteopenia
http://www.google.com/search?q=osteopenia&hl=en&qscrl=1&nord=1&rlz=1T4ADFA_ enUS417US433&prmd=imvns&source=lnms&tbm=isch&sa=X&ei=768NUPqZBqbg0QG Fg8H6Aw&ved=0CEgQ_AUoAQ&biw=960&bih=414

Google images of Bone Mineral Density
http://www.google.com/search?q=bone+mineral+density&hl=en&qscrl=1&nord=1&rlz =1T4ADFA_enUS417US433&prmd=imvns&tbm=isch&tbo=u&source=univ&sa=X&ei= qqn1T5qBBKX50gHZ-pDRBg&ved=0CHgQsAQ&biw=960&bih=414

Arthritis, Gout, and Chronic Pain

Adegbenga A. Bankole, MD

Phyllis Brown Whitehead, PhD, APRN, ACHPN

INTRODUCTION

Rheumatism and arthritis are common names ascribed to aches and pains. Some of these aches and pains represent significant rheumatologic disease, but not all patients with joint symptoms need to be seen by a specialist. This chapter will help in understanding common rheumatologic problems and in determining when specialist help is needed. Care of patients involving specialists is more expensive when compared with that involving nonspecialist care. However, studies looking at specialty care showed that ambulatory care for osteoarthritis (OA) or low back pain was associated with improvement in functional status at slightly higher costs when compared with nonspecialty care.

As the population ages, rheumatology (rheuma: flows as a river or stream, logy: study of) becomes increasingly important as most of the rheumatologic diseases are lifelong. Once a noncurable rheumatologic disease has been diagnosed, the burden of that disease will be carried into later life. Rheumatologic illnesses are also very commonly diagnosed in older people, and one in five adults in the United States has reported being diagnosed with some form of arthritis.

Most rheumatologic conditions are more common in women, who comprise 60% of all those diagnosed with OA. Studies have also shown that most patients seen by rheumatologists are also female. This can partly be explained by the fact that women live longer than men. The age distribution in patients with a rheumatology-based diagnosis follows a standard distribution with the peak age range being 50 to 60 years of age. It has been estimated that one in five visits to a primary care doctor is related to rheumatic/musculoskeletal disease (Bitton, 2009; Vanhoof et al., 2002).

In the older adult, treatment may have to be tempered as a result of coexisting renal, cardiac, and gastrointestinal (GI) disorders as well as the increased potential for medication complications and drug–drug interactions. Older individuals are on more medications; each additional medication increases the risk of adverse events, complications, and interactions.

Rheumatologic illnesses, like all other illnesses, have both direct costs in relation to the cost of medical care, including the cost of patient visits as well as medications. The costs of medications have increased with the advent of the biological drugs. Surgical procedures such as joint replacement may be needed as a result of the disease. The indirect costs are less well known, but have also been looked at from a pharmacoeconomic viewpoint. The impact of rheumatoid arthritis (RA) on annual loss productivity due to sick leave amounted to 14 to 17 days/patient/year.

To date, there are no known preventive strategies for RA. Once the diagnosis is made, the above therapies are initiated to prevent pain and progression of the disease. For those individuals with a positive family history, tobacco use is strongly discouraged.

OSTEOARTHRITIS

Osteoarthritis is the most common form of joint disease seen in humans. Owing to the nature of the disease, it more commonly affects weight-dependent and most heavily used joints such as the hip, knee, and spine (Bitton, 2009).

On account of the cumulative nature of OA, it is considered ubiquitous in the geriatric population and the prevalence clearly increases with increasing age. About 10% of people over the age of 60 are disabled as a result of OA. While OA is less common in persons under 40 years old, current studies suggest that 75% of people over 65 years old have OA (Hunter, 2011).

The economic burden of OA on society is enormous (Bitton, 2009). Approximately one third of direct OA expenditures are used for medications, while hospitalization costs account for nearly half of the direct costs. Only about 5% of OA patients undergo hospitalization, with the inpatient stay accompanying joint replacement accounting for the vast majority of this. Indirect costs for OA are also high, largely as a result of work-related losses and home care costs (Hunter, 2011).

Studies have shown that culture influences the patient's choice of therapy. African Americans and other minorities are less likely to have invasive therapies such as surgery. While Asians would rather tolerate pain than report it, they are therefore less likely to be treated.

Screening and Risk Factors

There are no screening tests for OA. The American College of Rheumatology (ACR) has developed clinical and radiographic (articular and periarticular) criteria for the diagnosis (Primer on Rheumatic Diseases, n.d.). Osteoarthritis is a chronic polyarticular, noninflammatory degenerative condition most commonly affecting the weight-dependent joints. The joints affected can change over time. Pain and nodules are the primary symptoms of OA. Osteoarthritis should be considered an articular and a periarticular disease. Osteoarthritis can be primary or secondary (e.g., from trauma, infections, and inflammatory arthritis). Changes noted on imaging, most commonly on x-rays, are the hallmarks of the disease. Magnetic resonance imaging (MRI) shows the periarticular changes better than plain radiographs and computed tomography.

The common risk factors for OA include repetitive motion, strain, old age, joint trauma, and obesity. Osteoarthritis is also associated with mechanical occupations and individuals involved in contact sports. Recently, genetic factors have been linked to OA, and significant research is currently being done in this field. Other risk factors include gender (certain joints are more commonly affected among women) and race/ethnicity.

Although we no longer think of OA as a "wear and tear" disease, this explanation is easily understood by patients. Osteoarthritis is medically best considered as a failure of the joint, or as resulting from excessive mechanical stress applied to a joint that is susceptible to OA.

Presentation of Disease

The core symptom of OA is pain; however, the nature and severity of the pain vary with patients and the joints involved. Osteoarthritic pain is localized, tends to be related to the motion at the affected joint, and is accompanied by a relatively short duration of stiffness after a period of inactivity. There may be swelling, particularly if the knee joint is affected; the swelling may not be associated with history of warmth or redness. Although osteoarthritic nodules are commonly seen in small joints of fingers (proximal and distal interphalangeal) and feet, OA is also common to the knee and lower back joints. Knee and hand OA are more common among women. In the knees, symptoms of OA are often more pronounced on the medial aspect owing to the anatomy of the meniscus and the insertion of the vastus medialis. Conversely, inflammatory arthritis symptoms are common in the proximal interphalangeal joints (PIPJ), distal interphalangeal joints (DIPJ), wrist, and feet. The patient's general appearance, weight, mobility, and ability to perform activities of daily living help clinicians to determine the impact of the disease. In patients with OA, there is mild-to-firm swelling along the joint line with crepitus that may be audible in bigger joints. Other clinical presentations include joint instability, muscle atrophy, and limited range of motion.

Treatment and Management

The goal of treatment is to control symptoms, prevent disease progression, minimize disability, and improve quality of life. Although patients with OA are seen frequently by practitioners, long-term disability remains a major issue outcome. While existing therapies help to reduce symptoms, they are not effective in treating OA, as patients still experience substantial pain and functional impairment after treatment. Therefore, there has been a shift in therapy toward prevention of progression of the disease.

Management of OA includes various techniques and principles, both nonpharmacological and pharmacological (Seed et al., 2011). Osteoarthritis is best treated in early cases by nonspecialist doctors and at advanced stages by a specialist (orthopedics and or rheumatology). Multiple considerations for clinicians are outlined in Table 13.1.

Medication Management

Topical Therapy. Topical nonsteroidal anti-inflammatory drugs (NSAIDs) and capsaicin are alternatives for patients reluctant to use oral medications or who have contraindications to systemic agents. Topical medications are most effective in limited disease and are used as an adjunct to systemic therapy (Sun et al., 2007). Topical NSAIDs, capsaicin, or Lidocaine 5% patches are also useful alternatives. Studies have shown that the pain relief with these topical agents is comparable to oral celecoxib (tablet or capsule) 200 mg daily (Kivitz et al., 2008).

TABLE 13.1 • General Care of Osteoarthritis

- **Patient education** is a crucial step as this improves compliance with management. Patient education fosters good understanding of the disease and the use of nonpharmacological steps.

- **Weight loss** is of great importance and should be emphasized to patients. Every pound in weight loss reduces the pressure on the knees by 4 to 6 pounds. Weight loss not only improves symptoms but also reduces the progression of OA by reducing joint load and subsequent damage.

- **Proper shoes** that are comfortable and well fitting reduce joint load and help with symptoms. Other foot hygiene steps include aesthetics and insoles as needed.

- **Physical/occupational therapies** have been best studied in knees, back, and hands arthritis. They help to reduce symptoms, morbidity, and improve function in patients. Studies have shown that almost any physical activity helps. In addition, therapies such as Tai Chi, acupuncture, and massage have been shown to be effective. The aim of physical and occupational therapies is to improve range of motion, strengthen muscle, and enhance aerobic capacity.

- **Assistive devices** help to reduce the risk of falls and joint damage. Canes are often used in contralateral hip to reduce the impact of pressure force on the affected hip by as much as 50%. As helpful as assistive devices are, patients affected with OA are often reluctant to use them.

Nonopioid Analgesia. Acetaminophen tablet is effective for mild-to-moderate pain associated with OA. Studies have shown that it can reduce overall pain related to OA, it is more effective than placebo in trials, and should be the initial drug therapy.

NSAIDs are superior to acetaminophen in both patient- and physician-reported studies. However, in the geriatric population, other comorbid factors may influence the choice of NSAIDs, even if NSAIDs are considered safe to use. NSAIDs have consistently demonstrated efficacy for pain relief in OA. All NSAIDs, including cyclooxygenase-2 (COX-2)–selective agents, are equally effective for pain relief in OA among older adults; COX-2 selective agents would be a safer choice, especially for long-term use. COX-2 agents have been shown to benefit older patients who are at high risk for peptic ulcer disease or GI bleeding; the GI-protective benefits may not be evident in patients who are taking aspirin (Silverstein et al., 2000).

Opioid Analgesics. The ACR recommends that opioid analgesics should only be used in patients not controlled by or in patients who are unable to tolerate other treatment options for OA (Primer on the Rheumatic Diseases, n.d.). The use of narcotics or opioid for OA is better accomplished in a pain management clinic.

Intra-articular Injections. These are a nonsurgical alternative treatment for OA. They can be used as an adjunct to oral agents or if the patient is unable to use other treatment options (Bellamy et al., 2006).

Glucocorticoid Injections. All forms of parenteral steroids have shown to be effective. The choice and dose of corticosteroids used have been well studied and the general consensus is to inject as little as possible and at a maximum of every 3 months. Triamcinolone acetonide 40 mg knee injection every 3 months for up to 2 years has been used intra-articularly to control OA pain with minimal side effects (Raynauld et al., 2003).

Hyaluronate Injections. Hyaluronate injection has just been currently approved only for knee OA by the Food and Drug Administration (FDA). In recent times, the use of hyaluronate has increased greatly because full therapy can be achieved with a single injection, compared with the series of three weekly injections, which is the way it was used in the past.

Surgical Management

Surgical management is the last line of treatment for OA, but is effective in patients with intractable symptoms. Surgical interventions include total joint arthroplasty and joint lavage and debridement. Although joint lavage and debridement have been used, there is no evidence of its relieving pain or improving function better than the nonsurgical treatments. If surgery is needed, it should not be delayed as the goal is to preserve and restore function. Preoperative functional status is often used to predict the outcomes of the joint surgery (Primer on the Rheumatic Diseases, n.d.).

GOUT

Gout is an inflammatory arthritis caused by the deposition of monosodium urate crystals in synovial fluid and other tissues. It is the most prevalent form of inflammatory arthropathy in the older adult (De Leonardis et al., 2007). The prevalence and incidence of gout have risen over time owing to an increase in risk factors such as diet, alcohol consumption, metabolic syndrome, hypertension, obesity, diuretic use, and chronic renal disease. In the United States, the total prevalence of gout is about 5.2/1,000 and growing. The total incidence of gout is 1.4 in women and 4.0 in men per 1,000 person-years (Edward & Michael, 2010). An estimated 6.1 million adults in the United States have gout. Gout is an independent risk factor for cardiovascular diseases (Edward & Michael, 2010). Gout in minorities seems to occur at younger mean age at onset and among individuals who are less educated. Tophaceous gout is more common among minorities, with a higher number of tophi and larger tophi size (higher uric acid burden). High incidence of gout-related diseases such as hypertension, diabetes, and obesity has also been reported among the underrepresented (Vázquez-Mellado et al., 2006).

Gout has been split into two clinical types:

1. Elderly-onset gout (EOG) is a new onset gout in people 65 years and older. EOG frequently presents with subacute polyarticular symptoms and may persist as chronic symptoms. In EOG, atypical joint involvement is also very common, and it is not uncommon to have symptoms small joints of the hands. EOG can also present in a pseudo-rheumatoid–like picture. Tophi (a deposit of crystalline uric acid or other substances) is also noted in unusual locations. There is also an increase in the percentage of females affected by EOG (De Leonardis et al., 2007). Some people may have tophi without an acute attack of gout.
2. Typical middle-age gout presents as an acute monoarticular inflammatory arthritis seen in men, with the lower limbs more commonly affected.

Screening and Risk Factors

The ACR states that the diagnosis can also be presumed on the basis of clinical symptoms. Definitive diagnosis of gout is made by crystal examination from joint fluid; however, other diagnoses should also be ruled out. The definitive diagnosis is needed as other crystal-induced arthropathies and infections may present in a very similar fashion.

Hyperuricemia is the most important risk factor for the development of gout. Most people with asymptomatic hyperuricemia do not go on to develop gout, but the relative risk of developing gout increases with higher uric acid levels. The risk of developing gout is about 30% over 5 years in people with uric acid levels of over 10 mg/dl, but is less than 1% in patients with uric acid of less than 7 mg/day (Saag & Choi, 2006; Wise, 2007).

Gender and age are the major risk factors. Gout polyarticular is more prevalent in middle-aged men and postmenopausal women. On average, women develop gout about 7 to 10 years after their male counterparts. By the age of 60, 50% of newly diagnosed gout patients are women. Clustering is seen in certain families, and twin studies show high heritability for both uric acid production and renal clearance of uric acid, indicating a genetic predisposition. Defects in uric acid transporters have also been noted.

Diet is a major risk factor for gout; high consumption of fructose, meat, and seafood has been associated with an increased risk of gout. Alcohol use not only increases the risk of gout but can also trigger a gout attack (Saag & Choi, 2006). However, diets high in purine-rich vegetables have not been linked with gout. Metabolic syndrome, renal disease, and medications such as diuretics use and cyclosporine increase the risk of gout. However, consumption of dairy products and large quantities of coffee has a protective effect.

Gout in minorities seems to occur at a younger age and among individuals who are less educated. The minorities also have a longer disease course and tophaceous gout is also more common among this population. Minorities also have a higher incidence of metabolic syndrome such as hypertension, diabetes, and obesity, which increases the incidence of gout and vice versa (Vázquez-Mellado et al., 2006).

Clinical Presentation

Acute Gout

Acute gout presents as a sudden onset of severe pain in one or more joints. The pain typically lasts between 7 and 14 days and can be disabling. There are asymptomatic periods between these acute attacks. The most common joints involved are the first metatarsophalangeal (podagra), metatarsal, ankle, or knee joints. Pain, erythema, and swelling are the hallmark signs with pain often such that even the light touch of socks or bed linen cannot be tolerated.

Chronic Tophaceous Gout

Chronic gout involves polyarticular symptoms between attacks. It is characterized by crystal deposition (tophi) in soft tissues or joints. Tophi can occur in the helix of the ear, the olecranon process, and over the interphalangeal joints. This type of gout can be destructive and is often associated with chronic pain. The most important risk factors for the development of tophaceous gout are untreated acute gout and hyperuricemia. A study suggests that the majority of persons with untreated gout will develop tophi (Gutman, 1973).

Differential Diagnosis of Acute Gout

The two conditions most commonly confused with gout are pseudogout (calcium pyrophosphate deposition disease) and septic arthritis. The joint distribution of pseudogout is typically different from gout as it is more likely to affect the knee, wrist, or first metatarsophalangeal joint (MTPJ).

Besides the location, another approach to differentiate between pseudogout and septic arthritis is through analysis of the joint crystals. Septic arthritis is also associated with a fever, an elevated WBC, with white cells, and bacteria on the Gram stain of the joint fluid.

Treatment and Management

Older patients with gout are best treated the same way as people with renal impairment (El-Zawawy & Manndell, 2010) and under the care of a specialist. Barriers against treatment include lack of patient education, presence of comorbid conditions, communicant use of multiple medications, and cognitive decline (Ene-Stroescu & Gorbien, 2005).

Acute Gout

For acute attacks, the aim is to stop the attack as soon as possible (Saag & Choi, 2006). NSAIDs, colchicine, and glucocorticoids are the most effective groups of medications for acute gout. The choice of drug, dose, and duration depends on factors such as patient allergies and coexisting medical problems. NSAIDs and colchicine are first-line agents for acute attacks. Colchicine can be used for both acute treatment and prevention of further attacks of gout. The current recommendation is low-dose colchicine (1.8 mg over 1 hour) taken as early as possible to control acute gout, and then colchicine 0.6 mg once a day thereafter (Richette & Bardin, 2010). Various studies comparing NSAIDs have shown that there is no significant difference in the effectiveness of different NSAIDs (Schumacher et al., 2002). NSAIDs and colchicine are contraindicated if the glomerular filtration rate is less than 50 ml/minute (Aronoff et al., 1994). In such situations, glucocorticoids are used. Glucocorticoids are very effective in the treatment of acute gout, but the side effects have to be carefully considered. The choice of medications (oral or intra-articular) used to treat gout depends on the patient's preference and the number of joints involved. Recently, newer drugs such as interleukin-1 antagonists have been used, but these are prescribed only by the specialists.

Chronic Tophaceous Gout

If the serum uric acid can be reduced below 6 mg/dl, gout attacks become very rare (Zhang et al., 2006). The overall goal is to reduce the uric acid level to 6 or under after the onset of acute attack. Urate-lowering therapy should not be started during acute attacks, but rather between 2 and 4 weeks after the acute attack. Uric acid–lowering treatment should be started once there are at least two gout attacks in 1 year, or the uric acid level is above 12, or the patient has tophi (Zhang et al., 2006).

Prevention

It is important to stop further attacks with a prophylactic drug as starting urate-lowering therapy increases the risk of gout attacks in the first 3 months (Richette & Bardin, 2010; Zhang et al., 2006). Gout attacks triggered by urate-lowering drugs are more severe and prolonged compared with those in patients with spontaneous attacks. Colchicine 0.6 mg daily or twice daily is generally recommended for prophylaxis; this dose may be adjusted in the older adult and in cases of renal and hepatic impairment (Neogi, 2011; Saag & Choi, 2006). Although there are recommendations for colchicine dosing based on renal clearance, little has been reported in the literature in this regard but the ACR recommends that colchicine should be avoided if the glomerular filtration rate is less than 50 ml/minute (Aronoff et al., 1994).

Xanthine Oxidase Inhibitors

Xanthine oxidase inhibitor class of drugs blocks the synthesis of uric acid and can therefore be used in both overproduction and under-excretion of uric acid. It is the most common class of drug used. Allopurinol is a typical example of xanthine oxidase inhibitors, with the dose ranging from 100 to 800 mg daily. The dose of allopurinol should be tapered to the renal function of the patient. Febuxostat is a newer agent and has a dose range of 40 to 80 mg once a day. As febuxostat and allopurinol are in the same class, they should not be used together (Neogi, 2011; Saag & Choi, 2006).

Uricosuric Agents

Uricosuric group of medications blocks renal tubular urate reabsorption, thereby lowering the uric acid levels in patients who are under-excretors of uric acid. Patients who have uric acid stones should not be given these drugs.

Probenecid is the most common example and is typically used in doses of 500 mg twice a day. Probenecid should be avoided in patients with stages 4 and 5 chronic kidney disease (CKD) and used with caution in the older adult. The standard starting dose is 250 mg daily and if renal function is normal, can be increased by 500 mg/month to a maximum of 2 to 3 g daily.

Uricase Agents

This class of drugs breaks down the uric acid to allantoin, thus reducing the uric acid level. Pegloticase (a modified porcine recombinant uricase) is used in chronic gout refractory to other treatments. Pegloticase can only be prescribed by specialists.

RHEUMATOID ARTHRITIS

The prevalence and incidence of RA increases up to age 85, and the mean age of diagnosis is 60. The prevalence of RA in the United States in persons aged 60 and older is around 2% (Vanhoof et al., 2002). Old age and postmenopausal status have been associated with severe RA (Tutuncu & Kavanaugh, 2007). The disease is generally more prevalent among women, Mexican Americans, people with less education, and among patients who are 70 years and older. Tobacco use is also strongly associated with severe RA, and questions about tobacco use should be included in the assessment of RA. Two types of RA common among older adults are elderly-onset RA and adult-onset RA.

Elderly-Onset RA

Elderly-onset RA has its onset in adults aged 60 years or older. It is commonly seen in women and presents acutely with elevated inflammatory markers, debilitating morning stiffness, and pain commonly in the upper extremities (Tutuncu & Kavanaugh, 2005). The physical examination is marked by synovitis, particularly in larger joints.

Adult-Onset RA

Adults-onset RA starts before age 60 and may persist into later years. Examination may reveal both articular and systemic findings. The joint findings include both active polyarticular synovitis and deformities in both the upper and the lower extremities. Systemic findings may include rheumatoid lung, vasculitic ulcers, or peripheral neuropathy either from the RA or from medications used to treat them (Tutuncu & Kavanaugh, 2005).

The disease is generally more prevalent among women, Mexican Americans, people with less education, and among patients who are 70 years and older. Tobacco use has been shown to be strongly associated with severe RA.

Screening and Risk Factors

Diagnosis is more difficult in the older adult as the prevalence of autoantibodies (including the rheumatoid factor and anti-CCP antibody) increases with age and can be seen in people without rheumatic illnesses. Inflammatory markers (erythrocyte sedimentation rate [ESR] and C-reactive protein [CRP]) often used to monitor activity in RA are of limited value in older patients as elevation is common in advanced age. This may be due to age itself or concomitant disease conditions unrelated to RA. Imaging including x-rays and MRI of the affected joints may show stigmata of RA (Majithia et al., 2009).

Pathophysiology

The risk factors for RA are multifactorial, with genetics and environmental factors playing major roles in the disease (Primer on the Rheumatic Diseases, n.d.). The most important genetic risk factor is related to human leukocyte antigen (HLA) typing and a shared epitope has been noted to increase susceptibility and severity of RA. The shared epitope is rarely tested for in clinical practice. One environmental factor closely associated with RA is cigarette smoking, and this may increase the incidence and severity of RA (Primer on the Rheumatic Diseases, n.d.).

Clinical Presentation

Patients present with inflammatory symptoms, including insidious onset joint pain, swelling, redness, warmth, and stiffness. Joint stiffness is often worse in the morning and improves with use; this differentiates RA from degenerative arthritis with its worsening symptoms during activities. The symptoms and signs tend to be symmetrical, involving the small joints of the hands and feet and normally lasting for more than 6 weeks if it is not treated (Primer on the Rheumatic Diseases, n.d.; Kellys' Textbook of Rheumatology, n.d.). Any joint can be affected, but RA is commonly seen in smaller joints. The typical rheumatoid deformities and/or extra-articular complications are rare at the onset of the disease.

Although extra-articular complications are rare, it can affect any organ in the body and should be looked for during the history and physical examination. Skin nodules, eye dryness, Sjögren syndrome, and vasculitic changes in the skin should also be observed. Other clinical presentations include scleritis, episcleritis, and scleromalacia perforans. Rheumatoid nodules can also be found on extensor surfaces or pressure points. Patients with RA tend to have a long history of the disease and are normally rheumatoid factor positive. RA may also affect internal organs such as the heart and lungs, and RA-related nodules can be worsened by methotrexate use. Vasculitis can also affect internal organs, and it is common in erosive RA, among patients with a long history of the disease, and those with circulating cryoglobulins. Rheumatoid lung disease may take the form of pleural disease, lung fibrosis, RA nodules, and pulmonary hypertension (Kellys' Textbook of Rheumatology, n.d.).

Treatment

Treatment is a little harder in older patients as they have other comorbid problems and may have organ dysfunctions that may affect medication choice and tolerability. Age-related changes in pharmacokinetic parameters, altered tissue responsiveness, and an increased overall frequency of adverse drug events also play an important role in choice and doses of medications used. The aim of treatment is to control symptoms and progression of the disease. Patients need to be followed up both for the complications from medications used and for the disease process.

Symptomatic Therapy

NSAIDs and Low-Dose Prednisone. Low-dose prednisone and NSAIDs are used to control the symptoms of RA. People over the age of 65 have a much higher risk of toxicity with NSAIDs including upper GI bleeding. The risk of GI bleeding increases with concurrent use of prednisone or anticoagulants. Renal impairment is also common in people 65 years or older on NSAIDs, diuretics, angiotensin-converting enzyme inhibitors and patients with hypertension and congestive heart failure. Cyclo-oxygenase-2 (COX-2) specific inhibitors (COXIBs) are safer than NSAIDs in people 65 years and above (Silverstein et al., 2000). Low-dose prednisone is associated with osteoporosis, infection, glucose intolerance, GI erosive disease, and hypertension.

Disease-Modifying Antirheumatic Drugs (DMARD). DMARDs are normally used in combination with each other; normally two or three DMARDs are needed to control RA and could take several months to have effect. It is therefore important that symptoms be controlled when DMARDs are started. DMARDs are divided into two groups—nonbiological drugs and biological drugs (Ranganath & Furst, 2007; Saag et al., 2008).

Nonbiological Drugs. Nonbiological DMARDs cannot be used safely in patients with renal or hepatic compromise and need close monitoring to prevent or detect side effects early.

- Hydroxychloroquine is the most common nonbiological DMARD used and is considered one of the safest. It is always used in combination with other DMARDs. Hydroxychloroquine can cause skin rash and there is a risk of retinal toxicity. In general, people on hydroxychloroquine should have a retinal exam yearly.
- Methotrexate was one of the first effective DMARDs used. It is now recognized as the first-line agent for RA. Common side effects include oral ulcers, bone marrow suppression, and hepatic impairment. Rarer side effects include worsening nodules and lung disease. The mechanism of action is still not clearly understood, but the use of folic acid supplement reduces the risk of side effects.
- Leflunomide is also commonly used in place of methotrexate and was approved by the FDA in September 1998. It is a daily medication and has similar side effects. Close monitoring is also needed to ensure the patients remain well.
- Azathioprine is less commonly used, but can be very effective. Its main disadvantage is that it is not safe in patients taking xanthine oxidase inhibitors.
- Sulfasalazine is quite cheap, readily available, and it does require multiple doses in a 24-hour period. Common side effects include skin rash, GI irritation, and hemolytic problems.

TABLE 13.2 · Biological Drugs

Tumor Necrosis Factor–alpha Inhibitors (TNF inhibitors)
Examples of TNFs include etanercept, adalimumab, and infliximab. These were the first biological medications on the market. There are many other TNF inhibitors on the market now. They should be used by specialists only. They are given intravenously or subcutaneously by patient preference.

Interleukin-1 Inhibitors
This is approved for RA, but as it is a daily injection, it is not used as commonly as some of the other biological drugs.

Interleukin-6 Inhibitors
This is a relatively new line of therapy, and only Tocilizumab is currently clinically used. This drug is as effective as the TNF inhibitors, but is given intravenously. They do, however, have additional side effects and need very close monitoring.

B and T cell Costimulation Blocker
Currently, Abatacept is the only agent available, and it seems to have the best side effects profile.

B Cell Depleting Therapy
Rituximab is the only one that is currently available and is considered the last medication to be used in difficult-to-control RA.

Janus-Associated Kinases Inhibitors
Tofacitinib is currently the newest medication in our armory, and is an oral biological, administered b.i.d. As it is very new, long-term safety data need to be monitored.

Biological DMARD. This group of drugs has proven to be useful in the treatment of RA. Biological drugs allow for three or more drugs to be used to control RA. It could be safely used to treat RA among patients with concomitant disease conditions such as liver and renal disease and even for people on hemodialysis. All biological drugs have immunosuppression as their major side effect, which puts patients at risk for infections. Biological medications are mostly given parenterally (Saag et al., 2008), though in late 2012 a new class of oral biological drug was approved by the FDA (Table 13.2).

CHRONIC PAIN MANAGEMENT

Pain management is a crucial component of caring for the older patient, and it can be challenging to overcome the many barriers and misperceptions that exist in providing good pain management for elders. Despite these obstacles, nurses have created, preserved, as well as implemented best practices to minimize patients' pain and suffering. Older persons are vulnerable as they require careful assessment and treatment approaches to ensure safe and adequate pain management.

Presently, the senior population is the fastest growing segment of the world's population, with an estimated number of people worldwide 65 years and older at 506 million as of 2008, and this number is expected to increase to 1.3 billion by 2040 (Kaye et al., 2010). In 2008, individuals aged 65 and older accounted for 12.8% (38.9 million) of the total population in the United States, with 5.7 million people 85 years and older (Blumstein & Gorevic, 2005; Kaye et al., 2010). Persistent pain affects about 100 million Americans, which is more than the total number of adults affected by heart disease, cancer, and diabetes combined (Institute of Medicine of the National Academies [IOM], 2011).

Pain is prevalent among older individuals, increases with age, and is often undertreated (Kaye et al., 2010). The prevalence of pain among elders 65 years or older is estimated to be as high as 67% to 80% (Davis & Srivastava, 2003). Musculoskeletal conditions are the most common cause of pain for the older person, with 50% of individuals aged 65 years or greater having arthritic pain and 80% experiencing back pain at some point during their lifetime (Fitzcharles et al., 2010). Advanced cancer is a common cause of pain, with roughly 80% of cancer patients experiencing pain (Mercadante & Arcuri, 2007); one study estimated 25% to 40% of older patients with cancer having daily pain. In nursing homes, 45% to 80% of residents have pain that impairs their functionality, and half of these residents have daily pain (Davis & Srivastava, 2003). Additionally, more than 50% of postoperative patients have severe pain (Sauaia et al., 2005). Each of these epidemiologic data underscore the need for effective treatment of pain in the older adult patient.

Unrelieved pain has a significant impact on the physical, cognitive, emotional, and social functioning of the older individual (Hanks-Bell et al., 2004; Pautex et al., 2009). Poorly managed pain leads to decreased cognitive function and attention span, insomnia, immobility, increased depression, and mood disturbances, including apathy, anorexia, fear, social isolation, and increased health care expenditures (Abad et al., 2008; Davis & Srivastava, 2003; Hanks-Bell et al., 2004; Mitchell, 2001). Physical function is impaired related to decreased activity and ambulation, leading to deconditioning, gait disturbances, and injuries from falls (Hanks-Bell et al., 2004). Yet it is clearly documented that despite the high prevalence and serious consequences of pain in the older population, pain continues to be overlooked and untreated (Kaye et al., 2010; Chodosh et al., 2004; Pergolizzi, 2007).

Barriers to acceptable pain management in the older adult can be categorized into three sources: the patient, the health care community, and society in general (Hanks-Bell et al., 2004). Individual barriers include cognitive impairment, fatalism, denial, fear of being considered a bad patient if pain is reported, fear of adverse reactions, fear of loss of independence, fear of addiction and/or tolerance, fear of worsening of disease progression, saving medications until they "really need them," cultural barriers such as language difficulties, and financial restraints. Barriers related to health care providers include lack of knowledge and time, misconceptions of pain management and potential adverse effects upon the older patient, fear of opioids, fear of legal and regulatory scrutiny, and lack of competence in assessing cognitively impaired individuals. Finally, societal barriers comprise cost, time, and cultural bias regarding the aging population and opioid use (Davis & Srivastava, 2003; Hanks-Bell et al., 2004).

It is important to understand the complexities of pain to adequately assess and treat it in the geriatric population. There is no objective measurement of pain (Pasero & McCaffery, 2007). Pain cannot be quantified or disproved; it is subjective and individual. "Pain is whatever the experiencing person says it is, existing whenever he says it does" (Pasero & McCaffery, 2007). The International Association for the Study of Pain defines pain as "an unpleasant sensory and emotional experience associated with actual or potential tissue damage, or described in terms of such damage" (International Association for the Study of Pain [IASP], 2012). Pain management in the older patient is a multifaceted undertaking requiring a holistic approach that addresses physical, emotional, spiritual, and social domains of the person.

Pathophysiology

With the normal aging process, there is a steady decline of homeostatic mechanisms and organ system function (Kaye et al., 2010). A reduction in both cardiac index and renal function of

1% per year begins after the age of 40. There is a 1 ml/minute/year decrease in creatinine clearance (Kaye et al., 2010). Cardiac function changes include a stiffening vasculature with increased blood pressure and reduced myocardial reserve. In addition, reduced renal and hepatic function lead to a prolongation of medication circulation, uptake, and distribution (Pergolizzi et al., 2007). Decreased serum albumin may lead to diminished drug binding and increased levels of unbound medications (Blumstein & Gorevic, 2005). Furthermore, aldosterone and renin release are reduced owing to decreased sympathetic innervation of juxtaglomerular cells of the kidneys of the mature patient, leading to increased risk of hyperkalemia especially with the use of NSAIDs (Davis & Srivastava, 2003). Even though the structure and function of the kidneys declines, its clinical function appears to be mostly maintained in the healthy older patient with a few exceptions (Kaye et al., 2010). However, this inevitable reduction of the glomerular filtration rate can increase the half-life of those medications that are primarily eliminated by the kidneys, resulting in a higher risk of toxicity and drug-related adverse events (Pergolizzi et al., 2007). The creatinine clearance should be used when dosing medications for the mature patient and, if it cannot be calculated or measured, then a 40% reduction from the normal renal function should be assumed (Blumstein & Gorevic, 2005).

Several hepatic changes are seen, including decreased hepatic blood flow, decreased hepatic mass, and decreases in the monooxygenases and cytochrome enzymes, particularly P450 (Kaye et al., 2010; Davis & Srivastava, 2003; Pergolizzi et al., 2007). Prolonged clearance of medications may occur with an aged liver (Kaye et al., 2010). Decreased first pass metabolism and blood extraction are related to prehepatic dysfunction and secondary to lower GI absorption and/or poor blood flow (Kaye et al., 2010). Hepatic metabolism may be reduced up to 30% to 40%, increasing oral bioavailability of certain opioids by reducing hepatic extraction (Davis & Srivastava, 2003; Pergolizzi et al., 2007). Liver function tests may be within normal limits despite these changes (Kaye et al., 2010). For elders with chronic hepatic disease, medication dosage reduction or longer dosing intervals are required to prevent drug accumulation (Pergolizzi et al., 2007).

Increased body fat associated with aging increases the volume of distribution of lipophilic medications, delaying both elimination and the onset of drug action without altering serum concentrations. Furthermore, plasma concentrations of hydrophilic medications are increased due to reduced volume of distribution, which secondarily enhances drug diffusion to receptor sites (Davis & Srivastava, 2003). Lower volumes of distribution increase the peak plasma levels of morphine, increasing the risk of adverse events for elders (Pergolizzi et al., 2007). Since the older patient tends to have multiple comorbidities often resulting in polypharmacy, the potential for pharmacokinetic and pharmacodynamic drug–drug interactions is greatly increased (Davis & Srivastava, 2003).

There are numerous central nervous system alterations that occur with aging. Subcortical and cortical atrophy decrease potential receptor sites, receptor affinity, and synthesis of neurotransmitters such as acetylcholine, dopamine, GABA, and norepinephrine (Davis & Srivastava, 2003; Fitzcharles et al., 2010). There is a decrease in the density of drug receptors, an increase for potential interactions between the different receptors, and changes in the signal transduction pathways that are activated following drug binding in the older patient (Blumstein & Gorevic, 2005). Cerebral blood flow, especially in neocortex, hippocampus, locus ceruleus, and substantia nigra is reduced up to 28% in the older patient (Davis & Srivastava, 2003; Fitzcharles et al., 2010). Neurons of the older patient are less likely to be rejuvenated after cell death and are instead replaced by proliferating glial cells (Davis & Srivastava, 2003; Fitzcharles et al., 2010; Kaye et al., 2010). Additionally, the number of dendritic synapses, cell receptors, and intracellular enzymes declines (Kaye et al., 2010;

Davis & Srivastava, 2003). These changes predispose the older person to reduced drug tolerance and drug-induced delirium, each of which may contribute to opioid resistance and lead to uncontrolled pain (Davis & Srivastava, 2003). Neurologic disease and dysfunction, including dementia, strokes, Parkinson disease, and other movement disorders, are common in the older adult. These problems may alter the expression of pain, resulting in poor assessment and treatment of pain (Davis & Srivastava, 2003; Fitzcharles et al., 2010; Kaye et al., 2010).

Decreased salivary formation in the older patient combined with salivary reduction caused by the multiple medications with anticholinergic properties delays the absorption of sublingual tablets. Peristalsis reduction increases the risk of constipation, nausea, and vomiting from pain medications. Elders are also at high risk for orthostatic hypotension when taking adjuvants such as tricyclic antidepressants owing to the age-associated diminished baroreceptor response (Davis & Srivastava, 2003).

In summary, there are many physiological changes in organ function that occur with the aging process. Complicating these changes are numerous comorbidities resulting in polypharmacy that increase the risk of drug interactions and adverse events. These complex, multifactorial effects often lead to a narrowing of the therapeutic window and increased difficulty in balancing these barriers with proper analgesia for the health care provider caring for the older adult.

Acute and Chronic Pain and Presentation

There are several ways to classify pain, including acute pain (postoperative or trauma pain resolving usually within a few weeks to several months), cancer pain, and persistent or chronic pain (pain lasting greater than 3 months) such as OA or diabetic neuropathy (Kean et al., 2008; Mitchell, 2001; Pasero & McCaffery, 2007; Peterson, 2007). Another way to classify pain is based on the pathology, with nociceptive pain, neuropathic pain, or a combination of both. Nociceptive pain involves the normal neural processing of noxious stimuli, which includes transduction, transmission, perception, and modulation; it can be further subdivided into somatic (bone: achy and localized) and visceral (organ: crampy and diffuse) pain (Pasero & McCaffery, 2007). Neuropathic pain is the abnormal processing of sensory input by the peripheral or central nervous system (Ahmad & Goucke, 2002; Pasero & McCaffery, 2007). The older patient may experience either of these types of pain. The treatment is tailored to the type of pain, so it is imperative to characterize the pain correctly. As with younger patients, swift assessment and management of acute pain can minimize and often prevent the development of persistent pain in the older population.

The older patient tends to report pain less frequently, possibly because of several factors, including alterations in the sensorineural apparatus and the presence of stoicism or hesitancy to voice pain. The older patient may actually experience pain more often than younger patients since they are less likely to complain or report it. Furthermore, no physiological pain perception reducing alterations have been shown in the older patients (Mercadante & Arcuri, 2007). Some studies suggest that as we age, there is an impaired function of the Aδ-fibers (transmission of localized and rapid pain) and decreased transmission of pain sensations, while the function of the C-fibers is preserved (delayed and blunted response to painful stimuli), impairing nociceptive perception and modulation of pain, perhaps explaining the increased prevalence of persistent pain and coexistence of multiple types of pain in the older adult (Fitzcharles et al., 2010).

Pain threshold refers to the lowest stimulus intensity noticed by the patient that triggers a painful sensation (Ciampi et al., 2011). Current research suggests that older patients have higher thermal and mechanical pain thresholds than younger patients. Thus, they have higher pain thresholds and lower tolerances to painful stimuli, resulting in a flattening of the interval between onset of pain and the point where the pain becomes unbearable (Ciampi et al., 2011). Studies are now clearly indicating that there is an increase in pain thresholds with advancing age (Kaye et al., 2010).

Screening and Risk Factors

A thorough pain assessment of the older patient is key to early identification of pain and is the first step in the treatment. Since the nurse is often the first clinician to hear or observe a patient's report of pain, it is crucial for nurses to perform a comprehensive pain assessment in the older adult. A comprehensive pain assessment includes a thorough pain history, a complete physical examination, and, as indicated, laboratory or other diagnostic procedures (American Society of Pain Management Nursing, 2010; Hanks-Bell et al., 2004; Pasero & McCaffery, 2007).

An accurate pain assessment consists of patient's age, past medical, surgical, and pain histories, medications (what has and has not worked), allergies, adverse reactions to medications, hearing and visual impairments, financial issues, limitations or access to treatment, and cognitive and functional status (Hanks-Bell et al., 2004; Kaye et al., 2010). Assessment of the patient's level of function and independence, including activities of daily living such as eating, bathing, dressing, managing money, preparing meals, and ambulation, is part of an integral pain evaluation (Ahmad & Goucke, 2002; Hanks-Bell et al., 2004; Kaye et al., 2010).

Clinical manifestations of pain in older patients are often complex and multifactorial, making a thorough pain assessment even more crucial. Furthermore, disease conditions such as depression, poor health and memory, and psychosocial concerns contribute to the complexity of assessment and treatment. The clinician's communication and interpersonal skills are essential in assessing for pain in the older adult (Hanks-Bell et al., 2004; Kaye et al., 2010).

The patient's self-report remains the only reliable indicator of the existence and intensity of pain and its intensity even among the cognitively impaired. The pain assessment should be completed regularly and in a systematic manner with questions about onset, duration, quality/character, intensity, location, alleviating and aggravating factors, and impact on mood and sleep. Additionally, it is important to allocate more time to perform the pain assessment and to simplify questions to Yes or No answers for the cognitively impaired older adults. Cognitively impaired older adults may also demonstrate increased vocalizations like moaning or crying and behaviors such as grimacing, irritability, and guarding (Ahmad & Goucke, 2002; Hanks-Bell et al., 2004; Kaye et al., 2010; Pasero & McCaffery, 2007; Rao & Cohen, 2004). Family members and caregivers can provide insight into the cognitively impaired individual's pain (Ahmad & Goucke, 2002; Hanks-Bell et al., 2004; Kaye et al., 2010; Rao & Cohen, 2004). While physiological responses such as increased heart rate and blood pressure are a good measure of pain, they are poor indicators of pain in the nonverbal patient. Pain diaries may be helpful in ongoing management of pain for some patients (Kaye et al., 2010; Pasero & McCaffery, 2007).

Several standardized tools are available to assist with pain assessment. The numerical analogy scale and verbal descriptors are frequently used to assess pain intensity, whereas the visual analogy scale should be used with caution, with older patients reporting difficulty in completing (Kaye et al., 2010; Pasero & McCaffery, 2007). The McGill Pain Questionnaire has evidence of validity and reliability, and can be used to assess the sensory, affective, evaluative, and various components of pain for all ages, including the older adult. The Pain Thermometer and the Faces Pain Scale are other options that depend on visual acuity, so they may need to be enlarged for visually impaired patients.

Important to note is that cognitively impaired patients may not be able to distinguish between pain and mood with the Faces Pain Scale. The Checklist on Nonverbal Pain Indicators, The Assessment of Discomfort in Dementia Protocol, and the Pain Assessment in Advanced Dementia are behavioral tools that can aid in assessing pain of the cognitively impaired older patient (Kaye et al., 2010; Pasero & McCaffery, 2007). Behavioral tools may provide a number, but it is important to note that the number may not equate to the patient's self-report of pain intensity.

A complete physical examination is important; the clinician should pay special attention to the site of pain and surrounding areas. With the high prevalence of musculoskeletal pain in the older patient, the physical examination should focus on a thorough musculoskeletal and neurological examination. Additionally, the clinician should perform a cognitive, social, functional, and psychiatric assessment in conjunction with appropriate laboratory and diagnostic tests. With the complexity of pain assessment in geriatric patients, a multidisciplinary approach is often required to have the greatest chance of success (Kaye et al., 2010; Pasero & McCaffery, 2007). The pain team might include a nurse, pain management physician, psychologist or psychiatrist, a physical therapist, massage therapist, and interventionist.

Treatment

Nonopioids

On the basis of the 2009 American Geriatric Society recommendations, acetaminophen should be considered to be the first line of pharmacological treatment for mild-to-moderate pain, especially for musculoskeletal pain, since it is not associated with significant GI bleeding, adverse renal effects, or cardiovascular toxicity. It is important to educate patients on the maximum safe dose (<4 g/daily) of acetaminophen from all sources or medications used by the patient (Ickowicz, 2009; Reid et al., 2011). When maximum recommended doses are avoided with acetaminophen, the risk of hepatic toxicity is minimal for older adults with normal liver function, but in patients with liver failure, it is absolutely contraindicated (Ickowicz, 2009).

Even though NSAIDs are effective for chronic inflammatory pain such as OA and lower back pain, this group of medications and cyclooxygenase-2 inhibitors (COX-2) should be considered with extreme caution and in highly selective elders in view of the risks of GI bleeding, adverse renal effects, and cardiovascular toxicity. Patient selection criteria should involve determining when other safer therapies have failed, evidence of ongoing therapeutic goals not being met, and continuing assessment of risks and complications outweighing therapeutic benefits. Active peptic ulcer disease, CKD, and heart failure are considered absolute contraindications for use of NSAIDs and COX-2 inhibitors (Ickowicz, 2009; Kaye et al., 2010). The history of peptic ulcer disease, of concomitant use of corticosteroids or of selective serotonin reuptake inhibitors, hypertension, and *Helicobacter pylori* are considered relative contraindications for use of NSAIDs. Older adults taking nonselective NSAIDs should use a proton pump inhibitor or misoprostol for GI protection, not take more than one NSAID or COX-2 at any time, and be routinely assessed for GI and renal toxicity, hypertension, heart failure, and other drug–drug interactions (Ickowicz, 2009; Kaye et al., 2010).

Opioids

Opioid analgesic medications are an essential component of effective management of moderate-to-severe pain in the older patient (Collyott & Brooks, 2008; Ickowicz, 2009; Kaye et al., 2010). With the evidence that the use of NSAIDs and COX-2 inhibitors may result in serious and life-threatening adverse effects, a new interest in the safe and effective use of opioids has surfaced (American Geriatrics Society [AGS], 2012; Ickowicz, 2009). Opioids act mostly on the central nervous system, but also act secondarily on the peripheral system, decreasing the perception of pain (Mercadante & Arcuri, 2007). Unlike NSAIDS, most opioids do not have maximum doses and can be titrated until pain is relieved or adverse effects occur (Ickowicz, 2009; Kaye et al., 2010; Mercadante & Arcuri, 2007).

The following guidelines are suggested for opioid use in older patients. The oral route is the preferred administration route with a strong recommendation to avoid intramuscular injections because of variability of medication uptake, potential for injection site abscess, and patient discomfort (Hanks-Bell et al., 2004). Patients with frequent or continual pain on a daily basis may be managed with around-the-clock opioid dosing aimed at achieving a steady state of the opiate medication. When using long-acting opioid medications, breakthrough pain should be anticipated, assessed, and prevented or treated using short-acting immediate release opioid medications (Ickowicz, 2009; Kaye et al., 2010). Additionally, a bowel regimen should be initiated with the use of scheduled and/or as needed opioids to prevent constipation, the most common adverse effect (Mercadante & Arcuri, 2007).

Maximal safe doses of acetaminophen or NSAIDs should not be exceeded when using fixed dose opioid combination agents, and when possible, these combination agents should be avoided with pure one agent opioid medications being preferred with separate use of acetaminophen and NSAIDs to avoid adverse effects (Ickowicz, 2009; Kaye et al., 2010). Potential opioid-induced adverse effects such as nausea, pruritus, constipation, respiratory depression, sedation, urinary retention, and myoclonus should be anticipated, assessed for, and treated as indicated to minimize the risk to the patient (Ickowicz, 2009; Kaye et al., 2010). If severe adverse effects persist beyond 24 to 48 hours and despite active treatment, an opioid rotation may be considered (Mercadante & Arcuri, 2007). Patients taking opiates should be reassessed for ongoing attainment of therapeutic goals, adverse effects, and safe and responsible medication use (Ickowicz, 2009; Kaye et al., 2010).

Morphine is a commonly used opioid and has been shown to be effective in comparison with oxycodone, hydromorphone, fentanyl, or methadone. Morphine has several active metabolites such as morphine-3-glucuronide (M3G), morphine-6-glucuronide (M6G), and normorphine that can contribute to neurotoxicity, especially in older adults with renal impairment (Pergolizzi et al., 2007). There are very few, if any, studies on the effects of the opioids on elders. Buprenorphine appears to provide effective analgesia regardless of age (Pergolizzi et al., 2007; Vadivelu & Hines, 2008). Methadone should be used with caution and only with experienced clinicians owing to the long half-life. Tramadol is a synthetic opioid that inhibits central reuptake of serotonin and norepinephrine and has been shown to be effective and well tolerated in elders. Tramadol should not be used in combination with monoamine oxidase inhibitors or selective serotonin reuptake inhibitors and may lower the patient's seizure threshold (Pergolizzi et al., 2011).

A common fear of opioid use is addiction, which is very rare in older patients (AGS, 2012; Kaye et al., 2010; Mercadante & Arcuri, 2007). Although providers should remain vigilant about the potential for misuse and abuse of opioids in all patients, older patients have a significantly lower risk of opioid misuse and abuse. Some research suggests that underuse of opioids is a major problem in older adults (AGS, 2012; Reid et al., 2011). Opioids are a vital element of a multimodal treatment strategy of minimizing pain among older adults and should not be avoided.

Adjuvants

Several medications developed for purposes other than pain have been found to be helpful in managing pain. These classes include antidepressants, anticonvulsants, and other agents that alter neural membrane potentials, ion channels, cell surface receptor sites, synaptic neurotransmitter levels, and other neuronal processes involved in pain signal processing. Patients with neuropathic pain, fibromyalgia, and refractory persistent pain (back pain, headaches) should be considered for adjuvant medications (Ickowicz, 2009). Tertiary tricyclic antidepressants such as amitriptyline, imipramine, and doxepin should be avoided due to high risk of anticholinergic effects and cognitive impairment (Ickowicz, 2009; Kaye et al., 2010; Mercadante & Arcuri, 2007).

Adjuvants may be used alone, but often their analgesic effects are improved with combinations of other pain medications and nonpharmacological approaches (AGS, 2012; Kaye et al., 2010; Mercadante & Arcuri, 2007). Providers should always start with the lowest possible dose and increase slowly, depending on response and adverse effects, with the understanding that some adjuvants have a delayed onset and therapeutic benefits are slow to develop; thus adequate trials should be allowed before discontinuation of seemingly ineffective treatment (AGS, 2012; Kaye et al., 2010; Mercadante & Arcuri, 2007). The American Geriatrics Society Panel on the Pharmacological Management of Persistent Pain in Older Persons has provided a comprehensive list of recommended medications for pain for the population of older adults (Ickowicz, 2009).

Nonpharmacological Interventions

Effective pain management involves a multimodal approach to treatment, including psychological interventions such as cognitive behavioral therapy and biofeedback for older patients (Ciampi et al., 2011; Davis & Srivastava, 2003; Halaszynski, 2009). Older adults have been shown to benefit from transcutaneous electrical nerve stimulation, massage, and application of heat and cold (Ciampi et al., 2011). Physical activity programs such as walking and aquatic therapy have also been shown to reduce pain, especially among patients suffering with chronic low back pain (Ciampi et al., 2011). Pain coping strategies may involve relaxation, prayer, music, pet therapy, and attention diversion strategies (Delacorte et al., 2011; Kaye et al., 2010). Interventional modalities such as nerve blocks, chemical neurolysis, radiofrequency lesioning, cryoneurolysis, neuroaugmentation, and neuraxial drug delivery may be helpful (Dalacorte et al., 2011; Kaye et al., 2010; Pautex et al., 2009). As indicated, surgical interventions such as joint replacements to alleviate the source of pain should be considered.

Cultural Considerations

It is accepted that ethnic groups express pain and suffering differently. For example, the Chinese culture maintains that pain is an essential component of life and is a trial or sacrifice that must be endured; thus individuals with this background may not report pain until it is unbearable. Furthermore, the Asian older patients may prefer Asian medicines and acupuncture instead of analgesics (Pasero & McCaffery, 2007). Owing to the numerous cultural and individual differences that clinicians may encounter, it is crucial to seek information from patients and family members regarding specific cultural beliefs and values for integration into a pain management plan. Teaching materials in the patient's own language should be sought as well as certified interpreters (Pasero & McCaffery, 2007). It is also important to note that studies reveal that African American, Asian, and Hispanic patients are less likely to be treated or undertreated for pain as compared with Caucasian patients (Bernabei et al., 1998; Pasero & McCaffery, 2007).

Prevention

Early identification of pain in the older population is key to minimizing suffering. Aggressive pain assessment and ongoing reassessment must be integrated into the routine interaction with older patients. In fact, if acute pain is managed early and aggressively, persistent pain can be either minimized or eliminated. Unfortunately, elders are undertreated owing to the many factors previously discussed, resulting in pain syndromes and other complications associated with pain. Additionally, pharmacological adverse effects can be minimized or avoided with a proactive approach that includes the initiation of a bowel regimen and close reassessment for these adverse effects. Polypharmacy should also be addressed early, thus minimizing potential adverse effects and potential complications such as falls.

Patient Education

The beliefs of older adults regarding pain, addiction, self-ability to manage one's pain, and psychological reactions to pain must be assessed for a tailored or individualized educational program (Edwards et al., 2011). Unfortunately, current studies suggest that patient education on medications such NSAIDs and opioids is not adequate, especially in the areas of side effects and the dangers of polypharmacy (Taylor et al., 2012). Education is an important aspect of self-management of one's pain and must involve caregivers and family members (Fitzcharles et al., 2010). It is crucial for clinicians to provide effective and culturally competent education for the older patients. If the cause of pain is known, education on progression as well as pharmacological and complementary treatment options should be shared. Patient education should include benefits and risks, anticipated adverse effects, prevention and management options, goals of care, costs, and resources available to assist with self-management of care (Fitzcharles et al., 2010; Mercadante & Arcuri, 2007).

Structured educational programs such as the Arthritis Foundation–sponsored educational program have been found to improve knowledge and compliance (Fitzcharlese et al., 2010). Enhanced communication between clinicians and patients, routine follow-up care, group education, and medication reviews by pharmacists along with individualized medication counseling by clinicians have been shown to improve compliance and pain control among the older adults (Kaye et al., 2010). Additionally, clinicians must be knowledgeable about pain assessment and mechanisms such as diagnoses, disease progression, medications, current research, and misperceptions of pain as part of the normal aging process among older adults (Hanks-Bell et al., 2004; Kean et al., 2008).

REFERENCES

Abad, V. C., Sarinas, P. S., & Guilleminault, C. (2008). Sleep and rheumatologic disorders. *Sleep Medicine Reviews, 12,* 211–228.

Ahmad, M., & Goucke, C. R. (2002). Management strategies for the treatment of neuropathic pain in the elderly. *Drugs & Aging, 19*(12), 929–945.

American Geriatrics Society. (2012). Statement on the use of opioids in the treatment of persistent pain in older adults. Retrieved from http://www.americangeriatrics.org/files/documents/Opioid_Statement_April_2012.pdf

American Society of Pain Management Nursing. (2010). *Core curriculum for pain management nursing* (2nd ed.). Dubuque, IA: Kendal Hunt Professional.

Aronoff, G., Brater, D. C., Schrier, R., & Bennett, W. M. (1994). Use of drugs in patients with renal insufficiency. Workshop report. *Blood Purification, 12,* 14–19.

Bellamy, N., Campbell, J., Robinson, V., Gee, T., Bourne, R., & Wells, G. (2006). Intraarticular corticosteroid for treatment of osteoarthritis of the knee. The Cochrane Collaboration. *Cochrane Database of Systematic Reviews,* (2), CD005328.

Bernabei, R., Gambassi, G., Lapane, K., Landi, F., Gatsonis, C., Dunlop, R., ... Mor, V. (1998). Management of pain in elderly patients with cancer. *Journal of the American Medical Association, 279*(23), 1877–1882.

Bitton, R. (2009). The economic burden of osteoarthritis. *American Journal of Managed Care, 15*, S230–S235.

Blumstein, H., & Gorevic, P. D. (2005). Rheumatologic illnesses: Treatment strategies for older adults. *Geriatrics, 60*(6), 28–35.

Buenaver, L. F., & Smith, M. T. (2008). Sleep in rheumatic diseases and other painful conditions. *Current Treatments Options in Neurology, 9*, 325–336.

Chodosh J., Solomon D. H., Roth C. P., Chang J. T., MacLean, C. H., Ferrell, B. A., ... Wenger, N. S. (2004). The quality of medical care provided to vulnerable older patients with chronic pain. *Journal of the American Geriatrics Society, 52*(5), 756.

Ciampi de Andrade, D., Vieira de Faria, J. W., Caramelli, P., Alverenga, L., Galhardoni, R., Siqueira, S. R., ... Teixeira, M. J. (2011). The assessment and management of pain in the demented and non-demented patient. *Arquivos de Neuro-psiquiatria, 69*(2B), 387–394.

Collyott, C. L., & Brooks, M. V. (2008). Evaluation and management of joint pain. *Orthopaedic Nursing, 27*(4), 246–250.

Dalacorte, R. R., Rigo, J. C., & Dalacorte, A. (2011). Pain management in the elderly at the end of life. *North American Journal of Medical Sciences, 3*(8), 348–354.

Davis, M. P., & Srivastava, M. (2003). Demographics, assessment and management of pain in the elderly. *Drugs & Aging, 20*(1), 23–57.

De Leonardis, F., Govoni, M., Colina, M., Bruschi, M., & Trotta, F. (2007). Elderly-onset gout: A review. *Rheumatology International, 28*(1), 1–6.

Edwards, R. R., Cahalan, C., Mensing, G., Smith, M., & Haythornthwaite, J. A. (2011). Pain catastrophizing, and depression in the rheumatic diseases. *Nature Reviews Rheumatology, 7*, 216–224.

El-Zawawy, H., & Mandell, B. (2010). Managing gout: How is it different in patients with chronic kidney disease? *Cleveland Clinic Journal of Medicine, 77*(12), 919–928.

Ene-Stroescu, D., & Gorbien, M. J. (2005). Gouty arthritis: A primer on late-onset gout. *Geriatrics, 60*(7), 24–31.

Fitzcharles, M. A., Lussier, D., & Shir, Y. (2010). Management of chronic arthritis pain in the elderly. *Drugs & Aging, 27*(6), 471–490.

Gutman, A. B. (1973). The past four decades of progress in the knowledge of gout, with an assessment of the present status. *Arthritis & Rheumatism, 16*, 431–445.

Halaszynski, T. M. (2009). Pain management in the elderly and cognitively impaired patient: The role of regional anesthesia and analgesia. *Current Opinion in Anesthesiology, 22*, 594–599.

Hanks-Bell, M., Halvey, K., & Paice, J. A. (2004). Pain assessment and management in aging. *Online Journal of Issues in Nursing.* http://www.nursingworld.org/MainMenuCategories/ANAMarketplace/ANAPeriodicals/OJIN/TableofContents/Volume92004/No3Sept04/ArticlePreviousTopic/PainAssessmentandManagementinAging.html

Hunter, D. J. (2011). Lower extremity osteoarthritis management needs a paradigm shift. *British. Journal of Sports Medicine, 45*(4), 283–288.

Ickowicz, E. (2009). American geriatrics society panel on pharmacological management of persistent pain in older persons. *Journal of the American Geriatrics Society, 57*, 1331–1346.

Institute of Medicine of the National Academies. (2011, June). Relieving pain in America: A blueprint for transforming prevention, care, education, and research. Retrieved from http://www.iom.edu/~/media/files/report%20files/2011/relieving-pain-in-america-a-blueprint-for-transforming-prevention-care-education-research/pain%20research%202011%20report%20brief.pdf

International Association for the Study of Pain. (2012). Retrieved from http://www.iasp-pain.org/AM/Template.cfm?Section=Pain_Definitions&Template=/CM/HTMLDisplay.cfm&ContentID=1728

John H. Klippel. Primer on the Rheumatic diseases. Thirteenth Edition. Publisher Springer.

Kaye, A. D., Baluch, A., & Scott, J. T. (2010). Pain management in the elderly population: A review. *Ochsner Journal, 10*, 179–187.

Kean, W. F., Rainsford, K. D., & Kean, I. R. L. (2008). Management of chronic musculoskeletal pain in the elderly: Opinions on oral medication use. *Inflammopharmacology, 16*(2), 53–75.

Kelly's Textbook of Rheumatology Vol 1&2. Eight edition. Publisher Saunders.

Kivitz, A., Fairfax, M., Sheldon, E. A., Xiang, Q., Jones, B. A., Gammaitoni, A. R., & Gould, E. M. (2008). Comparison of the effectiveness and tolerability of lidocaine patch 5% versus celecoxib for osteoarthritis-related knee pain: Post hoc analysis of a 12 week, prospective, randomized, active-controlled, open-label, parallel-group trial in adults. *Clinical Therapeutics, 30*(12), 2366–2377.

Majitha, V., Peel, C., & Geraci, S. A. (2009). Rheumatoid arthritis in elderly patients. *Geriatrics, 64*(9), 22–28.

Mercadante, S., & Arcuri, E. (2007). Pharmacological management of cancer pain in the elderly. *Drugs & Aging, 25*(9), 761–776.

Mitchell, C. (2001). Assessment and management of chronic pain in elderly people. *British Journal of Nursing, 10*(5), 296–304.

Neogi, T. (2011). Clinical practice. Gout. *New England Journal of Medicine, 364*(5), 443–452.

Pasero, C., & McCaffery, M. (2007). *Pain assessment and pharmacologic management.* St. Louis, MO: Elsevier.

Pautex, S., Herrmann, F. R., Le Lous, P., & Gold, G. (2009). Improving pain management in elderly patients with dementia: Validation of the Doloshort observational pain assessment scale. *Age and Ageing, 38*(6), 754–757.

Pergolizzi, J., Boger, R. H., Budd, K., Dahan, A., Erdine, S., Hans, G., … Sacerdote, P. (2007). Opioids and the management of chronic severe pain in the elderly: Consensus statement of an International Expert Panel with focus on the six clinically most often used World Health Organization step III opioids (buprenorphine, fentanyl, hydromorphone, methadone, morphine, oxycodone). *Pain Practice: Official Journal of World Institute of Pain, 8*(4), 287–313.

Peterson, E. L. (2007). Fibromyalgia: Management of a misunderstood disorder. *Journal of the American Academy of Nurse Practitioners, 19*(7), 341–348.

Ranganath, V., & Furst, D. (2007). Disease-modifying antirheumatic drug use in the elderly rheumatoid arthritis patients. *Rheumatic Disease Clinics of North America, 33*, 197–217.

Rao, A., & Cohen, J. (2004). Symptom management in the elderly cancer patient: Fatigue, pain and depression. *Journal of the National Cancer Institute Monographs,* (32), 150–157.

Raynauld, J. P., Buckland-Wright, C., Ward, R., Choquette, D., Haraoui, B., … Pelletier, J. P. (2003). Safety and efficacy of long-term intraarticular steroid injection in osteoarthritis of the knee: A randomized, double-blind, placebo-controlled trial. *Arthritis & Rheumatism, 48*(2), 370–377.

Reid, M. C., Bennett, D. A., Chen, W. G., Eldadah, B. A., Farrar, J. T., Ferrell, B., … Zacharoff, K. L. (2011). Improving the pharmacologic management of pain in older adults: Identifying the research gaps and methods to address them. *Pain Medicine: Official Journal of World Institute of Pain, 12*(9), 1336–1357.

Richette, P., & Bardin, T. (2010). Colchicine for the treatment of gout. *Expert Opinion on Pharmacotherapy, 11*(17), 2933–2938.

Roddy, E., & Doherty, M. (2010). Gout. Epidemiology of gout. *Arthritis Research & Therapy, 12*, 223.

Saag, K. G., & Choi, H. (2006). Epidemiology, risk factors, and lifestyle modifications for gout. *Arthritis Research & Therapy, 8*(Suppl. 1), S2.

Saag, K., Teng, G. G., Patkar, N. M., Anuntiyo, J., Finney, C., Curtis, J. R., … American College of Rheumatology. (2008). American College of Rheumatology 2008 recommendations for the use of nonbiologic and biologic disease-modifying antirheumatic drugs in rheumatoid arthritis. *Arthritis Care & Research, 59*(6), 762–784.

Sauaia, A., Min, S., Leber, C., Erbacher, K., Abrams, F., & Fink, R. (2005). Postoperative pain management in elderly patients: Correlation between adherence to treatment guidelines and patient satisfaction. *Journal of the American Geriatrics Society, 53*(2), 274–282.

Schumacher, H. R., Boice, J. A., Daikh, D. I., Mukhopadhyay, S., Malmstrom, K., Ng, J., … Molina, J. (2002). Randomised double blind trial of etoricoxib and indomethacin in treatment of acute gouty arthritis. *British Medical Journal, 324*, 1488–1492.

Seed, S. M., Dunican, K. C., & Lynch, A. M. (2011). Treatment options for osteoarthritis: Considerations for older adults. *Hospital Practice, 39*(1), 62–73.

Silverstein, F. E., Faich, G., Goldstein, J. L., Simon, L. S., Pincus, T., Whelton, A., … Geis, G. S. (2000). Gastrointestinal toxicity with celecoxib vs nonsteroidal anti-inflammatory drugs for osteoarthritis and rheumatoid arthritis: The CLASS study: A randomized controlled trial. Celecoxib Long-term Arthritis Safety Study. *Journal of the American Medical Association, 284*(10), 1247–1255.

Sun, B. H., Wu, C. W., & Kalunian, K. C. (2007). New developments in osteoarthritis. *Rheumatic Disease Clinics of North America, 33*, 135–148.

Taylor, R., Lemtouni, S., Weiss, K., & Pergolizzi, J. V. (2012). Pain management in the elderly: An FDA safe use initiative expert panel's view on preventable harm associated with NSAID therapy. *Current Gerontology and Geriatrics Research.* doi:10.1155/2012/196159

Tutuncu, Z., & Kavanaugh, A. (2005). Rheumatic disease in the elderly: Rheumatoid arthritis. *Clinics in Geriatric Medicine, 21*(3), 513–525.

Tutuncu, Z., & Kavanaugh, A. (2007). Rheumatic disease in the elderly: Rheumatoid arthritis. *Rheumatic Disease Clinics of North America, 33*, 57–70.

Vadivelu, N., & Hines, R. L. (2008). Management of chronic pain in the elderly: Focus on transdermal buprenorphine. *Journal of Clinical Interventions in Aging, 3*(3), 421–430.

Vanhoof, J., Declerck, K., & Geusens, P. (2002). Prevalence of rheumatic diseases in a rheumatological outpatient practice. *Annals of the Rheumatic Diseases, 61*, 453–455.

Vázquez-Mellado, J., Cruz, J., Guzmán, S., Casasola-Vargas, J., Lino, L., & Burgos-Vargas R. (2006). Severe tophaceous gout. Characterization of low socioeconomic level patients from México. *Clinical and Experimental Rheumatology, 24*(3), 233–238.

Wise, C. (2007). Crystal-associated arthritis in the elderly. *Rheumatic Disease Clinics of North America, 33*, 33–55.

Zhang, W., Doherty, M., Bardin, T., Pascual, E., Barskova, V., Conaghan, P., … Zimmermann-Gòrska, I. (2006). EULAR evidence based recommendations for gout. Part II: Management. Report of a task force of the EULAR Standing Committee for International Clinical Studies Including Therapeutics (ESCISIT). *Annals of the Rheumatic Diseases, 65*(10), 1312–1324.

CHAPTER 13: IT RESOURCES

Websites

American College of Rheumatology
　http://www.rheumatology.org/practice/clinical/patients/index.asp
Arthritis Foundation
　http://www.arthritis.org/
Arthritis Today
　http://www.arthritistoday.org/
Arthritis.com
　http://www.arthritis.com/
The PubMed Health references below include causes, incidence, risk factors, symptoms, signs and tests, treatment, medications, preventions, and references.
Osteoarthritis from PubMed Health
　http://www.ncbi.nlm.nih.gov/pubmedhealth/PMH0001460/
Gout from PubMed Health
　http://www.ncbi.nlm.nih.gov/pubmedhealth/PMH0001459/
Rheumatoid Arthritis from PubMed Health
　http://www.ncbi.nlm.nih.gov/pubmedhealth/PMH0001467/
The Mayo Clinic references below include definitions, symptoms, causes, risk factors, complications, tests and diagnosis, treatments and drugs, alternative medicines, and prevention.
Osteoarthritis from Mayo Clinic
　http://www.mayoclinic.com/health/osteoarthritis/DS00019/
Gout from Mayo Clinic
　http://www.mayoclinic.com/health/gout/DS00090
Rheumatoid Arthritis from Mayo Clinic
　http://www.mayoclinic.com/health/rheumatoid-arthritis/DS00020/tab=InDepth
Osteoarthritis from MedicineNet.com
　http://www.medicinenet.com/osteoarthritis/article.htm
Gout Pictures Slideshow taken from MedicineNet.com
　http://www.medicinenet.com/gout_pictures_slideshow/article.htm
Rheumatoid Arthritis Pictures Slideshow taken from MedicineNet.com
　http://www.medicinenet.com/rheumatoid_arthritis_pictures_slideshow/article.htm
Osteoarthritis Pictures Slideshow taken from MedicineNet.com
　http://www.medicinenet.com/osteoarthritis_overview_pictures_slideshow/article.htm
International Association for the Study of Pain
　http://www.iasp-pain.org

American Nurse Today—Managing Chronic Pain in the Elderly
  http://www.americannursetoday.com/article.aspx?id=7084
When Seniors have Chronic Pain
  http://pain.about.com/od/whatischronicpain/a/elderly_and_pain.htm
WebMD—Treating Pain in the Elderly
  http://www.webmd.com/pain-management/treating-pain-elderly
American Geriatrics Society—Pharmacological Management of Persistent Pain in Older Persons
  http://www.americangeriatrics.org/health_care_professionals/clinical_practice/
  clinical_guidelines_recommendations/persistent_pain_executive_summary/
Nursing Standard of Practice Protocol: Pain Management in Older Adults
  http://consultgerirn.org/topics/pain/want_to_know_more

PDF Documents

Office Management of Chronic Pain in the Elderly
  http://geriatricsrotation.uchicago.edu/internal/documents/Chronicpain.pdf
The International Association for the Study of Pain—Facts on Pain in Older Persons
  http://www.iasp-pain.org/AM/Template.cfm?Section=2006_2007_Pain_in_Older_
  Persons1&Template=/CM/ContentDisplay.cfm&ContentID=3611
Adult Measures of Pain: The McGill Pain Questionnaire (MPQ), Rheumatoid Arthritis Pain
  Scale (RAPS), Short-Form McGill Pain Questionnaire (SF-MPQ), Verbal Descriptive Scale
  (VDS), Visual Analog Scale (VAS), and West Haven-Yale Multidisciplinary Pain Inventory
  (WHYMPI)
  http://onlinelibrary.wiley.com/doi/10.1002/art.11440/pdf
McGill Pain Questionnaire
  http://www.ama-cmeonline.com/pain_mgmt/pdf/mcgill.pdf
The Assessment of Discomfort in Dementia
  http://prc.coh.org/PainNOA/ADD_D.pdf

Videos

Rheumatoid Arthritis (2008) (3:53 minutes)
  http://youtu.be/0uwx64YaxSk
Rheumatoid Arthritis: Part 1 (2008) (28:41 minutes)
  http://youtu.be/djZfEi-ztVQ
Chronic Rheumatoid Arthritis in the Knee taken from About.com (1:42 minutes)
  http://video.about.com/arthritis/Chronic-Rheumatism-Knee.htm
Osteoarthritis taken from MedlinePlus (2012)
  http://www.nlm.nih.gov/medlineplus/ency/anatomyvideos/000092.htm
Gout: Patrick's Story (2010) (1:59 minutes)
  http://www.nhs.uk/conditions/Gout/Pages/Introduction.aspx
Body Invaders: Gout (2009) (3:23 minutes)
  http://youtu.be/YVYvM4BhQBE
Assessing Chronic Pain in the Cognitively Impaired (2012) (1:30 minutes)
  http://youtu.be/g13gKXuYQSw

Seniors and Chronic Pain (3 minutes)
   http://youtu.be/2HgVAH5pf50
New Pain Guidelines for the Elderly (2 minutes)
   http://youtu.be/HVZbXHgteyA
Pain and Suffering in the Elderly Parts 1 to 4 (15 minutes each), Charlotta Eaton, MD (2011)
   http://youtu.be/dC7e1zcuZyA
   http://youtu.be/bhuuFYXvmCU
   http://youtu.be/7XYOyidX_Ng
   http://youtu.be/xs_p-8aJJDs

Images

Google images of Osteoarthritis
   http://www.google.com/search?q=osteoarthritis&hl=en&rlz=1T4ADFA_enUS417US433&
   prmd=imvns&source=lnms&tbm=isch&sa=X&ei=pCgQUNvMB4X20gG95YDgDw&ved=
   0CEwQ_AUoAQ&biw=853&bih=529
Google images of Gout
   http://www.google.com/search?q=gout&source=lnms&tbm=isch&sa=X&ei=m6mnUYysB8rh
   0QHgnICQDg&sqi=2&ved=0CAcQ_AUoAQ&biw=1024&bih=564
Google images of Rheumatoid Arthritis
   http://www.google.com/search?q=rheumatoid+arthritis&source=lnms&tbm=isch&sa=X&ei=
   5amnUdKNKZC40AHO7IHQDA&sqi=2&ved=0CAcQ_AUoAQ&biw=1024&bih=564
Google images of Pain and Older Adults
   http://www.google.com/search?q=pain+and+older+adult&source=lnms&tbm=isch&sa=X&ei=
   BKqnUdvmHJK00AGOuYGQAQ&ved=0CAcQ_AUoAQ&biw=1024&bih=564

Kidney Disease

Jill Bass, DNP, RN, GCNS-BC
Aubrey L. Knight, MD

INTRODUCTION

With aging, each organ system faces senescent changes; the urogenital system is no exception. From the increased prevalence of infections of the urinary tract to the ever-increasing average age at which individuals undergo renal replacement therapy, primary care and geriatric providers, on a daily basis, are faced with dealing with disorders of the urogenital system. Currently, nearly 50% of patients on hemodialysis are older than 65 years. The prevalence of the two primary diseases that lead to End Stage Renal Disease (ESRD), hypertension and diabetes mellitus (DM), increases substantially with age. In addition, anatomic and physiological changes in the urogenital system increase the likelihood of urinary incontinence (UI) and urinary tract infections.

In this chapter, we will discuss chronic kidney disease (CKD) and UI. Urinary tract infections will be discussed in the chapter dedicated to infectious diseases. CKD and UI are not only prevalent but also expensive. According to the United States Renal Data Set 2011 Annual Report, 8.5% of Medicare beneficiaries aged 65 and over have recognized CKD (United States Renal Data Set, n.d.). This percentage rises to 12.8% among African Americans. In 2009, Medicare expenditures for persons with CKD totaled $34 billion, representing 6.4% of the entire Medicare budget. The data on UI are less clear as this is often a problem that does not come to the attention of the health care or health insurance industries. It is estimated that 25% to 30% of US adults will experience UI at some point in their lives. Older adults with UI have greater individual annual health care costs compared with nonincontinent persons of similar age (Griebling, 2009), and the presence of UI is associated with a dramatic reduction in overall and health-related quality of life in older adults (Ko et al., 2005). The most recent estimate of societal cost, including diagnosis, treatment, and purchase of absorbent products, is based on 2000 information and was estimated to be $14 billion. The actual number is likely much higher.

CHRONIC KIDNEY DISEASE

Definition and Staging

According to the National Kidney Foundation, one in nine Americans have kidney disease (National Kidney Foundation [NKF], n.d.). Because the disease is relatively symptom free until late in the disease, the majority do not know they have the disease. The prevalence of CKD increases with increasing age.

The Aging Kidney

The aging kidney decreases in size accompanied by several anatomic changes. There is glomerular hypertrophy and focal or segmental glomerulosclerosis. In addition, tubules show evidence of atrophy and dilatation with an increased number of tubular diverticulae. These diverticulae are thought to play a role in the increased incidence of urinary tract infections in the older adult as bacteria can be harbored in the diverticulae (Lindeman & Goldman, 1986). There is renal arteriolar hyalinosis and other forms of aging vascular changes similar to those found in other organ systems. These anatomic changes result in an inevitable decline in renal function with aging. While serum creatinine does not decline with age, more accurate measures of renal function show a progressive decline in renal function after age 40. Sodium balance is also altered with age; this alteration along with the Western diet that is high in sodium partially accounts for the high prevalence of hypertension in the older adult.

Acute Kidney Injury and Reversibility

Acute kidney injury (AKI) is the rapid loss of kidney function over a short period, and it leads to the accumulation of toxins and waste products as well as dysregulation in electrolyte balance. Older adults are very susceptible to AKI for a variety of reasons, including sepsis, dehydration, medications, and trauma. AKI is associated with increased morbidity and mortality, especially in the older adult (Schmitt et al., 2008). AKI is defined by increases in creatinine to levels as little as 1.5 times the baseline creatinine, and even increases that small are associated with functional or morphologic alterations in the kidney (Khalil et al., 2008). The causes of AKI can be conveniently divided into prerenal cause, intrinsic renal causes, and postrenal causes.

Prerenal AKI

Prerenal AKI is due to renal hypoperfusion and is classically caused by hypovolemia or as a result of blood loss, sepsis as a result of insensible losses, heart failure, or liver failure. Medications such as nonsteroidal anti-inflammatory drugs (NSAIDs) and angiotensin-converting enzyme inhibitors/angiotensin II receptor blockers (ACEIs/ARBs) are also implicated in prerenal AKI.

Intrinsic AKI

Intrinsic AKI is a condition due to direct injury to the kidney and is further categorized on the basis of the predominant location of the injury. There are four broad categories of intrinsic AKI: acute tubular necrosis (ATN), acute interstitial nephritis (AIN), glomerulonephritis, and acute vascular disorders with direct damage to the kidney.

Acute Tubular Necrosis (ATN).   ATN is the most common form of AKI. Conditions leading to ATN include sepsis, dehydration, perioperative hypotension, especially in the setting of cardiac or vascular surgery, severe hemolysis, rhabdomyolysis, and the direct toxic effects of medications or contrast media. The most commonly encountered medications that can cause ATN include aminoglycosides, amphotericin B, and chemotherapeutic drugs such as cisplatin. Contrast-induced nephrotoxicity (CIN) is a frequently encountered cause of ATN in older adults. In addition to age, the risk of CIN increases with volume depletion, concomitant DM, and volume of contrast administered. The primary means of preventing CIN include minimizing the amount of contrast and assuring good hydration status before and during interventions that require contrast.

ATN is the result of ischemic injury to the tubular epithelial cells with resulting apoptosis and necrosis. Clinically, there may be anuria or oliguria with elevation in the blood urea nitrogen (BUN) and creatinine.

Acute Interstitial Necrosis (AIN).   The classic triad of fever, rash, and eosinophilia accompanied by sterile pyuria, WBC casts, hematuria, and proteinuria are the hallmark findings in AIN. Hypersensitivity to medications is the most common cause of AIN. Antibiotics, specifically penicillins, cephalosporins, and sulfonamides, and NSAIDs are the most frequently encountered culprits. Treatment consists of discontinuation of the offending drug with return to normal renal function and resolution in proteinuria in weeks to months.

Acute Glomerulonephritis.   AKI from glomerulonephritis occurs from a variety of causes. When secondary to infections, prognosis is generally good, even in the older patient. Other progressive forms of glomerulonephritis carry a poor prognosis and often lead to renal failure. In addition to laboratory evidence of renal failure, there is acute hypertension, hematuria, proteinuria, and red blood cell casts. Serologic studies reveal elevations in various acute phase reactants. Kidney biopsy is often needed to confirm the diagnosis.

Acute Renal Vascular Disease.   AKI can be caused by renal artery thromboembolism, renal vein thrombosis, renal artery dissection, or diffuse renal vascular atherosclerosis. The first three are large vessel disease and often present with acute flank pain, hematuria, oliguria, and elevated serum lactate dehydrogenase. Diffuse renal vascular atherosclerosis is a more insidious disorder and often progresses in an asymptomatic manner. It is also more common in older adults and is less likely to be reversible.

Postrenal AKI

Postrenal AKI due to bladder outlet obstruction is common, especially in older men due to benign prostatic hyperplasia (BPH), and can result in diminished renal function. Postrenal AKI may present with anuria (complete obstruction) or oliguria (partial obstruction). In addition to BPH, causes of postrenal AKI include nephrolithiasis, pelvic neoplasms, retroperitoneal masses, urethral strictures, bladder messes or neurogenic bladder.

Evaluation and Treatment of AKI

The first step in the evaluation of AKI is to categorize properly the condition as prerenal, intrinsic, or postrenal. Serum chemistries and urinalysis are to include urine sediment evaluation, urine

TABLE 14.1 • Differential Findings in AKI

Measure	Prerenal	Intrinsic	Postrenal
BUN/Creatinine	>20:1	<15:1	Nonspecific
Urine osmolality	>500	<350	Nonspecific
Urine sodium	<20	>40	Nonspecific
Urine microscopy	Nonspecific	Epithelial cells or casts	Nonspecific
Postvoid residual	Low or normal	Low or normal	Elevated (>150 ml)

chemistries (sodium and creatinine), and evaluation of bladder volume either with insertion of a urinary catheter or bladder sonogram. Table 14.1 details the differentiating findings.

When AKI is due to prerenal causes, prompt volume repletion and discontinuation of medications or toxins causing the renal failure will often return renal function to normal. The challenge with prerenal AKI occurs when there is concomitant heart or liver failure, which requires extra care in managing the volume status.

Once intrinsic AKI is identified, the clinician needs to classify the condition further so as to know how to progress with therapy. In general, supportive therapy and removal of potential inciting agents form the primary interventions. While corticosteroid use is controversial with AIN, it is a mainstay in treating acute glomerulonephritis. In addition, immunosuppressive therapy and plasmapheresis might be of benefit in certain causes of glomerulonephritis. In addition to these supportive and therapeutic options, renal replacement therapy with intermittent hemodialysis or peritoneal dialysis might be necessary.

Treatment of postrenal AKI consists of rapid relief of obstruction with bladder catheter for lower tract disease and ureteral stents or percutaneous nephrostomy tubes for upper tract processes. Careful monitoring of the fluid status and electrolytes is necessary.

Prognosis/Reversibility

AKI in the older adult is associated with increased morbidity and mortality. While renal function recovery is possible, a recent meta-analysis suggests that 31% of older individuals with AKI failed to recover renal function (Schmitt et al., 2008). Older patients with AKI, even if there seems to be recovery in renal function, should be followed very closely and should be considered at high risk for recurrent AKI. The 2-year mortality rate in the older patient with AKI is 29% (Ishani et al., 2009).

Stages of CKD

CKD is defined as the presence of structural or functional abnormalities of the kidney with or without laboratory evidence of a reduction in glomerular filtration rate (GFR). The staging nomenclature was developed several years ago by the National Kidney Foundation for use in communication, clinical practice, and research. The staging is based on known kidney disease and the estimated glomerular filtration rate (eGFR). Most laboratories now report the eGFR based on the serum creatinine and mathematical formulae. The gold standard is to measure directly the GFR by measuring insulin clearance. This is both time consuming and impractical. There are three calculations that can be employed. The Cockcroft–Gault equation (CGE) is the most commonly employed. This calculation tends to overestimate GFR. A more accurate estimate of GFR can be obtained using the modification of diet in renal disease (MDRD) equation. The MDRD equation and may give a falsely elevated GFR as a result of fluctuations in fluid balance. The most accurate calculation is the Chronic Kidney Disease Epidemiology Collaboration (CKD-EPI) formula. The CKD-EPI formula is extremely complicated; the result can be easily obtained using a Web-based calculator found at: http://www.nephron.com/MDRD_GFR.cgi. The Cockcroft–Gault eGFR and MDRD formulae are as follows:

$$\text{Cockcroft–Gault eGFR} = \frac{(140 - \text{age}) \times (\text{Wt in kg}) \times (0.85 \text{ if female})}{72 \times S_{cr}}$$

MDRD eGFR $= 186 \times (S_{cr})^{-1.154} \times (\text{age})^{-0.203} \times 1.212$ (if the patient is black) $\times 0.742$ (if the patient is female)

While these can be calculated personally, there are multiple Web-based calculators available to plug in the variables and obtain an eGFR. As the formulae indicate, normal GFR varies with age, sex, and size. The peak GFR is 120 to 130 ml/minute/1.73 m^2 in young adults and decreases by approximately 1 ml/minute/1.73 m^2/year after age 30 (NKF, 2002).

As we will discuss in more detail later, the National Kidney Foundation and other organizations employ the classification to guide preventive and treatment strategies. Table 14.2 gives the criteria for and some characteristics of the various stages. Markers of kidney damage include proteinuria, microalbuminuria, persistent hematuria, and cellular casts.

Cultural Considerations

While hypertension and DM have a slightly higher prevalence in certain ethnic minorities, ethnic and racial minority status does not significantly increase the risk of CKD in persons with these diseases who are older than 60 (Vassalotti et al., 2007).

TABLE 14.2 · Stages of CKD

Stage	Description	eGFR[a]/ACR[b]	ICD-9/ICD-10
1	Kidney damage with normal or increased GFR	≥90/≥30[c]	585.1/N18.1
2	Kidney damage with mildly decreased GFR	60–89/≥30[c]	585.2/N18.2
3	Moderately decreased GFR	30–59	585.3/N18.3
4	Severely decreased GFR	15–20	585.4/N18.4
5	Kidney failure	<15	585.5/N18.5

[a]Estimated Glomerular Filtration Rate (MDRD formula):
GFR $= 186 \times (S_{cr})^{-1.154} \times (\text{age})^{-0.203} \times 1.212$ (if patient is black) $\times 0.742$ (if patient is female).
[b]Urinary albumin/creatinine ratio.
[c]Plus presence of markers of kidney damage.

Screening and Risk Factors

Screening and Surveillance Guidelines

While routine screening with urinalysis, serum creatinine to estimate GFR, or urine albumin/creatinine ratio to detect proteinuria are not recommended for healthy adults, annual screening for CKD is recommended by the American Diabetes Association (ADA, 2011) for diabetics, by the National Kidney Foundation for those at risk (Kidney Disease Outcomes Quality Initiative, 2007), by the Joint National Committee on Hypertension for patients with hypertension (Chobanian et al., 2003), and the American Heart Association for patients with cardiovascular disease (Brosius et al., 2006). The US Preventive Services Task Force concludes that "evidence is insufficient to balance the benefits and harms of routine screening for CKD in asymptomatic adults (Moyer, 2012).

The serum creatinine is an insensitive measure of kidney function, especially in the older adult and those with low body mass. Most laboratories will provide an eGFR with routine chemistry profiles.

Proteinuria can be an indicator of kidney disease. Dipstick protein indicators are insensitive measures of proteinuria and should not be employed as a form of CKD screening. If a dipstick protein is positive, it should be repeated and if persistent should lead to more accurate tests determining the proteinuria. The urinary protein/creatinine ratio is the better indicator of proteinuria and should be less than 200 mg/g. A protein/creatinine ratio of greater than 3,000 mg/g is indicative of nephritic syndrome, the most common cause of which is diabetes.

The urinary albumin/creatinine ratio is the measurement that can lead to the diagnosis of microalbuminuria. The normal albumin/creatinine ratio is less than 30 mg/g, meaning patients with albumin/creatinine ratios between 30 and 300 mg/g are classified as having microalbuminuria. Those with ratios greater than 300 mg/g are classified as having macroalbuminuria. As indicated in Table 14.2, microalbuminuria is the abnormality that most often defines stages 1 and 2 CKD.

Diabetes

Diabetic nephropathy is most often defined by the presence of protein. Diabetics who progress from micro- to macroalbuminuria have an increased likelihood of developing ESRD. Data from 2006 reveal that diabetes was the most common cause of ESRD in North America and accounted for 44.4% of cases (United States Renal Data System [USRDS], 2008). The rates are increasing and at an alarming rate in the population over age 65. Despite this, surveillance, preventive measures, and CKD care is suboptimal. Pathologically and clinically, there is no difference in the diabetic nephropathy of those with type 2 DM and type 1 DM. The injury is noted in the renal parenchyma as well as the vasculature. Patients with DM who develop diabetic nephropathy will do so within 5 to 10 years of diagnosis depending on the time of diagnosis and the medical attention. This time may be shortened in persons with late onset type 2 DM, likely secondary to kidney senescence (Zhou et al., 2007). The American Diabetes Association recommends an annual test to assess albumin excretion starting at diagnosis in all type 2 diabetics and starting at the fifth year after diagnosis for type 1 diabetics. In addition, in their Executive Summary: Standards of Medical Care in Diabetes (2012), they recommend yearly estimates of GFR in order to stage the level of CKD.

Hypertension

CKD is a major comorbidity among older patients with hypertension. Data from the National Health and Nutrition Examination Survey indicate that 77% of persons over the age of 60 have both conditions. Hypertension is an independent risk factor for the development of CKD. Blood pressure should be measured with each encounter and at least yearly. The Seventh Joint National Committee on Prevention, Detection, Evaluation, and Treatment of High Blood Pressure (JNC 7) has defined criteria for classification of hypertension (Chobian et al., 2003). Hypertension is defined as a blood pressure of greater than 140/90 with prehypertension defined as a blood pressure greater than 120/80. Once the diagnosis is confirmed, lifestyle modification with or without treatment is aimed at lowering the blood pressure to normal ranges in an effort to minimize the complications. As with diabetes, the eGFR should be determined in order to determine and classify the level of CKD.

Other Risk Factors

Although DM and hypertension are the most common causes of CKD, there are other risk factors. The most common conditions, other than diabetes and hypertension that increase the likelihood of developing CKD, include autoimmune disease, exposure to certain toxins (lead, cadmium, arsenic, mercury) or drugs (aminoglycosides, NSAIDs, contrast medium), nephrolithiasis, and recurrent urinary tract infections.

Prevention

The prevention of CKD begins with recognition of and appropriate screening for the risk factors. In individuals identified as being at risk, lifestyle modifications and surveillance should be undertaken. Diabetics should strive for blood sugar and HbA1C control, and patients with hypertension toward blood pressure control. Patients placed on potentially nephrotoxic medications or who undergo studies with contrast media should follow kidney damage preventive instructions. Once CKD has been identified, measures to prevent progression to higher stages of CKD should be undertaken. Table 14.3 details some of the strategies to be undertaken.

Presentation

Initial Presentation

CKD is typically a silent condition on presentation. The diagnosis usually occurs in the process of the standard guidelines for care in the two major conditions that pose a risk to progression to CKD, DM, and hypertension. Occasionally, and most likely in patients who have renal trauma or who have been exposed to nephrotoxic substances, patients will present with signs and symptoms of AKI. Once the AKI is reversed, there may be evidence of CKD. AKI can present with decreased or absent urine output possibly accompanied by mental slowing or frank delirium and edema. When AKI is identified, there may be other symptoms present that serve to assist in identifying the potential cause of the renal insufficiency. For instance, AKI in the presence of acute or chronic back pain might lead the clinician to consider multiple myeloma or renal/extrarenal masses.

TABLE 14.3 • Strategies for Management Aimed at Prevention of Progression of CKD

Stage	Management
1	Quantify proteinuria Manage BP—goal <130/80 mm Hg Initiate ACEI or ARB
2	Consider statins Tight glucose control (in diabetics)-HbA1C <7
3	Screen for anemia Screen for calcium, phosphorus, and PTH abnormalities Monitor electrolytes and albumin Aggressively manage lipids
4	Manage BP, glucose, lipid levels, anemia, calcium/phosphorus status Monitor nutrition, electrolyte balance, and fluid status Prepare for dialysis or transplantation
5	Initiate dialysis

Work-up of New Onset CKD

We have previously discussed the suggested work-up and surveillance plan for patients with diabetes and hypertension who have or are at risk for developing CKD. In patients who do not have these two conditions, it is the clinician's task to determine not only the stage of the CKD but also the underlying condition that led to the kidney damage. The work-up should, therefore, include a careful history and review of systems, paying particular attention to the family history, presence of recent infections or rash, and any symptoms during urination. On physical examination, the clinician should pay particular attention to the following:

- Ophthalmoscopic exam looking for hypertensive or diabetic retinal disease.
- Cardiovascular exam looking for carotid or abdominal bruits, evidence of ventricular hypertrophy, edema, diminished peripheral pulses.
- Abdominal exam looking for bladder distension or abdominal or flank tenderness.
- Musculoskeletal exam looking for arthritic changes or synovitis.
- Skin exam looking for a rash or skin changes indicative of an autoimmune disease.

An initial laboratory evaluation might include:

- Comprehensive metabolic profile—in order to get the eGFR as well as the baseline hepatic function and electrolytes.
- CBC—looking for evidence of an infection or the presence of anemia or eosinophilia.
- Serum or urine electrophoresis if amyloidosis or multiple myelomas are suspected.
- Serum complement C3 and C4 if suspicious for poststreptococcal or membranoproliferative glomerulonephritis.

Other more specific serologic tests and the conditions a positive result might indicate are detailed in Table 14.4. Imaging studies such as renal ultrasound or abdominal computed tomography might be indicated depending upon the clinical situation.

TABLE 14.4 · Chronic Renal Conditions Associated with Abnormal Lab Tests

Abnormal Laboratory Test	Condition
Abnormal serum or urine electrophoresis	Light chain deposition disease Multiple myeloma Amyloidosis
Decreased serum complement C3 or C4	Poststreptococcal glomerulonephritis Membranoproliferative glomerulonephritis Lupus nephritis
Positive Antinuclear Antibody (ANA)	Lupus nephritis
Positive antiglomerular basement membrane antibody test	Goodpasture syndrome Rapidly progressive glomerulonephritis
Positive antineutrophil cytoplasmic antibody test	Wegener granulomatosis
Positive hepatitis B, hepatitis C, HIV serology	Viral associated glomerulopathies

Signs and Symptoms Suggestive of Progression

Progression of CKD is more often recognized by serial determinations of eGFR than by signs and symptoms. However, a sudden change in the level of consciousness or cognitive state, increasing edema, or decreased urine output might be indicative of progression.

Treatment

Management

Once CKD has been diagnosed, management is aimed at preventing progression and treating the common associated clinical conditions. Patients should be made aware of the factors that can lead to progression and complications and should be encouraged to implement lifestyle modifications accordingly. Because of the increased risk of cardiovascular complications, patients should be encouraged to quit smoking, modify their diet, and treat lipids according to standard evidence-based guidelines. Patients should be made aware of nephrotoxic medications (see Table 14.5) and should be encouraged to ask prior to starting any medication, OTC remedy, or nutritional supplement. Acetaminophen should be the analgesic of choice for the treatment of pain, especially in individuals with stage 3 or higher CKD. Nonsteroidal anti-inflammatory agents may be used, but only with monitoring of renal function.

Blood Pressure

Among antihypertensive agents, ACEIs or ARBs have the most prospective data evaluating outcomes. Both classes have a demonstrated effect in improving cardiovascular outcomes and in delaying progression of nephropathy. Target blood pressure should be 130/80 or less based on the JNC-7 recommendations.

TABLE 14.5 · Commonly Used Medications that Need Dosage Modifications in CKD

Drug	Dose Adjustment		
	eGFR >50	eGFR 10–50	eGFR <10
ACEIs	100%	75%	25%–50%
Acetaminophen	Every 4 h	Every 6 h	Every 8 h
Acyclovir	100%	100%	200 mg every 12 h
Amoxicillin	100%	100%	50%–75%
Atenolol	100%	50%	25%
Ciprofloxacin	100%	50%–75%	50%
Fentanyl	100%	75%	50%
Fluconazole	100%	50%	50%
Gabapentin	100%	50%	25%
Glyburide	100%	Avoid	Avoid
H2 blockers (cimetidine, famotidine, ranitidine)	100%	75%	25%
Metformin	100%	Avoid	Avoid
Metoclopramide	100%	75%	50%
Morphine	100%	75%	50%
Nitrofurantoin	100%	Likely ineffective	Avoid
Spironolactone	100%	100%	Avoid
Trimethoprim/Sulfamethoxazole	Every 12 h	Every 18 h	Every 24 h

Glycemic Control

In diabetic patients, glycemic control is thought to delay the onset of CKD and, when CKD is already present, to slow the progression of disease. A recent study, by the ADVANCE Collaborative Group (2008), with subjects of an average age of 66 showed a 10% relative reduction in major cardiovascular outcomes and a 21% reduction in incidence of diabetic nephropathy over 5 years in subjects whose HbA1C was 6.5% compared with controls of 7.3%. As renal function declines, care should be taken in treating diabetes; doses of oral hypoglycemic agents and insulin may need to be reduced in order to prevent hypoglycemia (Biensenbach et al., 2003).

Lipids

Patients with CKD should be considered at very high risk for cardiovascular events and thus should be offered statin therapy to an LDL-C goal of less than 70 mg/dl (European Association for Cardiovascular Prevention & Rehabilitation et al., 2011).

Anemia

As CKD progresses from stage 3 to stage 4, there is a marked increase in the prevalence of a low hemoglobin. Beginning with stage 3 CKD, CBC, reticulocyte count, and assessment of iron stores should be obtained yearly. When the Hgb is less than 10 g/dl, an erythrocyte stimulating agent should be given to a target Hgb between 10 and 12 g/dl.

Bone Health

As the renal function declines, metabolic derangements result in disordered bone function. There is decreased phosphate excretion and poor conversion of Vitamin D3 to active forms. These changes result in hyperphosphatemia, hypocalcemia, and skeletal resistance to parathyroid hormone (PTH). In an effort to minimize the skeletal effects of these derangements, dietary phosphate should be restricted to 800 to 1,000 mg/day. Calcium carbonate should be prescribed in order to maintain bone health and to serve as a phosphate binder. In addition, 25-hydroxyvitamin D levels should be checked and normalized.

Fluid Status

Indications for Nephrology Consultation. Nephrology consultation is indicated when the eGFR is less than 30 ml/minute/1.73 m^2. Other circumstances where nephrology consultation might prove helpful include unexplained decrease in the eGFR, refractory proteinuria, anemia of CKD, resistant hypertension, or refractory hyperkalemia despite treatment. The National Kidney Foundation has a suggested multidisciplinary care plan for CKD available at www.kidney.org/professionals/KDOQI/cap.cfm.

Indications for Renal Replacement Therapy (RRT). RRT, in the form of hemodialysis (HD), continuous ambulatory peritoneal dialysis (CAPD), continuous cyclic peritoneal dialysis (CCPD), or renal transplantation, offers improved survival. The choice of the modality of RRT depends on patient choice, comorbidities, social support, and age. Unfortunately, studies of these therapies in the older adult with functional disabilities do not show significant improvements in functional outcomes (Cook & Jassal, 2008; Lo et al., 2008).

The choice of the most appropriate modality for RRT can be very difficult. Among older adults, there seems to be better survival in HD versus either form of peritoneal dialysis (Vonesh et al., 2006). Kidney transplantation is generally accepted as the best option for RRT, even in persons aged 70 and older (Rao et al., 2007). In this review, older transplant recipients enjoyed a 41% decreased mortality risk when compared with age-matched patients in a transplant waiting list. Despite this, the rate of transplantation among older adults remains low.

Patient Education

Prevention of Progression

Patients should be supplied with information about the disease, the value of monitoring, and the known interventions to prevent progression. Patients should also be aware of medications and remedies that are potentially nephrotoxic.

Advance Care Planning in the Context of CKD

Even though RRT carries the promise of overcoming renal failure, overall outcomes are pessimistic in the older adult. CKD, especially when accompanied by comorbidities, in the older patient should prompt the clinician to have conversations with patients about the trajectory of the disease and preferences. Older patients may elect to forego RRT or to stop dialysis once begun. Providers must be prepared to counsel patients and to assist in the provision of the best end-of-life strategy for patients who refuse RRT.

URINARY INCONTINENCE

UI is the involuntary loss of urine of sufficient amount to be a social or health problem. Although a common symptom, it can be both costly and lead to disability and is not a normal part of aging. It affects 10 million adults in the United States, and more than 200 million people worldwide have issues related to UI (Nabel, 2011). Approximately 15% to 30% of adult women experience UI at some time in their life, with increasing prevalence with advancing age. Men are also affected by UI more significantly with aging and changes in health status. The economic costs of UI for the nation have been estimated to be more than $15 billion annually. Increasing awareness and acceptance of UI as a significant medical issue crossing boundaries of age, gender, and social status has led to improved therapies although the cure for UI remains elusive (Phillips, 2004).

Secondary but significant costs include skin breakdown, infection related to rashes and ulcers, urinary tract infections, anxiety, depression, low self-esteem, and social isolation (Blott). Approximately half of the nursing home residents experience UI; this may be a causative factor in nursing home placement. Economic costs for nursing home residents are close to $5 billion annually and include costs associated with staffing, laundry, and supplies. UI often leads to falls related to urge to toilet and difficulty with mobility or mechanical failures due to loss of urine, leading to unsafe ambulation. Fractures secondary to falls or slippage in urine will significantly impact health, and placement for rehabilitation. Other health issues with cleanliness secondary to leakage and continual maceration of the perineal skin may increase infection rates and may contribute to the loss of independence if the home situation declines past the acceptable or it becomes unsafe for the individual to continue living alone.

Incontinence issues impact the individual both psychologically and physiologically. Changes in work or personal life may occur with frequency of trips to the toilet interrupting meetings or family times. Intimacy may become embarrassing owing to urine leakage and may lead to increased isolation (Mayo Clinic, 2011). Ten percent to 24% of sexually active women with pelvic floor disorders have reported coital incontinence during either penetration or orgasm (Karlovsky, 2009). The negative impact may lead to depression, social isolation, and altered relationships, and may lead to caregivers feeling frustrated on account of time and care needs of the individual with incontinence (Blott, 2006).

Definitions

Definitions of UI include the loss of bladder control ranging in severity from occasionally leaking during coughing, sneezing, or activities that place pressure on the abdomen to having an urge to urinate that is sudden or of strength that prevents getting to the toilet in a timely fashion. UI is not a disease; rather it is a symptom. The International Continence Society Standardization

Committee defines UI as "a condition in which involuntary loss of urine is a social or hygienic problem and is objectively demonstrable" (Bates et al., 1979). UI may be a complaint of involuntary loss of urine without a specific etiology or may be a multifactorial syndrome, especially in the older individual (DuBeau, 2012).

Pathophysiology

Several physiological processes must be coordinated for micturition to occur. In order to regulate bladder volume, information from somatic and autonomic nerves is sent to the spinal cord, and motor output to the detrusor, sphincter, and bladder musculature is adjusted accordingly. Exerting an inhibitory influence is the cerebral cortex, while the brainstem coordinates relaxation of the urethral sphincter and contraction of the detrusor muscle. While the bladder fills, sympathetic nerves lead to closure of the bladder neck and relaxation of the bladder dome, and inhibit parasympathetic tone. Somatic innervations maintain tone in the pelvic floor and striated periurethral muscles.

As sympathetic and somatic tones in the bladder and periurethral muscles diminish, leading to decreased urethral resistance, urination occurs. At the same time, cholinergic parasympathetic tone increases to result in contraction of the bladder. When bladder pressure exceeds urethral resistance, micturition occurs. The normal bladder capacity is 300 to 500 ml with initial urge to void usually occurring when bladder volumes are between 150 and 300 ml. When there is a disruption in micturition physiology or functional ability to toilet, incontinence occurs (Nabel, 2011).

Becoming especially problematic after 50 years of age, UI may be viewed as a normal part of aging, a minor inconvenience, or a major life change. Often UI is underdiagnosed in both sexes, as it may be viewed as too embarrassing to present, or health care providers may fail to ask. The senescent changes within the urogenital system account for increased frequency and delayed awareness of the urge to urinate. With aging, mobility issues may make the physical process of getting to the toilet more problematic. Aging of the bladder muscle leads to a decrease in its capacity to store urine and increase symptoms of an overactive bladder. If there is also blood vessel disease, such as secondary to diabetes or hypertension, the risk for UI increases. Postmenopausal women produce less estrogen, a necessary hormone for the health of the bladder and urethra, resulting in thinning and drying of the skin in the vagina or urethra. These women may experience deterioration of the tissues of the bladder and urethra, increasing issues such as UI. As the uterus and bladder are supported by many of the same muscles and ligaments, surgeries such as hysterectomy may damage the supporting pelvic floor muscles leading to incontinence. Pregnancy may lead to weakened and stretched pelvic muscles and continue to be problematic after delivery. Studies have varied as to the effect of age of first pregnancies, effect of the number of pregnancies, and familial history of UI. The impact of age on UI appears to lessen by age 50 (Rortveit & Hunskaar, 2006). It is estimated that between 16% and 22% of the adult population experience UI, with the greatest prevalence across all age groups being in women and with incidence increasing with age.

With aging, men experience an increase in lower urinary tract symptoms (LUTS), including frequency, urgency, and nocturia related to an overactive bladder and leading to UI. Men tend to show a more sudden onset, especially apparent after age 60, while women tend to have a more gradual increase but have episodes of incontinence at an earlier age (Srulevich & Chopra, 2009). In older males, incontinence may occur with enlargement of the prostate gland as in benign prostatic hyperplasia (BPH) or due to inflammation of the prostate gland (prostatitis). Incontinence may be a side effect of treatments—surgery or radiation—for prostate cancer and may be a sign or symptom of bladder cancer or bladder stones. Conditions that interfere with nerve signals involved in bladder control, such as multiple sclerosis, Parkinson disease, stroke, brain tumor, or a spinal injury may cause UI in both males and females. Obstruction secondary to stones in the kidneys, bladder, or ureters may lead to overflow incontinence (Mayo Clinic, 2011). Research suggests that older men with UI are more likely to be institutionalized, thereby resulting in a major impact on quality of life and an increased risk of mortality (Nuotio et al., 2003).

Presentation of disease in older adults is frequently different from that in younger individuals (Nuotio et al., 2003). UI may be an acute or chronic condition. To evaluate acute UI it is helpful to utilize the DIAPPERS mnemonic (Delirium, Infection, Atrophic urethritis and vaginitis, Pharmaceuticals, Psychologic disorders, especially depression, Excessive urine output, Restricted mobility, Stool impaction), as developed and published by N. Resnick in 1984. Ruling out treatable causes of UI will direct the approach for chronic or established conditions. Although UI is common, it is not a part of the normal aging process despite its presentation as a symptom for a large number of older individuals. The impact of UI is greatest in the oldest age groups with those 65 to 69 years old reporting UI impact in approximately 14%, with 90- to 95-year-olds impacting 27% and for those over 95 years approximately 38% (Shamliyan et al., 2007). The at-risk population for incontinence includes individuals with immobility, impaired cognitive ability, multiple medications, morbid obesity, and other medical conditions, including estrogen depletion and pelvic muscle weakness.

Types of Incontinence

The presentation of incontinence varies with the type of incontinence. Incontinence is commonly identified on the basis of such symptoms as urge, stress, overflow, functional, mixed, or total. Characteristics and treatments may vary depending on the type of incontinence.

Urge incontinence is a sudden, intense urge to urinate followed by involuntary loss of bladder control and leakage. Often the urge to urinate occurs, but the ability to do so is lost or arrival at the bathroom is delayed, leading to leakage or urination occurring beyond the control of the individual. This type of UI is caused by an overactive detrusor and is associated with frequency and nocturia. The detrusor instability may be due to loss of cortical inhibition of the voiding reflex following a stroke or dementia or secondary to local bladder irritation perhaps due to cystitis.

Stress incontinence is the loss of urine when pressure is exerted on the abdomen secondary to coughing, sneezing, laughing, exercising, or heavy lifting. It is associated with urethral hypermobility or intrinsic sphincter deficiency. This is more frequent when the sphincter muscle of the bladder is weakened following pregnancy, childbirth and menopause in women or removal of the prostate gland in men. The weakness of the pelvic floor muscles allows the proximal urethra and base of the bladder to push out of the pelvis during periods of increased abdominal pressure, resulting in leakage of urine. The urethral sphincter fails to remain closed during bladder filling or periods of exertion. Studies have found that in older women, a higher BMI has an association with stress UI, but not necessarily with urge UI (Shamliyan et al., 2007; Jackson et al., 2004). Increasing BMI was found in some studies of the 40- to 60-year-old female to be associated with urge UI (Dolan et al., 2009; Shamliyan et al., 2007).

Overflow incontinence is associated with either a contractile bladder or a bladder outlet obstruction. It is more common in older men, especially when constriction of the urethra by an enlarged prostate gland allows the constant dribble of urine with an inability to fully empty the bladder. This may be experienced with or without the feeling of urgency. Usually there is incomplete bladder emptying secondary to impaired detrusor contractility or bladder outlet obstruction. In females, contributing factors may be pelvic organ prolapse, trauma from pelvic fracture, complications of urologic procedures, and fistulae (Nabel, 2011). This is more frequent with a damaged bladder, blocked urethra, or nerve damage from diseases such as diabetes, multiple sclerosis or spinal cord injury. In males, overflow incontinence is also associated with tumors of the prostate gland surrounding the urethra. Often referred to as overactive bladder, this type of incontinence is a symptom syndrome consisting usually of urgency, frequency, and nocturia, with or without urge incontinence. There may also be the feeling of continuous leakage, although dribbling experienced is usually of small amounts of urine (DuBeau, 2012). Detrusor hyperactivity with impaired contractility (DHIC) may occur in frail older persons with a combination of detrusor function being both underactive and overactive. Usually DHIC is characterized by urgency, and PRV would be elevated. Frequently DHIC is misdiagnosed as stress UI if triggered by stress maneuvers since it shares similar symptoms (Abrams et al., 2010; Resnick et al., 1996).

Functional incontinence is a frequent presentation in older adults who reside in nursing homes or facilities. As frailty increases, immobility issues in community-dwelling individuals experiencing incontinence. Resulting from a physical or mental impairment or unwillingness to perform toileting (Werner, 2012), such patients may be prevented from getting to the toilet in a timely fashion. In the case of functional incontinence, the ability of the individual to respond appropriately to the body cues to void is hampered. This may be due to mental or physical hindrances to necessary manipulation of clothing or ability to find the appropriate location. Often, this type of incontinence is seen in persons with normal voiding systems but impediments that prevent or complicate reaching the toilet. Since the sensation of urge to void may occur closer to sphincter relaxation, the confined individual requiring assistance to toilet may have incontinence almost coincidentally with calling for assistance if they are cognitively able to recognize the signals.

Mixed incontinence is experiencing symptoms of more than one type of UI. Most often, mixed incontinence combines a bladder and urethral dysfunction, leading to a combination of stress and urge incontinence. Generally, this is defined as detrusor overactivity with impaired urethral function. This may first be noted as a slow stream of urine flow, usually compared with previous performance. In women with the complaint of incontinent symptoms, this is the most common type identified (Nabel, 2011).

Total incontinence is a term sometimes used in describing continuous leaking or urine that occurs during the day and night, or the periodic uncontrollable leaking of large volumes of urine (Mayo Clinic, 2011). Common causes of total incontinence include pelvic disease, postsurgical, neurologic issues, and post childbirth. Other causes can include damage to nerves due to spinal deformity as with scoliosis, trauma to the spinal cord or neurologic diseases such as multiple sclerosis or amyotrophic lateral sclerosis. Females also may experience total incontinence following repeated surgeries for stress incontinence with complete scarring of the urethra. Treatment may involve a sling procedure. In males following radical prostatectomies for prostate cancer, total incontinence may occur. Treatment will depend on the cause and must be tailored to the individual with the awareness that it may not always result in complete elimination of the UI. If a fistula is present, surgery may be required to close the fistula and prevent further leakage. Diversion of the urinary tract may be required if the fistula cannot be closed. For some individuals, implantation of an artificial sphincter may be created (Werner, 2012).

Cultural Considerations

Most epidemiological studies have been conducted with White females, and owing to methodological differences, it is difficult to directly compare these studies with one another or with the limited number of studies of varying racial or ethnic groups sampled. Studies that have investigated culture and UI have found that non-Hispanics have higher rates of incontinence than Hispanics (38% to 31%). Whites and Indians had higher rates of UI than did Asians and Blacks (Shamliyan et al., 2007). The majority of studies conducted in White male populations also use different survey methodologies, including methods for estimating prevalence. One study in the United States did find that Black males had a higher rate or UI (21%) compared with non-Hispanic White men (16%) and Mexican-American men (14%). Another cross-cultural study found that American Indians and Whites had higher rates of UI than either Blacks or Asians (Mardon et al., 2006).

Being a nation populated by many cultures, sensitivity to and awareness of race and culture must be part of the clinical practice. Common barriers to seeking medical advice for incontinence was an embarrassment and assuming UI to be a normal aging process for most of the population (El-Azab & Shaaban, 2010). There have been studies that indicate differences in incontinence prevalence between Black (14.6%) and White women (33.1%). This study compared continence system functions to determine relative contributions of urethral sphincteric function and urethral support to incontinence. The significant finding was that Black women with reports of incontinence had an 11% higher bladder pressure during maximal cough despite similar resting bladder pressures. They had higher urethral closure pressures compared with White women. However, Black women were less likely than White women to have UI secondary to urethral function (Bump, 1993). Race is not found to be significantly associated with the quality of life outcome scores although incontinence frequency was worse for Caucasians and African Americans but not for Asian Americans or Hispanics (Stacj-Lempinen et al., 2003). Life impact of incontinence in the Study of Women's Health Across the Nation (SWAN) (Sampselle et al., 2002) and a study by Bogner (2004) each suggest that the life impact of incontinence may be greater for Hispanics and African Americans than for Caucasians. Thom's research investigated the prevalence of stress and urge incontinence, and findings indicated low levels of stress and urge incontinence for Asian American women, while White and Hispanic women reported high levels of both. Black women reported less stress incontinence than all other groups, but had the highest prevalence of urge incontinence (Thom et al., 2006).

Progression of UI in males usually indicates that, when men become incontinent they develop urge or other types of UI; but those with urge UI alone either stayed as urge UI or developed mixed UI (Herzog et al., 1990). UI studies using samples of both males and females over 65 years of age and residing in Long Term Care facilities (LTC) tend to have combined group information for prevalence and varying definitions for UI. These may indicate daytime incontinence only, at least two episodes in the past 2 weeks, or urine loss twice in a month, and may be self-report or report of the staff, but range from 30% to 77% of the population with some degree of UI. Further variation occurs depending on when UI information was collected in relation to the admission to LTC. Prevalence rates tend to increase with advancing age in both men and women, and in populations of various regions, sampling may indicate conflicting findings. On admission, one study found higher prevalence in Blacks (71%) compared with Whites (64%), but more similar prevalence rates after admission (78% to 74%) (Boyington et al., 2007).

Screening

Initially screening should begin with simply starting the conversation. Whether initiated by the patient or the health care provider, it is important to ask during the medical history whether there are any symptoms indicating loss of bladder control. Simple questions about continence may lead to discussion of a topic that is often not the primary reason for the visit yet has a significant impact on life. It is wise for patients to be prepared for the assessment by having written down their symptoms, any noted causes of UI they are aware of, and anything tried that reduces the episodes of UI. During the evaluation, the health care provider will want to know when the symptoms were first experienced, whether the episodes have been occasional or continuous, and how severe the patient finds the symptoms. Patients should be encouraged to keep a simple bladder diary for 3 to 7 days before the evaluation to help to provide a graphic order to the symptoms. The diary should include a column for food and liquids consumed as dietary choices and hydration can affect urine output and incontinence. If the diary and related questions are not known before the appointment, it would be wise to obtain a bladder diary to assist with screening. A simple questionnaire can distinguish between urge and stress incontinence (Palmer, 2004).

Urinalysis can be completed on a fresh-voided urine specimen to assess the individual with UI in order to determine whether the incontinence is associated with a urinary tract infection (UTI). If infection is present, it should be treated and cleared before further evaluation with diagnostic evaluations can be initiated to rule out other causes of UI. The urinalysis will suggest not only infection but also inflammation, and further studies may be necessary to rule out tumor or stones if there are other symptoms such as hematuria or pyuria. Blood tests may be needed to measure renal function, electrolytes, blood glucose, and serum calcium for exclusion of other conditions that may cause UI.

Bladder Scan/Postvoiding residual (PVR) is a useful test in the evaluation of UI. The PVR is best accomplished using a straight catheterization of the urinary bladder following the attempt to complete voiding. Portable bladder scanning and pelvic ultrasonography are safe and accurate alternative methods of estimating the urine remaining in the bladder post voiding. For evaluation purpose, a PVR of less than 50 ml is considered normal. A PRV greater than 150 to 200 ml is abnormal and indicates the need for further evaluation. This may be accomplished by a repeat PVR or urologic evaluation. If the PVR is over 300 ml, further renal function studies should be conducted. In males with high PVR, bladder outlet obstruction should be considered (Clemens, 2011).

Postmenopausal estrogen insufficiency occurs in women, resulting in thinning and drying of skin in the vagina and urethra. Incontinence can be aggravated when these tissues deteriorate. Some women find relief of symptoms through the application of low-dose, topical estrogen in the form of a vaginal cream, ring, or patch as this helps to rejuvenate tissues in the urethra and vaginal areas (Mayo Clinic, 2011).

Medications and chronic conditions: Men or women who have had diabetes for years may develop nerve damage that may affect bladder control. The history of stroke, Parkinson disease, and multiple sclerosis all affect the brain and nervous system and can cause problems with adequate bladder emptying. Spinal cord injury with interruption of nerve signals required for bladder control will affect bladder emptying. Along with the medical condition, the individual will be prescribed many medications that may cause or increase the incidence of incontinence. A careful medication review and selection of medications with the lowest potential for increasing incontinence is an essential function of the health care provider.

Risk Factors

Risk Factors of UI include sex, age, smoking, being overweight, and the presence of other disease conditions. Sex or gender is a risk factor as women are more likely than men to have stress incontinence related to individual history of pregnancy, childbirth, menopause, and the normal female anatomy. Some studies find that daughters of mothers with stress UI have a higher prevalence of stress UI (71.4%) than age-matched controls (40.3%). Also, UI symptoms appeared 7 years earlier in families with reported incontinence than in families without incontinence history (Ertunc et al., 2004). Men with prostate gland issues have an increased risk of urge and overflow incontinence.

Age normally leads to decreased muscle strength of the bladder and urethra. Muscle strength weakens with aging and leads to a reduction in the amount that the bladder can hold. Sphincter control may also contribute to leakage. Having bladder tolerance for a smaller amount of urine increases the risk of loss of control.

Being obese or overweight causes increased pressure on the bladder and surrounding muscles. These muscles weaken and allow leakage of urine from the bladder with the occurrence of coughing or sneezing. Studies have found that in older women with a higher BMI, there is an association with stress UI, but not necessarily with urge UI (Jackson et al., 2004). Increasing BMI was found in some studies of the 40- to 60-year-old female to be associated with urge UI (Brown et al., 1999).

Smoking increases episodes of incontinence and puts stress on the urinary sphincter, leading to stress incontinence. Smoking also increases the risk of overactive bladder by causing increased bladder contractions. There are some studies that indicate dose–response relationships between the numbers of cigarettes smoked in both former and current smokers and the development of UI (Hannestad et al., 2003).

Other diseases, such as kidney disease or diabetes, may increase the risk for incontinence (Mayo Clinic, 2011). Prevalence of UI is higher in frail community-dwelling older adults with an impaired cognitive status. Over age 75 years, a 70% increase in development of UI was found in persons with memory problems (Ostbye et al., 2004). Depression is another risk factor for UI that has been studied, with some studies indicating that urge incontinence ranges from 23% to 81% (Maggi et al, 2001; Stenzelius et al., 2004).

Prevention

Prevention of stress incontinence may include identification of the issues of bladder control. Weight loss or dietary changes may help to alleviate symptoms. Avoidance of straining that places extra pressure on the abdomen may prevent some episodes. Control of risk factors, thereby preventing the development of UI, is better than treatment options. Coping techniques for UI, including pads and liners, are purchased at the individual's cost and are not reimbursable.

Prevention of overflow incontinence may relate to treatment of underlying medical issues that have precipitated changes in position of the bladder or controlling structures. Adequate hydration continues to be important in stress, urge, and overflow incontinence in order to reduce bladder spasms. Maintaining physical activity and muscle strength are important in prevention of development of UI in both men and women.

Presentation

While UI is a common symptom in the older population, it often adversely affects physical and psychosocial functioning and ultimately quality of life. The strong association between UI and depression has been seen as discussed in quality of life issues for cultural considerations. UI has been associated with decreased quality of life, leading to more depression. Depressed individuals rate their UI symptoms as significantly more severe than that of nondepressed individuals.

Symptoms of UI may occur following childbirth or surgical procedures or with aging and immobility issues. One of the dangers of UI is that it becomes accepted as a chronic condition and managed rather than being discussed with the health care provider or seeking a remedy.

Treatment

With cure being defined as complete absence of UI, the impact on quality of life is dependent on the impact of the incontinent episodes as perceived by the individual. The most common measure by health care providers of treatment efficacy is the reduction in UI episodes. Initial treatment for incontinence may be aimed at simply reducing the number of incontinent episodes. As the quality of life issue may be more related to the timing or inconvenience of UI such as nocturia or leakage with exercise, reduction in the number of episodes may not be perceived as an effective treatment, while methods that lead to improvement in the timing or time between toileting or less UI interference with activities may provide a greater impact.

Stepwise treatment strategies should be part of the plan of care discussed with the patient. Usually it is wise to start with the least invasive treatments (lifestyle changes, behavioral care, medications) and then advance to treatments that are more invasive. Correcting factors that contribute to UI, especially in the older adult, should be the initial focus. Comorbid conditions, functional impairment that interfere with toileting independence, and medications that are prescribed for one condition but contribute to UI issues may need to be evaluated and eliminated.

Treatment for incontinence presents many challenges. Using indwelling catheters, diapers, pads, and condom catheters for coping, while preventing serious complications, may lead to complications such as infections and wounds secondary to bacterial growth and increased cost of care. Wounds under the covering of pads and diapers allow greater exposure to bacteria for extended periods of time, and wounds may increase in size or severity. Out-of-pocket cost will vary as many of the products are not covered by Medicare. Cost-effectiveness analysis has focused mainly on medication treatments, but with few studies available to draw conclusions, especially in the use or cost of products in LTC facilities. The consumer is left with the vast majority of costs and the decisions of which product they can afford and will allow the greatest quality of life. This care also impacts partners or caregivers if help is required to manage urination. Developing a plan, providing assistance, and remaining active provides the best option for quality of life and management of incontinence.

Lifestyle changes include many common sense strategies. These include adequate fluid consumption up to two liters daily. Dietary changes, including the avoidance of caffeinated beverages, alcohol, carbonated beverages, and, for some individuals sensitive to them, the elimination or reduction of citrus, tomato products, spicy foods, artificial sweeteners, chocolate, or sugar, may reduce the frequency of UI episodes. For nocturnal incontinence, minimizing fluid intake in the evening may be beneficial; increasing physical activity may improve muscle control and strength and lead to weight reduction. Weight reduction can decrease episodes of stress UI. Treatment of constipation or cough symptoms may also improve UI.

An early step in treatment for incontinence includes documenting continence issues using a bladder diary. There may be a pattern that is evident to the health care practitioner that will assist in providing a more direct plan for the care. During this time, it is often recommended that toileting occur at regular timed intervals. Using or developing a habit called timed voiding may eliminate or reduce UI incidence. As control is regained, the individual is encouraged to extend the time interval between scheduled trips to the toilet.

Another behavioral treatment includes strengthening the pelvic and bladder muscles. While pelvic exercises to prevent incontinence in women after childbirth have been encouraged since 1922, the initial method, no longer recommended, was to begin urinating and cut off the flow of urine and then retain the urine as long as possible. In 1948, Arnold Kegel introduced what has commonly been called Kegel exercises with biofeedback for pelvic muscles to strengthen stretched or atrophic muscles, specifically the pubococcygeus. This muscle contributes to the support and sphincteric control of the pelvic viscera, and its function is essential to maintain the tone of both smooth and striated pelvic muscles. Vaginal examination would reveal that the tissues between the palpating finger and the symphysis or rami of the os pubis are thin and of poor quality, indicating atrophied perivaginal muscular structures. The therapy included learning to contract the pubococcygeus voluntarily. This contraction is repeated several times daily to strengthen the muscles. The ability to visualize the muscle contractions greatly increased the success rate of this simple management strategy. His invention of the perineometer allowed a woman to measure both the strength and the duration of the exercise and enabled more effective exercise of the pelvic muscles. Using the perineometer to measure vaginal pressure along with the Kegel exercises two to three times daily, he claimed a 93% success rate in control of incontinence in women following childbirth (Kegel, 1948).

Along with medical conditions there is an abundance of medications used for treatment. Not only must the side effects of each medication be considered, but also the side effects of other medications being taken by the individual must be assessed, as the greater the number of medications the higher the likelihood of drug–drug interactions. Some of the frequently used medications for incontinence are alpha blockers (ex: tamsulosin, silodosin, terazosin, and doxazosin), antimuscarinic drugs (ex: oxybutynin, tolterodine) or combinations of both types of medications. Anticholinergics are often used to calm an overactive bladder and are helpful for urge incontinence. Possible side effects of these medications include dry mouth, constipation, blurred vision, and flushing, so for some individuals the treatment may be more of a problem than the UI. Some tricyclic antidepressants (Imipramine) may be used to treat mixed incontinence. Duloxetine, another antidepressant, may be used to treat stress incontinence (Mayo Clinic, 2011).

There are other medical devices available to treat incontinence in women. Urethral inserts act as a plug to prevent leakage. Usually worn only for prevention during specific activities, they are not meant to be used 24 hours a day. These work best for women who have predictable episodes of incontinence, such as during sports events. The device is inserted before the activity and removed before urination. A pessary is a stiff ring inserted into the vagina and worn all day to help hold up the bladder and prevent urine leakage. The pessary is most beneficial if UI is due to a prolapsed bladder or uterus. This device needs to be regularly removed and cleaned.

Some of the interventional therapies include bulking material injections into tissues surrounding the urethra. This helps to keep the urethra closed, therefore reducing UI episodes. Repeat injections are usually required; these must be done in a doctor's office with minimal anesthesia. Injections of Botox into the bladder muscle have not yet been approved by the Food and Drug Administration (FDA), but may benefit overactive bladder. Complications include urinary retention severe enough to require self-catheterizations. Again, repeat injections are needed. Sacral nerve stimulators, a device that resembles a pacemaker, is implanted under the skin in the buttock with a wire connected to a sacral nerve. Painless electrical pulses stimulate the nerve and help control the bladder. Tibial nerve stimulators are approved for treatment of overactive bladder symptoms. These pulses travel along the tibial nerve to the sacral nerve, where they assist in controlling overactive bladder symptoms (Mayo Clinic, 2011).

Surgical procedures may be useful for returning the bladder to its normal position after childbirth. There are retropubic suspensions and also two types of sling procedures commonly used. For males, there is an artificial urinary sphincter option.

Retropubic suspension uses sutures to support the bladder neck with attachment to strong ligaments within the pelvis. This procedure is often done along with abdominal procedures, such as hysterectomy. Sling procedures use the individual's own fascia to cradle the bladder neck. This sling is then attached to the pubic bone or tied in front of the abdomen just above the pubic bone. Another type of sling is the mid-urethral sling that is performed as an outpatient procedure. This uses a synthetic mesh placed midway along the urethra. There are two general types. Using specially designed needles, the surgeon positions the synthetic tape under the urethra and pulls the ends of the tape through incisions behind the pubic bone or by the sides of the vaginal opening and then adjusts the tapes to provide the proper amount of urethral support (National Kidney & Urologic Diseases Information Clearinghouse [NKUDIC], 2011). Prior to any surgical intervention, careful and complete information must be evaluated as to the cause of the incontinence, potential risks of procedures, and probable benefits.

A device, shaped like a doughnut implanted around the neck of the bladder, may be particularly helpful for men with weakened urinary sphincters following treatment of prostate cancer or an enlarged prostate gland. This artificial urinary sphincter is fluid filled and keeps the urinary sphincter shut tight until the individual is ready to urinate. At that time, it presses a valve implanted under the skin, causing the ring to deflate and allowing urine to flow from the bladder. Referral to a urologist is necessary for more complicated incontinence issues. With male incontinence, if there is a history of prior surgery or pelvic radiation, pelvic pain, severe LUTS, evaluation by a urologist is essential. Recurrent urologic infections, severe incontinence, abnormal prostate exams, and elevated prostate specific antigen (PSA) levels also warrant a more specialized evaluation. Further tests, such as cystoscopy or imaging studies of the urinary tract, may be necessary for complete evaluation and careful planning.

Considering that incontinence issues increase with age, it is important to assess risk–benefit of procedures with quality of life issues before establishing the plan of care. Careful consideration of the issues that are most troubling to the individual will assist the health care provider in adequately addressing the treatment plan.

Patient Education

Prevention of UI may involve lifestyle changes. UI may increase owing to habits that can be altered such as the following: Alcohol acts as a diuretic and bladder stimulant, causing an increased urge to urinate. Overhydration over a short period increases the amount of urine that the kidneys secrete and that the bladder has to store. Caffeine is a diuretic and stimulates the bladder to empty. Other beverages, such as carbonated drinks, tea and coffee–with or without caffeine, artificial sweeteners–corn syrup, and foods or beverages high in spice, sugar, and acid, may increase bladder spasms. Medications prescribed for other conditions, such as heart medications, blood pressure treatments, sedatives, muscle relaxants, and many other medications may contribute to bladder control problems. UTIs can irritate the bladder, increasing strong urges to urinate. These infections may present with other signs and symptoms such as burning sensation during urination, or foul smell to the urine. Constipation, with nerves in the rectum located near the bladder, can cause nerves to be overactive, increasing urinary frequency. Further, this can interfere with bladder emptying and may cause overflow incontinence (Mayo Clinic, 2011).

Patient Education Components for Providers

Tests and procedures may include completion of a bladder diary as a record of liquid intake, when and how much urine is eliminated, and documentation of urge or incontinent episodes as well as a urinalysis to rule out signs of infections, traces of blood, or other abnormalities that may indicate a disease processes. A blood test will be sent for analysis to check for various chemicals and substances that may indicate a potential cause of incontinence. Further testing might include a PVR measurement either by catheterization or by ultrasound test to determine the amount of urine remaining in the bladder after emptying. PVR is not recommended for the evaluation of men with mild to moderate symptoms and suspected of having BPH. It may, however, be useful in the evaluation of men with more severe symptoms of BPH prior to initiating or following failure of antimuscarinic medications for overactive bladder symptoms. Measurement of PVR can be beneficial when dealing with spinal cord injuries, neurological diseases except dementia, recurrent UTIs, history of prior urinary retention episodes, or severe constipation. When the individual is already receiving high doses of multiple medications with potential to suppress detrusor contractility, PVR may supply additional insight. Persons with DM with potential for peripheral neuropathy may find PVR information beneficial to help determine bladder function (Clemens, 2011). Pelvic ultrasound may be used to view parts of the urinary tract to check for abnormalities. This test uses sound waves and is a noninvasive way to obtain an image of the kidneys, ureters, bladder, and urethra. A Bladder **Stress test** includes visualization while coughing or bearing down to observe for loss of urine.

Urodynamic testing is not recommended for UI screening. Although urodynamics are the physiological diagnostic "gold standard," they are expensive and invasive, and require special equipment and training. More importantly, they are not usually necessary to make the diagnosis. Using a catheter inserted into the bladder through the urethra and filling the bladder with water allows measurement and pressure in the bladder at rest and during filling to help measure bladder strength and urinary sphincter health. Cystogram is a contrast-enhanced x-ray of the bladder that is taken during catheterization and that displays images on a series of x-rays during micturition. Cystoscopy is a fiberoptic examination of the urethra and bladder to investigate and potentially remove abnormalities in the urinary tract.

In summary, it is important to consider quality of life issues with the assessment of UI. As UI incidence increases with age, it is important to evaluate other chronic conditions that may contribute to or worsen secondary to treatment options for the individual. Medications that may be beneficial for treatment of UI may contribute to problems with other conditions. Conversely, heart and blood pressure medications, sedatives, and muscle relaxants are some of the common medications used to treat other conditions that may contribute to bladder control issues. Determining the importance of various aspects of UI will allow the health care provider to treat the symptoms most problematic to the individual and not simply leading to a reduction in incontinence episodes. Maintaining good overall health, avoiding risk factors, and maintaining a healthy weight range may help alleviate symptoms of overactive bladder and eliminate or reduce UI episodes.

REFERENCES

Abrams, P., Andersson, K. E., Birder, L., Brubaker, L., Cardozo, L., Chapple, C.,…Wyndaele, J. J. (2010). Fourth International Consultation on Incontinence Recommendations of the International Scientific Committee: Evaluation and treatment of urinary incontinence, pelvic organ prolapse, and fecal incontinence. *Neurourology and Urodynamics, 29,* 213.

ADVANCE Collaborative Group. (2008). Intensive blood glucose control and vascular outcomes in patients with type 2 diabetes. *New England Journal of Medicine, 358,* 2560–2572.

American Diabetes Association. (2011). Standards of medical care in diabetes-2011. *Diabetes Care, 34*(Suppl. 1), S11–S61.

American Diabetes Association. (2012). Executive summary: Standards of medical care in diabetes—2012. *Diabetes Care, 35*(Suppl. 1), S4–S10.

Bates, P. E., Bradley, W. E., Glen, E., Griffiths, D., Melchior, H., Rowan, D., & Hald, T. (1979). The standardization of terminology of lower urinary tract function. *Journal of Urology, 121,* 551–554.

Biensenbach, G., Raml, A., Schmekal, B., & Eichbauer-Sturm, G. (2003). Decreased insulin requirement in relation to GFR in nephropathic type 1 and insulin treated type 2 diabetic patients. *Diabetic Medicine, 20,* 642–645.

Blott, E. (2006). Urinary incontinence. In J. Fitzpatrick & M. Wallace (Eds.), *Encyclopedia of nursing research* (2nd ed., pp. 614–615). New York, NY: Springer.

Bogner, H. (2004). Urinary incontinence and psychological distress in community-dwelling older African Americans and Whites. *Journal of the American Geriatrics Society, 52*(11), 1870–1874.

Boyington, J. E., Howard, D. L., Carter-Edwards, L., Gooden, K. M., Erdem, N., Jallah, Y., & Busby-Whitehead, J. (2007). Differences in resident characteristics and prevalence of urinary incontinence in nursing homes in the southeastern United States. *Nursing Research, 56*(2), 97–107.

Brosius, F. C., III, Hostetter, T. H., Kelepouris, E., Mitsnefes, M. M., Moe, S. M., Moore, M. A.,…Wilson, P. W. (2006). Detection of chronic kidney disease in patients with or at increased risk of cardiovascular disease: a science advisory from the American Heart Association Kidney And Cardiovascular Disease Council; the Councils on High Blood Pressure Research, Cardiovascular Disease in the Young, and Epidemiology and Prevention; and the Quality of Care and Outcomes Research Interdisciplinary Working Group: developed in collaboration with the National Kidney Foundation. *Circulation, 114*(10), 1083–1087.

Brown, J. S., Grady, D., Ouslander, J. G., Herzog, A. R., Varner, R. E., & Posner, S. F. (1999). Prevalence of urinary incontinence and associated risk factors in postmenopausal women: Heart and estrogen/progestin replacement study (HERS) research group. *Obstetrics & Gynecology, 94*(1), 66–70.

Bump, R. C. (1993). Racial comparisons and contrasts in urinary incontinence and pelvic organ prolapse. *Obstetrics & Gynecology, 81,* 421–425.

Chobanian, A. V., Bakris, G. L., Black, H. R., Cushman, W. C., Green, L. A., Jones, D. W.,…National High Blood Pressure Education Program Coordinating Committee. (2003). The seventh report of the Joint National Committee of the Joint National Committee on Prevention, Detection, Evaluation, and Treatment of High Blood Pressure: The JNC 7 report. *Journal of the American Medical Association, 289*(19), 2560–2572.

Clemens, J. Q. (2011, November 16). Urinary incontinence in men. Retrieved from http://www.uptodate.com/contents/urinary-incontinence-in-men?

Cook, W. L., & Jassal, S. V. (2008). Functional dependencies among elderly on hemodialysis. *Kidney International, 73,* 1289–1295.

Dolan, L. M., Casson, K., McDonald, P., & Ashe, R. G. (1999). Urinary incontinence in Northern Ireland: A prevalence study. *British Journal of Urology International, 83*(7), 760–766.

DuBeau, C. (2012). Epidemiology, risk factors, and pathogenesis of urinary incontinence. Retrieved from www.uptodate.com/contents/epidemiology-risk-factors-and-pathogenesis-of-urinary-incontinence

El-Azab, A. S., & Shaaban, O. M. (2010). Measuring the barriers against seeking consultation for urinary incontinence among Middle Eastern women. *BMC Women's Health, 10,* 3.

Ertunc, D., Tok, E. C., Pata, O., Dilek, U., Ozdemir, G., & Dilek, S. (2004). Is stress urinary incontinence a familial condition? *Acta Obstetricia et Gynecologica Scandinavica, 83*(10), 912–916.

European Association for Cardiovascular Prevention & Rehabilitation, Reiner, Z., Catapano, A. L., De Backer, G., Graham, I., Taskinen, M. R.,…ESC Committee for Practice Guidelines (CPG) 2008-2010 and 2010-2012 Committees. (2011). ESC/EAS Guidelines for the management of dyslipidaemias: The Task Force for the management of dyslipidaemias of the European Society of Cardiology (ESC) and the European Atherosclerosis Society (EAS). *European Heart Journal, 32,* 1769–1818.

Griebling, T. L. (2009). Urinary incontinence in the elderly. *Clinics in Geriatric Medicine, 25*(3), 445–457.

Hannestad, Y. S., Rortveit, G., Daltveit, A. T., & Hunskaar, S. (2003). Are smoking and other lifestyle factors associated with female urinary incontinence? The Norwegian EPINCONT Study. *BJOG: International Journal of Obstetrics & Gynecology*, *110*(3), 247–254.

Herzog, A. R., Diokno, A. C., Brown, M. B., Normolle, D. P., & Brock, B. M. (1990). Two-year incidence, remission, and change patterns of urinary incontinence in noninstitutionalized older adults. *Journal of Gerontology*, *45*(2), M67–M74.

Ishani, A., Xue, J. L., Himmelfarb, J., Eggers, P. W., Kimmel, P. L., Molitoris, B. A., & Collins, A. J. (2009). Acute kidney injury increases risk of ESRD among elderly. *Journal of the American Society of Nephrology*, *20*(1), 223–228.

Jackson, R. A., Vittinghoff, E., Kanaya, A. M., Miles, T. P., Resnick, H. E., Kritchevsky, S. B., . . . Brown, J. S. (2004). Urinary incontinence in elderly women: Findings from the Health, Aging, and Body Composition Study. *Obstetrics & Gynecology*, *104*(2), 301–307.

Karlovsky, M. E. (2009). Female urinary incontinence during intercourse (coital incontinence): A review. *The Female Patient*, *34*, 32–36.

Kidney Disease Outcomes Quality Initiative. (2007). KDOQI clinical practice guidelines and clinical practice recommendations for diabetes and chronic kidney disease. *American Journal of Kidney Diseases*, *49*(2 Suppl. 2), S12–S154.

Kegel, A. H. (1948). A nonsurgical method of increasing the tone of sphincters and their supporting structures. Retrieved from http://www.dothekegel.com/arnie/index.html

Khalil, P., Murty, P., & Palevsky, P. M. (2008). The patient with acute kidney injury. *Primary Care: Clinics in Office Practice*, *35*(2), 239–264.

Ko, Y., Lion, S. J., Salmon, J. W., & Bron, M. S. (2005). The impact of urinary incontinence on quality of life of the elderly. *American Journal of Managed Care*, *11*, S103–S111.

Lindeman, R. D., & Goldman, R. (1986). Anatomic and physiologic age changes in the kidney. *Experimental Gerontology*, *21*, 379–406.

Lo, D., Chiu, E., & Jassal, S. V. (2008). A prospective pilot study to measure changes in functional status associated with hospitalization in elderly dialysis-dependent patients. *American Journal of Kidney Diseases*, *52*(5), 956–961.

Maggi, S., Minicuci, N., Langlois, J., Pavan, M., Enzi, G., & Crepaldi, G. (2001). Prevalence rate of urinary incontinence in community-dwelling elderly individuals: The Veneto study. *Journals of Gerontology Series A: Biological Sciences & Medical Sciences*, *56*(1), M14–M18.

Mardon, R. E., Halim, S., Pawlson, L. G., & Haffer, S. C. (2006). Management of urinary incontinence in Medicare managed care beneficiaries: Results from the 2004 Medicare Health Outcomes Survey. *Archives of Internal Medicine*, *166*(10), 1128–1133.

Mayo Clinic. (2011). Urinary incontinence. Retrieved from http://www.mayoclinic.com/health/urinary-incontinence/DS00404

Moyer, V. A. (2012). Screening for chronic kidney disease: U. S. Preventive Services Task Force recommendation statement. *Annals of Internal Medicine*, *157*(8), 567–570.

Nabel, N. A. (2011). Emergency treatment of urinary incontinence. Retrieved from http://emedicine.medscape.com/article/778772-overview

National Kidney & Urologic Diseases Information Clearinghouse. (2011). Retrieved from National Institute of Diabetes and Digestive and Kidney Diseases, National Institutes of Health website, http://kidney.niddk.nih.gov/kudiseases/pubs/uiwomen/

National Kidney Foundation. (n.d.). Retrieved from http://www.kidney.org/kidneydisease/ckd/index.cfm#facts

National Kidney Foundation. (2002). K/DOQI clinical practice guidelines for chronic kidney disease: Evaluation, classification, and stratification. *American Journal of Kidney Diseases*, *39*(2 Suppl. 1), S1–S266.

Nuotio, M., Tammela, T. L., Luukkaala, T., & Jylhä, M. (2003). Predictors of institutionalization in an older population during a 13 year period: The effect of urge incontinence. *Journals of Gerontology Series A: Biological Sciences & Medical Sciences*, *58*(8), 756–762.

Ostbye, T., Seim, A., Krause, K. M., Feightner, J., Hachinski, V., Sykes, E., & Hunskaar, S. (2004). A 10 year follow up of urinary and fecal incontinence among the oldest old in the community: The Canadian Study of Health and Aging. *Canadian Journal on Aging*, *23*(4), 319–331.

Palmer, R. M. (2004). Urinary incontinence. In E. Nabel (Ed.), *ACP medicine* (pp. 5–10). Retrieved from http://wwwacpmedicine.com/acp/chapters/ch0809.htm

Phillips, B. B. (2004). Skip to the loo, my darlin': Urinary incontinence 1850—present. *Geriatric Nursing*, *25*(2), 74–80.

Rao, P. S., Merion, R. M., Ashby, V. B., Port, F. K., Wolfe, R. A., & Kayler, L. K. (2007). Renal transplantation in elderly patients older than 70 years of age: Results from the Scientific Registry of Transplant Recipients. *Transplantation*, *83*(8), 1069–1074.

Resnick, N. M., Brandeis, G. H., Baumann, M. M., DuBeau, C. E., & Yalla, S. V. (1996). Misdiagnosis of urinary incontinence in nursing home women: Prevalence and a proposed solution. *Neurourology & Urodynamics*, *15*, 599.

Rortveit, G., & Hunskaar, S. (2006). Urinary incontinence and age at the first and last delivery: The Norwegian HUNT/ EPINCONT study. *American Journal of Obstetrics and Gynecology, 195*(2), 433–438.

Sampselle, C. M., Harlow, S. D., Skurnick, J., Brubaker, L., & Bondarenko I. (2002). Urinary incontinence predictors and life impact in ethnically diverse perimenopausal women. *Obstetrics & Gynecology, 100*(6), 1230–1238.

Schmitt, R., Coca, S., Kanbay, M., Tinetti, M. E., Cantley, L. G., & Parikh, C. R. (2008). Recovery of kidney function after acute kidney injury in the elderly: A systematic review and meta-analysis. *American Journal of Kidney Diseases, 52*(2), 262–271.

Shamliyan, T., Wyman, J., Bliss, D. J., Kane, R. L., & Wilt, T. J. (2007). Prevention of urinary and fecal incontinence in adults. *Agency for Healthcare Research and Quality*, Publication No. 08-E003.

Srulevich, M., & Chopra, A. (2009). Urinary incontinence in older men. *Clinical Geriatrics, 15*(9), 38–45.

Stacj-Lempinen, B., Hakala, A. L., Laippala, P., Lehtinen, K., Metsänoja, R., & Kujansuu, E. (2003). Severe depression determines quality of life in urinary incontinent women. *Neurolourology & Urodynamics, 22*(6), 563–568.

Stenzelius, K., Marriasson, A., Hallberg, I. R., & Westergren, A. (2004). Symptoms of urinary and faecal incontinence among men and women 75+ in relations to health complaints and quality of life. *Neurourology & Urodynamics, 23*(3), 211–222.

Thom, D. H., van den Eeden, S. K., Ragins, A. I., Wassel-Fyr, C., Vittinghof, E., Subak, L. L., & Brown, J. S. (2006). Differences in prevalence of urinary incontinence by race/ethnicity. *Journal of Urology, 175*(1), 259–264.

U. S. Renal Data System. (n.d.). Annual data report. Retrieved from www.usrds.org/atlas.aspx

U. S. Renal Data System. (2008). *USRDS 2008 annual data report*. Bethesda, MD: National Institutes of Health, National Institute of Diabetes, Digestive, and Kidney Disease.

Vassalotti, J. A., Stevens, L. A., & Levey, A. S. (2007). Testing for chronic kidney disease: A position statement from the National Kidney Foundation. *American Journal of Kidney Diseases, 50*(2), 169–180.

Vonesh, E. F., Snyder, J. J., Foley, R. N., & Collins, A. J. (2006). Mortality studies comparing peritoneal dialysis and hemodialysis: What they tell us? *Kidney International, 70*, S3–S11.

Werner, S. L. (2012). Total incontinence. [A newsletter from Werner- Francis Urology Associates]. Retrieved from http:// www.wmfurology.com/total.htm

Zhou, X. J., Laszik, Z. G., & Silva, F. G. (2007). Anatomical changes in the aging kidney. In J. F. Macias-Nunez, J. S. Cameron, & D. G. Oreopoulos (Eds.), *The aging kidney in health and disease* (pp. 39–54). New York, NY: Springer.

CHAPTER 14: IT RESOURCES

Websites

National Kidney Foundation
  http://www.kidney.org/

United States Renal Data System
  http://www.usrds.org/

National Kidney and Urologic Diseases Information Clearinghouse (NKUDIC)
  http://kidney.niddk.nih.gov/

National Institute of Diabetes and Digestive and Kidney Diseases
  http://www2.niddk.nih.gov/

About Chronic Kidney Disease
  http://www.kidney.org/kidneydisease/aboutckd.cfm

Is Chronic Kidney Disease in Older People a New Geriatric Giant?
  http://www.futuremedicine.com/doi/abs/10.2217/ahe.11.58

Chronic Kidney Disease—More Common in Older Adults
  http://www.agewell.com/health/45-bowling-chronic-kidney-disease-more-common-in-older-adults.aspx

Prediction, Progression, and Outcomes of Chronic Kidney Disease in Older Adults
  http://jasn.asnjournals.org/content/20/6/1199.full

Chronic Kidney Disease and the Elderly—a Fatal Combination?
http://www.ausmed.com.au/blog/entry/chronic-kidney-disease-and-the-elderly-a-fatal-combination
Chronic Kidney Disease—HealthyPeople.gov
http://www.healthypeople.gov/2020/topicsobjectives2020/overview.aspx?topicId=6
Kidney Failure and the Elderly
http://www.eldercarelink.com/Other-Resources/Health/kidney-failure-in-the-elderly.htm
Prognosis of Renal Failure in Elderly Patients
http://www.kidneyfailureweb.com/prognosis/280.html
Urinary Incontinence—Mayo Clinic
http://www.mayoclinic.com/health/urinary-incontinence/DS00404/DSECTION=symptoms
Types of Urinary Incontinence
http://www.mayoclinic.org/urinary-incontinence/types.html
Elderly Urinary Incontinence
http://nursing-homes.aplaceformom.com/articles/elderly-urinary-incontinence
Incontinence and Bladder Control
http://www.agingcare.com/Articles/An-Overview-of-Urinary-Incontinence-96655.htm
Acute Kidney Injury
http://www.renal.org/clinical/guidelinessection/AcuteKidneyInjury.aspx
Acute Tubular Necrosis—Medline
http://www.nlm.nih.gov/medlineplus/ency/article/000512.htm
Acute Tubular Necrosis—Medscape
http://emedicine.medscape.com/article/238064-overview
Acute Tubular Necrosis—Overview
http://www.umm.edu/ency/article/000512.htm
CKD-EPI & MDRD Study Equation Calculator (With SI Units)
http://www.nephron.com/MDRD_GFR.cgi
MDRD renal function calculator
http://nkdep.nih.gov/professionals/gfr_calculators/idms_con.htm
GFR Calculator
http://www.davita.com/gfr-calculator/
National Institute for Diabetes, Digestive, and Kidney Diseases
http://www2.niddk.nih.gov/
Patient education materials from the National Kidney Disease Education Program
http://nkdep.nih.gov/patients/index.htm

PDF Documents

National Chronic Kidney Disease Fact Sheet (2010)
http://www.cdc.gov/diabetes/pubs/pdf/kidney_Factsheet.pdf
Chronic Kidney Disease in Adults: UK Guidelines for Identification, Management and Referral
http://www.renal.org/ckdguide/full/ukckdfull.pdf
Managing Urinary Incontinence in Older People
http://www.sld.cu/galerias/pdf/sitios/gericuba/manejo_incontinenecia_urinaria.pdf
United States Renal Data System 2010 Annual Data Report
http://www.usrds.org/2010/pdf/v1_00a_intros.pdf

Urinary Retention Protocol Algorithm
http://www.sjhlex.org/documents/Nursing/urinary_retention_protocol_algorithm_
letter_061808.pdf

Videos

Chronic Kidney Disease (2012) (2:39 minutes)
http://youtu.be/2H3zYq2zqy8
Diagnosing Chronic Kidney Disease (2010) (4:43 minutes)
http://youtu.be/k4eK8LrrSCQ
Stages of Chronic Kidney Disease (2012)
How do you know which stage of CKD you're in? Learn how to find out with DaVita's GFR
Calculator. (3:37 minutes)
http://youtu.be/zTxICCqywuI
Kidney Disease—Causes and Treatment of Kidney Failure (2013)
In this animation, the functioning of the kidneys and the symptoms of kidney disease are
explained. It tells about how kidney failure develops and what treatment can be applied.
(2:48 minutes)
http://youtu.be/BodnYcHGtiA
Educating Elderly Patients with Chronic Kidney Disease (2013) (1:21 minutes)
http://youtu.be/qwAd1R3Zgt4
I've Got a Secret: Identifying and Treating Urinary Incontinence in the Elderly (2011) (46:24
minutes)
http://youtu.be/sFgy6aHAFQo
Urinary Incontinence Causes, Symptoms and Treatment (2010)
This video features Doctor Charles Feinstein, a nationally renowned urologist, who
specializes in the treatment of Urinary Incontinence in woman. In this video Doctor
Feinstein talks about the causes, symptoms and treatment for Urinary Incontinence in
women. (15:07 minutes)
http://youtu.be/ZAMi4CGYHLU
Acute Tubular Necrosis Lecture (2012)
Acute tubular necrosis is caused by ischemia or direct toxic effect of medications on the renal
tubules in the kidney. (16:30 minutes)
http://youtu.be/ZhqrIXyM0PU
Histopathology Kidney—Acute Tubular Necrosis from Ethylene (2007) (3:36 minutes)
http://youtu.be/ajCG3sIe2iw

Images

Google images of Chronic Kidney Disease
http://www.google.com/search?q=Chronic+Kidney+Disease&hl=en&biw=1011&bih=214&
um=1&ie=UTF-8&tbm=isch&source=og&sa=N&tab=wi&ei=I_yhUf7SCfG10AHbgoHYCw
Mayo Clinic images for Urinary Incontinence
http://www.mayoclinic.com/health/urinary-incontinence/DS00404/TAB=multimedia

Septicemia and Infection

Mazen Madhoun, MD
Tanya Sigmon, MPAS, PA-C

INTRODUCTION

Infection is the primary cause of death in one third of individuals aged 65 years and older and is a contributor to death for many others. Infection also has a marked impact on morbidity in older adults, either exacerbating underlying illnesses or initiating functional decline. Multiple biologic, cultural, and societal factors account for the increased susceptibility of older adults to infection, and their poorer outcomes when infected. These factors also alter the presentation of infectious syndromes in older adults and may necessitate treatment modifications. In this chapter, we will discuss the factors that serve to put older individuals at particular risk for infection and will discuss four of the most common infections encountered in the geriatric population: sepsis, urinary tract infection (UTI), *Clostridium difficile* colitis, and skin and soft tissue infections. Pneumonia is discussed in the pulmonary disease chapter.

RISK FACTORS

Fundamental alterations in quantitative and qualitative immune response occur with aging and initiate a process that has been called immune senescence. Immune function is further compromised by the increasing number of concomitant medical problems that occur with aging. Impaired immunity correlates more with an individual's disease burden than chronologic age. Older adults who have chronic diseases (e.g., diabetes, chronic obstructive pulmonary disease [COPD], or heart failure) are more susceptible to common infections and exhibit poorer vaccine responses than those who do not have underlying health issues.

Multiple age-related changes contribute to decreased protection from infection in older adults. These changes include:

- Alterations in the barriers posed by the skin, lungs, and gastrointestinal tract (and other mucosal linings), permitting invasion by pathogenic organisms.
- Changes in cellular and humoral immunity, including decreases in specific cell populations, loss of the proliferative capacity of immune cells, and decreased production of specific cytokines (e.g., IL-2) that leads to increased risk of intracellular pathogens. Impaired signal transduction after cytokine binding is also associated with impaired defense against fungal and viral pathogens (Castle et al., 2007; Weiskopf et al., 2009).
- Decreased antibody response to vaccines, related to reductions in toll-like receptors and senescence of CD8$^+$ T cells (Goronzy et al., 2001).
- Reductions in immunoglobulin production and naive B cells (Pfister et al., 2006).

The risk of infection is further exacerbated by communal residence or other social institutions for older persons in developed nations, such as daycare programs or senior centers. Institutionalization is a major risk factor not only for acquiring disease in general, but for acquiring disease due to antibiotic resistant organisms. Methicillin-resistant *Staphylococcus aureus* (MRSA), vancomycin-resistant enterococci (VRE), fluoroquinolone-resistant *Streptococcus pneumoniae*, and multiply-resistant gram-negative bacilli are more frequent causes of infection among institutionalized older patients than those who are community-dwelling (Bradley, 1999; Kupronis et al., 2003; O'Fallon et al., 2009). Antibiotic resistance is fostered in the nursing home setting by debilitated hosts, proximity of residents, and persistent antibiotic pressure. A Canadian study found that 8% to 17% of nursing home residents were taking antibiotics at any given time, that 50% to 70% were exposed to antibiotics over the course of one year, and that 22% to 89% of this antibiotic use was inappropriate (Loeb et al., 2001).

DIAGNOSIS AND MANAGEMENT

It has been known for centuries that older adults can have a severe infection in the absence of typical signs or symptoms. Fever, the cardinal feature of infection, is absent in 30% to 50% of frail, older adults, even in the setting of serious infections like pneumonia or endocarditis (Henschke, 1993; Musgrave & Verghese, 1990). The blunted febrile response in older adults is due to changes in multiple systems responsible for thermoregulation: Shivering, vasoconstriction, hypothalamic regulation, and thermogenesis by brown adipose tissue are all impaired with advanced age.

Baseline body temperature is often lower than 37°C in older adults. Postmenopausal women have lower basal body temperatures than premenopausal women, and the presence of dementia, dependence in activities of daily living (ADLs), or a low body mass index ($<20 \, kg/m^2$) also increase the risk of lower body temperatures. Since signs of infection are commonly atypical in the older population, a rise in temperature from baseline becomes an important indicator of infection (Norman, 2000).

In addition to the frequent lack of fever, infections in older adults may be associated with a nonspecific decline in baseline functional status such as increased confusion, falling, and anorexia. For some seniors, exacerbations of underlying illness (e.g., atrial fibrillation) may be the predominant feature of infection.

Cognitive impairment further contributes to the atypical presentation of infections in older adults, reducing the capacity to communicate symptoms. Clinicians must be ready to pursue objective assessments such as laboratory and radiologic evaluations at a lower threshold in cognitively impaired patients, unless advanced directives and goals of care indicate otherwise.

Fever

Relatively healthy, community-dwelling older adults may be appropriately managed utilizing conventional definitions of fever. Fevers greater than 38°C (100.4°F) indicate a potential for serious infection, while hypothermia relative to baseline body temperatures may signify severe infection or even sepsis.

Revision of parameters used to identify "fever" in frail older patients has been suggested, owing to their altered febrile response. Fever in frail older patients may be considered as one or more of the following:

- Single oral temperature greater than 37.8°C (100°F)
- Persistent oral or tympanic membrane temperature greater than 37.2°C (99.0°F)
- Rectal temperature greater than 37.5°C (99.5°F)
- Rise in temperature of greater than 1.1°C (greater than 2°F) above baseline temperature (Castle et al., 1993; High et al., 2009; Norman, 2000).

Fever of Unknown Origin

Fever of unknown origin (FUO) is a classic medical syndrome defined as temperature greater than 38.3°C (101°F) for at least 3 weeks and undiagnosed after 1 week of medical evaluation. The differential diagnosis of FUO in older patients differs from that in younger.

Roughly a third of older patients with FUO have treatable infections (e.g., intra-abdominal abscess, bacterial endocarditis, tuberculosis, perinephric abscess, or occult osteomyelitis). Endocarditis and tuberculosis are more common in older adults than in younger patients (Tal et al., 2002).

- Giant cell arteritis (GCA, also known as temporal arteritis) and polymyalgia rheumatica (PMR) account for 19% of all FUO in the older population (Mourad et al., 2003). The evaluation of FUO in patients age greater than 60 years should include a rheumatological evaluation, including early temporal artery biopsy, particularly if the erythrocyte sedimentation rate or liver enzymes are elevated.
- Malignancy, particularly lymphoma, was a more common cause of FUO in older adults; more recent series suggest malignant disease as a cause of FUO occurs with similar frequency in old and young adults, perhaps because of the ability to establish a diagnosis by more aggressive imaging/CT scanning before patients reach FUO definitions (Ely et al., 2003). In both young and older adults, non-Hodgkin lymphoma accounts for the majority of cases.
- Rare causes of FUO in the older adult include drug fever, deep venous thrombosis with or without pulmonary embolism, and hyperthyroidism.

ANTIBIOTIC MANAGEMENT

The distribution, metabolism, and excretion of many drugs are altered with age. Of all the pharmacokinetic changes observed with advanced age, the most important is the decrease in the glomerular filtration rate (GFR) that occurs with aging. The simple rule "start low, go slow" is appropriate for dosing most medications in older patients. However, an important cautionary note must be sounded regarding certain antimicrobials (e.g., fluoroquinolones) that have concentration-dependent activity. Higher doses of these antibiotics are more effective and less likely to engender resistance. Thus, it is important that older adults with a serious infection receive a first antibiotic dose at the highest level with known safety profile, with subsequent dosing to maintain drug levels in the therapeutic range. This may take extra care in older adults in whom calculated creatinine clearance becomes less reliable with age.

When possible, drug levels should be monitored to avoid toxicity or subtherapeutic dosing. This is particularly important for levels of antibiotics that have a narrow therapeutic index, such as aminoglycosides, with heightened concern in patients with a reduced GFR.

Patient adherence to prescribed medications may be limited owing to many factors that are more common in older adults, including poor cognitive function, impaired hearing or vision, polypharmacy, medication side effects, and economic issues (inability to afford medications).

The choice of an initial antibiotic is not different from that in younger patients for most routine infections. However, special consideration is indicated for older adults who reside in an institution where multidrug resistant organisms are prevalent. Additionally, broader initial coverage may be appropriate in seriously ill older adults in whom sepsis, severe pneumonia, or other life-threatening infections are suspected since outcomes (mortality, length of ICU stay) are improved when the initial antibiotic regimen is effective against the infecting organism or organisms. Older individuals are more likely to have infections from more than one source (e.g., genitourinary or gastrointestinal, in addition to respiratory or skin sources). Thus, coverage should be broad until the infecting organisms are identified.

Prompt institution of antibiotics may be particularly relevant to outcomes in older adults when pneumonia is diagnosed. Data suggest that delaying initiation of therapy for 8 or more hours after admission to the hospital is associated with an increased risk of mortality. Since this study did not evaluate outcomes in younger patients, it is not known whether the effect of delayed antibiotic initiation is more relevant in older compared with younger patients (Meehan et al., 1997).

Just as prompt and appropriate use of antibiotics is important, the overuse and inappropriate use of antibiotics carries risks. Overuse of antibiotics can lead to antibiotic resistance, adverse reactions, and secondary infections, including *Clostridium difficile* and *Candida albicans* infections.

Antibiotic Drug Interactions

Antibiotic interactions occur with many medications commonly prescribed for older adults, particularly those drugs with a narrow therapeutic index. Significant interactions with commonly prescribed antibiotics are seen for:

- Digoxin
- Warfarin
- Oral hypoglycemic agents
- Theophylline
- Antacids and H_2 receptor antagonists
- Lipid lowering agents
- Lipophilic beta-blockers and non-dihydropyridine calcium channel blockers

The direction of the interaction may be hard to predict, and may even be biphasic (e.g., rifampin increases concentrations of some drugs initially, but induction of hepatic enzymes may lead to reduced drug concentrations in a few days). Atrophic gastritis, a common entity in older adults, and use of H_2-blockers or proton pump inhibitors can reduce the absorption of some antibiotics (e.g., itraconazole). Drug interactions, such as fluoroquinolones and antacids, may also reduce absorption.

INFECTION IN LONG-TERM CARE FACILITIES

Bacterial infections are common and rates of antibiotic use are particularly high in long-term care facilities. Khandelwal and colleagues (2012) described the 10 situations in long-term care for which antibiotics are often prescribed but rarely necessary. These include the following:

- Positive urine culture in an asymptomatic patient
- Urinalysis or culture for cloudy or malodorous urine
- Nonspecific symptoms or signs not referable to the urinary tract
- Upper respiratory infections
- Bronchitis, not in the setting of COPD
- Suspected or proven influenza without a secondary infection
- Respiratory symptoms in a terminal patient with dementia
- Skin wounds without cellulitis, sepsis, or osteomyelitis
- Small localized abscess without significant cellulitis
- Decubitus ulcer in a terminal patient

McGeer and colleagues, in 1991, proposed a set of criteria for surveillance of infections in the nursing home. Criteria included constitutional criteria for infection (Table 15.1). These criteria are intended to recognize that older patients and, in particular, frail older patients can have infections and present in unusual ways while also standardizing the language of consideration of infection. Providers should not simply use "not acting right" as the criteria for searching for or treating infections.

TABLE 15.1 • Definitions for Constitutional Criteria in Residents of Long-Term Care Facilities

A. Fever
 1. Single oral temperature >37.8°C (>100°F), OR
 2. Repeated oral temperatures >37.2°C (99°F) or rectal temperatures >37.5°C (99.5°F), OR
 3. Single temperature >1.1°C (2°F) over baseline from any site (oral, tympanic, axillary)
B. Leukocytosis
 1. Neutrophilia (>14,000 leukocytes/mm³), OR
 2. Left shift (>6% bands or ≥1,500 bands/mm³)
C. Acute change in mental status from baseline (all criteria must be present)
 1. Acute onset
 2. Fluctuating course
 3. Inattention, AND
 4. Either disorganized thinking or altered level of consciousness
D. Acute functional decline
 1. A new 3-point increase in total ADL score (range 0–28) from baseline, based on the following 7 ADL items each scored from 0 (independent) to 4 (dependent)
  a. Bed mobility
  b. Transfer
  c. Locomotion within the facility
  d. Dressing
  e. Toilet use
  f. Personal hygiene
  g. Eating

From Stone, N. D., Ashraf, M. S., Calder, J., Crnich, C. J., Crossley, K., Drinka, P. J.,... Bradley, S. F. (2012). Surveillance definitions of infections in long-term care facilities: Revisiting the McGeer criteria. *Infection Control and Hospital Epidemiology, 33*(10), 965–977, with permission.

SPECIFIC INFECTIONS

Bacteremia and Sepsis

According to the American College of Chest Physicians and the Society of Critical Care Medicine, the term bacteremia denotes the presence of bacteria in the blood (Bone et al., 1992). It does not say anything about the host response to the bacteria. Conversely, sepsis is determined by the response to infection. Even though every patient with bacteremia does not have sepsis, the syndrome is likely under-recognized in the older adult, partly owing to the lack of typical manifestations of systemic inflammatory response syndrome (SIRS) (see Table 15.2).

Epidemiology

It is estimated that there are 2,500 cases of sepsis per 10,000 persons aged 85 and above (Martin et al., 2006). In a retrospective study using the National Hospital Discharge Survey, Martin et al determined that persons aged 65 and older were 13 times more likely to have sepsis when compared with younger individuals (Martin et al., 2006).

Bacteremia carries a poor prognosis with advanced age. For example, nosocomial gram-negative bacteremia has a mortality rate of 5% to 35% in young adults, and 37% to 50% in older adults. Factors contributing to increased mortality in older adults include the use of invasive devices such as intravenous or urinary catheters, presence of coexisting disease, reduced immune response mechanisms leading to more prolonged inflammation, and a greater incidence of end

TABLE 15.2 · Definitions of Sepsis, Bacteremia, and Related Disorders

Disorder	Definition
Infection	Microbial phenomenon characterized by an inflammatory response to the presence of microorganisms or the invasion of normally sterile host tissue by those organisms. A pathologic process caused by the invasion of normally sterile tissue or fluid or body cavity by pathogenic or potentially pathogenic microorganisms.
Bacteremia	Presence of bacteria in the blood.
SIRS	The systemic inflammatory response to a variety of clinical insults exhibited by at least two of the following: (1) temperature >38°C or <36°C, (2) heart rate >90 beats/min, (3) respiratory rate >20 breaths/min with a $PaCO_2$ <32 mm Hg, and (4) WBC >12,000/mm^3 or <4,000/mm^3 or >10% immature (band) forms.
Sepsis	SIRS and documented or suspected infection
Severe sepsis	Sepsis associated with organ dysfunction, hypoperfusion, or hypotension. Hypoperfusion and perfusion abnormalities may include, but are not limited to, lactic acidosis, oliguria, or an acute alteration in mental status.
Septic shock	Sepsis complicated by hypotension (i.e., SBP <90 mm Hg or MAP <60 mm Hg) despite adequate fluid resuscitation.

Abbreviations: MAP, mean arterial pressure; SBP, systolic blood pressure; SIRS, systemic inflammatory response syndrome; WBC, white blood cells.
From Bone, R. C., Balk, R. A., Cerra, F. B., Dellinger, R. P., Fein, A. M., Knaus, W. A., ... Sibbald, W. J. (1992). Definitions for sepsis and organ failure and guidelines for the use of innovative therapies in sepsis: The ACCP/SCCM Consensus Conference Committee. American College of Chest Physicians/Society of Critical Care Medicine. *Chest, 101*(6), 1644–1655, with permission.

organ damage in the face of a septic episode (e.g., acute respiratory distress syndrome or acute kidney injury) (Pien et al., 2010).

Pathogenesis

Escherichia coli is the most frequently isolated pathogen among older patients with community-acquired bacteremia (Diekema et al., 2002). This is, at least in part, due to gastrointestinal and, even more frequently, genitourinary sources of bacteremia being the more common source of the bacteremia. This trend continues to increase throughout the eighth and ninth decades of life. Age does not necessarily increase the likelihood of endocarditis or osteomyelitis, but these infections will also frequently result in bacteremia.

With the increasing rates of colonization and infection and the resulting antibiotic use comes the problem of antibiotic resistant bacteria. This is a particular problem in nursing homes.

Risk Factors

Older persons are at greater risk for bacteremia or sepsis as a result of three primary factors. As mentioned previously, immune senescence increases the risk of infection as well as of sepsis. Secondly, older persons have higher rates of such chronic illnesses as COPD, diabetes mellitus, cancer, chronic kidney disease requiring hemodialysis, and heart failure. With aging comes a greater risk of malnutrition and poor performance status, again increasing the risk of infection. Older persons with chronic skin wounds such as venous stasis ulcers, arterial ulcers, and pressure ulcers are at risk for bacterial contamination of the wound with bacteremia and sepsis often resulting. In addition, because aspiration is more common with increasing age, older persons at risk for aspiration can become bacteremic from the aspiration.

Finally, there are iatrogenic factors at play that increase the risk of infection and sepsis. Both short- and long-term institutionalization increase the risk of infection. Older individuals, especially those confined to institutions, are at greater risk for indwelling urinary catheters. The presence of an indwelling urinary catheter is the most common source of bacteria single highest risk of infection and sepsis in older adults. Other procedures and instrumentation, in addition to indwelling urinary catheters, carry the risk of introducing bacteria and resulting infection and sepsis.

Clinical Presentation

When compared with young adults, older patients with bacteremia are less likely to have chills or sweating, and fever is frequently absent. Similarly, vital sign changes may also be more subtle. Hypothermia and hypotension may be clues to bacteremia or sepsis. Older persons are less likely to generate a heart rate response to stress; tachycardia is a less reliable sign than in younger persons; however, older adults with infection frequently present clinically with nonspecific clinical findings such as delirium, somnolence, anorexia, generalized weakness, or falls. Because of the nonspecific nature of these findings, as well as the high frequency of comorbid conditions such as dementia and cerebrovascular disease, older adults with infection can present a diagnostic challenge to the clinician.

Older persons are at greater risk for death due to bacteremia and sepsis, primarily due to the higher likelihood of concomitant organ dysfunction. For those who survive sepsis, there is often a functional decline.

Evaluation

There have been limited studies to guide providers on the triggers to collect blood cultures and, in particular, demonstrating the utility of blood cultures in the long-term care setting. With that being said, patients with indwelling vascular catheters, including peripherally inserted central catheters (PICC) and hemodialysis catheters, who have symptoms suggestive of bacteremia or sepsis should have blood cultures obtained and, in certain circumstances, have the line removed with the tip cultured.

Treatment

The key to successful treatment of bacteremia and sepsis, regardless of the age of the patient, involves adequate antimicrobial coverage and removal of the source of the infection. In addition, because the sepsis syndrome is often accompanied by detrimental effects of the inflammatory response on end organs, efforts to eliminate or minimize these effects need to be undertaken.

By definition, the diagnosis of bacteremia and sepsis depends on the presence of a positive blood culture. The culture result and antibiotic sensitivities will guide the clinician toward the proper antibiotic selection. However, in the case of the sepsis syndrome, one cannot wait until the culture and sensitivity results, thus necessitating the use of empiric antibiotics. Antibiotic administration should not be delayed longer than one hour after sepsis is suspected (Dellinger et al., 2004). The empiric antibiotic selected should have a broad spectrum and should be used until such time as a more targeted antibiotic can be selected based on the culture and sensitivity result. The length of treatment will be determined by the source of the infection, with bacteremia resulting from endocarditis or osteomyelitis necessitating lengthy intravenous antibiotic course of treatment.

When there is a source of infection, such as a catheter or device, necrotic tissue, or abscess, these should be removed or addressed. When the source of infection is less obvious, diagnostic studies should be performed to identify potential sources of infection.

All patients with severe sepsis or septic shock will need fluid resuscitation. Some may require blood products and pressor agents such as dopamine. Mechanical ventilation may be required during the initial resuscitation, particularly in patients who develop acute respiratory distress syndrome (ARDS). Prophylactic measures to prevent deep venous thrombosis (DVT) and stress ulcers should also be considered. Finally, delirium occurs very commonly in the older adult with infection. The balance between sedation and analgesia and delirium can be difficult; therefore, medications that are known to cause delirium should be discontinued.

Urinary Tract Infection

UTI is the most common infection in adults aged 65 and over. The incidence rate approaches 10% in women and 5.3% in men over the age of 80. UTIs are the second most common infection for those who reside in the community and the number one cause of infection for those who reside in a long-term care facility or are hospitalized (Foxman & Brown, 2003). Gram-negative bacilli (e.g., *E. coli*, *Enterobacter* spp., *Klebsiella* spp., *Proteus* spp.) are most common, but there is an increase in more resistant isolates such as *Pseudomonas aeruginosa*, and gram-positive organisms, including enterococci (*Enterococcus fecalis* and *Enterococcus faecium*), coagulase-negative staphylococci and *Streptococcus agalactiae* (group B strep), when compared with young adults.

UTIs can involve several distinct entities, including asymptomatic bacteriuria, symptomatic infections, lower tract UTIs such as cystitis (infection of the bladder), and upper tract UTIs such as pyelonephritis (infection of the kidneys). As a result of their ability to cause renal damage, upper tract UTIs are considered more serious than lower tract UTIs. When a UTI develops, it is usually from bacteria that have colonized the urethra, vagina, or perianal area.

Asymptomatic Bacteriuria

Asymptomatic bacteriuria (ASB) is a common phenomenon in older adults, occurring in up to 6% to 16% of women in the community and 25% to 54% of women who reside in a nursing home (Juthani-Mehta, 2007). This is in part due to physiological changes that occur with aging, including decreased estrogen in women and decrease in the bactericidal activity of prostatic secretion in men. The preponderance of evidence suggests that routine screening for or treatment of ASB is not recommended in older persons (Abrutyn et al., 1994; Nicolle et al., 1983, 1987; Ouslander et al., 1995). The exception to this recommendation suggests that screening for and treatment of bacteriuria is recommended before transurethral resection of the prostate and before other urologic procedures where mucosal bleeding is expected (Nicolle et al., 2005). There are no good studies on the prevention of ASB, and treatment does not decrease the prevalence of bacteriuria at 6 months (Boscia et al., 1987).

Diagnosis of UTI

The diagnosis of UTI requires the combination of significant bacteriuria ($\geq 10^5$ colony-forming unit [CFU]/ml) associated with genitourinary symptoms. The difficulty arises in the cognitively impaired individual who is unable to describe symptoms referable to the urinary tract. The most common pathogens are gram-negative organisms, most commonly *E. coli*. In the 20% that are not gram-negative, the most common organisms are Enterococcus or MRSA.

Evaluation

Clinical guidelines from the Infectious Diseases Society of America for evaluation of infection in older residents of long-term care facilities advise that urinalysis and urine cultures should not be ordered for asymptomatic individuals (High et al., 2009). The McGeer surveillance guidelines for UTIs in the long-term care setting are detailed in Table 15.3 (Stone et al., 2012). Diagnostic testing should be reserved for residents with fever, dysuria, gross hematuria, worsening incontinence, or suspected bacteremia. There is some evidence for using dipstick urine tests as a first line in gauging whether or not to order full urine culture or to begin presumptive antibiotic treatment awaiting culture results (Arinzon et al., 2009).

UTIs are also categorized as uncomplicated or complicated. Uncomplicated UTIs are defined as those that occur when patients do not have any functional or structural abnormalities of the urinary tract that would inhibit the flow of urine or normal voiding mechanism. Complicated UTIs may involve the lower or upper urinary tract and occur in situations in which there are functional or structural abnormalities of the urinary tract that inhibit the normal flow or urine or defense mechanisms. Stone formation, indwelling catheters, prostatic hypertrophy, obstruction, cancer, or neurologic conditions are common causative effects in complicated UTIs.

Infections often present in a subtle fashion in older adults. Diagnosis of a UTI in these patients relies on clinical signs (e.g., altered mental status) and symptoms, supported by laboratory data.

TABLE 15.3 • Surveillance Definitions for UTIs

A. For residents without an indwelling catheter (both criteria 1 and 2 must be present)
1. At least one of the following
   a. Acute dysuria or acute pain, swelling, or tenderness of the testes, epididymis, or prostate
   b. Fever or leukocytosis (see Table 15.1) and at least one of the following localizing urinary tract subcriteria
      i. Acute costovertebral angle pain or tenderness
      ii. Suprapubic pain
      iii. Gross hematuria
      iv. New or increase in incontinence
      v. New or marked increase in urgency
      vi. New or marked increase in frequency
   c. In the absence of fever or leukocytosis, then two or more of the following localizing urinary tract subcriteria
      i. Suprapubic pain
      ii. Gross hematuria
      iii. New or increase in incontinence
      iv. New or marked increase in urgency
      v. New or marked increase in frequency
2. One of the following microbiologic subcriteria
   a. At least 10^5 colony-forming unit (CFU)/ml of no more than two species of microorganisms in a voided urine specimen
   b. At least 10^2 CFU/ml of any number of organisms in a specimen collected by in-and-out catheter
B. For residents with an indwelling catheter (both criteria 1 and 2 must be present)
1. At least one of the following sign or symptom subcriteria
   a. Fever, rigors, or new-onset hypotension, with no alternate site of infection
   b. Either acute change in mental status or acute functional decline, with no alternate diagnosis or leukocytosis
   c. New-onset suprapubic pain or costovertebral angle pain or tenderness
   d. Purulent discharge from around the catheter or acute pain, swelling, or tenderness of the testes, epididymis, or prostate
2. Urinary catheter specimen culture of at least 10^5 CFU/ml of any organism(s)

From Stone, N. D., Ashraf, M. S., Calder, J., Crnich, C. J., Crossley, K., Drinka, P. J., ... Bradley, S. F. (2012). Surveillance definitions of infections in long-term care facilities: Revisiting the McGeer criteria. *Infection Control and Hospital Epidemiology, 33*(10), 965–977, with permission.

Urine cultures in infected older patients may have lower colony counts (10^2 to 10^3 CFU/ml) compared with 10^5 CFU/ml in younger patients. Therapeutic antibiotic "trials" are not recommended in order to minimize potential drug toxicity, drug–drug interaction, superinfection, and antimicrobial resistance.

In the case of individuals of either sex who are unable to provide adequate urine specimen for culture, an in-and-out catheterization should be performed. The urine culture should always be obtained before initiating antibiotic therapy.

Risk Factors for UTI

Older adults are at increased risk for UTIs. Also at risk are persons with urinary obstruction and reflux, individuals with neurogenic disorders that impair bladder emptying, and men with diseases of the prostate. Instrumentation and urinary catheterization are the most common predisposing factors for nosocomial UTIs. UTIs are also more common in women with diabetes than in women without the disease. Several factors that predispose the older adult to UTIs are poor bladder emptying due to immobility, bladder outflow obstruction caused by prostatic hyperplasia or kidney stones, bladder ischemia caused by urine retention, senile vaginitis, constipation, and diminished bactericidal activity of urine and prostatic secretions.

As mentioned previously, ASB is common in the senior adult population. With the use of chronic catheters, rates are even higher, with about 85% for condom catheters and nearly 100% for indwelling catheters having bacteriuria (Juthani-Mehta, 2007). The most common uropathogen in ASB of the older population is *E. coli*, although at a lower rate than in patients with symptomatic UTIs. Numerous studies suggest that there is no clinical benefit when ASB is treated, but treatment can lead to significant side effects, expense, and potential for selection of resistant organisms. Thus, treatment is not recommended, even in the presence of white blood cells in the urine.

Prevention

In postmenopausal women with recurrent UTIs, intravaginal estradiol therapy has been shown to reduce the number of episodes (Raz & Stamm, 1993). Antibiotic prophylaxis may have a role, although the literature demonstrates increased rates of resistance with the use of antibiotic prophylaxis (Matthews & Lancaster, 2011). The use of cranberry juice or capsules, at doses of 100 to 500 mg of cranberry concentrate daily, have been shown in several studies to reduce the incidence of UTIs (Jepson & Craig, 2008; Matthews & Lancaster, 2011; McMurdo et al., 2009). The most effective means of preventing UTIs in women and men is avoiding the use of an indwelling catheter and removal of the catheter as quickly as possible when placement is mandated.

Treatment

Cystitis. When true UTI is documented in an older woman, therapy is based on the location of infection (upper versus lower tract disease) and likely causative agent. Lower tract UTIs (cystitis), characterized by dysuria, frequency, and urgency are often treated with short courses of antibiotics (for 3 to 5 days) in young women. A systematic review comparing antibiotic course duration (single day, 3 to 6 days, or 7 to 14 days) for uncomplicated symptomatic lower UTI in older women found that 3- to 6-day courses were sufficient for treatment. Most recent guidelines recommend the use of nitrofurantoin (Macrobid), Bactrim, and monurol (Fosfomycin) as first-line treatment, leaving the Quinolones as second-line treatment (Lutters & Vogt-Ferrier, 2008). Fosfomycin comes in a 3-g-per- dose packet. For uncomplicated UTI, one 3-g dose may be all that is needed. As long as the symptoms associated with the UTI have resolved, there is no need for a test of cure urinalysis and culture.

UTI in older men is frequently caused by concomitant prostate disease (primarily hyperplasia) or functional bladder impairment, such as poor bladder emptying due to diabetes with peripheral neuropathy. Studies on the optimal duration for the treatment of cystitis in men are less clear, with the recommended duration of treatment between 7 and 14 days (Nicolle, 2009). In men who have recurrent UTI thought secondary to a prostatic origin, the duration of treatment should be 6 to 12 weeks (Nicolle, 2009).

Acute Pyelonephritis. Upper tract UTI (pyelonephritis) is typically characterized by fever, chills, nausea, and flank pain often accompanied by lower tract symptoms although, as with all infections, presentation in older adults may be more subtle. The primary pathogen for pyelonephritis remains *E. coli*, though this bacterium accounts for a lower percentage in the older population compared with a younger population (Matthews & Lancaster, 2011).

The location for treatment will depend on the severity of symptoms, the ability to tolerate oral medications, the living conditions, and the ability of the patient to comply. In general, upper tract infection requires longer courses of therapy than lower tract infection. Because of the excellent bioavailability of many antibiotics, particularly the fluoroquinolones, intravenous therapy is not essential if the patient can tolerate oral medications, is not septic, and the infecting organisms are sensitive to oral agents.

When intravenous therapy is needed, the ability of the facility or home care services to provide and administer the drugs becomes paramount. The older patient should be hospitalized when the nature of the therapy exceeds the capability of the institution to meet that need. The choice of intravenous antibiotic will depend on the resistance pattern of the community. In general, the length of therapy should be 10 to 14 days for acute pyelonephritis. The intravenous delivery can be changed to the oral route when the patient is able to tolerate oral medications. In addition to antibiotics, older patients with acute pyelonephritis often require attention to fluid status and may require other, more aggressive, means to treat septic shock.

Catheter-Associated UTI. For the patient with an indwelling catheter, a urine sample should be attained from the catheter port, not the collection bag. Symptomatic patients with an indwelling urethral catheter in place for greater than 2 weeks should have the catheter replaced, and the urine collected from the new catheter. A catheter-associated UTI (CA-UTI) is defined by a properly collected urine sample that grows greater than or equal to 10^3 CFU/ml (Matthews & Lancaster, 2011). The organisms are similar for CA-UTI, so treatment choices are similar to what was described above. The duration of treatment can depend on the response of the patient, with 7 days being adequate for patients who respond quickly. Patients with a more delayed response may require 10 to 14 days of treatment (Matthews & Lancaster, 2011).

Clostridium Difficile

C. difficile is the most common cause of antibiotic-associated diarrhea, the most common cause of infectious diarrhea on the health care setting, and a main cause of the health care–associated infections (Aslam et al., 2005; Cohen et al., 2010). The incidence of *C. difficile* colitis nearly doubled between 2000 and 2005, with the majority of cases in the older populations (Janka & O'Grady, 2009). *C. difficile* may be asymptomatic, but if symptoms are present, they may range from mild diarrhea to life-threatening pseudomembranous colitis. The mainstay of treatment for many years has been Flagyl and oral vancomycin. However, the recently released Fidaxomicin (Dificid) and the experimental drug, Cadazolid, are showing promise.

Major risk factors for *C. difficile* include recent exposure to antimicrobial agents, recent hospitalizations, and advanced age. Mature adult patients often receive broad-spectrum antimicrobial agents to treat the various infections they experience. In addition, owing to comorbidities, they are likely to be hospitalized for longer periods. Residents of long-term care facilities are at even greater risk for the same reasons as well as the limited ability to isolate them in a private room.

Immune system function declines with age, and changes in fecal flora occur. Older persons have an increased incidence of initial and recurrent infection, appear to be at risk for more severe infection, and have a higher mortality rate. In hospitalized older patients, the incidence of *C. difficile* is 5 to 10 times higher than the incidence of younger patients (Simor, 2010).

C. difficile is a gram-positive, anaerobic, spore-forming, toxin-producing rod with a characteristic odor of horse feces and can exist in the vegetative or spore state. After a patient with *C. difficile* has been discharged from a hospital room, spores can survive up to 40 days (Dubberke & Wertheimer, 2009). The bacterium exists in a vegetative (active) or spore (dormant) state.

Toxin production is associated with clinical disease. The two main toxin-producing strains are Toxin A and Toxin B, which lead to the production of tumor necrosis factor, release proinflammatory interleukins, and cytokines. The toxins increase vascular permeability, resulting in watery diarrhea, colitis, and pseudomembranous formation.

Pathogenesis

Human transmission of *C. difficile* is primarily via the fecal–oral route. However, in the health care setting, environmental contamination plays an important role. Spores are excreted in the feces of patients infected with the bacteria. Infection may spread after the hands of patients and health care workers, the main source of transmission, become contaminated with *C. difficile*, and the spores are orally ingested.

Fomites are also a source of transmission. *C. difficile* has been cultured from toilets, bedding and bed rails, furniture, telephones, floors, windowsills, and medical equipment (Simor, 2010). Once ingested, spores are able to survive the gastric acid of the stomach and then become vegetative and pathogenic in the colon. Toxin production is greatest when most of the *C. difficile* population is in vegetative form, and it is lowest when mainly spores are present (Kee, 2012).

Epidemiology

Approximately 3% of adults are colonized with *C. difficile* and without symptoms. In hospitals, 20% to 30% of adults are colonized, and in long-term care facilities, this frequency may be as high as 50% (Salkind, 2010). In the United States, it is estimated that there are approximately 500,000 cases of *C. difficile* per year in hospitals and long-term care facilities (Rupnik et al., 2009).

The recent increase in the prevalence and virulence of *C. difficile* can be attributed to a new hypervirulent strain of *C. difficile* that has been associated with several outbreaks during the past decade. This strain has developed resistance to all fluoroquinolones.

Risk Factors

The primary risk factor for *C. difficile* infection (CDI) is antibiotic exposure. The precipitating event for *C. difficile* colitis is disruption of the normal flora of the colon, with broad-spectrum antibiotics often causing the disruption. All antibiotics have the potential to promote CDI; however, certain antibiotics disrupt large bowel flora more than others. Clindamycin, broad-spectrum penicillins (particularly Augmentin), second- and third-generation cephalosporins, and, most recently, fluoroquinolones have been implicated most frequently. The longer the duration of antibiotic therapy and the greater the number of antibiotics, the greater the risk of *C. difficile*.

The other major risk factors include recent stay in a hospital or nursing home and older age. Other risk factors include immunosuppression, multiple and severe underlying diseases, sharing a hospital or nursing home room with a patient with *C. difficile*, use of gastric acid suppressing agents (e.g., proton pump inhibitors and H_2-receptor antagonists), use of antineoplastic agents, and use of enemas (Kee, 2012).

Symptoms

In patients exhibiting symptoms, the most common symptom is diarrhea while taking or shortly after finishing a course of antibiotics, although it may occur as long as 8 weeks after therapy has ended. The diarrhea is watery, non-bloody, and characteristically foul smelling. This is often the only symptom; patients may have up to 10 bowel movements per day. Other features include typical signs and symptoms of colitis, including abdominal cramps, fever, leukocytosis, leukocytes in the feces, hypoalbuminemia, polymorphonuclear pseudomembranes visualized by endoscopy, and colonic wall thickening.

Older adults may have an atypical clinical presentation, making diagnosis more challenging. Fever may not be present, but when fever is present in older patients, it may indicate a more severe infection. Acute confusion or altered mental status may be the first symptom. Other non-specific symptoms of infection may be seen, including weakness, anorexia, weight loss, frequent falls, and loss of physical functional capacity.

Evaluation and Diagnosis

C. difficile is diagnosed when symptoms (usually diarrhea) are present and either a stool test is positive for C. difficile toxins or toxigenic C. difficile or with pathology by colonoscopy revealing pseudomembranous colitis. Stool culture is impractical due to the slow turnaround time. Recent guidelines recommend a two-step approach to diagnosing CDI. This approach first uses enzyme immunoassay to detect glutamate dehydrogenase, also known as C. difficile common antigen, and then uses the cell cytotoxicity assay or toxigenic culture to confirm glutamate dehydrogenase positive stool specimens (Kee, 2012).

Prevention

To prevent the spread of CDI, health care workers and visitors should use gloves and gowns when entering the room of a patient with CDI, and should wash their hands with soap (antimicrobial soap) and water after contact with patients. Alcohol-based hand sanitizers are ineffective against C. difficile spores. Patients with CDI should be isolated in a private room if available; if not available, each patient in a room should be provided with a dedicated commode. These precautions should be taken until the diarrhea resolves.

Treatment

Asymptomatic carriers should not be treated. When treating patients with symptomatic CDI, all antibiotics that might have contributed to the infection should be discontinued. This step alone may resolve mild infections. In patients in whom antibiotic treatment cannot be stopped and in those with more severe disease, active treatment is necessary. If antibiotic discontinuation is not possible, agents that are less frequently or rarely associated with CDI (e.g., ampicillin, sulfonamides, erythromycin, tetracycline, penicillin, and antistaphylococcal penicillin, or a first-generation cephalosporin) should be considered.

Antimotility agents such as loperamide should not be used as that can impair response and increase the risk of toxic megacolon, a common complication of CDI. The primary antibiotics effective in the treatment of CDI treatment are metronidazole and vancomycin. Metronidazole has long been considered the first line of treatment, with vancomycin being reserved mainly for severe or refractory cases. The primary reason to limit the use of vancomycin is the concern of its overuse leading to VRE. Several trials have found that recurrence rates following therapy with metronidazole or vancomycin are similar (15% to 25%); more recent reports, however, have suggested that recurrence rates with metronidazole in frail adults may be as high as 50% (Cohen et al., 2010; van Nispen tot Pannerden et al., 2011). The recent FDA approval of fidaxomicin (Difcid) in 2011 has provided an alternative to metronidazole and vancomycin for the treatment of *C. difficile*–associated diarrhea in adults. Fifty percent of patients in controlled clinical trials were aged greater than 65 years, and 31% were greater than 75 years (U.S. Food and Drug Administration, 2011). There are no contraindications to the use of fidaxomicin; however, there is a warning that the drug should not be used for systemic infections. Fidaxomicin is a macrolide antibiotic; the approved dosage is 200 mg orally twice daily with or without food. No clinically significant drug interactions have been identified with fidaxomicin. The most common adverse reactions observed during clinical trials were nausea (11%), vomiting (7%), abdominal pain (6%), gastrointestinal hemorrhage (4%), anemia (2%), and neutropenia (2%).

Recent guidelines recommend metronidazole and/or vancomycin, depending on the severity (mild to moderate, severe with no complications, or severe with complications) and episode (initial, first recurrent, or second recurrent) (see Table 15.4). Mild to moderate CDI is defined as leukocytosis with a white blood cell count of less than or equal to 15,000/µl or a serum creatinine level less than 1.5 times the premorbid level. Severe CDI is defined as a leukocytosis with a WBC count greater than 15,000/µl or a serum creatinine level greater than 1.5 times the premorbid level, and if hypotension, shock, ileus, or megacolon are present, it is considered complicated, severe CDI (Cohen et al., 2010).

TABLE 15.4 · Clinical Practice Guideline Recommendations for *Clostridium difficile* Infections

Initial episode, mild or moderate WBC <15k and <50% decrease serum Cr	Metronidazole 500 mg by mouth three times per day for 10–14 days
Initial episode, severe WBC >15k and >50% decrease serum Cr	Vancomycin 125 mg by mouth four times per day for 10–14 days
Initial episode, severe, complicated WBC >15k and >50% decrease serum Cr Evidence of sepsis or toxic megacolon	Hospitalization Metronidazole 500 mg intravenously every 8 hr plus: – vancomycin 125 mg by mouth or nasogastric tube four times per day (consider adding rectal instillation of vancomycin if complete ileus)
First recurrence	Metronidazole 500 mg by mouth three times per day for 10–14 days
Second recurrence	Oral vancomycin in a tapered and/or pulsed regimen; various regimens have been used and are similar to the following: 125 mg q.i.d. for 10–14 days, then 125 mg b.i.d. for one week, then 125 mg daily for a week, then 125 mg every 2–3 days for 2–8 weeks

From Dubberke, E. R., & Wertheimer, A. I. (2009). Review of current literature in the economic burden of *Clostridium difficile* infection. *Infection Control and Hospital Epidemiology, 30*(1), 57–66, with permission.

Oral metronidazole monotherapy is recommended for initial mild to moderate episodes or for first recurrence. Metronidazole is not recommended for recurrent disease or for long-term use. Oral vancomycin monotherapy is recommended for initial severe episodes or for second recurrence. For initial episodes of severe, complicated CDI, intravenous metronidazole plus vancomycin orally or by nasogastric tube (rectal vancomycin can be added if a complete ileus is present) is recommended (Janka & O'Grady, 2009).

Skin and Soft Tissue Infections

The aging skin loses some of its protective capacity, and thus the likelihood for skin breakdown as well as for skin infection increases. While a skin wound does not inevitably lead to bacterial overgrowth and infection, this complication should be a primary concern in managing skin wounds. Systemic antibiotic use, in the absence of signs of deep infection, does not prevent infection. In fact, such a practice leads to an increased incidence of complications of antibiotics, antibiotic resistance, and greater difficulty in treating should a true bacterial infection develop.

Risk Factors

Risk factors for skin infection can be divided into two categories, risk factors for skin breakdown and risk factors for infection once the skin has been compromised. With aging, the skin becomes more fragile and thus more susceptible to breakdown. In addition, obesity, venous or lymph stasis, recent skin trauma, and skin conditions such as eczema are risk factors for bacterial overgrowth. Older patients are more susceptible to skin fragility as well as to conditions that result in a greater likelihood of tissue hypoxia, such as obesity and venous stasis. Risk factors for skin infection include urinary and fecal incontinence, the use of antibiotics for infections elsewhere, and overall improper attention to open wounds. Pressure ulcers are more common with aging; risk factors for pressure ulcers include immobility, incontinence, PVD, (Peripheral Vascular Disease) diabetes mellitus, and dementia.

Clinical Presentation

When managing skin wounds, providers should assure that the wound is actively infected prior to administering systemic antibiotics. The practice of obtaining culture and sensitivity studies on wounds that do not show signs of infection should be discouraged as this will result in inappropriate use of antibiotics. There are a number of systemic signs that point toward infection, including increased size of the wound, poor wound healing, odor, erythema, warmth, pain, and exudative drainage. Studies vary on the number or extent of such signs that should trigger a culture and the use of systemic antibiotics. In a European study, redness, malodor, pain and delayed healing, or deterioration of the wound were the signs that pointed to infection (Cutting et al., 2005). Inherent in this study is the importance of close monitoring of the wound over time.

Prevention

The best way to prevent skin infections is to maintain the integrity of the skin. Edema should be prevented or minimized by aggressive medical management and/or the use of compression stockings. In addition, such interventions as attending to macerated feet with good foot care or antifungals, good care of surgical wounds and other open areas in an effort to prevent infection, and prevention of maceration of sacral skin in patients with urinary incontinence can help to prevent skin and soft tissue infections. Finally attention to comorbid factors such as glucose control in diabetics, obesity, and tobacco use can be of value.

When a patient is in a health care setting and the skin is infected or colonized with MRSA, isolation and/or the use of appropriate infection control procedures is important in preventing spread to other patients.

Treatment

For toxic appearing patients or those who are septic, the initial treatment needs to be intravenous. Milder cases can safely be treated with oral antibiotics. Antimicrobial therapy must be effective against streptococci and *S. aureus.* For culture-proven MRSA or in patients with a recent history of and MRSA infection, initial treatment should include vancomycin, linezolid, or daptomycin. Typical courses of antibiotic therapy might range from 5 to14 days depending upon the severity of the infection. Transition from intravenous to oral therapy can occur as the patient improves clinically. For deep infections, abscesses, and necrotizing fasciitis, the hallmark of treatment involves surgical drainage or other intervention.

REFERENCES

Abrutyn, E., Mossey, J., Berlin, J. A., Boscia, J., Levison, M., Pitsakis, P., & Kaye, D. (1994). Does asymptomatic bacteriuria predict mortality and does antimicrobial treatment reduce mortality in elderly ambulatory women? *Annals of Internal Medicine, 120,* 827–833.

Arinzon, Z., Peisakh, A., Shuval, I., Shabat, S., & Berner, Y. N. (2009). Detection of urinary tract infection (UTI) in long-term care setting: Is the multireagent strip an adequate diagnostic tool? *Archives of Gerontology and Geriatrics, 48,* 227–231.

Aslam, S., Hamill, R. J., & Musher, D. M. (2005). Treatment of *Clostridium difficile*-associated disease: Old therapies and new strategies. *Lancet Infectious Diseases, 5*(9), 549–557.

Bone, R. C., Balk, R. A., Cerra, F. B., Dellinger, R. P., Fein, A. M., Knaus, W. A.,…Sibbald, W. J. (1992). Definitions for sepsis and organ failure and guidelines for the use of innovative therapies in sepsis: The ACCP/SCCP Consensus Conference Committee, American College of Chest Physicians/Society of Critical Care Medicine. *Chest, 101*(6), 1644–1655.

Boscia, J. A., Kobasa, W. D., Knight, R. A., Abrutyn, E., Levison, M. E., & Kaye, D. (1987). Therapy vs no therapy for bacteriuria in elderly ambulatory nonhospitalized women. *JAMA: The Journal of the American Medical Association, 257,* 1067–1071.

Bradley, S. F. (1999). Issues in the management of resistant bacteria in long-term-care facilities. *Infection Control and Hospital Epidemiology, 20*(5), 362.

Castle, S. C., Uyemura, K., Fulop, T., & Makinodan, T. (2007). Host resistance and immune responses in advanced age. *Clinics in Geriatric Medicine, 23*(3), 463.

Castle, S. C., Yeh, M., Toledo, S. D., Yoshikawa, T. T., & Norman, D. C. (1993). Lowering the fever criterion improves detection of infections in nursing home residents. *Aging—Immunology and Infectious Diseases, 4,* 67.

Cohen, S. H., Gerding, D. N., Johnson, S., Kelly, C. P., Loo, V. G., McDonald, L. C.,…Wilcox, M. H. (2010). Clinical practice guidelines for *Clostridium difficile* infection in adults: 2010 update by the Society for Healthcare Epidemiology of America (SHEA) and the Infectious Diseases Society of America (IDSA). *Infection Control and Hospital Epidemiology, 31*(5), 431–444.

Cutting, K. F., White, R. J., Mahoney, P., & Harding, K. G. (2005). Clinical identification of wound infection: A Delphi approach. In European Wound Management Association (Ed.), *Position document: Identifying criteria for wound infection.* London, England: MEP.

Dellinger, R. P., Carlet, J. M., Masur, H., Gerlach, H., Calandra, T., Cohen, J.,…Levy, M. M. (2004). Surviving sepsis campaign guidelines for management of severe sepsis and septic shock. *Critical Care Medicine, 32*(3), 858–873.

Diekema, D. J., Pfaller, M. A., & Jones, R. N. (2002). Age-related trends in pathogen frequency and antimicrobial susceptibility of bloodstream isolates in North America: SENTRY Antimicrobial Surveillance Program, 1997–2000. *International Journal of Antimicrobial Agents, 20*(6), 412–418.

Dubberke, E. R., & Wertheimer, A. I. (2009). Review of current literature in the economic burden of *Clostridium difficile* infection. *Infection Control and Hospital Epidemiology, 30*(1), 57–66.

Ely, E. W., Angus, D. C., Williams, M. D., Bates, B., Qualy, R., & Bernard, G. R. (2003). Drotrecogin alfa (activated) treatment of older patients with severe sepsis. *Clinical Infectious Diseases, 37*(2), 187.

Foxman, B., & Brown, P. (2003). Epidemiology of urinary tract infections: Transmission and risk factors, incidence, and costs. *Infectious Disease Clinics of North America, 17*(2), 227.

Goronzy, J. J., Fulbright, J. W., Crowson, C. S., Poland, G. A., O'Fallon, W. M., & Weyand, C. M. (2001). Value of immunological markers in predicting responsiveness to influenza vaccination in elderly individuals. *Journal of Virology, 75*(24), 12182.

Henschke, P. J. (1993). Infections in the elderly. *Medical Journal of Australia, 158*(12), 830.

High, K. P., Bradley, S. F., Gravenstein, S., Mehr, D. R., Quagliarello, V. J., Richards, C., & Yoshikawa, T. T. (2009). Clinical practice guideline for the evaluation of fever and infection in older adult residents of long-term care facilities: 2008 update by the Infectious Diseases Society of America. *Clinical Infectious Diseases, 48*(2), 149.

Janka, J., & O'Grady, N. P. (2009). *Clostridium difficile* infection: Current perspectives. *Current Opinion in Critical Care, 15*, 149–153.

Jepson, R. G., & Craig, J. C. (2008). Cranberries for preventing urinary tract infections. *Cochrane Database of Systematic Reviews,* (1), CD001321.

Juthani-Mehta, M. (2007). Asymptomatic bacteriuria and urinary tract infection in older adults. *Clinics in Geriatric Medicine, 23*(3), 585.

Kee, V. R. (2012). *Clostridium difficile* infection in older adults: A review and update on its management. *American Journal of Geriatric Pharmacotherapy, 10*(1), 14–24.

Khandelwal, C., Lathren, C., & Sloane, P. (2012). Ten clinical situations in long-term care for which antibiotics are often prescribed but rarely necessary. *Annals of Long-Term Care: Clinical Care and Aging, 20*(4), 23–29.

Kupronis, B. A., Richards, C. L., & Whitney, C. G., Active Bacterial Core Surveillance Team. (2003). Invasive pneumococcal disease in older adults residing in long-term care facilities and in the community. *Journal of the American Geriatrics Society, 51*(11), 1520.

Loeb, M., Simor, A. E., Landry, L., Walter, S., McArthur, M., Duffy, J.,…McGeer, A. (2001). Antibiotic use in Ontario facilities that provide chronic care. *Journal of General Internal Medicine, 16*(6), 376.

Lutters, M., & Vogt-Ferrier, N. B. (2008). Antibiotic duration for treating uncomplicated, symptomatic lower urinary tract infections in elderly women. *Cochrane Database of Systematic Review.* Retrieved from http://summaries.cochrane.org/CD001535/antibiotic-duration-for-treating-uncomplicated-symptomatic-lower-urinary-tract-infection-in-elderly-women

Martin, G. S., Mannino, D. M., & Moss, M. (2006). The effect of age on the development and outcome of adult sepsis. *Critical Care Medicine, 34*(1), 15–21.

Matthews, S. J., & Lancaster, L. W. (2011). Urinary tract infections in the elderly population. *American Journal of Geriatric Pharmacotherapy, 9*, 286–309.

McGeer, A., Campbell, B., Emori, T. G., Hierholzer, W. J., Jackson, M. M., Nicolle, L. E.,…Wang, E. E.-L. (1991). Definitions of infection for surveillance in long-term care facilities. *American Journal of Infection Control, 19*, 1–7.

McMurdo, M. E., Agro, I., Phillips, G., Daly, F., & Davey, P. (2009). Cranberry or trimethoprim for the prevention of recurrent urinary tract infections? A randomized controlled trial in older women. *Journal of Antimicrobial Chemotherapy, 63*, 389–395.

Meehan, T. P., Fine, M. J., Krumholz, H. M., Scinto, J. D., Galusha, D. H., Mockalis, J. T.,…Fine, J. M. (1997). Quality of care, process, and outcomes in elderly patients with pneumonia. *JAMA: The Journal of the American Medical Association, 278*(23), 2080.

Mourad, O., Palda, V., & Detsky, A. S. (2003). A comprehensive evidence-based approach to fever of unknown origin. *Archives of Internal Medicine, 163*(5), 545.

Musgrave, T., & Verghese, A. (1990). Clinical features of pneumonia in the elderly. *Seminars in Respiratory Infections, 5*(4), 269.

Nicolle, L. E. (2009). Urinary tract infections in the elderly. *Clinics in Geriatric Medicine, 25*, 423–436.

Nicolle, L. E., Bjornson, J., Harding, G. K., & MacDonell, J. A. (1983). Bacteriuria in elderly institutionalized men. *New England Journal of Medicine, 309*, 1420–1425.

Nicolle, L. E., Bradley, S., Colgan, R., Rice, J. C., Schaeffer, A., & Hooton, T. M. (2005). Infectious Diseases Society of America guidelines for the diagnosis and treatment of asymptomatic bacteriuria in adults. *Clinical Infectious Diseases, 40*, 643–654.

Nicolle, L. E., Mayhew, W. J., & Bryan, L. (1987). Prospective randomized comparison of therapy and no therapy for asymptomatic bacteriuria in institutionalized elderly women. *American Journal of Medicine, 83*, 27–33.

Norman, D. C. (2000). Fever in the elderly. *Clinical Infectious Diseases, 31*(1), 148.

O'Fallon, E., Schreiber, R., Kandel, R., & D'Agata, E. M. (2009). Multidrug-resistant gram-negative bacteria at a long-term care facility: Assessment of residents, healthcare workers, and inanimate surfaces. *Infection Control and Hospital Epidemiology, 30*(12), 1172.

Ouslander, J. G., Schapira, M., Schnelle, J. F., Uman, G., Fingold, S., Tuico, E., & Nigam, J. G. (1995). Does eradicating bacteriuria affect the severity of chronic urinary incontinence in nursing home residents? *Annals of Internal Medicine, 122*, 749–754.

Pfister, G., Weiskopf, D., Lazuardi, L., Kovaiou, R. D., Cioca, D. P., Keller, M.,…Grubeck-Loebenstein, B. (2006). Naive T cells in the elderly: Are they still there? *Annals of the New York Academy of Sciences, 1067*, 152.

Pien, B. C., Sundaram, P., Raoof, N., Costa, S. F., Mirrett, S., Woods, C. W.,…Weinstein, M. P. (2010). The clinical and prognostic importance of positive blood cultures in adults. *American Journal of Medicine, 123*(9), 819.

Raz, R., & Stamm, W. E. (1993). A controlled trial of intravaginal estriol in postmenopausal women with recurrent urinary tract infections. *New England Journal of Medicine, 329*, 753–756.

Rupnik, M., Wilcox, M. H., & Gerding, D. N. (2009). *Clostridium difficile* infection: New developments in epidemiology and pathogenesis. *Nature Reviews. Microbiology, 7*, 526–536.

Salkind, A. R. (2010). *Clostridium difficile*: An update for the primary care clinician. *Southern Medical Journal, 103*, 896–902.

Simor, A. E. (2010). Diagnosis, management, and prevention of *Clostridium difficile* infection in long-term care facilities: A review. *Journal of the American Geriatrics Society, 58*, 1556–1564.

Stone, N. D., Ashraf, M. S., Calder, J., Crnich, C. J., Crossley, K., Drinka, P. J.,…Bradley, S. F. (2012). Surveillance definitions of infections in long-term care facilities: Revisiting the McGeer criteria. *Infection Control and Hospital Epidemiology, 33*(10), 965–977.

Tal, S., Guller, V., Gurevich, A., & Levi, S. (2002). Fever of unknown origin in the elderly. *Journal of Internal Medicine, 252*(4), 295.

U.S. Food and Drug Administration. (2011, April 5). *Anti-Infective Drugs Advisory Committee briefing document: DIFICID (fidaxomicin) tablets* (NDA 201699). Optimer Pharmaceuticals. Retrieved from http://www.fda.gov/downloads/AdvisoryCommittees/CommitteeMeetingMaterials/Drugs/Anti-InfectiveDrugsAdvisoryCommittee/UCM249354.pdf

Van Nispen tot Pannerden, C. M., Verbon, A., & Kuipers, E. J. (2011). Recurrent *Clostridium difficile* infection: What are the treatment options? *Drugs, 71*, 853–868.

Weiskopf, D., Weinberger, B., & Grubeck-Loebenstein, B. (2009). The aging of the immune system. *Transplant International, 22*(11), 1041.

CHAPTER 15: IT RESOURCES

Websites

American Society for Microbiology
www.asm.org

What Is Septicemia?
http://www.wisegeek.com/what-is-septicemia.htm#slideshow

Sepsis (Blood Infection) and Septic Shock
http://www.webmd.com/a-to-z-guides/sepsis-septicemia-blood-infection

Septicemia
http://www.nlm.nih.gov/medlineplus/ency/article/001355.htm

Prevention of Healthcare-Associated Infections
http://www.ahrq.gov/research/findings/evidence-based-reports/gaphaistp.html

Elderly Urinary Tract Infections
http://www.aplaceformom.com/articles/elderly-urinary-tract-infection

Urinary Tract Infections in the Elderly
http://www.agingcare.com/Articles/urinary-tract-infections-elderly-146026.htm

Urinary Tract Infection—Adults
http://www.nlm.nih.gov/medlineplus/ency/article/000521.htm

Optimal Management of Urinary Tract Infections in Older People
http://www.ncbi.nlm.nih.gov/pmc/articles/PMC3131987/

Urinary Tract Infections in Older Adults: Current Issues and New Therapeutic Options
http://www.medscape.com/viewarticle/586757

Urinary Tract Infection in Older Adults
http://journals.lww.com/nursing/Fulltext/2012/04000/Urinary_tract_infection_in_older_adults.25.aspx

Urinary Tract Infection (UTI) and Dementia
http://www.alzheimers.org.uk/site/scripts/documents_info.php?documentID=1777

Urinary Tract Infections (UTIs) in Older Adults
http://www.emedicinehealth.com/urinary_tract_infections_utis_in_older_adults-health/article_em.htm

Mayo Clinic—*C. difficile*
http://www.mayoclinic.com/health/c-difficile/DS00736

Clostridium Difficile Colitis—Overview
http://www.webmd.com/digestive-disorders/tc/clostridium-difficile-colitis-overview

Clostridium Difficile Colitis
http://emedicine.medscape.com/article/186458-overview

Clostridium Difficile Colitis Diet
http://www.drdahlman.com/clostridium-difficile-colitis-diet.shtml?gclid=CPLcl_m5srcCFcaj4AodJ3gAOw

Patient Information: Skin and Soft Tissue Infection (cellulitis)
http://www.uptodate.com/contents/skin-and-soft-tissue-infection-cellulitis-beyond-the-basics

PDF Documents

Inpatient Care for Septicemia or Sepsis: A Challenge for Patients and Hospitals
http://www.cdc.gov/nchs/data/databriefs/db62.pdf

Videos

Band Cells, Nucleated Red Blood Cells, and Septicemia Video (2012)
Process of bacterial infection in the blood (septicemia) and resultant production of band cells and nucleated red blood cells by the bone marrow. Reviews various stages in white blood cell and red blood cell maturation in the bone marrow. (4:24 minutes)
http://youtu.be/sFBlRAq4Mpc

Urinary Tract Infection, Elderly Can be more Susceptible. Why? (2010)
About millions of people are diagnosed with urinary tract infection. Almost every day the only reason for confinement is having simple colds that lead to this kind of infection. The reason is simply by ignoring them, left untreated and unhealthy habits. Women are generally more susceptible than men; however, the elderly can be at great risk. There are certain factors why elderly people can acquire this kind of infection. Presented by www.cranberryurinary-tract.com (3 minutes) http://youtu.be/Bo-rMLziomA

C. difficile Infection (2012)

C. difficile bacteria normally live in the bowel, but when normal balance of bacteria is disturbed by antibiotics, these bugs can grow out of control and cause an infection of the colon and severe diarrhea. (11:27 minutes)

http://youtu.be/EP3iezk8Sj4

Medical School—*Clostridium Difficile* Infection (2013)

This video is a discussion of the types of *C. difficile*, pathogenesis, diagnosis, and treatment of *C. difficile* colitis. (6:52 minutes)

http://youtu.be/j9j8RqG2j2Q

Skin and Soft Tissue Photo Review—John Green, MD (2012)

A Fast-paced photo review of Skin and Soft Tissue Infections (45 minutes)

http://youtu.be/_qe3Pg2Yl_c

Cellulitis—a Patient Education Video (2012)

Cellulitis is a common skin and soft tissue infection usually caused by strep and staph bacteria. In this video, we discuss the treatment and management in a way that makes it simple for our patients to understand. (4:17 minutes)

http://youtu.be/YSik5lUmBGE

Images

Google images for Septicemia

http://www.google.com/search?q=septicemia&source=lnms&tbm=isch&sa=X&ei=3kqhU fuzMrGz4APtyIHoBw&sqi=2&ved=0CAcQ_AUoAQ&biw=1011&bih=227

Google images for Urinary Tract Infection

http://www.google.com/search?q=urinary+tract+infection+and+older+adults&source= lnms&tbm=isch&sa=X&ei=lU2hUeDIAbbh4APUpYG4Cg&ved=0CAcQ_AUoAQ& biw=1011&bih=214

Google images of *Clostridium Difficile* Colitis

http://www.google.com/search?hl=en&site=imghp&tbm=isch&source=hp&biw=1011& bih=214&oq=Clostridium+Difficile+Colitis+&gs_l=img.12..0i24l10.2065.2065.0.4586 .1.1.0.0.0.0.28.28.1.1.0...0.0...1ac.1.14.img.vYhQBcnEG6w&q=Clostridium%20Difficile% 20Colitis

Google images of Skin and Soft Tissue Infections

http://www.google.com/search?q=skin+and+soft+tissue+infections&source=lnms& tbm=isch&sa=X&ei=fvKhUbLiAdbG4AOW74HYBA&sqi=2&ved=0CAcQ_AUoAQ& biw=1011&bih=214

Anemia and Leukemia

Julia D'Amora, DO
Soheir S. Boshra, MD, FAAFP, CMD

INTRODUCTION

Our goal in geriatric medicine is to reduce the duration and limit the complications of the most common afflictions seen in the older adult. This chapter will cover two such common conditions, anemia and leukemia. Both of these hematological disorders have increased incidence with age. This makes them important areas to study so as to reduce the morbidity associated with aging. This chapter will review common geriatric causes of anemia, consequences of anemia, and a rational workup for anemia with respect to the geriatric population. It will also look at the most prevalent types of leukemia seen in older adults and discuss when and who needs to be treated.

ANEMIA

The World Health Organization (WHO) defines anemia as hemoglobin less than or equal to 12 g/dl for women and less than or equal to 13 g/dl for men (Guralink et al., 2005). The NHANES III study found that the prevalence of anemia increases with age. Anemia was found in 9.5% of individuals greater than 65 years and continues to increase to the point of greater than 20% over the age of 85. The prevalence is higher for African American populations compared with Caucasians (Guralnik et al., 2004). More important than the actual prevalence is the increase in debility, quality of life, and mortality associated with anemia. The most common causes of anemia in the older adult are nutritional, anemia of chronic renal disease/inflammation, and unexplained anemia divided fairly evenly into thirds (Guralnik et al., 2004).

Assessment of Anemia

The WHO guidelines for anemia deem a workup necessary for anyone with hemoglobin below 13 g/dl for men and 12 g/dl for women. Once anemia is determined, the next step is to evaluate the mean cellular volume (MCV). As with younger individuals, the MCV often guides the next appropriate lab work. In the older population, however, the MCV is not as helpful since the geriatric population will often have multiple nutritional deficiencies occurring simultaneously.

To fully evaluate a patient with anemia, a complete history and physical is performed. It should focus upon identification of a bleeding source, history of long-standing or hereditary anemia, alcohol use, and sequelae of chronic illnesses. All older adults who present with a clinical challenge deserve a current medication review. Special emphasis should be placed upon medications that cause suppression of blood cells or increased risk of bleeding.

The laboratory evaluation starts with a reticulocyte count to determine a hypoproliferative anemia versus an anemia of acute loss of red blood cells. If the reticulocyte count is low, this is suggestive of a hypoproliferative anemia. The differential diagnosis includes nutritional deficiencies such as iron deficiency, B_{12}/folate deficiency, anemia of chronic disease/inflammation, and myeloplastic anemia. If the reticulocyte count is elevated, this would indicate increased loss of red blood cells seen with acute hemorrhage or hemolytic anemia. In most geriatric cases, the reticulocyte count is normal to low, and the most common causes are poor nutrition and inflammation.

Anemia with a Nutritional Cause

Iron Deficiency Anemia (IDA)

The main tests needed to evaluate IDA include total serum iron, total iron binding capacity (TIBC), and ferritin. From the iron and TIBC values, the percent transferrin saturation can be derived. The total iron is a direct measure of the number of iron molecules in the blood. The TIBC is a calculated number that gives an estimate of the amount of iron being transported throughout the body. In iron-deficient states, the body attempts to maximize its carrying capacity and the TIBC rises. The third test is ferritin. Ferritin is the best way to measure the body's storage supply of iron. It must be used with caution, as it is an acute phase reactant. This means ferritin will be elevated in any acute inflammatory state. In the iron-deficient state, with all the iron stores depleted, the ferritin is low. Table 16.1 lists the most frequently encountered laboratory abnormalities in IDA.

An iron-deficient state will become iron-deficient anemia through a predictable course. As the amount of iron is depleted through either decreased intake or increased loss, the body will first use up its iron stores, causing a low ferritin level. The total iron, TIBC, percent transferrin saturation, and hemoglobin level will all remain within normal ranges until the iron stores are depleted.

TABLE 16.1 · Lab Values Consistent with IDA

- Low MCV
- Low serum iron
- High TIBC
- Low serum ferritin
- Low % transferrin saturation

Secondly, as the body realizes that the stores have become depleted and less iron is being moved, the TIBC will rise to help the body move more iron. With more binding molecules and less iron to be bound, the percent transferrin will begin to decrease. The third and final phase affects the actual synthesis of red blood cells. As the body loses its building block of iron in the construction of red blood cells, the cells tend to become hypochromic in appearance. If the iron is not replaced, the hemoglobin and MCV will begin to decrease.

Causes of IDA. The two causes of iron deficiency are (1) limited intake or absorption and (2) loss of iron from bleeding. In the older adult, either one or both may be occurring. Specific nutritional issues, poor diet, and decreased appetite are seen in association with medications and comorbid conditions such as congestive heart failure, dementia, and depression. Besides causing alterations in taste and appetite, some medications limit the absorption of iron. Many acid-reducing agents, often used by the older adult, cause elevated gastric pH and interfere with iron metabolism. Losses from the gastrointestinal tract such as occult malignancy and vascular malformations are common. If the losses are greater than can be compensated for through intake and absorption of iron, anemia will develop. Gastrointestinal tract blood losses may also be from inflammatory bowel disease, hemorrhoids, and gastritis. Non–gastrointestinal tract blood loss may occur through hematuria, epistaxis, tumor in other locations, menorrhagia, multiple blood draws, and surgery.

Treatment of IDA. Once IDA has been found, along with a search for its etiology, replacement with elemental iron should be started. There are three different types of ferrous iron supplements, each containing different amounts of elemental iron. The Centers for Disease Control and Prevention (CDC) recommends 180 mg of elemental iron each day. This may be given in divided doses. With respect to the older adult, the side effects of iron replacement may become intolerable. Constipation and nausea may be overwhelming, causing dehydration and weight loss. Dosing and duration, therefore, may need to be adjusted. To maximize the absorption, give iron on an empty stomach and avoid use with antacids. If the diagnosis of IDA is in doubt, a trial with iron is appropriate with continued close monitoring of hemoglobin levels for a therapeutic response.

If the hemoglobin is lower than 8 mg/dl and/or the patient is becoming clinically compromised, acute hospitalization and blood transfusion is an appropriate course of action. While a blood transfusion will improve the symptoms rapidly, the risk of volume overload, iron overload, infection, and transfusion reaction are always present (Bross et al., 2010).

Cobalamin (B_{12}) and Folate Deficient Anemia

Another common nutritional anemia in the older adult is vitamin B_{12} (cobalamin) deficiency. Studies report that as many as 30% to 40% of ill and/or institutionalized people are B_{12} deficient (Van Asselt et al., 2009). The Framingham study reported 12% community dwelling older adults have deficient levels of vitamin B_{12} (Lindenbaum et al., 1994). Low B_{12} levels have implications that reach beyond anemia. A low B_{12} level can cause dementia, neuropsychiatric disorders, and increased risk of cardiovascular events. The level of B_{12} is often measured with folate. Folate deficiency would indicate alcohol use and/or malnutrition, whereas B_{12} deficiency will often be associated with atrophic gastritis in the older adult. Both nutritional deficiencies will cause a macrocytic anemia in contrast to microcytic anemia of iron deficiency. Poor nutrition and medication-induced changes of gastric lining are ubiquitous in the older population.

Vitamin B_{12} can be measured either directly or indirectly. The direct measurement quantifies the serum B_{12} level while the indirect method measures the biochemical markers homocysteine or methylmalonic acid (MMA). The direct measurement is less reliable when the B_{12} levels are in the low normal range (less than 300 pmol/L). If the serum B_{12} levels fall within this indeterminate range, an elevated homocysteine or MMA level can help confirm a B_{12} deficiency.

Causes of B_{12} and Folate Deficiency. Some of the more common causes that contribute to the inability to properly absorb B_{12} include medications that cause an elevated pH. The most prevalent offenders include H_2 blockers, antacids, proton pump inhibitors, and biguanides. Other common reasons for low B_{12} levels are chronic alcoholism, previous gastric surgery, pancreatic exocrine failure, and chronic *Helicobacter pylori* infection.

Treatment of B_{12} and Folate Deficiency. B_{12} can be replaced by parenteral route or oral route. The more traditional method is the intramuscular parenteral route using 1,000 µg/day for 1 week, then 1,000 µg/week for 1 month, and then 1,000 µg/month until the underlying cause is corrected. Oral route can be just as effective, giving 1,000 µg/day until replaced or the underlying cause is corrected. B_{12} supplementation often remains lifelong in the older adult. Folate may be corrected with 1 mg oral supplementation daily until hematological correction or resolution of the underlying cause is achieved.

Iron deficiency and B_{12} deficiency may occur together and diagnostic criteria may be uncertain. As with iron deficiency, a trial of B_{12} replacement is always prudent because of the significant morbidity associated with B_{12} deficiency.

Anemia of Chronic Inflammation/Disease

Anemia of Chronic Inflammation

Anemia of chronic inflammation (ACI) is another major cause of anemia in the older adult. It is often confused with iron-deficient anemia because the laboratory values can be similar. The NHANES study estimated that 19.7% of all types of anemia in the older patient are associated with inflammation (National Vital Statistics Report, 2007). The inflammation may come from any source, but the result it has on the maturation of red blood cells is the same. A patient with a mild injury or surgical procedure will have an inflammatory response. The inflammatory condition will cause tissue hypoxia. The tissue hypoxia upregulates the glycoprotein erythropoietin (EPO). This is the protein that controls production of red blood cells. The younger, healthier response to tissue hypoxia is to increase EPO, which subsequently increases the production of red blood cells. However, the inflammatory response in the older adult is often prolonged and dysfunctional. This mechanism is not well understood but results in increased levels of tumor necrosis factor (TNF)-alpha and interleukin (IL)-6 in the plasma. In a study done by Faquin et al. (1992), it was found that when inflammatory cytokines such as those listed above are present, EPO response to hypoxia is markedly reduced. With this reduction in EPO production, the amount of red blood cells in circulation is decreased. In addition to EPO's poor response, inflammatory states limit the mobilization of iron from storage sites. This will result in a further drop in red cell production.

Conditions that cause ACI in the older adult include not only age but also acute or chronic infections, autoimmune disease, tissue injury from such things as fractures or decubitus ulcers, myocardial infarction, surgery, cancers, and renal disease. The anemia of chronic renal disease has its own relationship to EPO production that goes beyond the inflammatory state alone.

TABLE 16.2 · Lab Values Consistent with ACI
■ Low or normal MCV
■ Low total iron
■ Normal-to-low TIBC
■ Normal-to-elevated ferritin
■ Low % transferring saturation

The laboratory findings of anemia of chronic inflammatory disease and iron-deficient anemia are often overlapping. There are some differences, as listed in Table 16.2, that can be helpful in making a diagnosis.

ACI will have low serum iron like IDA owing to the poor mobilization of iron from the storage sites. However, one difference is that the stores are intact in ACI, making the ferritin levels normal to elevated. Both IDA and ACI can have microcytic or normocytic appearance to the red blood cells since both have decreased access to iron, the former due to lack of stores and the latter due to a lack of proper mobilization from the storage. This lack of mobilization also causes decreased transferrin saturation in ACI as it does in IDA. The high TIBC seen with IDA is not seen with ACI. With the storage being normal, the body has no need to increase the carrying capacity, so the TIBC is normal to low. It is common in older adults to have overlap of iron-deficient anemia and ACI. This can pose significant problems with management strategies.

Anemia of Chronic Kidney Disease

Chronic kidney disease is well known to cause a decrease in hemoglobin levels. As the kidney function declines, the anemia becomes more severe. The main mechanism is decreased production of EPO. Erythropoietin is produced in the pretubular cells of the kidney. As renal cells become less functional and less numerous, the hemoglobin predictably declines. Other chronic inflammatory illnesses as well as poor nutritional states so commonly found in the frail older adult further compromise the red blood cell production. Anemia (hemoglobin less than 11 g/dl) becomes more prevalent as the glomerular filtration rate (GFR) drops below 30 ml/minute/1.73 m^2. The proper determination of GFR in older patients can be difficult. There are multiple common causes of renal disease in the older adult. An in-depth discussion about this topic is covered in the renal section of this book.

Treatment of ACI. The treatment of ACI can be difficult and may require specialty consultation. The first course of action is to treat the underlying inflammatory process if possible. Treatment, for example, of rheumatoid arthritis with disease-modifying agents can increase hemoglobin levels (Weiss & Goodnough, 2005). It is not always possible to treat the underlying cause of inflammation in the majority of geriatric patients. Transfusions of packed red blood cells can be used, when necessary, to avoid life-threatening complications. Low cardiac output or hypoxia seen with congestive heart failure and chronic obstructive pulmonary disease may be reasons for transfusion. If anemia is mild, transfusion may not be necessary. It is also important to attempt to evaluate iron deficiency. Iron therapy is controversial in ACI, but in patients with low iron stores, it may help improve the anemia. It is important to make sure the iron stores (as measured with ferritin) are depleted before starting iron. If the ferritin is between 30 and 100 ng/ml, there is more likely to be an association with iron deficiency. Iron replacement in this case may improve the condition. If the ferritin is above 100 ng/ml, it is more likely associated with pure ACI. In this latter case, giving iron may be detrimental. An overload of iron stores has been shown to cause bacteremia and accumulation of toxic radicals, which cause an increase in cardiovascular events (Weiss & Goodnough, 2005).

The use of erythropoietic agents for anemia is most often seen in anemia of chronic kidney disease. It has also been approved for use in cancer patients getting chemotherapy and HIV-infected patients on myelosuppressive agents. These agents can improve quality of life for some older persons, and this option should not be excluded simply because of age. The use of erythro-poietic agents can, however, have significant morbidity and cost to older patients. A decision to use this therapy should be considered with the help of specialty consultation.

As discussed above, the most common cause of anemia in an older person is nutritional-based, including IDA, B$_{12}$, and folate deficiency. The second most common cause of anemia in-volves inflammation as it is related to comorbid conditions. Special consideration is given to anemia of chronic renal disease. The third most common cause of anemia is often referred to as "unexplained anemia." This would be a diagnosis of exclusion. Much controversy exists as to the definition of a complete anemia workup. The workup must be guided by the patient's physical and mental endurance to undergo an arduous evaluation. Many older adults and their families are reluctant to have a battery of painful, expensive, and often unhelpful tests performed. This may explain why so many anemic patients have no final diagnosis. It was reported in the NHANES III study that 33.6% of all anemic patients were considered "unexplained" (Guralnik et al., 2004). Research is ongoing in this area. The challenge remains in determining ACI from unexplained anemia. Studies looking at IL-6 levels and other inflammatory markers are ongoing. Measures of EPO levels are being evaluated to help determine endocrine renal defects. Protein-calorie malnu-trition may also be a culprit. The National Geriatric Research Consortium did a survey of anemia in the nursing home. The data collected from this survey have been used in several other studies aimed at answering the questions about unexplained anemia (Weiss & Goodnough, 2005).

Comorbidities and Anemia

Anemia can present alone or with other laboratory abnormalities. If an anemia is present with thrombocytopenia, leucopenia, or unexplained kidney or liver disease, a more extensive evalua-tion is warranted. Such things as myelodysplastic syndromes (MDS), multiple myeloma, or leu-kemia must be considered. These disorders are seen with other history and physical examination features suggestive of more serious illness. These features include splenomegaly, lymphadenopa-thy, unexplained fevers, weight loss, bone pain, or history of previous chemotherapy. When these features are seen, a bone marrow biopsy is indicated. Before such a test is undertaken, the goals of the patient and caregivers must be considered. In the presence of end-stage organ disease, the patient would be unlikely to tolerate or benefit from treatment. If the case warrants further inves-tigation, a bone marrow biopsy can differentiate among blood disorders. In the next section we will discuss the most common primary hematological disorders found in the geriatric population.

Myelodysplastic Syndromes

If an anemia is found that is not related to nutritional causes, blood loss, and inflammatory or renal conditions, further investigation may be undertaken. This is even more necessary if other cell lines are abnormal. If a patient is found to have neutropenia and/or thrombocytopenia in the absence of drug effects, severe infection, excessive alcohol use, liver disease, or current chemotherapy, examination of their peripheral blood smear and bone marrow biopsy are the next steps for proper evaluation. Often the results of both blood smear and bone marrow biopsy lead to a diagnosis of MDS. Myelodysplastic syndromes are a group of blood disorders associated with bone marrow dysfunction, causing ineffective hematopoiesis. The most severe types can transform into acute myeloid leukemia (AML).

The epidemiology of myelodysplasia is limited. It is thought to be underestimated at less than 10,000 cases per year in the United States. It is difficult to get accurate numbers owing to the need for bone marrow biopsy and the limited number of older adults willing or able to have this procedure. The mean age of diagnosis is 76 years with predominance in white males (Weiss & Goodnough, 2005). Survival rates are poor and span from months to years. The average survival is 20 months for any form of MDS.

Diagnosis of MDS

The changes in the peripheral blood will give some clues to the diagnosis of MDS. The red blood cells (erythroid cell line) will be macrocytic, the white blood cells (myeloid cell line) will be hypogranular with hypolobulated nuclei, and the platelets (megakaryocytes) will be agranular (Provan, 2003). In the bone marrow aspirate, the erythroid cells have an abnormal shape with abnormal chromatin patterns. Some types of MDS will have ring sideroblasts. These are immature red blood cells with a ring of iron granules. The platelets look small (micromegakaryocytes) and may be mononuclear. These changes in the bone marrow cause dysfunctional and ineffective hematopoietic cells (Provan, 2003).

Several classification criteria have been created over the years to diagnose and treat patients. The first was created by a group of French, American, and British pathologists. It is known as the FAB classification. The classification includes the percentage of blast cells (immature cells), the presence of ring sideroblasts, and the peripheral blood monocyte count. It was first created in 1976 and revised in 1982 (Greenberg et al., 1997; Provan, 2003).

The FAB classification includes refractory anemia (RA) with less than 5% blasts in the bone marrow. Refractory anemia with ring sideroblasts (RARS) is next with less than 5% blasts and greater than 15% sideroblasts found in bone marrow. The third class is refractory anemia with excessive blasts (RAEB). It has between 5% and 20% blasts in marrow. The fourth class is refractory anemia with excessive blasts in transition (RAEB-T) and contains 20% to 30% blasts with some in transition. The final class is chronic myelomonocytic leukemia (CMML) and contains greater than 20% blasts in marrow and many monocytes on peripheral blood smear.

The WHO has also developed its own classification of MDS. The categories help to identify more severe cases and guide treatment. They are based on the number of cell lines that are affected, genetic markers, and morphological changes on bone marrow biopsy. The presence of chromosomal changes confirms, without doubt, the presence of a true bone marrow dysfunction (Provan, 2003). The system looks for "clonal" chromosomal abnormalities in the bone marrow aspirate. A "clonal" chromosomal abnormality is the same abnormal process seen in more than one cell. One of the main chromosomal changes is on chromosome 5 with loss of its long arm "q" (5q syndrome). The 5q syndrome type is seen more in older women and has a low risk of transformation to AML. On the other hand, a deletion in chromosome 17 leads to worse survival and drug resistance. The changes made to further refine the FAB are listed below.

Differences between FAB and WHO. There are differences between FAB and WHO, and they are as follows:

- One cell line cytopenic for diagnosis of RA and RARS as long as other causes were ruled out and the dysplasia was greater than 6 months.
- The presence of cytogenic abnormalities.
- Acute leukemia was redefined as greater than 20% blasts in the bone marrow.
- CMML was reclassified as a mixed myelodysplastic and myeloproliferative disease by adding splenomegaly and constitutional symptoms (fever, weight loss).

Since the WHO, a third tool was derived using both FAB and WHO along with age and survival data. Greenberg and colleagues created the International Prognostic Scoring System (IPSS) in 1997.

The IPSS scoring system gives a score that ranges from 0 to 2.0, depending on the percentage of marrow blasts (0 would be less than 5% and up to 2.0 for 20% to 30% blasts). It also gives a 0 to 2.0 score for karyotype (a good karyotype is 0, and a poor karyotype is worth 1.0 point). The final score is for the number of cytopenias present. Zero to one gives a score of 0, and two or three cell lines down gives a score of 0.5. These scores are added together to use for prognosis. A low score between 0.5 and 1.0 gives you a survival without treatment of almost 6 years, while a score of greater than 2.5 gives a survival without treatment of only 0.4 year. This tool gives a numerical value to the types of MDS.

Treatment of MDS

Treatments for MDS range from supportive care with transfusions and erythropoietin therapy to chemotherapy and/or bone marrow transplant. The considerations for aggressive treatment include age less than 65 years, general fitness, severity, and stability of disease. Most treatment will be palliative in the older adult. The effects of chemotherapy with or without bone marrow transplant can cause more morbidity and mortality than supportive care. Some new processes in bone marrow transplant are less aggressive and are therefore better tolerated. These may prove to be an option in the future for geriatric patients. Until then, the mainstay of treatment for the geriatric population will be blood product transfusion and symptomatic treatment (Balducci et al., 2007).

LEUKEMIA

The diseases discussed below are the most common types of leukemia encountered in older adults. This is not an exhaustive list of the many different types of blood cancers found. It is true that most cancers do occur in older persons, leukemia being no exception. Leukemia can have widely varying courses and treatment options as compared with the younger population. Also, there are unique challenges in the diagnosis and treatment of leukemia in the older patient. This group tends to have a limited tolerance to chemotherapy, a higher risk of severe infections, and a higher burden of comorbid illnesses. We now discuss evaluation, treatment, and prognosis of AML, chronic lymphocytic leukemia (CLL), and multiple myeloma, as these are the most commonly encountered blood cancers in older adults.

Acute Myeloid Leukemia

AML is the most feared consequence of MDS. This is a severe form of leukemia that has a particularly poor prognosis in the older patient. It can occur *de novo* or as transformation from MDS. Its annual incidence is 2.4 per 100,000 and increases with age to reach 12.5 in 100,000 over the age of 65 years (Lowenberg et al., 1999). The mean age of presentation is 70 years (Estey & Dohner, 2006). It is defined by a rapid growth of immature white blood cells. The cells are arrested in their immature state, the myeloblast. These cells are dysfunctional and will build up in the marrow, leaving room for little else. The initial clinical presentation of AML can be confused for a multitude of other common geriatric illnesses. Fatigue, shortness of breath, palpitations, and multiple infections are all common early symptoms of AML. Other features include easy bruising, gum hypertrophy, petechial/purpura rash, bone and joint pain, splenomegaly, hepatomegaly, and rarely lymphadenopathy. Some patients may present as critically ill with serious hemorrhage or overwhelming sepsis.

The laboratory findings are remarkable for elevated white blood cell count and varying degrees of anemia and thrombocytopenia. A concerning finding of blasts on peripheral smear should lead one to consider a bone marrow biopsy for a definitive diagnosis. As defined by the WHO, leukemia can be diagnosed with greater than 20 leukemic blastic cells in the bone marrow and/or peripheral smear (Provan, 2004).

As with MDS, classification of AML is by morphology and genetic factors. It is the basis for treatment and prognosis. The WHO has four categories defined. The first category includes translocations and inversions of various chromosomes. The second category involves multiple cell line dysplasia; these are prior cases of MDS or MPD (myeloproliferative syndrome) that have transformed into AML. Older patients will fall into this category and unfortunately the prognosis is poor. The third group is AML with MDS related to prior treatment with chemotherapy. The fourth is AML not otherwise categorized.

Treatment of AML

Treatment with chemotherapy is poorly tolerated in the older adult with a survival of only months (Estey & Dohner, 2006). An older adult, as defined in most leukemia treatment studies, is one greater than 55 to 60 years old. These patients show increased drug resistance due to certain protein expressions found on the cells. Those over 60 years of age also have increased numbers of genetic variations that are associated with poor survival. Treatment is also less effective in MDS conversion cases, which make up many of the aged cases of AML.

Treatment of AML is done when a patient is thought to have good performance status, minimal organ dysfunction, and limited comorbidities (Zaretsky et al., 2008). For newly diagnosed and previously untreated patients over the age of 55 years, chemotherapy is recommended. Traditionally, an induction of high-dose chemotherapy with anthracycline or anthracenedione is given. The hope is to cause a complete remission. Those who survive the treatment and its toxicities and who are in complete remission go on to get consolidation therapy with low or intermediate dose cytarabine (Zaretsky et al., 2008). Stem cell transplants are not generally offered to those over 60 years old. For those patients who show poor performance, have multiple organ dysfunctions, and multiple comorbidities, a palliative approach is offered. The palliative treatment involves the use of low-dose cytarabine; it has less toxicity and is better tolerated, but this treatment option will not result in complete remission. In patients over 60 years old who receive full-dose chemotherapy treatment, complete remission occurs in about 50% to 60% and decreases with each decade a person ages. The rate of relapse of AML after complete remission is 80% to 90%. If an older person has the physical stamina to tolerate chemotherapy, the side effects of treatment, including bleeding and infections, often limits survivability. In several recent studies, the presence of dementia is being used as criteria for palliative treatment. However, there is no clear evidence for any one specific prognostic factor to guide treatment plans for older adults (Zaretsky et al., 2008).

In the older population, especially those over 75 years and/or who are living in long-term care settings, a palliative approach is more common. Some comfort can be given with blood product transfusions. This will help to relieve shortness of breath and palpitations. The use of narcotic pain medications will not only help pain but also relieve the symptoms of dyspnea and air hunger. Neutropenic precautions may help decrease infections, which are a common cause of morbidity and mortality. The most common infection sites include chest, perianal, oral, and skin, resulting from pseudomonas, HSV, Candida, and staphylococcus. Hemorrhage from the rectum, uterus, or nose is frequently seen and can be very distressing to the patient and family. Gum hypertrophy may also be a source of bleeding and discomfort, which limits oral intake. Pain level should be evaluated often and treated aggressively with narcotics (Provan, 2004).

Chronic Lymphocytic Leukemia

CLL is the most common type of adult leukemia in the Western world (Elter & Engert, 2006). The mean age of diagnosis is 72 years (National Cancer Institute, 2011). The true incidence of CLL in the population is unknown since it has few symptoms and likely goes undiagnosed. The incidence is estimated to be 2 to 4.5 per 100,000 in the general population (Kristinsson et al., 2009). It is seen more commonly in white men. In contrast to AML, CLL is well tolerated in the older population. Older patients have a slow progression of disease and will never need treatment. It is marked by elevated leukocytes on a complete blood count (CBC). Often, CLL is found incidentally during routine blood work or while evaluating another illness. Its pathophysiology is that of dysfunctional lymphocytes. These lymphocytes are mature in appearance on peripheral smear and bone marrow aspirate. The older lymphocytes accumulate in other locations as well. The accumulation of lymphocytes in other locations accounts for the physical findings of lymphadenopathy (usually painless and symmetrical), hepatomegaly, and splenomegaly. In some cases, the lymphocytes infiltrate the bone marrow to a greater degree, causing bone marrow failure. It is at this point that anemia and pancytopenia will appear.

Two staging systems exist to guide the prognosis and treatment of CLL. The two main systems are the Rai Modified Staging System and the Binet Clinical Staging System. The Rai system divides patients into low-, intermediate-, and high-risk groups. Low risk is defined as only lymphocytosis without any other findings. This group has a survival of over 13 years. They require only monitoring and not treatment. The intermediate group is divided into two categories, intermediate (I) and intermediate (II). Intermediate (I) is lymphocytosis and lymphadenopathy. Intermediate (II) has lymphocytosis and splenomegaly or hepatomegaly. The intermediate (I) group has a survival of 8 years and intermediate (II) has a survival of 5 years. High-risk disease is also divided into two groups. High grade (III), defined by hemoglobin of less than 11.0 g/dl, has a survival of 2 years, and high grade (IV) disease has thrombocytopenia less than 100×10^9 /L with a survival of 1 year. The Binet Clinical Staging has similar criteria and is divided into A, B, and C stages. Stage A is lymphocytosis with no other cell line abnormalities and less than three lymphoid regions enlarged. The survival is approximately 12 years. The B category is the same as A but with three or more lymphoid regions enlarged and has a survival of 5 years. The C stage has a hemoglobin of less than 10 g/dl and/or thrombocytopenia of less than 100×10^9 /L. The mean survival is only 2 years.

Treatments are considered on the basis of early versus advanced disease. Early disease of MDS is monitored and not treated. This would include Rai low and some intermediate groups as well as Binet A and B groups. If progression or change in disease pattern is detected, treatment may be indicated. Criteria for treatment often include hemoglobin less than 10 g/dl, platelets less than 100×10^9 /L, fatigue, fevers, night sweats, weight loss of 10% in 6 months and signs of progressive disease such as lymphocytes doubling in 12 months. Chemotherapy with alkylating agents like chlorambucil can improve survival, but cure is not thought to be possible with chemotherapy. Monitoring patients for recurrent infections and prompt treatment of infection is important. Monthly IV Ig may be offered to reduce infections.

CLL is considered an incurable disease. However, the majority of patients remain asymptomatic and die of other unrelated diseases. CLL progresses slowly with a 5-year survival rate of 78% for white males (Elter & Engert, 2006). Most patients can expect to live 5 to 10 years with CLL (Kristinsson et al., 2009).

Multiple Myeloma

Multiple myeloma is more common in the older population. The mean age of diagnosis is 69 years. The age-adjusted incidence is 5.7 per 100,000 people. Unlike the previously mentioned cancers, multiple myeloma affects the African American population to a greater degree than the white population. Its survival is poor with only a 40% survival rate at 5 years (National Cancer Institute, 2011). In multiple myeloma, a mutant form of single clone lymphocyte plasma cell leads to overproduction of antibodies. As a result of excess antibodies, tissue and bone damage takes place. The antibodies cause increased osteoclastic activity and decreased osteoblastic activity. This imbalance causes lytic (punched out) lesions of bone. As bone breaks down, it spills out its calcium, and the level of calcium in the blood rises. Multiple myeloma is marked by elevated serum calcium levels. With the increase in bone turnover causing elevated calcium and an increased number of circulating proteins from the plasma cells, the kidneys become overloaded, resulting in renal failure. The excess plasma cells will also affect the bone marrow production of red blood cells, resulting in anemia (Provan, 2004).

The combination of clinical features such as multiple infections, lethargy, and bone pain, with or without fractures, warrants investigation for possible multiple myeloma. Basic laboratory workup for multiple myeloma reveals a normocytic, normochromic anemia, elevated sedimentation rate, elevated serum calcium, elevated serum creatine, and proteinuria. A serum and urine electrophoresis reveals elevated concentrations of paraprotein, monoclonal protein (M protein) band. A paraprotein is an abnormal immunoglobulin produced by the tumor clone cells. Any one of the classes of immunoglobulins can be overproduced. Serum immunoglobulin of IgG greater than 30% g/L or IgA greater than 20% g/L are part of the diagnostic criteria for multiple myeloma. Other immunoglobulins are less common but can be seen in multiple myeloma. These include IgM, IgD, and IgE. In the urine, the finding of Bence Jones paraproteins is enough to make a diagnosis of multiple myeloma. A bone marrow aspiration is diagnostic if it has greater than 10% plasma cells. Plasmacytoma, a solid tumor of plasma cells in the soft tissue or bone, is also diagnostic of multiple myeloma.

The minimal diagnosis criteria to confirm a case of multiple myeloma includes greater than 10% plasma cells in bone marrow, clinical features, and at least one of the following: osteolytic lesions on bone survey, elevated serum paraprotein, or Bence Jones protein in the urine.

More common than a true diagnosis of multiple myeloma is the diagnosis of monoclonal gammopathy of undetermined significance (MGUS) reported to be 20 times more prevalent than multiple myeloma. An important difference between these two diseases is that MGUS requires only monitoring and no treatment. MGUS must be monitored because one quarter of the cases progress to multiple myeloma, macroglobulin anemia, amyloidosis, or lymphoma. The criteria for diagnosis must exclude the aforementioned diseases along with no clinical features of myeloma. MGUS will have less than 5% plasma cells on bone marrow, a stable M spike protein concentration of less than 30% g/L in the plasma, little or no paraproteins in the urine, and no bone lesions, anemia, hypercalcemia, or renal impairment.

Treatment for multiple myeloma targets cancer cells using chemotherapy and monitoring and managing hypercalcemia, bone pain, and renal failure. Chemotherapy is offered to those greater than 60 years of age in the form of alkylating agents (melphalan) with or without prednisone. Often, patients will achieve a plateau of disease and remain on maintenance therapy with interferon for up to 1 year. Close monitoring of symptoms and hematological markers is continued, and treatment is restarted if myeloma returns. Eventually, the myeloma will become resistant to treatment or patients will succumb to overwhelming infections and other sequelae of myeloma. During the course of chemotherapy, other treatments are used to help control pain, life-threatening infections, and electrolyte abnormalities.

Bone pain can be severe and is managed with opiates and local radiation of bone lesions. Surgical fixation of unstable bones helps pain control. Nonsteroidal anti-inflammatory medications are avoided due to the renal insufficiency. Magnetic resonance imaging should be done immediately if any severe back pain develops, especially if it is associated with neurological features. Spinal cord lesions leading to cord compression can develop, and the result may be devastating. These are often amenable to radiation treatment. Hydration is another key to prevent complications associated with myeloma. This will treat both the renal insufficiency and the hypercalcemia, both of which can be life threatening. Intravenous biphosphonates therapy and dialysis are used in severe hypercalcemia. Oral biphosphonates can be used to treat less severe pain and control hypercalcemia. Anemia is treated with transfusions and erythropoietin. The most common cause of death in multiple myeloma is infection, usually respiratory. Prompt diagnosis and treatment with broad-spectrum antibiotics is appropriate. In more advanced disease, fungal infection should be considered.

The combination of bone pain with or without fractures, increased calcium, renal failure, and anemia is the classic presentation of multiple myeloma. Some specific features leading to a more dismal outcome include the following: hemoglobin less than 8.5 g/dl, hypercalcemia, advanced bone lesions, high M protein production, renal insufficiency, low serum albumin, and elevated C-reactive protein. Also, on genetic analysis, a 13-q deletion is associated with worse outcomes (Provan, 2004).

SCREENING AND RISK FACTORS

Both anemia and leukemia are found with routine CBC. No recommendation has been made by the USPTF (United States Preventative Task Force) on CBC screening; however, it is so often done in the older population owing to comorbid illness. The risk factors for both anemia and leukemia are advanced age. Risk factors for anemia include poor nutrition, weight loss, renal and heart disease, or any chronic inflammatory state. An excessive alcohol intake is also a risk factor.

The main risk factor for the types of leukemia mentioned in this chapter is advanced age. AML risk increases with history of previous chemotherapy and exposure to such toxins as benzene and organic solvents (Provan, 2004). With AML there is some familial increased risk as there is with other types of cancers. Down syndrome appears to show a significant increased prevalence of AML. ALL (Acute Lymphocytic Leukemia) has shown some increased prevalence with exposure to herbicides and insecticides. Multiple myeloma risk increases with the male gender and the African American descent and is also more prevalent in obese patients (Provan, 2004).

PREVENTION

Anemia can be a consequence of poor diet and chronic illness. Basic prevention of heart disease, hypertension, and diabetes can decrease the chances of developing anemia related to chronic disease. Heart-healthy diet, exercise, and limitation of excessive alcohol are good practices to prevent the chronic illness that can lead to anemia. It is important to ask whether patients are having any limitation in getting or preparing food. This is unfortunately not a rare occurrence. Prevention of leukemia would involve limiting exposures to carcinogenic material, as discussed above, but otherwise there is no known prevention for leukemia.

PATIENT EDUCATION

Education about proper diet and exercise for the prevention of chronic disease is always beneficial. Limiting excessive alcohol may decrease the chances of nutritional anemia. Counseling about proper timing of medication such as iron supplementation can help maximize absorption and tolerance. Discuss with your patients the symptoms of anemia such as fatigue, weakness, and dyspnea. Patients may feel these are just normal aging changes. They may simply slow down activity to compensate for low blood counts.

REFERENCES

Balducci, L., Ershler, W. B., & Bennett, J. M. (2007). *Anemia in the elderly* (pp. 75–79). New York, NY: Springer.

Bross, M., Soch K., & Smith-Knuppel, T. (2010). Anemia in older persons. *American Family Physician, 82*(5), 480–487.

Elter, T., & Engert, A. (2006). Fludarabine in chronic lymphocytic leukemia. *Expert Opinion on Pharmacotherapy, 7*(12), 1641–1651.

Estey, E., & Dohner, H. (2006). Acute myeloid leukemia. *Lancet, 368*, 1894–1907.

Faquin, W. C., Schneider, T. J., & Goldberg M. A. (1992). Effect of inflammatory cytokines on hypoxia-induced erythropoietin production. *Blood, 79*, 1987–1994.

Greenberg, P., Cox C., & Lebeau, M. (1997). International scoring system for the prognosis in myelodysplastic syndromes. *Blood, 89*, 2079–2088.

Guralnik, J. M., Eisenstaedt, R. S., Ferrucci, L., Klein, H. G., & Woodman, R. C. (2004). Prevalence of anemia in persons 65 years and older in the United States: Evidence for high rate of unexplained anemia. *Blood, 104*(8), 2263–2268.

Guralnik, J. M., Ershler, W. B., Schrier, S. L., & Picozzi, V. J. (2005). Anemia in the elderly: A public health crisis in hematology. *Hematology American Society Hematology Educational Program*, 528–532.

Kristinsson, S. Y., Dickman, P. W., Wilson, W. H., Caporaso, N., Bjorkhdm, M., & Landgren, O. (2009). Improved survival in CLL in past decade: A population-based study including 11,179 patients diagnosed between 1973–2003 in Sweden. *Haematological, 94*(9), 1259–1265.

Lindenbaum, J., Rosenberg, I. H., Wilson, P. W., Stabler, S. P., & Allen, R. H. (1994). Prevalence of cobalamin deficiency in the Framingham elderly population. *American Journal of Clinical Nutrition, 60*, 2–11.

Lowenberg, B., Downing, J. R., & Burnett, A. (1999). Medical progress: Acute myeloid leukemia. *New England Journal of Medicine, 341*, 1051–1062.

National Cancer Institute. (2011). SEER Stat facts sheet: Chronic lymphocytic leukemia. Retrieved from http://seer.cancer.gov/statfacts/html/clyl.html

Provan, D. (2003). *ABC of clinical hematology* (2nd ed., Chapters 8 & 9). London: BMJ Books.

Provan, D. (2004). *Oxford hand book of clinical hematology* (2nd ed.). New York, NY: Oxford University Press.

Van Asselt, D. Z., Blom, H. J., Zuiderent, R., Wevers, R. A., Jakobs, C., van den Broek, W. J., . . . Hoefnagels, W. H. (2009). Clinical significance of low cobalamin levels in older hospitalized patients. *Netherlands Journal of Medicine, 57*, 41–49.

Weiss, G., & Goodnough, L. T. (2005). Anemia of chronic disease. *New England Journal of Medicine, 352*, 1011–1023.

Zaretsky, Y., Crump, M., Haynes, A. E., Imrie, K., Stevens, A., Meyer R. M., & Hematology Disease Site Group. (2008). *Treatment of acute myeloid leukemia in older patients: Guideline recommendations* (p. 65). Toronto, ON: Cancer Care Ontario (CCO) (Evidence-based series no. 6–14).

CHAPTER 16: IT RESOURCES

Websites

American Society of Hematology
  http://www.hematology.org/
Iron Disorders Institute
  http://www.irondisorders.org/
National Cancer Institute—Leukemia
  http://www.cancer.gov/cancertopics/types/leukemia
American Cancer Society—Acute Myeloid Leukemia (AML)
  http://www.cancer.org/cancer/leukemia-acutemyeloidaml/
Leukemia and Lymphoma Society
  http://www.lls.org/
WebMD—Types of Blood Disorders
  http://www.webmd.com/a-to-z-guides/blood-disorder-types-and-treatment
WebMD— Understanding Anemia— The Basics
  http://www.webmd.com/a-to-z-guides/understanding-anemia-basics
WebMD—Leukemia
  http://www.webmd.com/cancer/tc/leukemia-topic-overview
WebMD—Acute Myeloid Leukemia
  http://www.webmd.com/cancer/acute-myeloid-leukemia-symptoms-treatments
Mayo Clinic—Anemia
  http://www.mayoclinic.com/health/anemia/DS00321
Mayo Clinic—Iron Deficiency Anemia
  http://www.mayoclinic.com/health/iron-deficiency-anemia/DS00323
Mayo Clinic—Leukemia
  http://www.mayoclinic.com/health/leukemia/DS00351
Mayo Clinic—Acute Myelogenous Leukemia
  http://www.mayoclinic.com/health/acute-myelogenous-leukemia/DS00548

Mayo Clinic—Chronic Lymphocytic Leukemia
http://www.mayoclinic.com/health/chronic-lymphocytic-leukemia/DS00565
MedicineNet—Anemia
http://www.medicinenet.com/anemia/article.htm
MedicineNet—Leukemia
http://www.medicinenet.com/leukemia/article.htm
World Health Organization—Anemia
http://www.who.int/topics/anaemia/en/
Office on Women's Health—Anemia Fact Sheet
http://womenshealth.gov/publications/our-publications/fact-sheet/anemia.cfm
UpToDate—Anemia in the Older Adult
http://www.uptodate.com/contents/anemia-in-the-older-adult
Epidemiology of Anemia in Older Adults
http://www.ncbi.nlm.nih.gov/pmc/articles/PMC2572827/
Medscape—Anemia in Elderly Persons
http://emedicine.medscape.com/article/1339998-overview
American Family Physician—Anemia in Older Persons
http://www.aafp.org/afp/2010/0901/p480.html
WebMD—Tracking and Treating Anemia in Elderly Patients
http://www.anemia.org/professionals/feature-articles/content.php?contentid=344
WebMD—Iron Deficiency Anemia
http://www.webmd.com/a-to-z-guides/iron-deficiency-anemia-topic-overview
National Hematologic Diseases
Information Service (NHDIS)—Anemia of Inflammation and Chronic Disease
http://hematologic.niddk.nih.gov/anemiachronic.aspx
Kidney Disease: Improving Global Outcomes—(KDIGO) Clinical Practice Guideline for
Anemia in Chronic Kidney Disease
http://www.kdigo.org/clinical_practice_guidelines/anemia.php
Be The Match—Acute Myelogenous Leukemia (AML)
http://marrow.org/Patient/Disease_and_Treatment/About_Your_Disease/AML/Acute_
Myelogenous_Leukemia_(AML).aspx
Medscape—Chronic Lymphocytic Leukemia In the Elderly - Is the Game Plan Changing?
http://www.medscape.com/viewarticle/742137
CLL Topics Updates—How to Treat Elderly Chronic Lymphocytic Leukemia Patients
http://updates.clltopics.org/4371-how-to-treat-elderly-cll-patients
CANCER*Care*.org—Treatment Update: Multiple Myelomahttp://www.cancercare.org/
publications/12-advances_in_the_treatment_of_multiple_myeloma
Multiple Myeloma Research Foundation—Living with Multiple Myeloma
http://www.themmrf.org/living-with-multiple-myeloma/newly-diagnosed-patients/
what-is-multiple-myeloma/

Pdf Documents

Anemia and Chronic Kidney Disease
http://www.kidney.org/atoz/pdf/anemia.pdf

Videos

Unexplained Anemia in the Elderly (2011)
    Nathan Berger, MD, discusses unexplained Anemia of the Elderly at the Department of Medicine Grand Rounds. (49 minutes)
    http://youtu.be/HrXjKshiPIQ
Anemia (2011)
    Dr. Bob talks about anemia and how it affects your health. (1:40 minutes)
    http://youtu.be/1b4fhPFlyio
Leukemia (2010)
    This patient education video explains what leukemia is. It discusses the causes, symptoms, diagnosis, and treatment options and their risks. (6:30 minutes)
    http://youtu.be/FJOYAaygQFE
Acute Leukemia: What is "Acute Promyelocytic Leukemia" (APL)? (2011)
    http://www.dailymotion.com/video/xgg1ic_acute-leukemia-what-is-acute-promyelocytic-leukemia-apl_lifestyle
Leukemia Videos
    http://www.medpagetoday.com/HematologyOncology/Leukemia-Videos/

Images

Google images for Anemia
    http://www.google.com/search?q=anemia&hl=en&source=lnms&tbm=isch&sa=X&ei=1C6dUZa5JsXF4AOFo4DABQ&sqi=2&ved=0CAcQ_AUoAQ&biw=1024&bih=564
Google images of Leukemia
    http://www.google.com/search?q=leukemia&hl=en&source=lnms&tbm=isch&sa=X&ei=GTOdUZP8OrGq4AOTwYHgDQ&sqi=2&ved=0CAcQ_AUoAQ&biw=1024&bih=564
Leukemia images from the Mayo Clinic
    http://www.mayoclinic.com/health/leukemia/DS00351/TAB=multimedia

Pressure Ulcers

David M. Mercer, ACNP-BC, CWOCN, CFCN

INTRODUCTION

Health care providers are in the midst of a burgeoning health care paradigm shift. As the population over age 65 increases and the number of patients in long-term care climbs, the management of chronic disease is now a reality that few debate. Emphasis on disease management is shifting to coordination of care for chronic disease; this is an optimistic observation. The demographic realities of an increasing older population are expected to eclipse 90 million in 2060. This will be nearly 22% of the total population (United States Census Bureau, 2013).

As individuals age, the health of the skin undergoes changes that are often irreversible and unpredictable. Degenerative changes and metabolic changes associated with aging often present challenges for the health care provider regarding skin management and dermatological presentation. Systemic disease, lifestyle habits, medications, socioeconomic factors, climate, race, gender, nutrition, and culture contribute to the role of maintaining one's skin integrity (Jafferany et al., 2012). The importance of maintaining skin integrity for patients in the health care setting or the community cannot be underestimated. Skin, as our first line of defense in disease acquisition, is vital to the physiological and psychological well-being of many older adults. This chapter offers a review of the integumentary system with emphasis on the identification and management of pressure ulcers (PUs).

Few wounds evoke an emotional response and influence health care policy like those of PUs. A PU is localized injury to the skin and/or underlying tissue usually over a bony prominence, as a result of pressure, or pressure in combination with friction and shear. A number of contributing or confounding factors are also associated with PUs; the significance of these factors is yet to be completely understood (J. Black et al., 2007). PUs do not discriminate on the basis of age, gender, race, or setting. From infants to older adults, PUs are thought, by many, to be preventable and a significant problem in many health care settings (Lyder, 2003). The Institution for Healthcare Improvement estimated that PU treatment costs the United States health care system $11 billion per year (Bales & Duvendack, 2011). PUs are a major problem, and as health care reform reshapes the landscape of care delivery, hospitals and long-term care facilities are under more pressure to improve quality, save money, and prevent foreseeable injuries such as PUs. As a vulnerable population, older adults are at greatest risk for prolonged, uninterrupted pressure. Immobility is the most common reason for PU formation.

BASIC SKIN ANATOMY

The skin is the largest organ of the body. It is exposed at all times and susceptible to changes in the environment. Disruptions of the skin primarily fall into two categories: acute skin wounds or chronic wounds. Common acute skin injuries include trauma, burns, and surgeries. Further characterization of acute skin injuries pertains to the level of depth in the injury—partial-thickness or full-thickness injury. For example, minor sunburn or localized skin tear is considered to be a partial-thickness acute wound, whereas surgical incisions are often full-thickness acute wounds. The concepts of depth in wounds are best understood after a rudimentary discussion of normal physiology of skin.

Human skin is divided into two primary layers—epidermis (outermost layer) and dermis (innermost layer) (Fig. 17.1). These two layers are separated by a structure called the *basement membrane*. Beneath the dermis is a layer of loose connective tissue called the *hypodermis*. Major functions of the skin are protection, thermoregulation, aesthetic value, sensation, metabolism, and communication (Jacob et al., 1982). The average adult has approximately 6 lb (2.7 kg) of skin,

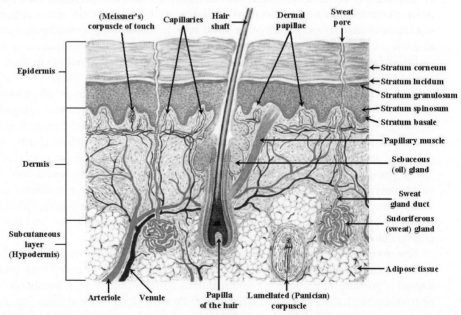

FIGURE 17.1. Basic skin anatomy of healthy intact skin. (From Lazaroff, M and Rollinson, D. The Anatomy of Hair. In: Forensics: An Online Textbook [online]. Retrieved from: http://shs2.westport.k12.ct.us/forensics/09-trace_evidence/splitting_hairs.htm#parts, with permission)

and it receives about a third of the body's circulating blood volume. The skin forms a protective barrier from the environment while maintaining homeostasis internally. There are numerous external appendages to one's skin—hair follicles, nails of the hand and foot, and sweat orifices. Remarkably, the skin has the ability to regenerate.

Epidermis

The epidermis, the outmost layer of the skin is avascularized and, with the exception of the palms of the hands and the soles of the feet, is quite thin. The epidermal layer is constantly being renewed with cellular turnover time ranging from 25 to 42 days. The epidermal layer is composed of stratified squamous epithelial cells, or keratinocytes, and divided into five layers. These layers, beginning from the outermost to the innermost, are the stratum corneum, stratum lucidum, stratum granulosum, stratum spinosum, and stratum basale. In the acute or chronic wound care context, wounds limited to the epidermal layer are considered *partial thickness* wounds.

Dermis

The dermis is the thickest tissue layer of the skin, with thickness ranging from 2 to 4 mm. It is vascularized and innervated. Depending on the location of the body, dermal thickness varies. For example, the dermis of the back is thicker than the dermis of the scalp. This is important as it pertains to PU formation because the location of pressure injury *matters*—PUs of the ear are likely to progress in a more rapid fashion because of the limited depths of skin tissue. In contrast, PUs of the thighs may develop more slowly through the stages owing to thicker dermal tissue.

The major proteins of the dermis are collagen and elastin. Collagen is the major structural protein in the dermis. Collagen is responsible for skin tensile strength, or clinically, the ability of the skin to withstand tear and shear forces. Elastin is a protein that provides skin with its elastic recoil and when abundant, keeps skin from being permanently reshaped to changes in the environment. The dermis also plays a role in immunology, whereas mast cells such as macrophages and lymphocytes are involved in bacterial surveillance at all times. Wounds extending through the dermis and beyond are considered *full-thickness* wounds.

NORMAL INTRINSIC VERSUS EXTERNAL VARIATIONS IN THE SKIN

Skin aging is characterized by concomitant physiological changes. For those that spend more time in sunnier climates, photoaging is more prominent on exposed parts of the skin (Hashizume, 2004). This would be classified as an environmental and extrinsic factor. Another extrinsic factor commonly overlooked is the role of smoking. Smoking increases the amount of free radicals that act as an accelerant on aging. Intrinsic factors are changes that occur from chronological aging and the body's normal metabolic aging process. This includes thinning of epidermis, diminished blood flow, and reduced collagen deposition, which leads to a reduction in elasticity. Moreover, there is a reduction in the skin's ability to fight bacterial invasion since immune function is also reduced as part of the normal aging process.

Other intrinsic changes in the skin of older adults include decreased epidermal turnover, resulting in skin roughness. There is marked reduction in skin lipids and barrier function making older skin more permeable to chemical substances such as stool or urine. The role of fecal and/or urinary incontinence is thought to be an independent risk factor for the formation of PUs

(Barrois et al., 2008; Berlowitz et al., 2001; Cakmak et al., 2009). There is smaller surface contact between the dermis and the epidermis, resulting in less nutritional transfer and poor adhesion between the dermis and the epidermis. Clinically, this is observed as skin wrinkles and susceptibility in the older adult for skin tears. Decreased sensory perception increases the tendency for injuries. Impaired thermoregulation makes older adults vulnerable to heat and cold. Reduced function of sweat glands places older adults at risk for overheating and heat stroke.

What is beyond the scope of this chapter yet highly influential in the treatment of geriatric skin conditions is the role of acute and chronic conditions or disease. Chronic kidney disease, diabetes, obesity, vascular disorders, vasculitides, nutritional disorders, cancer, fecal and/or urinary incontinence play a major role in the care of one's skin. The roles of medications on skin disease and the growing concern of polypharmacy for geriatrics is emerging science (Cheung, 2010). Skin care management of the older patient is challenging for most clinicians. However, most acute and chronic wounds can be improved with thoughtful attention and guideline-driven management.

ACUTE VERSUS CHRONIC WOUNDS

Case Vignette. Ms. X is an 85-year-old female who was admitted for treatment of an acute expanding aortic aneurysm. Her BMI was normal at 25, and her past medical history is significant for hypertension and a 60-pack/year history of smoking. She underwent endovascular repair of her aortic aneurysm approximately 3 weeks ago. Unfortunately, deployment of her stent graft to occlude the dissected aorta resulted in infarction of her spinal cord at the thoracic spine. She is now paralyzed from her mid-thoracic vertebrae down. Also resulting from this postoperative variance is urinary and fecal incontinence. The nurse contacts you, a primary care provider, to address her concerns of a developing redness of her sacrococcygeal skin. Upon examination, you see a fairly inflamed area of ulcerated skin over her coccyx. The epidermis appears intact although there is a distinct dark purple discoloration in the area of her sacrum (Fig. 17.2). The wound border is irregularly shaped. There is no drainage, and the patient is insensate or feels no pain from this wound.

Questions at this time for the clinician:

Is this an acute or chronic wound?
What risk factors predispose Ms. X to the development of this ulcer?
How long will it take for this wound to heal?

Acute Wound Healing Process

A wound is a disruption of normal anatomic structure and function (Lazarus et al., 1994). From our case vignette, it is important to distinguish the acute from the chronic wound. Indeed, this is an acute wound and injury to her coccyx, a PU. Any acute wound may turn chronic, and this distinction is rarely made in the clinical arena for many reasons. First, it is very difficult to link your history to the origins of a PU. Most patients do not know exactly when they occurred. In normal acute wound healing, the mechanism of injury must be removed or at least alleviated. In this case, pressure must be relieved and her skin examined to determine the extent of the damage. Thus, the first step in wound healing is for a person to mount an inflammatory response; hence, the *inflammation phase*. This phase begins the moment the tissue is injured as blood components spill into the site of the injury, triggering platelets to release clotting factors and essential growth factors. Integral to this phase is the stoppage of bleeding. This leads to the *proliferative* phase as

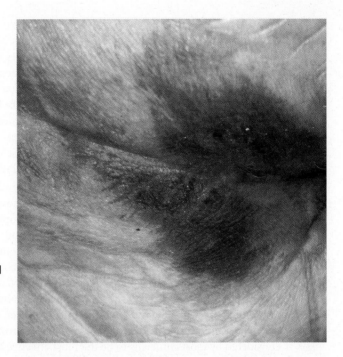

FIGURE 17.2. 85-Year-old female with prolonged immobility to sacral region. Note dark purple irregular wound indicative of deep tissue injury (bruise). (Photograph courtesy of David Mercer.)

macrophages, lymphocytes, angiocytes, and neurocytes are recruited to the area for the contracture and building of repaired skin. The goal of this inflammatory response is for the body to control bleeding and establish a clean wound bed. The final phase of wound healing is the remodeling phase and occurs in partial thickness wounds as reepithelialization is complete. The partial thickness wound when healed will take on the appearance as if no injury occurred. In contrast, in full thickness wound healing, scar tissue forms.

Most clinicians agree that in the absence of chronic disease or medications known to impair any of these phases (i.e., Prednisone) or nutritional compromise, acute wound healing will occur in a normal and orderly fashion. It is this *orderly fashion* that sets acute wound healing apart from that of a chronic wound. Any event or condition that interferes with this order can influence a wound's ability to heal. Most wounds of an acute nature in the absence of disorder can be expected to heal within 2 to 6 weeks. The most common acute wounds are trauma related, surgical, and burns.

Chronic Wound Healing Process

In contrast to the orderly fashion of acute wound healing, a *disorderly pattern* to wound healing is labeled a chronic wound. As with many steps that must occur for the body to form new skin, there are many aspects to healing that can be impaired, rendering a wound indolent or incompetent in progressing through the phases of normal wound healing. A chronic wound can be locked into a particular phase such as that of the *inflammation* phase. From our case vignette, Ms. X entered the hospital as a smoker, and she is now paralyzed from her middle back to her feet. Should she continue to smoke when she goes home, she will continue on the presumptive pathway of inducing vasoconstriction to her peripheral tissues, and together with her immobility, fecal and urinary incontinence, her chances of this ulcer healing in an orderly fashion have been reported to be less than 30% (Mian et al., 1991). The most common chronic wounds in the order of their prevalence are venous ulcers, diabetic ulcers, and PUs.

The increase in many systemic and chronic diseases in older adults contributes to the formation of PUs (Margolis et al., 2003). Many diseases will influence any of the phases of wound healing. For example, diabetes or stroke can cause neuropathy, impairing their ability to recognize a PU. This is particularly problematic in the heels or other areas of the feet. Congestive heart failure or chronic kidney disease may result in poor perfusion and chronic edema, also making skin disruption more likely. Neurological decline and conditions such as Alzheimer disease may cause emotional lability and agitation. Loss of self-control or of one's ability to independently control physical movement can lead to an increase in pressure, friction, and shear—widely known contributing factors in PU formation.

Case Vignette Summary. Ms. X, at 85 years of age and a life-time smoker, entered the hospital with a baseline risk for PU formation. A catastrophic variance in her treatment for aortic dissection caused paralysis, and now she is immobile, incontinent, and unable to turn herself without assistance. We have discovered an acute wound that is a PU, and unless caregivers are aggressive in preventing further injury to her sacrococcygeal skin, this ulcer will most certainly progress in a chronic, nonhealing wound. Given optimal care, including pressure relief, meticulous incontinence care, and aggressive nutritional intervention, this ulcer should heal in an orderly fashion in approximately one month's time. However, as we have discussed, any risk factor that is left unaddressed may influence this orderly approximation. Thus, prevention is critical and considered by most clinicians to be the most effective wound care intervention.

SCREENING FOR PRESSURE ULCERS

Most patients consider PUs to be avoidable (J. M. Black et al., 2011). Many regulatory agencies consider the acquisition of new PUs as "preventable" and "never events." In October 2008, Medicare addressed this issue directly and imposed a final rule that for certain hospital-acquired conditions considered preventable in the hospital setting, reimbursements would be withheld for their care. PUs were among these conditions. However, there is a lack of firm agreement, with the avoidable versus nonavoidable debate. The Wound, Ostomy, and Continence Association, a professional nursing society that promotes the care of individuals with wounds, published a 2009 position statement aimed at refuting the assumption that all PUs are avoidable (Wound, Ostomy, and Continence Nursing Society, 2009). The development of a PU can be complex and multifactorial (Berlowitz & Brienza, 2007). Despite a lack of consensus, it is just and ethical for all health care providers to consider all PUs as avoidable. However, wound care consultants anecdotally report that despite strict adherence to best practice, skin may "fail" as with multi-system organ dysfunction that commonly affects an individual's end-of-life care.

If we are to assume that PUs are avoidable, then there are known best practices with regard to assessment of risk. Consider any older patient over 65 with mobility and nutritional deficits at risk for PU formation. Additionally, normal variants of aging contribute to the risk of PUs. As clinicians, we must perform a local evaluation and a holistic assessment of each patient. Having a PU affects an individual's quality of life and in many ways will speak to their functional status and ability to perform the activities of daily living and maintain independence. As more attention is placed on the concept of the medical home, the future of patient care is expected (and wanted) by most patients to be self-directed (Backer, 2009). It is essential for practitioners to organize such care and pay close attention to the whole patient, and a thoughtful assessment of skin care is not only well received by most patients, but also appreciated.

There are numerous tools to assist the clinician in the assessment of PU risk. Most health care institutions that use PU risk assessment tools use either the Braden Scale or the Norton Scale, the Braden scale being the most widely used in the United States. The Norton scale score ranges from 5 to 20 points (Norton et al., 1962). It assesses five risk-based items: physical condition, mental condition, activity, mobility, and continence. A score of 14 or less is considered high risk. The Braden scale score ranges from 6 to 23 points and assesses risk according to six factors: sensory perception, skin moisture, activity levels, mobility, nutritional status, and the identification of friction and shear (Bergstrom, 2005). A score of less than 18 is considered at risk. Research has shown that predicting PUs risk in hospitalized patients occurs over 75% of the time after an interactive learning session on the Braden scale (Maklebust et al., 2005). Regardless of what risk assessment scale is used, it is imperative for the calculation of a score to drive preventative interventions. Hence, a Braden score of 16 may include a mobility sub-score of 3 (slightly limited mobility) and a moisture sub-score of 1 (constantly moist). Practitioners would be addressing PU risk by ensuring that moisture prevention or skin-related damage from moisture is minimized.

Case Vignette No. 2 Part A. Mr. Q enters your family practice clinic for a routine annual physical. You have been seeing him in your office for over 15 years. He is 90 years old, and his wife is reporting a gradual functional decline. "He sleeps in his chair all the time now," she states, and he is only eating "roughly half of his meals." She endorses a 15 lb (6.8 kg) weight loss for her husband over the past 2 months. His past medical history is significant for mild dementia and arthritis. When speaking to Mr. Q, you find him withdrawn and gaunt in appearance. He tells you that he does not feel much like eating anymore and agrees that sitting in the chair and watching sports is about all he can do at this point in his life. His wife is sad, very supportive, and wishes to help him in any way. She helps him to the bathroom every 4 hours and over the last 2 days noticed two breaks in his skin over his "buttocks." As part of your physical exam, you find two partial- to full-thickness skin lesions over bilateral ischial tuberosities. There is an erythematous wound border, and when you palpate the area, he briskly tells you to "get off that please!" There is a slight blood tinge on his underwear, and the ulcers have a yellow crusty appearance and are fairly dry.

Questions at this time for the clinician:

Assuming these are PUs, what stage are they and what caused them?
How can you help Mrs. Q assist her husband in preventing further injury?

ASSESSMENT OF PRESSURE ULCERS

It should be noted that in the context of health care settings there is a tendency for ancillary staff to stage all wounds regardless of their etiology. A wound on the top of one's foot that may be diabetic in origin, for example, is inadequately staged as a stage II ulcer. *Only PUs are staged.* This staging system is based on the identified level of skin injury over a bony prominence, or a known device that when removed has obviously caused the injury (i.e., oxygen tubing causing a pressure injury on the ear). There are six PU stages. In addition to the I–IV staging, the *deep tissue injury* and *unstageable* categories were added in 2007 by the National Pressure Ulcer Advisory Panel (2007) (Table 17.1). While this is not a universal system, it is most widely used in the United States. Importantly, PUs are not downstaged as they are healing. In other words, a stage IV PU that is healing and has depths

TABLE 17.1 · Stages of PU. Stage I–IV, Unstageable, and Deep Tissue Injury

National Pressure Ulcer Advisory Panel PU Staging System[a]

Stage I: Nonblanchable erythema

Intact skin with nonblanchable redness of a localized area usually over a bony prominence. Darkly pigmented skin may not have visible blanching; its color may differ from the surrounding area. The area may be painful, firm, soft, warmer or cooler as compared to adjacent tissue. Stage I may be difficult to detect in individuals with dark skin tones. May indicate "at risk" persons.

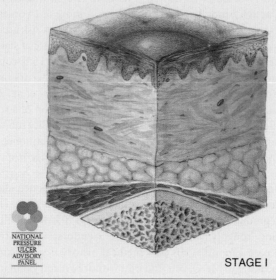

STAGE I

Stage II: Partial-thickness skin loss

Partial-thickness loss of dermis presenting as a shallow open ulcer with a red-pink wound bed, without slough. May also present as an intact or open/ruptured serum-filled or serosanguinous-filled blister. Presents as a shiny or dry shallow ulcer without slough or bruising[b]. This category should not be used to describe skin tears, tape burns, incontinence-associated dermatitis, maceration, or excoriation.

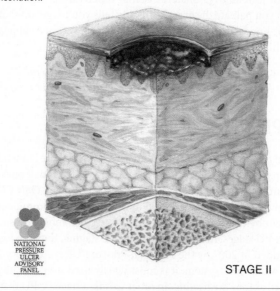

STAGE II

National Pressure Ulcer Advisory Panel PU Staging System[a]

Stage III: Full-thickness skin loss

Full-thickness tissue loss. Subcutaneous fat may be visible but bone, tendon, or muscles are *not* exposed. Slough may be present but does not obscure the depth of tissue loss. *May* include undermining and tunneling. The depth of a category/stage III PU varies by anatomical location. The bridge of the nose, ear, occiput, and malleolus do not have (adipose) subcutaneous tissue and category/stage III ulcers can be shallow. In contrast, areas of significant adiposity can develop extremely deep category/stage III PUs. Bone/tendon is not visible or directly palpable.

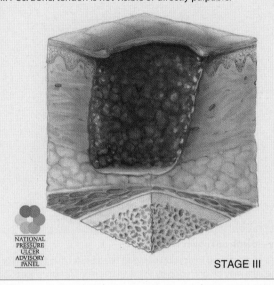

STAGE III

Stage IV: Full-thickness tissue loss

Full-thickness tissue loss with exposed bone, tendon, or muscle. Slough or eschar may be present. Often includes undermining and tunneling. The depth of a category/stage IV PU varies by anatomical location. The bridge of the nose, ear, occiput, and malleolus do not have (adipose) subcutaneous tissue, and these ulcers can be shallow. Category/stage IV ulcers can extend into muscle and/or supporting structures (e.g., fascia, tendon, or joint capsule) making osteomyelitis or osteitis likely to occur. Exposed bone/muscle is visible or directly palpable.

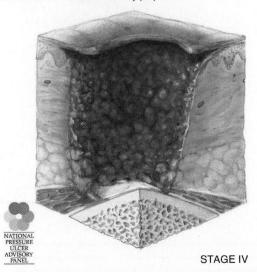

STAGE IV

(Continued)

National Pressure Ulcer Advisory Panel PU Staging System[a]

Unstageable: Full-thickness skin or tissue loss—depth unknown

Full-thickness tissue loss in which actual depth of the ulcer is completely obscured by slough (yellow, tan, gray, green, or brown) and/or eschar (tan, brown, or black) in the wound bed. Until enough slough and/or eschar are removed to expose the base of the wound, the true depth cannot be determined; but it will be either a category/stage III or IV. Stable (dry, adherent, intact without erythema or fluctuance) eschar on the heels serves as "the body's natural (biological) cover" and should not be removed.

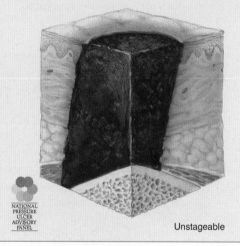

Unstageable

Suspected deep tissue injury—depth unknown

Purple or maroon localized area of discolored intact skin or blood-filled blister due to damage of underlying soft tissue from pressure and/or *shear*. The area may be preceded by tissue that is painful, firm, mushy, boggy, warmer, or cooler as compared to adjacent tissue. Deep tissue injury may be difficult to detect in individuals with dark skin tones. Evolution may include a thin blister over a dark wound bed. The wound may further evolve and become covered by thin eschar. Evolution may be rapid exposing additional layers of tissue even with optimal treatment.

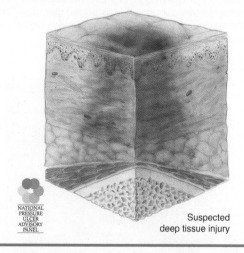

Suspected
deep tissue injury

[a]© National Pressure Ulcer Advisory Panel.
[b]Bruising indicates deep tissue injury.
From National Pressure Ulcer Advisory Panel, NPUAP Pressure Ulcer Stages/Categories retrieved from http://www.npuap.org/resources/educational-and-clinical-resources/npuap-pressure-ulcer-stagescategories/ and Pressure Ulcer Category/Staging Illustrations retrieved from http://www.npuap.org/resources/educational-and-clinical-resources/pressure-ulcer-categorystaging-illustrations/, with permission.

similar to stage II would be staged as *a healing stage IV* and not a stage II ulcer. It is, and will always be, a healing stage IV PU until total re-epithelialization and/or scar tissue has occurred.

The nomenclature for PUs varies widely in the literature and often we hear of PUs referred to as decubiti, bedsores, or pressure sores. Decubitus is perhaps the most widely known in the medical community. This is not only outdated but does not imply the true nature of injury in most PUs. A decubitus position is not necessary for one to develop a pressure injury. PUs may be caused by any object or device; thus, the term pressure ulcer is now contemporary.

Assessments of PUs include an approximation of size and appearance. In the clinical arena, there are instruments that have been developed and validated to assess the healing of PUs. One of the most widely used tools is called the Pressure Ulcer Scale for Healing (PUSH) tool. The PUSH tool is composed of three wound characteristics, namely, size of ulcer (length × width), exudate amount, and tissue type that are scored and summed to determine the level of healing of a PU (Stotts et al., 2001). In the home environment, clinicians have fewer tools to assist patients and care providers. The PUSH tool is clinically oriented and not geared to caregivers at home. Most caregivers resort to comments such as "it is getting worse" or "it is getting better" when speaking of wound care for their loved ones. Therefore, it is critical for clinicians to perform patient/caregiver assessments. A thoughtful analysis of a patient's/caregiver's beliefs, values, cultural influences, environment, and educational needs is critical to wound care planning. More research is needed to identify educational tools that are feasible, especially for use in the patient at home. Questions such as "how can we help you with this wound?" and "tell me what you see as the best outcome as we discuss care of this wound" are open ended and place the onus of responsibility on the patient to share his/her thoughts of the eventual management. Sometimes, the goal for some patients may not be wound healing at all but alleviation of pain and suffering (palliative). It is essential that we understand the needs and goals for each patient and family. An assessment of a PU must include physical characteristics and evaluation of infection, odor, drainage, pain, presence of undermining, and the condition of the surrounding skin.

Physical Characteristics

The color of the wound matters—bright pink and free of devitalized tissue is ideal and supportive for most wound healing to occur. Pallor indicates poor blood flow or nutritional compromise. Devitalized tissue is often black, yellow, crusty, or leathery and usually indicates a wound that is indolent and chronic. A dark red or bruise-like appearance to a wound may indicate further tissue hypoxemia or tissue damage that is actively occurring. Occasionally, muscle, bone, skin structures such as fascia, foreign bodies, hair, or other elements can be seen in a wound. A PU that is covered with nonviable tissue is, by definition, unstageable. A PU is staged only when you can see viable tissue and you know that pressure was a chief mechanism of injury.

Infection in a wound is often diagnosed clinically with the classic manifestations such as redness, pain, heat, swelling, foul odor, bleeding, and purulent material providing evidence of an infection (Dow, 2001). Wound cultures are often recommended by medical personnel, but their relatively clinical value is limited owing to the polymicrobial nature of most chronic wounds. Clinical infection should be considered with careful holistic assessment of each patient, noting the patient's past ability to heal, current health status, nutritional status, and characteristic of the wound and surrounding tissue. If a clinician suspects an infection, cultures are warranted, and their value is shown in the identification of superbugs, most notably methicillin-resistant *Staphylococcus aureus* (MRSA), vancomycin-resistant *Enterococcus* (VRE), or newly emerging strains such as *Klebsiella pneumoniae* (carbapenem-resistant Enterobacteriaceae [CRE]). Qualitative cultures should not be obtained as superficial swabs, but rather of any purulent material or using deeper tissue culture techniques.

Antibiotics are often given when a clinical suspicion for infection is noted in chronic wounds, their use directed at times on the basis of culture results. However, most chronic wounds such as PUs are colonized with some of the most common skin pathogenic bacteria; for example, *S. aureus*. Practicing clinicians should note that no clear consensus on antibiotic use and chronic wound care is available. All chronic wounds (including PUs) are colonized with bacteria. In the absence of bone infection (osteomyelitis) or soft tissue infection (cellulitis), antibiotics have not been shown to be definitively needed or effective in wound healing (O'Meara et al., 2001). Despite the lack of specific guidelines and the caution not to use antibiotics unless clearly warranted, patients are frequently treated with antibiotics for suspected wound infections. The implications of such practices are controversial; however, for clinical relevance, it should be noted that only patients who need antibiotics for their chronic wound should obtain antibiotics.

Case Vignette No. 2 Summary Part A. Mr. Q, in fact, has the emerging PUs of his bilateral ischial tuberosities. This is the most common site for PUs in patients who sit with unrelieved pressure for extended periods. His ulcers are dry, yellow, and crusted in appearance, making them *unstageable*. There is blood tinged on his underwear, and this implies local inflammation to the area. This is confirmed with the presence of significant pain that Mr. Q expresses after you palpate the ulcers. There is no soft tissue infection or marked inflammation of the periwound skin. Further exam and blood work do not imply that there is active infection, and thus, antibiotics are not initiated. A thoughtful discussion follows with Mrs. Q in the presence of her husband. His weight loss implies nutritional deficiencies, and this coupled with his sitting for a majority of a 24-hour period is critical for this patient in the formation of a PU. You discuss simple ways for him to increase protein and calories in his diet as well as ways to off-load his ischial tuberosities during the times he is sitting. His wife states that she will attempt to limit his sitting to "half a day" and add protein-rich supplements to his diet in the form of shakes. Wound care will be discussed in the following section, and we will pick up this discussion about what we are going to recommend for Mr. Q's wound treatment.

MANAGEMENT OF THE GERIATRIC PU PATIENT

The PU in the older adult is difficult to manage. As suggested, comorbid conditions and normal variants of aging make wound etiology multifactorial. For simplification, many older adults obtain PUs with three main etiological factors

1. Immobility
2. Moisture-related skin damage
3. Nutritional deficiencies

Care is directed at addressing each component and other factors that are realized after patient and caregiver assessment. Once identified, there are known clinical practices that are well documented, well researched, and clearly in the public domain to aid providers in making the best choices. A summary of some reputable guidelines is presented in Table 17.2.

Case Vignette No. 2 Part B. Mrs. Q asked you, the primary care provider, to recommend what to place on these wounds to prevent further problems and promote wound healing. She feels her

TABLE 17.2 · Guidelines for PU Prevention and Treatment

Guideline Title

Pressure Ulcer Treatment Recommendations. In: *Prevention and Treatment of Pressure Ulcers: Clinical Practice Guideline* (Whitney et al., 2006)

Pressure Ulcer: The Management of Pressure Ulcers in Primary and Secondary Care (National Institute for Health and Clinical Excellence, 2005)

Guidelines for Prevention and Management of PUs (Wound, Ostomy, and Continence Nurses Society, 2010)

Widely accessible in the public domain.

husband has been unable to care for himself at times, and she is taking on a more active role in some of the most basic daily activities of daily living. Some of these include, but are not limited to, toileting and choosing appropriate clothes for the day. With regard to toileting, she states her husband often has "accidents," and to remedy the situation, she has to pull-up briefs for him that he wears continuously. Having just noticed the PUs this past week, she had no idea what to put on them. Her husband says he has been cleaning the areas with hydrogen peroxide full strength. He was going to put a "salve" on it, but opted not to because he thought it would just get better letting some "air to it." Last night he took a bath and stated that "soaking it felt great."

Cleansing

Wound cleansing refers to the process of removing inflammatory contaminates from the wound surface. It is a critical step and is essential to create a milieu of orderly healing through the stages of normal wound healing. As suggested, the chronic wound as a PU may be locked into the inflammatory phase of healing, and wound bioburden is a significant step (among others) in the reversal of this inflammatory process.

Common household remedial therapies for wound healing are agents such as hydrogen peroxide or various alcohols. What patients often do not understand is that they are harming their wounds with these agents and doing little in the promotion of healing as these agents cause cell damage. Already, wounds are, by nature, pro-inflammatory. Critical to reversing this process and to promoting wound healing is choosing an agent that has a minimal toxicity profile to healthy tissue. It is vital to remove contaminates from the wound surface; however, this benefit must be weighed against the tendency for such agents to harm newly forming tissue or cellular growth. Wounds should be clean, moist, and free of devitalized tissue for orderly healing to occur. Despite evidence supporting the toxicity of agents such as hydrogen peroxide, acetic acid, hypochlorite, and iodine, Povidone-Iodine (Betadine), their use remains steadfast in the clinical arena. There is no scientific rigor supporting their use, yet clinicians rely on them despite decades of data that call for limiting their use (Atiyeh et al., 2009; Fernandez & Griffiths, 2012; Z. Moore & Cowman, 2008; Z. E. Moore & Cowman, 2005). Many practitioners rely on anecdotal evidence or more frequent, common sense approaches to managing a wound that is colonized with bacteria, and this often leads them to the path of antiseptics for cleansing the chronic wound.

Wound cleansing for an older adult at home can be accomplished with water or home-made preparations (two teaspoons of salt per four cups of boiled water) of normal saline. If the water is safe to drink, the water is safe for their wound. There are a number of enhanced wound cleaners on the market that offer surfactant technology, which serves to break bonds of wound contaminants, but again you run the risk of toxicity to newly and highly sensitive tissue. In general, rigorous research has shown that there are no agents superior to that of water or saline in the routine cleansing of most chronic wounds. A careful and thought out discussion with your patients over the role of cleaning wounds will help avoid many cost-ineffective practices surrounding wound cleansing.

Finally, the role of bathing or *soaking* is worth special mention and its relationship to cleaning. Chronic wounds require moisture in their support of healing, but excessive moisture is counterproductive in the orderly fashion of healing. Already, geriatric skin is less capable of accommodating changes in the environment and prone to dryness. Skin (wounds) allowed to soak become waterlogged much like the skin submerged in water for a prolonged period. For a wound, this condition is referred to as maceration, and this excessive moisture is not supportive in wound healing. It harms healthy cellular growth. Soaking and/or whirlpool bathing has been shown to decrease some of the devitalized overgrowth of wounds, but this perceived benefit must follow with the right wound therapy (dressing) and moisturization that promotes maintenance of wound hydration so that dryness and devitalization of the wound bed does not occur. Left open to air, most chronic wounds dry out, forming dry, necrotic eschar (scab) that rarely promotes the healing process.

Debridement

Debridement is the cornerstone for treating PUs that are not responding to conservative management. Debridement is performed to remove necrotic tissue, slough, and any nonviable components of the ulcer. The most important step in promoting wound healing and reducing the bacterial load in the chronic wound is the removal of all devitalized tissue. Bacteria proliferate in devitalized tissue (Rodeheaver, 2001). All dressing therapies are best directed toward accomplishing the goal of a clean wound bed that is prone to healing. Depending on the properties of a chosen therapy, debridement will be performed.

Before choosing a type of debridement, it is important to perform a holistic assessment of the patient and establish mutual goals of therapy. PUs are painful. Although necrotic tissue is devoid of viability and nerve conduction, once this tissue is removed you most certainly will excite healthy tissue rich in nerve innervations, and this may exacerbate pain in your patient. Choosing a therapy with this in mind is important as one begins wound therapy. Additional considerations for the older patient include noting the presence of medical comorbidities such as vascular disease. If the PU was on the calcaneus (heel), performing debridement without first establishing that the patient has adequate blood flow to heal a wound would be possibly harmful to the patient. In some cases, such patients should be referred to specialists for vascular studies prior to your intervention.

The presence of gross infection or palpable bone in a wound bed warrants further investigation and may be indicative of acute or chronic osteomyelitis. It is important for clinicians to realize that such patients may not be sick in the classic sense, exhibiting fever or chills or excessive wound pain. Older adults are much more likely to exhibit atypical responses to their wound infections such as confusion, decreased functional status, or even more vague, a reduced quality of life. Some PUs are present for months to years before patients seek medical attention. It is important to perform and identify a good historian (if not the patient) who can not only detail when the wound developed but also elicit any functional changes that have occurred as a result of the wound. It is not uncommon for caregivers to report that their loved ones never mentioned a wound and confess that they simply never knew that their family member has completely adapted their life around a wound like a PU.

Once the above considerations are considered, debridement should proceed and often falls into two categories, selective and nonselective. With selective debridement, only nonviable tissue is targeted and obtained. There is limited removal, if any, of viable tissue. In contrast, nonselective debridement involves the removal of viable tissue and nonviable tissue. In the latter, therapies deemed nonselective cannot distinguish between healthy and nonviable tissue. It is one of the ways that vendors are targeting future therapies. Techniques or dressings aimed at being very selective are promising, and we are seeing more and more dressings on the market targeting selective debridement and minimally traumatic to healthy tissue upon their removal. Debridement is commonly classified by what method or mechanism of action is used to accomplish selective and/or nonselective tissue from a wound.

The types of debridement seen in clinical practice include conservative sharp (bedside debridement or in-office with scissors, scalpel, curette), surgical (formal introduction of patient into an operative suite under sterile conditions), enzymatic (use of biologically active enzymes that cleave nonviable collagen, reducing necrotic tissue burden), mechanical (use of whirlpool, ultrasound mist therapy, wet-to-dry dressings, pressured lavage), autolytic (choosing a dressing that encourages a moist environment and the body's natural process of cleansing), and biological (the use of medical grade sterile farmed larvae, maggots) (Fig. 17.3).

As discussed, choosing the optimal technique for debridement of the wound is best made with the clinician, caregiver, and/or patient. In the absence of chronic disease or decrease in functional status (mobility), most wounds will heal through the autolytic process. Simply putting a Band-Aid, for instance, over a wound will promote autolytic debridement as compared with the wound that is left open to air. When a wound is full-thickness, the most common dressing that is called upon in clinical practice is one that is constructed—with cotton gauze or roll-type dressings. A full-thickness wound bed must be packed or filled so that dead space is allowed contact with the dressing that will nourish and moisturize it. Often, filling wounds is difficult as often seen with a stage III or IV ulcer. There can be undermining or tunneling that is not initially evident. It is important, however, to pack the entire wound or the risk increases for dead space and abscess formation. The application of such dressings might be aided with the careful guidance of a cotton swab applicator.

The wet-to-dry dressing continues to thrive in clinical practice although its name is actually more controversial. Clinical wound experts of wound care management promote moisture-associated wound healing. Classic wet-to-dry dressings of the past are no longer superior in that they are very nonselective in their debridement. True wet-to-dry dressings are placed in moist, and then allowed to dry within the wound bed. When removed, the dressings take necrotic tissue with them. However, there is significant pain and trauma to both the patient and the wound bed; hence, this method is no longer promoted nor supported in the literature today. However, wet-to-dry dressings have survived at least in name, and most clinicians use it as a synonym for moist-to-moist dressings. For the purposes of this discussion, moist-to-moist dressings are the gold standard therapy for most conservative chronic wound management. This involves moistening gauze with saline (or water in some instances), wringing it out completely and feeding it into the wound bed, and then a water-impermeable dressing is placed over this and adhered to the patient. The dressing is changed with a frequency that permits no drying of this dressing to the wound bed. If this occurs, gentle wound irrigation is instilled into the wound or water irrigation

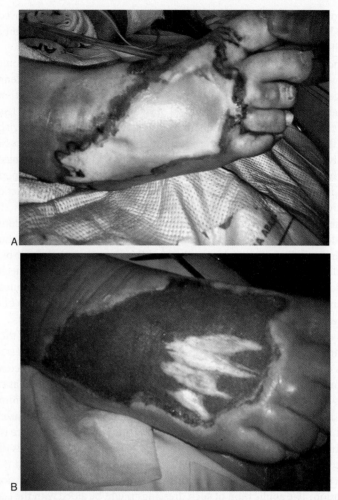

FIGURE 17.3. The debridement process. Note nonviable tissue in **(A)** prior to debridement strategy (a combination maggot biodebridement, conservative, sharp, enzymatic, and autolytic debridement used). A wound will only progress to **(B)** if and when devitalized tissue is removed. **A.** PU caused from foot pump pad in vulnerable patient. **B.** Same foot after debridement and wound healing therapies aimed at moist, clean, wound bed preparation. Healthy, robust granulation tissue with exposed tendons of foot (1 month allotted time). (Photographs courtesy of David Mercer.)

(take a shower before wound care) is performed so that the dressing can be atraumatically removed. Finally, this is followed with proper wound cleansing before the process is repeated.

Most wounds, such as PUs, require a combination approach to debridement. In other words, one may perform some conservative sharp debridement (low cost) in an office setting and then choose a dressing that is promoting moisture to the wound bed (autolytic debridement). For indolent wounds or wounds refractory to conservative debridement strategies, enzymatic (use of a proprietary ointment with suspended collagenases) debridement is available by prescription and covered by most health plans. However, enzymatic debridement is costly and most third-party payers may require preauthorization and/or approvals for use in acute or chronic wound management. Pulse lavage or whirlpool therapies are available in some wound care centers. This mechanical debridement is appropriate and helpful in some instances where large pressures are not easily managed with light irrigation. Finally, biological debridement is an outstanding method of debridement that is rich in history and clinical practice. Maggots have been used for centuries to clean wounds; however, such a therapy is difficult to apply and requires the formation of a cage-like dressing that remains in place for up to 48 hours. Many patients find it unacceptable at first; however, the most suitable patients are those such as the older adult, where more aggressive forms of debridement such as surgery may be contraindicated (Sherman, 2002).

Regardless of the type of debridement chosen, clinicians must decide on the most effective method that is cost effective, goal oriented, and least painful to the patient. Promotion of healthy tissue growth is vital to the wound healing milieu. Clinicians call this "wound bed preparation," and what we are preparing for is important and relevant to most victims of PUs, healing.

Dressing Selection

Once a wound is clean, it is essential to preserve a moist healing environment. Left open to air, most PUs of full-thickness depth will certainly become necrotic. There are so many dressings on the market today, so there is confusion as to which is best. There is no *one* dressing that is superior. The best dressing for a patient is the dressing that is cost effective, promoting the healing cascade, easy to place or remove, is not painful for the patient, atraumatic to the wound bed when removed, and that manages moisture. All PUs have patterns that must be considered when choosing a dressing type. Some PUs are very painful in some patients. Some PUs are very dry; others drain so often that they are hard to contain within a dressing. Some PUs start out clean and end up turning against the patient in a short time. Some PUs are actively getting worse (actively inflamed), others are healing with evidence of epithelial tissue bordering or overlay.

The most basic of dressings is the moist cotton gauze. Very controversial is the role of clean versus sterile technique. For most chronic wounds such as PUs, clean technique is most often employed (Barber, 2002). In most instances, asking the patient or caregiver to wash their hands before and after dressing procedures is adequate. Where patients obtain supplies is an additional challenge as wound care products are very expensive for those wishing to buy out-of-pocket. Medicare remains, for older adults, a primary payer supplies, and only when certain criteria are met will most patients obtain supplies that are prescribed. Every supplier will have paperwork that must be filled out; it is important to obtain such paperwork as part of your service to the patient. Even more difficult, every supplier has different criteria. Basic wound *care* with gauze, tapes, and cleansing solutions are often easiest to obtain with fundamental wound characteristics such as location of wound, length, width, and depth of wound, and the amount of wound drainage.

The advanced wound care market is emerging and expected to rise in the immediate future, driven by an increase in chronic wounds such as PUs. Estimates of the total advanced wound care market exceed 16 billion by 2023 (Visiongain, 2012). Advanced wound care comprises wound care products such as film dressings, foams, hydrocolloids, hydrogels, collagen, alginates, and many hybrids. Regardless of basic or advanced wound care strategies, the primary goal in PU management is optimization of the moist wound healing environment. Some of the most prevalent wound dressings in wound care centers today will be discussed below and included in Table 17.3.

TABLE 17.3 · Common Dressing Classifications and Vendor Examples

Dressing Type	Primary Dressing Examples
Hydrocolloid—ideal for wounds that are shallow with low-to-moderate levels of exudate	Duoderm (Conva-Tec, Skillman, New Jersey)
	Comfeel (Coloplast, Minneapolis, Minnesota)
	Exuderm Odorshield (Medline, Mundelein, Illinois)
	Restore (Hollister Inc, Libertyville, Illinois)
Alginate—ideal for wounds that are shallow or deep with moderate-to-heavy exudate. Many available in silver antimicrobial preparations	Kaltostat (Conva-Tec)
	SeaSorb (Coloplast)
	Restore Calcium (Hollister Inc.)
	Maxorb (Medline, Mundelein)
	Melgisorb (Molnlycke Healthcare, Norcross, Georgia)
Hydrofiber—ideal for wounds that are shallow or deep with moderate-to-heavy exudate. Available in regular or silver antimicrobial preparation	Aquacel (Conva-Tec)
Foams—ideal for wounds that are moderate-to-heavy exudate. Evidence-base emerging in prophylactic PU prevention. Many available in silver antimicrobial preparations	Alleyvn (Smith & Nephew, Andover, Massachusetts)
	Biatain (Coloplast)
	Mepilex Border (Molnlycke Healthcare)
	Restore Foam (Hollister Inc.)
	Tegaderm Foam (3M, St. Paul, Minnesota)
	Optifoam (Medline)
Films—ideal for superficial and shallow wounds with low exudate	OpSite (Smith & Nephew)
	Tegaderm (3M)
	Bioclusive (Johnson & Johnson, New Brunswick, New Jersey)
Hydrogels—ideal for wounds that are dry, containing slough and/or necrotic tissue Many available in silver antimicrobial preparations	IntraSite Gel (Smith & Nephew)
	SAF-Gel (Conva-Tec)
	Silvasorb Gel (Medline)
	Restore Hydrogel (Hollister Inc.)
Collagen—ideal for wounds that are dry and showing signs of poor wound healing with conservative therapy	Puracol Plus (Medline)
	Endoform (Hollister Inc.)

Dressings

Alginates

Alginate dressings are derived from different types of sterilized algae and seaweeds. These types of dressings are best used on PUs that have a large amount of wound drainage. They may be used on a variety of chronic wounds where moisture management or exudate control is considered critical. Alginates have natural hemostatic properties.

Hydrofibers

Hydrofiber dressings are soft, sterile, nonwoven (some are incorporating woven material within them to strengthen the fiber), pad or ribbon composed of sodium carboxymethylcellulose, which is incorporated in the form of a fleece held together by a needle bonding process. This is conformable and can absorb a large amount of wound fluid, such as exudate with bacteria. Once it interacts with wound fluid, it gels, creating a moist environment to support the healing environment. The gelling also renders the dressing less likely to adhere to the wound base.

Foams

Foam dressings are highly absorbent dressings generally made from a hydrophilic polyurethane foam. There are various absorption rates of the different foams on the market, and most companies distinguish themselves on claims of absorbency. Highly absorbent foams may allow the caregiver to change dressings less frequently. Foams that absorb exudate and keep it off the wound will aid in reducing maceration to a wound bed and fragile skin around the wound. It is best used in wounds that are heavily exudating. Most foam dressings are either stand-alone foams or foams incorporated into an adhesive dressing. Silicone adhesives are becoming more and more popular owing to their gentle qualities on fragile, older adult skin. Many foam adhesive dressings are being marketed today as PU prophylactic products. Such adhesive foams are placed over bony prominences of high-risk individuals such as older patients in acute or long-term care. The adhesive foam serves as a barrier to friction and shear, and aids in the ideal moisture climate of the sacral skin (urine or stool impermeable).

Hydrogels

Hydrogels are either dressings impregnated or free standing tubes of gel that consist of water-absorbing polymers. It is a synthetic dressing that is particularly good for PUs that are dry or necrotic or at risk for drying out. Hydrogels can be used as a wound filler in this regard, or there are dressings that have hydrogel impregnation designed to be placed directly over a superficially dry wound. It is composed mainly of water and emerged as a wound care modality when the relationship to moisture healing was popularized. It is most supportive in promoting a moist healing environment and autolytic debridement (Lay-Furrie, 2004).

Collagen

Collagen dressings employ the use of a carrier such as gels, pastes, or polymers. The collagen tends to be derived from bovine, porcine, equine, or avian sources, which is purified to render it nonantigenic. A given collagen dressing may contain ingredients, such as alginates and cellulose that can enhance absorbency, flexibility, moisture balance, and comfort. The primary goal of collagen-based dressings is to promote fibroblast production, hence supporting the wound healing cascade (Graumlich et al., 2003).

Hydrocolloids

Hydrocolloids are often opaque, and water-impermeable adherent dressing. The active surface of most hydrocolloids is gelatin, pectin, and carboxymethylcellulose together with other polymers and adhesives, forming a flexible wafer. They were among the first advanced wound dressings out on the market and have been used for many years. In contact with a shallow wound and exudate, the polymers absorb water and swell, forming a gel that is held within the structure of the adhesive matrix. This creates the moist environment conducive to healing. Hydrocolloids have become less popular as the emergence of more advanced wound care therapies has occurred. However, their use remains wide and their effectiveness well established (Darkovich et al., 1990).

Films

Film dressings are generally breathable, transparent, and water proof. They are flexible and self-adhesive and have been around for many years. Films dressings are not suitable where exudate control is an issue. Many do not absorb moisture, although some of the newer films on the market are incorporating polymer or acrylics within them offering some absorptive capacity. They do offer an effective barrier to infection and therefore protection of the wound. Films should be used cautiously in the older adult owing to their tendency for stronger adhesion and damage to skin upon their removal.

Most of the dressings above have both regular and antimicrobial versions. Unfortunately, the cost comparisons of silver versions from their regular counterparts are astronomical with silver versions costing, in some instances, hundreds more. Hence, when attempting to prescribe an advanced wound care dressing with silver technology, most payers seek justification for their use prior to their release, including evidence that other more conservative dressings have been employed. Adding to the confusion is limited unbiased evidence supporting their use. Antimicrobial properties generally conceived through the use of ionic silver technology.

Ionic silver is a broad and active antimicrobial agent. Silver dressings have a far lower propensity to induce microbial resistance than systemic antibiotics, making silver dressings a fairly rapidly emerging market in advanced wound care dressings. When ionic silver encounters bacterial cells, the silver ions damage the bacterial cell walls and interfere with DNA synthesis. It effectively kills the bacteria. Silver containing dressings are indicated in wounds (1) of patients who may be prone to infection (2) that have obvious bioburden (pus) (3) that have gross infection within the wound bed. It is important to note that silver technologies have emerged in the entire advanced wound care product arrays. Companies are attempting to stay competitive through the wedding of various technologies as well. For example, some companies are incorporating surgical dressing with hydrocolloid, hydrofiber, and silver technology all-in-one dressing. Their role in PU management is less known (Swezey, 2010).

The choice of optimal dressings depends on the wound. Host factors in the older adult add additional complexity in choosing the correct dressing. A patient confined to a sitting position for 23 hours a day will unlikely relieve pressure to adequately support wound healing. Use of high-cost dressings in these instances will likely not prove cost effective. Ask yourself what provocative measures caused this ulcer? What stage is this ulcer? What is the odor? How much drainage is coming from the wound? Are there external factors making it more moist (urinary incontinence)? Is it infected? The answers to these questions drive clinical decision making.

Alternative Therapies for Wound Healing

Negative pressure wound therapy (NPWT) is quite popular today and is used to treat a variety of wounds, including PUs. It is a process by which negative, sub-atmospheric pressure is distributed across the wound surface with the intent of accelerating wound healing. Currently, many industry leaders have versions of NPWT that incorporate either bacteriostatic gauze or foam as wound fillers. Each vendor markets and promotes proprietary pumps that deliver a constant or variable pressure within the wound bed after a leak-free wrapping is applied under clean or sterile conditions. NPWT's role in PU management mirrors that of any dressing. It must be chosen on the basis of characteristics of the wound and the patient's willingness to comply with therapy. Moreover, NPWT is geared for the insured patient or those on Medicare/Medicaid as out-of-pocket expense for NPWT is prohibitive for most patients. Its role in healing PUs is studied and remains an active research interest for providers (de Laat et al., 2011; Gupta & Ichioka, 2012). NPWT optimizes wound bed preparation as when therapy is initiated, a wound is rarely too dry or too moist—but just right. It actively removes potentially harmful exudate from the wound, and it elicits a cellular response through the action of the dressing on the wound surface. Further, it aids in the contraction of wounds and is supportive to them. When chosen wisely, NPWT has a promising role in the treatment of PUs.

Low-Frequency Ultrasonic Wound Therapy

The use of ultrasound (US) is emerging as a mainstay of therapy in the treatment of PUs. Popular therapies employ the use of a carrier (normal saline) that is combined with the low-frequency US that sends waves through the wound beds of PUs. Most promising is US in the treatment of deep tissue injuries where centers are using US to help stimulate healthy growth factors within the wound bed. Benefits of US include increasing blood flow to the area, removal of debris, and stimulation of growth factors promoting wound healing. The evidence of US is emerging and payers are signing on to the benefits of US in many parts of the country. However, more research is needed in this area in terms of providing US as a standard of care in the treatment of PUs (Baba-Akbari et al., 2006)

Hyperbaric Oxygenation

Topical hyperbaric oxygen therapy (THBO) is the administration of 100% oxygen while the entire patient is enclosed within a chamber at a pressure of 1.4 atmospheres absolute or greater (Kindwall & Whelan, 1999). THBO provides a regulated, pressurized oxygen flow directly to a wound. Supporters of THBO claim that oxygen is essential as it dissolves into tissue fluids, stimulates angiogenesis, and prevents bacterial proliferation. Use of THBO chambers is controversial as it pertains to PU treatment. The quality and rigor of studies have been questioned, making the evidence-base warranting their routine use in PU care equivocal (Kranke et al., 2012).

Electrical Stimulation

Electrical stimulation is defined as the use of an electrical current to transfer energy to a wound. The type of electricity that is transferred is controlled by the electrical source. Electrodes are usually placed over wet conductive medium, in the wound bed and on the skin a distance away from the wound. Most studies of this therapy involve treatment for stage III and IV PUs that have proved unresponsive to conventional therapy. Electrical stimulation may also be useful for recalcitrant stage II ulcers (Baker et al., 1996; Franek et al., 2012; Health Quality Ontario, 2009). A moist wound environment is required for electrical stimulation to function. A rationale for applying electrical stimulation is that it mimics the natural current of injury and will jump-start or accelerate the wound healing process.

It should be noted that the full gamut of alternative therapies are beyond the scope of this chapter. Many other modalities exist in the treatment of chronic wounds such as PUs, including the use of pharmaceuticals, nutraceuticals, skin substitutes, or herbal/botanical therapy. Older adults are increasing their knowledge as consumers of health care, and practitioners should be prepared to address questions of alternative therapies and, if necessary, find appropriate and fact-based information.

Support Surfaces

Support surfaces are defined as what the patient is either sitting on or lying on. For many practicing clinicians, it is an area of great confusion. PUs are caused by a myriad of factors, and the support surfaces our patients choose does matter. A wheelchair bound patient, for instance, on a poor cushion will be at increased risk for PU formation. However, many immobile patients cite poor mattresses or seating cushions as the reason they developed their PU. If this were true, many healthy patients without risk factors would obtain PUs. In short, a poor support surface does not *cause* a PU. Immobile patients, when on a poor support surface, are at increased risk for the development of a PU. This distinction is worthy of further explanation to your patient who enters your health care center claiming the need for a new support surface. Support surfaces alone do not treat patients; we do. It is necessary for the patient to assume accountability in the role of pressure redistribution. If not, he/she is utterly dependent on others or the quality of their support surfaces ability to protect them.

Support surfaces are intended to aid in the redistribution of pressure and prevention of friction, shear, and moisture for patients deemed at risk for PUs. By definition, all support surfaces must meet a clinical need for patients and be medically necessary as durable medical equipment. A prescription is often necessary. Surfaces are either static (high density foams/egg crates) or dynamic (use of pumps delivering air to cushions). The use of pumps to distribute air flow is considered low air-loss therapy.

Low air-loss systems assist in the management of the microclimate (moisture and heat) of the skin and are essentially blowing air on the skin at all times. Many have alternating pressure whereby, if more pressure is exerted over the sacrum, pressure will be released there (redistributed) and released to another location where pressure is not as great a concern. There are many therapies that serve as either overlays (over traditional mattresses), mattress replacement systems, or entire framed bed replacements.

Practitioners are recommended to visit CMS.gov for prescribing information as it pertains to support surfaces for older adults (Center for Medicare and Medicaid Services, n.d.). Most pertinent to clinicians is that support surfaces are just one piece of the puzzle in prevention and treatment of PUs. It is imperative for patients to continue a comprehensive mobility program even when positioned on a specialty support surface.

Role of Nutrition in PU Management

PUs and poor nutrition often coexist. There is a strong correlation between nutrition and PUs (Ayello et al., 1999; Thomas, 1997). A clinician can choose the most expensive dressing modality and design the most intricate prevention strategy possible, but without nutrition you are guaranteed to a cost-ineffective outcome. Primary care clinicians should include the basic biometrics of height and weight with emphasis on recent loss over a given time. Losing weight for the older patients should be regarded as abnormal unless patients are actively working toward that goal (refer to Chapter 10).

Older patients are often at risk for nutritional deficits. Declining functional status, social conditions, or mental conditions all play a role in nutrition. A thorough nutritional history is imperative, particularly with regard to protein and total calorie consumption. Is there a history of digestion problems? Does your older patient have adequate dentition at this stage in their lives? The role of routine laboratory findings is less than specific, although serum albumin levels are commonly thought to be determinants of wound healing potential. As the primary care provider, elicit whether the patient is motivated and capitalize on pertinent positives, rewarding individual strengths while offering empathic support with each identified issue. Dieticians and clinical support nutritionists are of great value and well versed in the prevention of PUs through optimizing nutrition. It is important for professionals to know about the issues and make appropriate referrals. For example, a referral to a local nutritionist should be very specific: "I would like to you meet Mr. Q, a 90-year-old male with a recent development of PUs. He is sitting for most of the day. I have contracted with him to become more mobile. He endorses a 15 lb. weight loss over the past few months. The patient and family are interested in learning better ways to increase his calories and protein." Thus, the care of the PU is multidisciplinary.

Case Vignette No. 2 Part B: Organization of Care. First, goals of care must be agreed upon. The family is vested in helping Mr. Q as they actively want to alleviate pain and suffering for him. Mr. Q is clearly decompensating clinically, and he is confined to a chair for a majority of the day. A compromise must be made with all parties that seek to limit the amount of pressure that he is creating on his ischial tuberosities. Off-loading strategies can be discussed with emphasis on pressure relief. Reinforce that cleaning his wounds is desirable, yet limit his time in the bath tub as wounds of this nature do not want to be oversaturated or waterlogged so as to prevent maceration and damage to newly forming tissue. His nutritional status is also a chief concern. If desired, prompt referral to a nearby nutritionist will be helpful in determining nutritional goals. His wounds are obviously worsening, as evidenced by the pain and active inflammation of the area (redness). Although there is no gross infection, you are concerned that the wounds are dry and necrotic in appearance. Moreover, you know that he is experiencing urinary incontinence and that this excessively moist environment may inhibit healthy skin barrier function. You understand these wounds are most certainly going to be chronic for him if you do not take action. You recommend that in tandem with a pressure relief strategy, a dressing over these areas will encourage removal of the devitalized tissue. Owing to pain, Mr. Q declines conservative sharp debridement, but he is amenable for a dressing. Due to the need for wound hydration, you chose a hydrocolloid dressing that can be cut to fit and placed over these areas. Such a dressing is robust and may withstand moisture from the top down (from incontinence), and you recommend a toileting regimen and pull-up briefs that wick moisture away from the skin. You instruct the family on how to cut the dressing and place directly over the dry ulcerations. Make it clear that the wound will become moister and often this scares patients at home as the healthy tissue emerges from the nonviable wound bed. Instruct them on clinical signs and symptoms of systemic and local infection, making them aware of more atypical presentations of infection in the aged. You will discuss with your administrative assistant where Mr. Q can obtain his supplies and agree to sign for Medicare paperwork that will be necessary for his dressings. Arrange for follow-up in a mutually agreed upon time (approximately 2 weeks) to determine progress. At that time, you will evaluate the clinical response to your recommendations and determine whether a specialty mattress may be a necessary component of his wound care prevention plan.

CONCLUSION

The older adult poses many challenges for the primary care provider. Comorbidities and normal variants of aging skin make the older adult a vulnerable population with regard to PU risk. When your patient enters the health care setting for the first time, he or she is but a puzzle, with many scattered pieces in random order. This chapter sought to align the pieces of that puzzle with regard to PU management for the geriatric patient. Pressure redistribution, dressings, support surfaces, and adjunct therapies are big pieces, but not all, in the puzzle of PU prevention and treatment. With expert assessment and interventions based on identification of risk factors, clinicians are in an optimal position to help the older adult. Older adults want to be at home. Clinicians play a pivotal role in managing comorbidities and demonstrating an understanding of basic wound principles. A holistic plan of care is primary, the most important treatment strategy being prevention.

REFERENCES

Atiyeh, B. S., Dibo, S. A., & Hayek, S. N. (2009). Wound cleansing, topical antiseptics and wound healing. *International Wound Journal, 6*(6), 420–430.

Ayello, E. A., Thomas, D. R., & Litchford, M. A. (1999). Nutritional aspects of wound healing. *Home Healthcare Nurse, 17*(11), 719–729.

Backer, L. A. (2009). Building the case for the patient-centered medical home. *Family Practice Management, 16*(1), 14–18.

Baba-Akbari Sari, A., Flemming, K., Cullum, N. A., & Wollina, U. (2006). Therapeutic ultrasound for pressure ulcers. *Cochrane Database of Systematic Reviews,* (3), 001275.

Baker, L. L., Rubayi, S., Villar, F., & Demuth, S. K. (1996). Effect of electrical stimulation wave form on healing of ulcers in human beings with spinal cord injury. *Wound Repair and Regeneration, 4*(1), 21–28.

Bales, I., & Duvendack, T. (2011). Reaching for the moon: Achieving zero pressure ulcer prevalence, an update. *Journal of Wound Care, 20*(8), 374.

Barber, L. A. (2002). Clean technique or sterile technique? Let's take a moment to think. *Journal of Wound, Ostomy, and Continence Nursing, 29*(1), 29–32.

Barrois, B., Labalette, C., Rousseau, P., Corbin, A., Colin, D., Allaert, F., & Saumet, J. L. (2008). A national prevalence study of pressure ulcers in French hospital inpatients. *Journal of Wound Care, 17*(9), 373–376.

Bergstrom, N. (2005). The Braden scale for predicting pressure sore risk: Reflections on the perioperative period. *Journal of Wound, Ostomy, and Continence Nursing, 32*(2), 79–80.

Berlowitz, D. R., Brandeis, G. H., Anderson, J. J., Ash, A. S., Kader, B., Morris, J. N., & Moskowitz, M. A. (2001). Evaluation of a risk-adjustment model for pressure ulcer development using the minimum data set. *Journal of the American Geriatrics Society, 49*(7), 872–876.

Berlowitz, D. R., & Brienza, D. M. (2007). Are all pressure ulcers the result of deep tissue injury? A review of the literature. *Ostomy Wound Management, 53*(10), 34–38.

Black, J., Baharestani, M., Cuddigan, J., Dorner, B., Edsberg, L., Langemo, D., . . . National Pressure Ulcer Advisory Panel. (2007). National Pressure Ulcer Advisory Panel's updated pressure ulcer staging system. *Dermatology Nursing, 19*(4), 343–349.

Black, J. M., Edsberg, L. E., Baharestani, M. M., Langemo, D., Goldberg, M., McNichol, L., . . . National Pressure Ulcer Advisory Panel. (2011). Pressure ulcers: Avoidable or unavoidable? Results of the National Pressure Ulcer Advisory Panel consensus conference. *Ostomy Wound Management, 57*(2), 24–37.

Cakmak, S. K., Gul, U., Ozer, S., Yigit, Z., & Gonu, M. (2009). Risk factors for pressure ulcers. *Advances in Skin & Wound Care, 22*(9), 412–415.

Center for Medicare and Medicaid Services. (n.d.). Medicare policy regarding pressure reducing support surfaces. Retrieved from http://www.cms.gov/Outreach-and-Education/Medicare-Learning-Network-MLN/MLNMatters Articles/downloads/SE1014.pdf

Cheung, C. (2010). Older adults and ulcers: Chronic wounds in the geriatric population. *Advances in Skin & Wound Care, 23*(1), 39–44.

Darkovich, S. L., Brown-Etris, M., & Spencer, M. (1990). Bio-film hydrogel dressing: A clinical evaluation in the treatment of pressure sores. *Ostomy Wound Management, 29*, 47–60.

de Laat, E. H., van den Boogaard, M. H., Spauwen, P. H., van Kuppevelt, D. H., van Goor, H., & Schoonhoven, L. (2011). Faster wound healing with topical negative pressure therapy in difficult-to-heal wounds: A prospective randomized controlled trial. *Annals of Plastic Surgery, 67*(6), 626–631.

Dow, G. (2001). Infection in chronic wounds. In D. Krasner, G. T. Rodeheaver, & R. G. Sibbald (Eds.), *Chronic wound care: A clinical source book for healthcare professionals* (3rd ed., p. 344). Wayne, PA: HMP Communications.

Fernandez, R., & Griffiths, R. (2012). Water for wound cleansing. *Cochrane Database of Systematic Reviews*, (2), CD003861.

Franek, A., Kostur, R., Polak, A., Taradaj, J., Szlachta, Z., Blaszczak, E., . . . Kucio, C. (2012). Using high-voltage electrical stimulation in the treatment of recalcitrant pressure ulcers: Results of a randomized, controlled clinical study. *Ostomy Wound Management, 58*(3), 30–44.

Graumlich, J. F., Blough, L. S., McLoughlin, R. G., Milbrandt, C. J., Calderone, C. L., Agha, S. A., & Shiebel, L. W. (2003). Healing pressure ulcers with collagen or hydrocolloid: A randomized, controlled trial. *Journal of the American Geriatrics Society, 51*(2), 147–154.

Gupta, S., & Ichioka, S. (2012). Optimal use of negative pressure wound therapy in treating pressure ulcers. *International Wound Journal, 9*(Suppl. 1), 8–16.

Hashizume, H. (2004). Skin aging and dry skin. *Journal of Dermatology, 31*(8), 603–609.

Health Quality Ontario. (2009). Management of chronic pressure ulcers: An evidence-based analysis. *Ontario Health Technology Assessment Series, 9*(3), 1–203.

Jacob, S. W., Francone, C. A., & Lossow, W. J. (1982). *Structure and function in man* (5th ed.). Philadelphia, PA: W.B. Saunders.

Jafferany, M., Huynh, T. V., Silverman, M. A., & Zaidi, Z. (2012). Geriatric dermatoses: A clinical review of skin diseases in an aging population. *International Journal of Dermatology, 51*(5), 509–522.

Kindwall, E. P., & Whelan, H. T. (1999). *Hyperbaric medicine practice* (2nd ed.). Flagstaff, AZ: Best Publishing.

Kranke, P., Bennett, M. H., Martyn-St James, M., Schnabel, A., & Debus, S. E. (2012). Hyperbaric oxygen therapy for chronic wounds. *Cochrane Database of Systematic Reviews*, (4), CD004123.

Lay-Flurrie, K. (2004). The properties of hydrogel dressings and their impact on wound healing. *Professional Nurse, 19*(5), 269-273.

Lazarus, G. S., Cooper, D. M., Knighton, D. R., Margolis, D. J., Pecoraro, R. E., Rodeheaver, G., & Robson, M. C. (1994). Definitions and guidelines for assessment of wounds and evaluation of healing. *Archives of Dermatology, 130*(4), 489–493.

Lyder, C. H. (2003). Pressure ulcer prevention and management. *JAMA, 289*(2), 223–226.

Maklebust, J., Sieggreen, M. Y., Sidor, D., Gerlach, M. A., Bauer, C., & Anderson, C. (2005). Computer-based testing of the Braden scale for predicting pressure sore risk. *Ostomy Wound Management, 51*(4), 40–42.

Margolis, D. J., Knauss, J., Bilker, W., & Baumgarten, M. (2003). Medical conditions as risk factors for pressure ulcers in an outpatient setting. *Age and Ageing, 32*(3), 259–264.

Mian, E., Mian, M., & Beghe, F. (1991). Lyophilized type-I collagen and chronic leg ulcers. *International Journal of Tissue Reactions, 13*(5), 257–269.

Moore, Z., & Cowman, S. (2008). A systematic review of wound cleansing for pressure ulcers. *Journal of Clinical Nursing, 17*(15), 1963–1972.

Moore, Z. E., & Cowman, S. (2005). Wound cleansing for pressure ulcers. *Cochrane Database of Systematic Reviews*, (4), CD004983.

National Institute for Health and Clinical Excellence. (2005). *Pressure ulcers: The management of pressure ulcers in primary and secondary care* (No. CG29). London, England: Author.

National Pressure Ulcer Advisory Panel. (2007). Pressure ulcer stages revised by the National Pressure Ulcer Advisory Panel. *Ostomy Wound Management, 53*(3), 30–31.

Norton, D., McLaren, R., & Exton-Smith, A. N. (1962). *An investigation of geriatric nursing problems in the hospital.* London, UK: National Corporation for the Care of Old People.

O'Meara, S. M., Cullum, N. A., Majid, M., & Sheldon, T. A. (2001). Systematic review of antimicrobial agents used for chronic wounds. *British Journal of Surgery, 88*(1), 4–21.

Rodeheaver, G. T. (2001). Wound cleansing, wound irrigation, wound disinfection. In D. Krasner, G. T. Rodeheaver, & R. G. Sibbald (Eds.), *Chronic wound care: A clinical source book for healthcare professionals* (3rd ed., p. 375). Wayne, PA: HMP Communications.

Sherman, R. A. (2002). Maggot conservative debridement therapy for the treatment of pressure ulcers. *Wound Repair and Regeneration, 10*(4), 208–214.

Stotts, N. A., Rodeheaver, G. T., Thomas, D. R., Frantz, R. A., Bartolucci, A. A., Sussman, C., . . . Maklebust, J. (2001). An instrument to measure healing in pressure ulcers: Development and validation of the pressure ulcer scale for healing (PUSH). *Journals of Gerontology Series A: Biological Sciences & Medical Sciences, 56*(12), M795–M799.

Swezey, L. (2010). Transparent film dressings. Retrieved from http://www.woundeducators.com/transparent-film-dressings/

Thomas, D. R. (1997). The role of nutrition in prevention and healing of pressure ulcers. *Clinics in Geriatric Medicine*, *13*(3), 497–511.

United States Census Bureau. (2013). Retrieved from http://www.census.gov/population/projections/

Visiongain. (2012). Advanced wound care: World market prospects 2013-2023. Retrieved from http://www.visiongain.com/Report/940/Advanced-Wound-Care-World-Market-Prospects-2013-2023

Whitney, J., Phillips, L., Aslam, R., Barbul, A., Gottrup, F., Gould, L., . . . Stotts, N. (2006). Guidelines for the treatment of pressure ulcers. *Wound Repair and Regeneration*, *14*(6), 663–679.

Wound, Ostomy, and Continence Nursing Society. (2009). *Avoidable versus unavoidable pressure ulcers: Position paper*. Retrieved from http://c.ymcdn.com/sites/www.wocn.org/resource/resmgr/docs/wocn-avoidable-unavoidable_p.pdf

Wound, Ostomy, and Continence Nurses Society. (2010). *Guidelines for prevention and managment of pressure ulcers*. Mount Laurel, NJ: Author.

CHAPTER 17: IT RESOURCES

Websites

National Pressure Ulcer Advisory Panel
  http://www.npuap.org/
Institute of Healthcare Improvement
  http://www.ihi.org/Pages/default.aspx
Mayo Clinic - Pressure Ulcers (Risk Factors)
  http://www.mayoclinic.com/health/bedsores/DS00570/DSECTION=risk-factors
Nursing Standard of Practice Protocol: Pressure Ulcer Prevention & Skin Tear Prevention
  http://consultgerirn.org/topics/pressure_ulcers_and_skin_tears/want_to_know_more
Preventive Skin Care for Older Adults
  http://www.medscape.com/viewarticle/531999
Older Adults' Knowledge of Pressure Ulcer Prevention: A Prospective Quasi-Experimental Study
  http://onlinelibrary.wiley.com/doi/10.1111/j.1748-3743.2011.00274.x/abstract
Pressure Ulcers, Causes, Diagnosis & Treatment – Clinical Key
  https://www.clinicalkey.com/topics/infectious-disease/pressure-ulcer.html
Pressure Ulcers – Support for Caregivers of Older Adults
  http://www.caregivercollege.org/scoa/?PressureSores.html
Pressure Ulcers
  http://www.cigna.com/individualandfamilies/health-and-well-being/hw/medical-topics/pressure-sores-tp17772.html
Repositioning Older People Every Three Hours Reduces Pressure Ulcers
  http://www.nursingtimes.net/nursing-practice/clinical-zones/older-people/repositioning-older-people-every-three-hours-reduces-pressure-ulcers/5031888.article
Pressure Ulcers: Decreasing the Risk for Older Adults
  http://www.gnjournal.com/article/S0197-4572(97)90356-6/abstract
Chronic Wound Care
  http://www.drugs.com/cg/chronic-wound-care.html
Wound Management
  http://www.health-first.org/hospitals_services/wound_faqs.cfm
Treating Chronic Wounds
  http://www.pennmedicine.org/woundcare/treatment.html
Chronic Wounds
  http://208.11.4.69/chronic.html

Wound Watch: Assessing Pressure Ulcers
   http://www.nursingcenter.com/lnc/static?pageid=844487
Pressure Ulcer Risk Assessment and Prevention: A Comparative Effectiveness Review
   http://effectivehealthcare.ahrq.gov/index.cfm/search-for-guides-reviews-and-reports/?page
   action=displayproduct&productid=926
Pressure Ulcer Scale for Healing (PUSH) Tool
   http://www.npuap.org/resources/educational-and-clinical-resources/push-tool/
Wound Dressings
   http://www.ncbi.nlm.nih.gov/pmc/articles/PMC1420733/
Nutrition and Pressure Ulcer Healing
   http://www.medscape.com/viewarticle/780833
Nutrition and Pressure Ulcers
   http://www.livestrong.com/article/301651-nutrition-pressure-ulcers/

Pdf Documents

Pressure Ulcers in Older Adults - ELDER CARE: A Resource for Interprofessional Providers
   http://www.reynolds.med.arizona.edu/EduProducts/providerSheets/Pressure%20
   Ulcers.pdf
A New Model to Identify Shared Risk Factors for Pressure Ulcers and Frailty in Older Adults
   http://www.rehabnurse.org/pdf/rnj311.pdf
The Role of Nutrition in Pressure Ulcer Prevention and Treatment: National Pressure Ulcer
   Advisory Panel White Paper
   http://www.npuap.org/wp-content/uploads/2012/03/Nutrition-White-Paper-Website-
   Version.pdf
Chronic Wound Care Guidelines
   http://www.woundheal.org/assets/documents/final%20pocket%20guide%20treatment.pdf
Assessment and Documentation of Pressure Ulcers
   http://www.healthinsight.org/Internal/events/Nursing_Home/Assessment_and_
   Documentation_Pressure_Ulcers%20_0110719_Color.pdf
Braden Scale for Predicting Pressure Ulcer Risk
   http://effectivehealthcare.ahrq.gov/index.cfm/search-for-guides-reviews-and-reports/?page
   action=displayproduct&productid=926
Using the PUSH Tool for Wound Assessment
   http://www.cfmc.org/files/nh/pushtool_frantz092603-rev.pdf
The Role of Nutrition in Pressure Ulcer Prevention and Treatment: National Pressure Ulcer
   Advisory Panel White Paper
   http://www.npuap.org/wp-content/uploads/2012/03/Nutrition-White-Paper-Website-
   Version.pdf

Videos

Pressure Ulcer Prevention – What Caring People Need to Know!
With a heightened focus on prevention, hospital and nursing home educators can use this new,
   19-minute training video for CNAs, nurses & family members to explain the causes and
   prevention of pressure ulcers.
   http://www.familyhealthmedia.com/ (19 minutes)

Gauze Wound Dressings (2010)

Some of the areas covered in the video: sterile gauze, ActCel hemostatic gauze, surgical gauze, fibers from gauze left in wound, removing gauze from healed wound, bandages, xeroform, tubular, mep, rolls, vaseline, pads, iodoform, quick clot combat, nu, invacare non adherent sterile gauze.

http://youtu.be/mon9-LXlh0A (5 minutes)

WoundEducators.com Videos

http://www.woundeducators.com/resources/videos/

Wound Care: Pressure Ulcers (2011)

http://youtu.be/jIztPN1X5Wg (8:30 minutes)

Pressure Ulcer Education (2011)

How to Identify and Prevent a Pressure Ulcer

http://youtu.be/QCW2R4vnzXc (6:30 minutes)

MDS 3.0 Wound Staging – Understand Wound Care

http://youtu.be/scRFI-g87Cs (8:30 minutes)

Understand Wound Care: Pressure Ulcers (2011)

http://youtu.be/jzu3PSRfY1w (3:15 minutes)

Images

Google images for Pressure Ulcers and Older Adults

http://www.google.com/search?q=pressure+ulcers+and+older+adults&source=lnms&tbm=isch&sa=X&ei=KJugUbv8MbCO0QHgqIDoDg&ved=0CAcQ_AUoATgK&biw=1011&bih=214

Mayo Clinic images for Pressure Ulcers

http://www.mayoclinic.com/health/bedsores/DS00570/TAB=multimedia

Image for PUSH Tool

http://www.google.com/search?q=push+tool&tbm=isch&tbo=u&source=univ&sa=X&ei=-EKhUYqpGvGn4AOL_YGoCA&sqi=2&ved=0CE0QsAQ&biw=1011&bih=214#facrc=_&imgrc=dEksbpvXDDnOyM%3A%3BMdz9ToorSYkOMM%3Bhttp%253A%252F%252Fwww.podiatricultrasound.com%252FPUSH%252520TOOL%252520Printed.jpg%3Bhttp%253A%252F%252Fwww.podiatricultrasound.com%252Fpush%252520tool%2525203.htm%3B664%3B800

Medication Safety

Eunyoung Lee, RN, ANP, ACNP, FNP, PhD, FAHA

INTRODUCTION

Medication safety in older adults is a priority when addressing health promotion, disease prevention, and clinical practice guidelines. Older adults commonly have three to four chronic diseases such as hypertension, diabetes, dyslipidemia, and chronic pain, requiring multiple drugs to treat them. Two national surveys have shown that 29% to 40% of adults aged 65 or older are taking five or more medications, and 40% of nursing home patients are taking nine or more medications. This is commonly known as polypharmacy. Additionally, adding new medication to treat symptoms caused by medications may lead to a prescribing cascade. The cognitive, physiological, and functional changes in older adults, combined with polypharmacy and the prescribing cascade among providers, can easily induce adverse drug effects which can lead to life-threatening incidents. Medication errors are now the sixth leading cause of death in the United States. Although older adults may be more susceptible to adverse drug effects, studies have shown that up to 88% of adverse drug events are related to medication errors and may be prevented.

This chapter aims to identify the major factors contributing to medication errors, and to increase awareness of drugs and their side effects in order to prevent drug errors in older adults. Useful tools will be provided to assist providers in the prevention of medication errors and to promote patient safety.

The Institute of Medicine (IOM)'s 1999 report, *To Err Is Human: Building a Safer Health System*, brought attention to the need for medication safety. As many as 98,000 patients in the United States had died of preventable medical errors such as adverse effects of medication, falls, injuries, burns, improper blood transfusions, wrong-site surgeries, pressure ulcers, resulting in a cost of $29 billion per year (IOM, 1999). According to the 2009 death/mortality data from the Centers for Disease Control and Prevention (CDC, 2011), preventable medical errors now rank as the

TABLE 18.1 · Leading Causes of Death

1. Heart disease: 599,413
2. Cancer: 567,628
3. Chronic lower respiratory diseases: 137,353
4. Stroke (cerebrovascular diseases): 128,842
5. Accidents (unintentional injuries): 118,021

Preventable Medical Errors: 98,000
6. Alzheimer disease: 79,003
7. Diabetes: 68,705
8. Influenza and pneumonia: 53,692
9. Nephritis, nephrotic syndrome, and nephrosis: 48,935
10. Intentional self-harm (suicide): 36,909

From Centers for Disease Control and Prevention. (2011). Deaths/mortality in the United States, 2009, National Center for Health Care Statistics at the Centers for Disease Control and Prevention. Retrieved from http://www.cdc .gov/nchs/data/nvsr/nvsr61/nvsr61_07.pdf. Kutner, M., Greenberg, E., Jin,Y., and Paulsen, C. (2006). HYPERLINK "http://nces.ed.gov/pubsearch/pubsinfo.asp?pubid=2006483" The Health Literacy of America's Adults: Results From the 2003 National Assessment of Adult Literacy (NCES 2006-483). U.S.Department of Education. Washington, DC: National Center for Education Statistics.

sixth leading cause of death in the United States, killing more Americans than pneumonia, breast cancer, traffic-related accidents, and HIV/AIDS (see Table 18.1).

Medication errors account for 5% to 10% of medical-related deaths (Kaiser Family Foundation, 2008). Adverse drug events are responsible for approximately 7,000 hospital deaths and 95,000 hospital admission each year in the United States (Weisbart, 2006), resulting in an annual cost of $3.5 billion (CDC, 2006). However, according to a report from the Agency for Healthcare Research and Quality (AHRQ) in 2001, approximately 28% to 95% of adverse drug effects are preventable. Similarly, several studies have estimated that approximately 50% to 88% of adverse drug events that occurred in older adults could have been prevented (Beijer & de Blaey, 2002; Gurwitz et al., 2005, 2008; *USA Today*, 2010). A recent meta-analysis (Hakkarainen et al., 2012) of 16 original studies in outpatients and 8 original studies in inpatients showed that 50% to 71% of adverse drug effects in outpatients and 45% of adverse drug effects in inpatients were preventable.

The 2007 IOM report, *Preventing Medication Errors,* estimated that 1.5 million preventable adverse drug events occur each year in the United States. In addition, the report stressed that adverse drug effects occur most often in the older adult population: between 380,000 and 450,000 adverse drug events occurring in long-term care facilities or nursing homes were preventable. Similarly, in a study of outpatient Medicare beneficiaries, Gurwitz and his colleagues (2003) reported that 530,000 preventable adverse drug events occur each year, indicating that more than one third of medication errors occur in the Medicare population (age 65 or older) in outpatient settings. The cost of treating preventable adverse drug events in those Medicare enrollees has reached more than $887 million per year (Field et al., 2005). A 2007 research report of the New England Healthcare Institute (NEHI) estimated that $2.4 trillion was spent on health care in the United States, of which one third could be saved without minimizing the quality of care if medication overuse and misuse as well as practice variation across the country were to improve (NEHI, 2009).

Older adults are the fastest growing segment of the population worldwide as well as in the United States. In 2009, approximately 39.6 million Americans were 65 years or older, representing 12.9% of the population of the United States. This number is expected to increase up to 72.1 million (19% of the population) by 2030 (Administration on Aging [AOA], 2013). These demographic realities of a national and global aging population indicate that with advancing chronic illnesses, more medications may be required particularly for hypertension, diabetes, and hyperlipidemia. Currently, 29% to 40% of older adults take 5 or more, and 17% to 19% take 10 or more, prescribed medications (Dwyer et al., 2010; Slone Epidemiology Center at Boston University, n.d.-b). This high prevalence of chronic disease, polypharmacy, and possible decreased cognitive function may double or triple the risk of medication misuse, overuse, or underuse. Indeed, seniors, along with children, are reported to be the most susceptible groups for adverse drug effects and medication errors (Budnitz et al., 2011; CDC, 2010; Slone Epidemiology Center at Boston University, n.d.-b).

Current trends in medicine encourage the early discharge of patients from the hospital once their acute problem is resolved in order to minimize hospital-acquired infections and to maximize an early return of physical and social functioning to pre-hospitalization level. However, an improper early discharge, inappropriate transitional care, and/or lack of self-management skills in patients with chronic disease can cause unanticipated readmission. In particular, older adults with low health literacy have a higher risk of improper medication use and missed follow-up visits, leading to the worsening of health outcomes. Thus, current health care processes stress the importance of a "client-focused care delivery system," empowering patients to manage their chronic disease, which has been shown to improve the quality and safety of patient health care and to reduce health care costs (National Network of Libraries of Medicine [NNLM], 2011).

CONTRIBUTING FACTORS TO MEDICATIONS SAFETY

Patient-Related Factors

Physiological, Cognitive, and Functional Changes

With aging, a decrease in physiological functions affects drug absorption, distribution, metabolism, and excretion, causing potentially excessive drug levels in the body that lead to adverse drug effects. A number of major physiological changes with aging may affect pharmacokinetics: decreased gastrointestinal motility, causing a decrease in drug absorption, decreased serum albumin and body fluids with increased body fat, causing an increase in drug distribution, decreased liver function, causing a decrease in drug metabolism, and decreased kidney function and glomerular filtration rate (GFR), causing a decrease in drug excretion. Additionally, there are fewer drug receptor sites, which decrease the response to drugs, and the above pharmacokinetic changes increase the adverse effects of the drugs (Buchholz, 2012). These changes place the older population at a two to three times higher risk of adverse drug reactions than other populations (Johnston, 2001).

Accompanying the physiological changes stated above, sensory changes such as poor hearing and low vision can also affect older adults' ability to understand and follow medication/medical device instructions. Further, a decrease in cognitive level such as memory loss, easy forgetfulness, or a decreased level of comprehension can make it harder to follow the instructions for taking medication. These physiological changes may also limit the functional level of older adults and impair their walking, performance of the activities of daily living (ADL), as well as their access to a pharmacy.

Health Literacy

Health literacy does not simply refer to reading ability. The U.S. Department of Health & Human Services [HHS] has defined health literacy as "the degree to which individuals have the capacity to obtain, process, and understand basic health information and services needed to make appropriate health decisions, as defined in Healthy People 2020" (Berkman et al., 2011, p. 13). For a patient to make decisions in the health care system, a complex group of skills is required to interpret documents, read and write prose (i.e., print literacy), use quantitative information (i.e., numeracy), and listen and speak effectively (i.e., oral literacy) (Berkman et al., 2011). These skills, required to understand and use health information, are directly related to choosing a healthy lifestyle, knowing how to seek and access medical care, taking advantage of preventive measures, making informed decisions, complying with therapeutic care plans such as medication adherence and follow-up appointments, and ultimately maintaining better individual/family health care outcomes.

In the 2004 report *Health Literacy: A Prescription to End Confusion,* the IOM highlighted the severity of health literacy issues in the US population. On the basis of a 2003 National Assessment of Adult Literacy, about 88% of the population in the United States was shown to have no proficiency in understanding and using health information to manage or improve their own health (IOM, 2004; Kirsch et.al., 1993; National Center for Education Statistics [NCES], 2006; NNLM, 2011; Parker & Kindig, 2006). Specifically, 36% of the population as well as 59% of adults aged 65 or older have below basic or marginal health literacy skills, indicating that they could not read or understand even basic materials such as prescription labels or could not fill out standard forms (NCES, 2006; see Fig. 18.1). These 2003 National Data on Health Literacy results (see resources on health literacy) indicate that health literacy in the United States had not improved much in the decade following a 1995 study (Williams et al., 1995), where two thirds (60%) of adults aged 60 and over in the United States had functionally inadequate or marginal health literacy skills.

The 2004 and 2011 *Literacy and Health Outcomes* reports from the AHRQ indicated that low health literacy is linked not only to higher use of hospitalization and expensive emergency services (Baker et al., 1998, 2002) but also to lower use of preventive care such as mammography, pap smear, or flu shot and a higher risk of taking medicines incorrectly (AHRQ, 2011; Bennet et al., 1998; Berkman et al., 2011; Scott et al., 2002). Relationships between health literacy and health outcomes have been demonstrated more clearly in patients with chronic diseases such as cancer, diabetes, asthma, and hypertension (Berkman et al., 2011). Low literacy has been shown to be strongly correlated with the improper use of a metered-dose inhaler (MDI) and frequent visits to the emergency department with an acute asthma attack (Williams et al., 1998). In patients with type 2 diabetes, inadequate health literacy has been shown to be an independent predictor

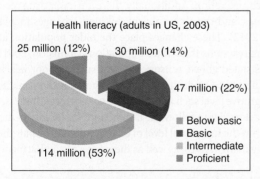
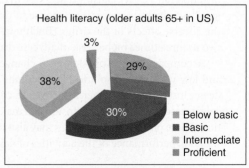

FIGURE 18.1. Health literacy statistics. (Data from National Center for Education Statistics. [2006]. *The health literacy of America's adults: Results from the 2003 National Assessment of Adult Literacy.* Washington, DC: U.S. Department of Education. Retrieved from http://nces.ed.gov/pubs2006/2006483.pdf)

of worse glycemic control and higher rates of retinopathy (Schillinger et al., 2002, 2003). Furthermore, in a study of Medicare patients aged 65 or over (Baker et al., 2007; Barclay, 2007), the unadjusted all-cause mortality rate among participants was strongly correlated with participants' literacy level: inadequate (39.4%), marginal (28.7%), and adequate health literacy (18.9%). Along with minorities (especially Hispanic and African Americans), low-income people, and people with chronic mental and/or physical health conditions, older adults are designated as a vulnerable population for low health literacy (National Patient Safety Foundation [NPSF], 2011). Low health literacy was consistently found to be an important mediator of health outcomes in those vulnerable populations, leading to worse health outcomes such as poor hemoglobin A1C control, or asthma symptom control (Baker et al., 1998, 2002; Berkman et al., 2011; NCES, 2006; NNLM, 2011; NPSF, 2011; Williams et al., 1998).

The IOM, in its 2004 *Health Literacy* report, highlighted the importance of health literacy, stating that the effort to improve quality and reduce costs and disparities cannot succeed without simultaneous improvement in health literacy. Low health literacy is one of the major risk factors for poor medication adherence. Therefore, in the aging population, the level of health literacy should be included as part of the patient assessment during each physician office visit to help patients and their families to understand and follow basic plans of care as well as medication administration instructions.

Poor Medication Adherence

According to the World Health Organization (NEHI, 2009), poor adherence is defined as any deviation from the prescribed course of medical treatment. Its related activities include (a) taking medicine at the wrong time, (b) taking incorrect doses, (c) not taking medicine at the proper time interval between doses, (d) stopping medicine when symptoms abate without following the physician's instruction, and (e) not refilling prescriptions on time.

One study has shown that one third to one half of Americans do not take their medications as prescribed (Osterberg & Blaschke, 2005). Poor medication adherence is a major contributor to poor patient safety as well as poor health outcomes in older adults, causing preventable loss of life, unnecessary hospitalization, or advancing disease. For example, in a study of patients with hypertension, patients taking antihypertensive medication with a medication adherence rate of less than 80% have a fourfold increased risk of cardiac events (Psaty et.al.,). In addition, health care costs related to nonadherence increases $100 billion each year in extra hospitalizations alone (NEHI, 2009).

Several investigations have identified some major contributors to poor patient medication adherence:

- Age itself is not a major risk factor for low medication adherence (Ho et al., 2006). Rather, low adherence is often found in patients under age 65 and with fewer comorbidities.
- The higher the number of prescribed medications, the higher the rates of adverse drug effects and nonadherence (Field et al., 2001).
- The frequency of doses (more than the twice-a-day dose schedule) and low health literacy were found to be significant contributors to poor patient outcomes (Odegard & Gray, 2008).
  - In a study of diabetes patients, Odegard and Gray (2008) observed that patients taking diabetes medication more than twice daily and/or having trouble reading the diabetes medication prescription label were significantly more likely to have a poorly controlled A1C level (defined as an A1C of >9.0%).

- Adherence rates when taking prescribed medications are lower in patients with chronic conditions than patients with acute conditions (Benner et al., 2002; Jackevicius et al., 2002; Kocurek, 2009). Adherence seems to be more challenging in patients with chronic diseases such as diabetes, asthma, and heart disease when the patient is asymptomatic, and the disease requires lifelong medication.
- In patients with chronic disease, the adherence rate drops from 80% at the initial phase of medication to 25% to 56% after 6 months to 20% after 5 years (Benner et al., 2002; Jackevicius et al., 2002; Kocurek, 2009).
  - One out of four patients with coronary artery disease was reported to have stopped taking medicine within 6 months (Jackevicius et al., 2002).
  - In a long-term study measuring the adherence rate of patients receiving statin drugs, adherence was shown to be nearly 80% within the first 3 months of treatment, but adherence dropped to 56% within 6 months, and 20% after 5 years (Benner et al., 2002).
  - In an online survey, one in five patients with diabetes reported they often skipped their medication (Kocurek, 2009).

In summary, major contributors to poor patient medication adherence include number of medications, frequency of doses, and presence of chronic disease; however, side effects or concerns about potential side effects, financial constraints, forgetfulness of refills and doses, disabilities, lack of belief that the medication will help, and cultural or religious beliefs were also identified as patient-related factors in poor patient adherence (Burley, 2007; Matz, 2011). Insufficient teaching time by the health provider, as well as lack of collaboration/communication with other providers, has been identified as provider-related factors resulting in poor patient adherence. Other factors include lack of transportation and family members' busy schedules (Burley, 2007).

Over-the-Counter Drugs

Studies have shown that about half of prescription drug users take at least one over-the-counter (OTC) medication and that older adults take an average of two to four nonprescription drugs daily (Johnston, 2001). OTC drugs have an advantage over prescription drugs in that they are cheaper and easier to access; improper use of over-the-counter drugs, however, can delay the adequate diagnosis of disease and its timely treatment. Inappropriate uses of OTC drugs or herbal/dietary supplements may cause the same major adverse effects as prescribed drugs, especially when a patient uses them for a long period. Patients often use a previously prescribed medication or a medication prescribed for another family member to treat similar symptoms without accurate diagnosis or proper consultation with a physician. The misuse of medication can lead to adverse drug effects and/or drug–drug or drug–herb interaction among prescribed drugs and OTC drugs, herbs, or dietary supplements.

Commonly used OTC drugs among older adults include laxatives, NSAIDS, antihistamines, sedatives, and H_2 blockers (often used for acid reflux treatment). It has been shown that about one third to one half of older adults use laxatives even though they do not have constipation (Johnston, 2001). Long-term use or inappropriate use of NSAIDS can cause severe gastrointestinal bleeding, and inappropriate use of sedating antihistamines, sedatives, and H_2 blockers can make elders excessively sedated and/or confused. OTC drugs in older adults should be used cautiously with the proper diagnosis of the problem, and inappropriate long-term use of OTC drugs should be avoided.

In addition to OTC drugs, the use of herbal or dietary supplements by older adults has increased in recent years, from 14% in 1998 (Kaufman et al., 2002) to 49% in 2006 (Qato et al., 2008). One study reported that three out of four patients took at least one prescription drug and one herbal or dietary supplement (Nahin et al., 2009). Eight commonly available and widely used herbs include St. John's wort, ginkgo biloba, echinacea, ginseng, garlic, saw palmetto, kava, and valerian root. Herbal or dietary supplements have been reported to be somewhat effective in controlling a particular symptom and thus help to reduce the number or doses of prescribed drugs (National Center for Complementary and Alternative Medicine [NCCAM], n.d.). For example, some studies have shown that Asian ginseng decreases blood glucose and improves immune function, and St. John's wort improves minor to moderate depression, anxiety, and/or sleep disturbance. However, users of herbal products should understand that just because a product is labeled "natural" it does not always mean it is safer. In fact, the many components of herbs may be unknown and are more complex than prescribed medicines (Adams et al., 2011). Further, drug–herb interactions have been found in quite a few herbs (Adams et al., 2011; Fugh-Berman, 2000; Wold et al., 2005), as described later in this chapter (see Table 18.4, in the "Drug–Herb Interactions" Section).

Despite the risk of serious adverse reactions to supplements, clinicians often neglect to ask patients about the use of herbs or dietary supplements; patients also do not voluntarily report the use of these non-prescribed supplements. Physicians should routinely elicit complete medication lists, including OTC drugs, dietary supplements, and herbs at each office visit. It is also recommended that patients consult with a physician prior to using a supplement or herb and that they start with a small dose, especially for those with chronic diseases.

Medication-Related Factors

Adverse Drug Reactions

Changes in physiological function such as a decrease in metabolism and clearance may make an older patient more susceptible to adverse drug reactions. In the older adult, the capacity to maintain homeostasis in response to physiological changes decreases, and even a small change in drug dosage may cause adverse side effects and can cause life-threatening events. For example, decreased function of the autonomic nervous system, venous return system, baroreceptor sensitivity, or heart contractility in an older patient often causes orthostatic hypotension. In an average individual, the maintenance of blood pressure with positional change occurs as a result of the combined mechanism of muscle contraction in the legs, with a one-way valve counteracting gravity in the venous system, and the autonomic nervous system causing increased heart rate, vascular contraction, and peripheral resistance (Bradley & Davis, 2003). Thus, even a small increase in the dose of antihypertensive drugs in older adults can intensify the vascular dilatation effect, leading to orthostatic hypotension and even life-threatening syncope.

Beijer and de Blaey's (2002) study showed that older adults are four times more likely to be hospitalized for adverse drug effects than younger adults. More specifically, according to the adverse-event data from the National Electronic Injury Surveillance System-Cooperative Adverse Drug Event Surveillance Project (2007 through 2009), nearly two thirds (65%) of hospitalizations for adverse drug events in older adults aged 65 or above were due to unintentional overdoses (Budnitz et al., 2011).

High-Alert Medication

The Institute for Safe Medication Practices (ISMP, 2011a and 2012) has identified medications that cause serious harm to patients when used in error and named them as high-alert medications (see Table 18.2). The 2012 ISMP's most current high-alert medication list includes 25

TABLE 18.2 • ISMP's High-Alert Medication Lists

Classes of Medication	Specific Medications
■ Adrenergic agonist, IV (e.g., EPINEPHrine) ■ Adrenergic antagonist, IV (e.g., metoprolol, labetolol) ■ Anesthetic agents, general, inhaled and IV ■ Antiarrhythmic agents, IV (e.g., amiodarone IV, lidocaine IV) ■ Antithrombic agents including heparin ■ Antiretroviral agents (e.g., efavirenz, lamiVUDine, raltegravir, ritonavir, combination)[a] ■ Cardioplegic solutions ■ Chemotherapeutic agents, parental ■ Chemotherapeutic agents, oral (excluding hormone agents) (e.g., cyclophosphamide, temozolomide)[a] ■ Dextrose, hypertonic, 20% or greater ■ Dialysis solution, peritoneal and hemodialysis ■ Epidural or intrathecal medications ■ Hypoglycemic agents, oral[a] (metformin,[a] glyburide) ■ Immunosuppressant agents (e.g., azaTHIOPRINE, cycloSPORINE, tacrolimus)[a] ■ Inotropic agents IV (e.g., digoxin) ■ Insulin,[a] subcutaneous and IV ■ Moderate sedation agents IV (e.g., midazolam[a]) ■ Moderate sedation agents, oral, for children (e.g., chloral hydrate liquid) ■ Liposomal forms of drug (e.g., liposomal amphotericin B) and conventional counterparts (e.g., amphotericin B desoxycholate) ■ Narcotics/opioids, all formulations[a] ■ Neuromuscular blocking agents (e.g., succinylcholine, rocuronium, vecuronium) ■ Parenteral nutrition preparations ■ Pediatric liquid medication that require measurement[a] ■ Pregnancy category X (e.g., bosentan, ISOtretinoin)[a] ■ Radiocontrast agents, IV ■ Sterile water for injection, inhalation, and irrigation (excluding pour bottles) in containers of 100 mL or more ■ Sodium chloride injection, hypertonic (more than 0.9% concentration)	■ carBAMzepine[a] ■ Chloral hydrate liquid, for sedation of children[a] ■ Heparin, including unfractionated and low-molecular-weight heparin ■ Magnesium sulfate injection ■ metFORMIN[a] ■ Methotrexate, oral, non-oncologic use[a] ■ Midazolam liquid, for sedation of children[a] ■ Nitroprusside sodium for injection ■ Potassium chloride for injection concentrate ■ Potassium phosphates injection ■ Promethazine, IV ■ Propylthiouracil[a] ■ Warfarin[a] ■ Epoprostenol (Flolan), IV ■ Opium tincture ■ Oxytocin, IV ■ Vasopressin, IV or intraosseous

The Institute for Safe Medication Practices (ISMP) has compiled two lists of "high-alert" drugs—one for the acute care setting and one for the community setting. This table combines the two ISMP lists.

[a]High-alert drugs used in the community/ambulatory setting. When prescribing these medications, extra precaution should be taken because these medications can cause serious patient harm when used in error.

Data from the Institute for Safe Medication Practices. *ISMP's list of high-alert medications* (copyright 2012). Retrieved from http://www.ismp.org/Tools/institutionalhighAlert.asp, with permission, and *ISMP's list of high-alert medications in community/ambulatory healthcare* (copyright 2011). Retrieved from http://www.ismp.org/communityRx/tools/ambulatoryhighalert.asp, with permission.

high-alert drug classes/categories as well as 10 specific high-alert medications, accessible on the ISMP website (see resources). ISMP's drug lists are similar to those of the 2011 National Committee on Quality Assurance (NCQA)'s High-Risk Medication Lists developed as part of the Healthcare Effectiveness Data and Information Set (HEDIS®) in that both identify high-risk drugs (i.e., medications causing severe problems with even small doses) to be avoided in the older population. However, the ISMP's drug lists are more extensive and incorporate practical considerations by including drugs that are commonly used by older adults in a community setting and that are reported to be related to a high frequency of adverse drug effects and related hospitalizations. Typical high-risk medications such as antiarrhythmic drugs, inotropic drugs, chemo/immunosuppressants, sedatives, and opioids are found on two high-risk medication lists. However, different from NCQA's high-risk medication lists, ISMP's high-alert drug lists also include warfarin, low-molecular-weight heparin, insulin, and oral agents for diabetes, commonly used in an outpatient/community setting and causing adverse drug events in the older adult.

In another study (Budnitz et al., 2011) of adverse events causing emergency hospitalization in the older adult, traditional high-risk medications as defined in NCQA's drug lists were found to be responsible for only 1.2% of hospitalizations; rather, 67% of those hospitalizations were caused by the single or combined use of the following four major types of medications, including warfarin (33.3%), insulin (13.9%), oral antiplatelet agents (13.3%), and oral hypoglycemic agents (10.7%). These medications are commonly used in a community setting for older adults with chronic disease. These results highlight the importance of improvement in the management of antithrombotic and antidiabetic drugs to reduce adverse drug events in the older adult. Johnston (2001) reported a study (Gerety, 1993) of adverse drug events in nursing homes, where it was observed that common medications causing numerous adverse drug effects in the older population include (a) cardiovascular drugs (36%), especially digoxin and furosemide, (b) central nervous system (CNS) drugs (19%), especially phenytoin, (c) analgesics (13%), especially ibuprofen, and (d) aspirin (7%).

Adverse drug effects in patients can be direct and/or indirect. Direct adverse drug effects in the older population may range from discomfort to severe gastrointestinal bleeding, falls/injuries, and delirium. Indirect adverse drug effects include unsatisfactory health outcomes resulting from noncompliance with medication instructions. One study reported that adverse drug effects mostly occur during a monitoring phase rather than a prescribing phase, indicating lack of self-management skills of diseases and medications by patients (Budnitz et al., 2011). Appropriate patient education along with the establishment of a supportive patient–provider relationship and frequent careful monitoring for adverse effects can promote medication adherence and minimize or avoid adverse drug effects and preventable emergency hospitalizations due to unintentional drug overdoses, especially when a patient is using a "high-alert medication."

The 2012 Beers Criteria

Because several medications may cause serious side effects, including falls, delirium/agitation, anticholinergic adverse effects (e.g., blurred vision, constipation, urinary retention) or bleeding, they have been identified as most likely ineffective in or poorly tolerated by older adults. *The 2012 Beers Criteria* identified 53 individual medications or classes of medication that are best avoided by patients over 65 years of age (American Geriatrics Society [AGS] 2012 Beers Criteria Update Expert Panel, 2012). In 2011, The AGS updated the Beers Criteria for Potentially Inappropriate Medication Use in Older Adults and incorporated updated evidence and information provided by stakeholders and experts. Nineteen medications and medication classes included in the 2003 criteria (Fick et.al., 2003) were dropped from the 2012 update as a result of insufficient evidence or new evidence evaluated by the panel. The *2012 Beers Criteria* cover three primary areas (AGS, 2011; AGS 2012 Beers Criteria Update Expert Panel, 2012):

1. Criteria for Potentially Inappropriate Medication Use in Older Persons: Independent of Diagnoses or Conditions
2. Criteria for Potentially Inappropriate Medication Use in Older Persons due to Drug–Disease/Syndrome Interaction
3. Criteria for Potentially Inappropriate Medication Use in Older Persons: Drugs to be Used with Caution

The first category includes medications that are potentially inappropriate for older people in most cases because they either pose high risks of adverse effects or appear to have limited effectiveness and because there are alternatives available to these medications. New inclusions in the *2012 Beers Criteria* in this category include glyburide, sliding-scale insulin, and megestrol. The second category includes medications that are potentially inappropriate for older people who have certain diseases because these medications may exacerbate specified health problems. New inclusions in this category are thiazolidinediones or glitazones with heart failure, acetylcholinesterase inhibitors with history of syncope, selective serotonin reuptake inhibitors with falls and fractures. The third category includes medications to be used with caution in older adults. The drugs in this category include 14 medications and classes. These medications emphasize the incorporation of the clinician's judgment to consider the risks and benefits of the medication for the unique condition of each individual, although its use may be associated with more risks than benefits in older people in general.

Where alternatives are available, the use of medications identified in the *2012 Beers Criteria* should be avoided as much as possible. The most current Beers criteria are available in a special AGS report (AGS 2012 Beers Criteria Update Expert Panel, 2012). The Therapeutic Research Center (2007) has provided a list of alternatives to these Beers Criteria Medications (see Resources on Medication Safety).

The major drug classifications included in the *Beers Medication Lists* pose a high risk of one or more of the following adverse effects: falls, delirium/confusion, anticholinergic adverse effects, and gastrointestinal bleeding. In particular, the adverse drug effects of falls, delirium, and confusion lead to an increased risk of fall-related injuries or fractures. Several studies have shown that the use of anticholinergic and sedative medications is closely associated with impaired mobility and cognitive function, in high-functioning, community-based older adults (Hilmer et al., 2007, 2009). Wilson et al.'s (2011) study also observed an interesting finding, namely, that the total number of medications does not increase impaired performances once sedatives and anticholinergics are excluded.

Common Drugs Causing Falls. According to the Beers lists (Therapeutic Research Center, 2007), major medications frequently causing falls or fractures include

- CNS depressants, especially long-acting benzodiazepines (e.g., diazepam, chlordiazepoxide) or large doses of short-acting benzodiazepines (e.g., Ativan, Xanax) and other sedative-hypnotics (e.g., barbiturate)
- Anticholinergics, including SSRI and tricyclic antidepressants (TCA) with active metabolites (e.g., Elavil, Tofranil)
- Analgesics (e.g., Demerol)
- Muscle relaxants (e.g., Prozac).

Additionally, anticonvulsants, antipsychotics, and sedating antihistamines (e.g., Benadryl, Atarax) were shown to increase the risk of falls. Diminished response ability to maintain homeostasis, characterized by orthostatic hypotension, increases the risk of falls and fractures in older adults, along with delayed body reaction to protect the body at the time of falls or injuries. Several cardiac medications such as alpha 1 antagonists (e.g., doxazosin, terazosin), nifedipine, and clonidine for the acute treatment of hypertension, type 1a anti-arrhythmics (i.e., sodium-channel blockers), and digoxin also slightly increase the risk of falls primarily due to hypotension. However, studies support that chronic use of most antihypertensives, including beta blockers, is not associated with the increased risk of falling (Heitterachi et al., 2002; Leipzig et al., 1999; Liu et al., 1995; Riefkohl et al., 2003). It should be noted, however, that orthostatic hypotension from the use of antihypertensives is often found in individual cases.

Common Drugs Causing Delirium/Confusion or Agitation. Any changes in body condition, caused by infection, medication, and/or even by environmental changes, may result in confusion in older adults. Studies have shown that medication is the most common cause of potentially reversible cognitive impairment. Demented patients, however, are more prone to drug-induced delirium. Common drug offenders causing delirium include (a) anticholinergics such as TCAs, long-life SSRI (e.g., Prozac daily dose), sedating antihistamines (e.g., Benadryl, Atarax), (b) potential CNS stimulants, and (c) others such as cimetidine, steroids, nonsteroidal anti-inflammatory drugs (NSAIDs), urinary drugs (e.g., Detrol, Ditropan), and analgesics (e.g., Demerol, Talwin) (AGS 2012 Beers Criteria Update Expert Panel, 2012; Kancelbaum, 2011; Riefkohl et al., 2003).

Common Drugs Causing Anticholinergic Activity. Anticholinergic-related adverse effects include memory impairment, confusion, hallucination, dry mouth, constipation, urinary retention, impaired sweating, and tachycardia. Thus, anticholinergic medications have been designated in the *Beers Criteria 2012* as drugs that should be avoided for older patients. One study measured the in vitro anticholinergic activity in 107 medications commonly used in older adults. At normal adult doses, significantly elevated anticholinergic activity was observed with TCA antidepressants (e.g., amitriptyline, nortriptyline), SSRI antidepressants (e.g., paroxetine), anticholinergic agents (e.g., atropine), antipsychotics (e.g., thioridazine, chlorpromazine, clozapine), antispasmodics (e.g., dicyclomine), antihistamines (e.g., diphenhydramine), and drugs that act on the genitourinary system (e.g., oxybutynin) (Chew et al., 2008). In older adults who already have poor gastrointestinal motility or impaired urinary function, and/or a decline in cognitive function, the use of medications having an anticholinergic effect, especially those identified in the *Beers Criteria*, can exacerbate pre-existing problems and cause serious adverse effects. Indeed, in a population study of 6,912 men and women aged 65 or older, patients taking anticholinergic medication were more likely to have cognitive decline and dementia; these cognitive changes improved with discontinuation of the medication (Carrière et al., 2009).

Common Drugs Causing Bleeding. Older people are more likely to use anti-inflammatory drugs on a long-term basis to control chronic inflammatory responses and/or chronic pain or to reduce the risk of thrombotic vascular disorder. In general, long-term use of non-COX-selective NSAIDs should be avoided in the older adult because there is a high risk that they may cause gastrointestinal bleeding, renal failure, high blood pressure, or heart failure (Therapeutic Research Center, 2007). The tendency to bleed increases, especially when non-COX-selective

NSAIDs are concurrently used with warfarin. The use of small doses should be considered with caution, however, when long-term treatment is required for the unique needs of an individual patient and when the benefit of their use outweighs its risk per an expert's judgment.

Drug–Disease Interactions.   Several drugs may interact adversely with the underlying disease of the patient. Such drug–disease interactions can place the older patient at risk for rehospitalization or other adverse events. One study reported that there was an increased risk of admission owing to the development of congestive heart failure (CHF) among older patients who had been taking NSAIDs (Heerdink et al., 1998). Common drug–disease interactions, supported by several studies (AGS 2012 Beers Criteria Update Expert Panel, 2012; Johnston, 2001; Therapeutic Research Center, 2007), are described below.

- NSAIDs, COX-2 inhibitor or steroids, as well as calcium channel blockers (CCB) may exacerbate CHF.
- Urinary retention may occur when a patient with benign prostate hypertrophy (BPH) uses decongestants or anticholinergics.
- Constipation may be worsened by calcium, anticholinergics, or CCBs.
- Neuroleptics and quinolones (e.g., Levaquin) may lower seizure thresholds.
- Long-term use of steroids may trigger or worsen osteoporosis or diabetes.

Polypharmacy.   Polypharmacy is defined as the use of five or more medications by a patient (Ferner & Aronson, 2006). A national population study, Slone Survey Report 2006, showed that for the last decade, the percentage of adults in the United States taking 5 or more or 10 or more medications has continuously increased up to 12% and 7%, respectively (Fig. 18.2) (Slone Epidemiology Center at Boston University, n.d.-b).

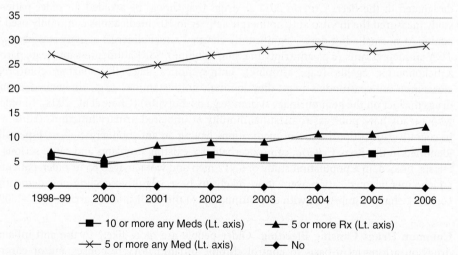

FIGURE 18.2. Medication use in adults aged 18 or more (%). (From Slone Epidemiology Center at Boston University. [n.d.]. *Patterns of medication use in the United States 2006: A report from the Slone survey.* Boston, MA: Slone Epidemiology Center at Boston University, with permission. Retrieved from http://www.bu.edu/slone/files/2012/11/SloneSurveyReport2006.pdf)

Polypharmacy is commonly found in the older adult in whom chronic disease such as hypertension, diabetes, dyslipidemia, and chronic pain alone or in combination, are common. In a US survey study of 3,005 community adults between 57 and 85 years of age, an average of 81% of participants were taking at least one prescription drug, and about 36% of older patients aged 75 to 85 years used five or more medications (Qato et al., 2008). Studies have shown that the average number of prescribed medicines in the older population is 5.7, increasing to 7 among nursing home patients. Similarly, in a recent study by Dwyer and colleagues (2010), the results of the 2004 National Nursing Home Survey showed that around 40% of nursing home residents took nine or more medications concurrently.

Polypharmacy is a major contributor to medication errors and adverse medication events in older adults, leading to emergency hospitalization or life-threatening incidents (Tinetti, 2004; Kohn et al., 2000; Weisbart, 2006). Adverse drug events increase dramatically with age, coupled with polypharmacy. Office visits for adverse drug events have been shown to increase from 9% of the population per year at ages between 25 and 44 to as high as 56.8% between ages 65 and 74 (Weisbart, 2006; Zhan et al., 2005). One study showed that polypharmacy is an independent risk factor for hip fracture in older adults related to increased potential exposure to CNS medication, leading to a higher risk of falling (Lai et al., 2010).

Prescribing Cascades. A prescribing cascade occurs when a new drug is prescribed to treat an unrecognized adverse effect of an existing drug rather than stopping the drug causing the adverse effect. Often, this new medication can cause another adverse effect, which can trigger adding another new and potentially unnecessary treatment. The sequence of events eventually causes more drug–drug interactions and potential harm to patients. This phenomenon often occurs in older adults who have chronic diseases and use multiple drugs, especially when the drug-induced symptom is similar to symptoms of the aging process (American Society of Consultant Pharmacists [ASCP], n.d; Rochon & Gurwitz, 1997).

Commonly found examples of prescribing cascades are described below.

- Increased use of anti-Parkinson therapy (e.g., levodopa) to treat extrapyramidal symptoms arising from metoclopramide (Reglan) (Avorn et al., 1995) or antipsychotics (Rochon et al., 2005).
- Increased use of drugs to treat "overactive bladder" (e.g., oxybutynin) arising from the use of cholinesterase inhibitors (e.g., donepezil, rivastigmine, galantamine), which was used to treat Alzheimer's disease. Over half of those using cholinesterase inhibitors were shown to receive a bladder anticholinergic drug (Gill et al., 2005).
- Increased use of antihypertensive drugs to treat sodium and water retention, which are often adverse effects of the use of NSAIDs in long-term NSAID users. In the study of Gurwitz et al. (1994), 66% of NSAID users were started on new antihypertensive drugs.

Drug–Drug Interactions. The prescribing cascade and polypharmacy in older adults pose a high risk of drug–drug interactions. These problems are exacerbated when multiple physicians are involved and/or when the patient uses multiple pharmacies. Drug–drug interactions may occur when one drug interrupts the absorption of other medication, when two drugs compete with each other to bind to and distribute transporting proteins, when one drug competes with another drug to use the P450 system for metabolism of the drug, or when one drug alters the excretion rate of the other. Among two competing drugs, these interactions may lead to the reduced effectiveness of one medication or to an increased adverse drug effect or toxicity of the displaced drug (Eldesoky, 2007; Kane et al., 2009; McLean & Le Couteur, 2004). Warfarin, hypoglycemic drugs such as glyburide, antidyslipidemic drugs such as statins, antacids, or H_2 blockers, and antihypertensive drugs are all commonly used to manage chronic diseases. Drug–drug interactions commonly found among the above drugs (Flockhart, 2007; Johnston, 2001; Kane et al., 2009; Romero et al., n.d.) are described in Table 18.3 and should be considered by a health provider prescribing the medications. Furthermore, when new symptoms develop in older adults, the adverse effects of existing medicines or a drug–drug interaction should be considered unless there is specific evidence for the diagnosis of a new disease.

Drug–Food Interactions. The absorption and metabolism of drugs may be affected by food. Cytochrome P450 (CYP3A4), which is responsible for the metabolism of more than 50% of clinical pharmaceuticals, has been shown to be a key enzyme in drug–food interactions (Fujita, 2004). When food requires the use of the same CYP3A4 enzyme used for medications to be metabolized and broken down, the CYP3A4 system is overloaded and cannot metabolize the medications, resulting

TABLE 18.3 · Common Drug–Drug Interactions

Drug–Drug Interaction Mechanism	Example of Drugs	Potential Effects
Altered absorption	Antacids + digoxin, antipsychotics, phenytoin, iron, or ciprofloxacin	Antacids may diminish effectiveness of important medication
Altered absorption (uncertain)	Digoxin + clarithromycin	Clarithromycin potentiates absorption of digoxin, causing toxicity
Displacement from binding proteins	Warfarin (higher affinity) + oral hypoglycemic agents + other highly protein-bound drugs	Can cause increased hypoglycemic effects
Altered metabolism: CYP 450 3A4 system inhibitor	Statins + CYP 450 3A4 inhibitors (azole antifungal agents, macrolide antibiotics such as erythromycin, and clarithromycin, ciprofloxacin; not azithromycin)	Increases toxicity of statins
Altered metabolism: CYP 450 3A4 system inhibitor effect	Antihistamine, CCB (calcium channel blocker) + CYP 450 3A4,5,7 inhibitor (antifungals, erythromycin, clarithromycin, SSRIs)	Increases toxicity of antihistamines or CCB
Altered metabolism: CYP 450 2C19 inhibitor effect	Plavix + CYP 450 2C19 inhibitors (e.g., cimetidine, omeprazole, fluoxetine (SSRI), fluconazole, ketoconazole)	Decreases effectiveness of Plavix
Altered metabolism: affect warfarin metabolism and reduce clotting factor	Warfarin + ciprofloxacin	Increases risk of bleeding
Altered excretion	Diuretics + lithium	Increases toxicity of lithium
Pharmacological antagonism	Anticholinergics (for bladder control) + cholinesterase inhibitors	Decreases effectiveness of either medication
Pharmacological synergism (severe)	Alpha1-blockers + antihypertensives	Increases risk of hypotension
Pharmacological synergism (moderate)	ACEI or NSAIDS or SSRI + sulfonylurea	ACEI increases hypoglycemic effect of sulfonylurea

in an increase in the level of the medication in the blood. Examples of drug–food interactions affecting CYP3A4 are interactions of grapefruit juice with felodipine and cyclosporine, and of red wine with cyclosporine. The following describes common drug–food interactions and the relevant recommendations related to them (Drugs.com, n.d.-a, n.d.-b; Fernstrom, 2006; University of Rochester Medical Center, 2005).

- **Grapefruit juice** is the most common food causing drug–food interactions. Grapefruit juice can cause drug–food interactions with around 50 medications, including CCBs, statins, erectile dysfunction medications (e.g., sildenafil, tadalafil), SSRI (e.g., fluvoxamine, sertraline), anxiolytics (e.g., alprazolam, triazolam, midazolam), antibiotics (e.g., clarithromycin, erythromycin), and warfarin.
- **Dairy products** should be avoided with the use of some antibiotics (e.g., tetracycline, ciprofloxacin, quinolone), anti-medications, and iron supplements because the calcium in dairy products will bind with these medicines and slow the drug absorption process.
- **Red wine and hard cheese** contain "tyramine" that acts the same way on the brain as the antidepressants called "monoamine oxidase inhibitors (MAOIs)" such as Parnate. The concurrent use of a tyramine-containing food with MAOIs will cause hypertensive crisis symptoms, characterized by high temperature, seizure, and high blood pressure.
- **Vitamin D** is often given as a dietary supplement. The concurrent use of Vitamin D with other CYP450 3A4 inducers (e.g., barbiturates, certain anticonvulsants such as phenytoins, rifampin, isoniazid) reduces the circulating levels of active Vitamin D.
- **Vitamin K-containing foods** (Dark-green vegetables such as green tea, spinach, kale, broccoli) promote blood clotting, counteracting blood thinners such as warfarin. Thus, the intake of a large amount of Vitamin K–containing food can potentially reduce the effectiveness of warfarin. However, eating a small amount of Vitamin K–containing food does not cause a problem.
- **Alcohol** affects and potentiates the effectiveness of antidepressants, sleeping pills, antihistamines, sedatives, some antibiotics, and warfarin. The concurrent use of alcohol with those medications should be avoided.
- **Cranberry Juice** can potentiate the effectiveness of warfarin. Avoid the concurrent intake of cranberry juice and warfarin.
- **Ciprofloxacin (Cipro)** absorption will be decreased when taken with vitamins or minerals that contain calcium, magnesium, zinc, or iron.
- **Alendronate (Fosamax)** must be taken on an empty stomach, or it will not be absorbed.

Drug–Herb Interactions. In a survey study of the use of 22 herbal supplements in 269 patients aged 60 or more, potential drug–herb interactions were found for 10 of the 22 supplements (Wold et al., 2005). Concurrent use of St. John's wort with CNS depressants, opioids or antidepressants can cause severe sedation. Ginkgo biloba extract can increase the potential risk of bleeding when taken with warfarin (Adams et al., 2011; Fugh-Berman, 2000). Common drug–herb interactions are described in Table 18.4.

Prescriber/System-Related Factors

Poor Communication/Practices: The Patient–Provider Relationship

Studies have consistently shown that the quality of the patient–provider relationship is associated with better adherence to medication and treatment plans and health outcomes (Beach et al., 2006; Davis et al., 2005; Flach et al., 2004; Flocke et al., 2002) and can also improve the patient's health

TABLE 18.4 · Common Herbs and Common Drug–Herb Interactions

Common Herbs	Primary Therapeutic Effects	Drug–Herb Interaction
Echinacea	Decreases the duration of cold; Increases immunity	■ Interacts with amiodarone and anabolic steroids → possible liver toxicity
St. John Wort	Reduces depression symptoms	■ Interacts with CNS depressants, antidepressants (SSRI, TCA) → increases sedation effects and causes serotonin syndrome ■ Interacts with warfarin → reduces the effect of warfarin
Ginkgo	Improves memory, reduces dizziness	■ Interacts with ASA, heparin, NSAIDs, warfarin → increases bleeding potential
Garlic	Reduces blood cholesterol, reduces blood pressure, anticoagulation	■ Interacts with insulin, oral hypoglycemic agents → increases hypoglycemic effects
Ginseng	Relieves stress, enhances immune system, decreases fatigue	■ Interacts with insulin, oral hypoglycemic agents → increases hypoglycemic effects

literacy (Dennis et al., 2012). In a study (Beach et al., 2006) of vulnerable patients with HIV, like the mentally ill, the physically disabled, or minorities, the patient's perception of being "known as a person," *patient-centeredness*, is shown to be significantly and independently associated with a higher rate of receiving highly active antiretroviral therapy (HAART). Davis et al. (2005) observed that, in his study of patients with chronic headache, if patients felt that their provider fully discussed their problem, their headache issues were likely to be resolved after one year.

Limited time to provide information at office visits has always been a barrier to providers' ability to listen to and engage with patients, to provide sufficient patient education, and to involve patients in a plan of care. In older adults with low health literacy, failure to provide sufficient information that the patient can understand commonly occurs, resulting in a direct impact on medication adherence, self-management of chronic disease, and health care outcomes. Based on the previous evidence, every current health care system highlights a patient-centered medical home model. Involving and empowering patients in their plan of care is very important in older patients who have chronic diseases such as hypertension, CHF, diabetes, dyslipidemia, and/or chronic pain related to degenerative disease.

Poor Communication/Practices among Health Care–Related Staff

Poor handwriting has always been a major cause of miscommunication and has led to medication errors. A 1979 study (Anonymous, 1979) estimated that one third of all prescribers' handwriting is illegible (Jenkins & Vaida, 2007). Although today many hospitals and clinics require electronic medical charting, which helps enormously to avoid this problem, there are many clinics and nursing homes in rural and underserved areas where paper charts continue to be used. In those cases, it is highly recommended to clearly type prescriptions rather than use *italics*. Along with poor handwriting, inappropriate use of abbreviation is another major contributor to medication errors. The ISMP (2013) has developed a complete list of error-prone abbreviations, symbols, and dose designations to be avoided. Table 18.5 describes some examples of such problematic abbreviations designated as official "Do Not Use" list by Joint Commission (2010), along with advice on how to alternately and

TABLE 18.5 · Official "Do Not Use" List

Do Not Use	Potential Problem	Use Instead
U, u (unit)	Mistaken for "0" (zero), the number "4" (four) or "cc"	Write "unit"
IU (International Unit)	Mistaken for IV (intravenous) or the number 10 (ten)	Write "International Unit"
Q.D., QD, q.d., qd (daily) Q.O.D., QOD, q.o.d, qod (every other day)	Mistaken for each other Period after the Q mistaken for "I" and the "O" mistaken for "I"	Write "daily" Write "every other day"
Trailing zero (X.0 mg) Lack of leading zero (.X mg)	Decimal point is missed	Write X mg Write 0.X mg
MS MSO$_4$ and MgSO$_4$	Can mean morphine sulfate or magnesium sulfate Confused for one another	Write "morphine sulfate" Write "magnesium sulfate"

Applies to all orders and all medication-related documentation that is handwritten (including free-text computer entry) or on pre-printed forms.
© The Joint Commission, 2013. From Facts about the official "do not use" list. Retrieved from http://www.jointcommission.org/assets/1/18/Do_Not_Use_List.pdf, with permission.

correctly write the prescription. Emergency situations often require a verbal order prior to a written order to manage the deteriorating conditions of patients in a timely manner. However, the intense and noisy environments surrounding the ordering health provider/prescriber and other staff at the scene of an emergency can distract or interrupt clear communication face-to-face or over the phone, resulting in medication errors. "Call out" when verbally ordering the medications in emergency situations, or "read back" when receiving the order are very effective communication skills and should be utilized every time to confirm the order and minimize/avoid medication errors.

Additionally, similar drug names can trigger medication errors, particularly when the prescription is handwritten. Lists of often-confused drug names have been determined (ISMP, 2011b), based on the reports of the Institute for Safety Medication Practices' National Medication Errors Reporting Program (ISMP NMERP). Examples of confused drug names include Buspiron-Bupropion, Celebrex-Cerebyx-Celexa, Clonidine-Klonopin-Clonazepam, Lamictal-Lamisil, and Zyprexa-Zantac-Zyrtec. Many of these confused medications have different indications for use. Thus, as a safe medication practice, ISMP has suggested that prescribers provide the indication for each medication on the prescription pad in writing or by using a drug indication checkbox.

Lack of Systematic/Cultural Support for Safety

The Safety Culture refers to "the extent to which individuals and groups will commit to personal responsibility for safety, act to preserve, enhance and communicate safety concerns, strive to actively learn, adapt, and modify (both individually and organizationally) behavior based on lessons learned from mistakes, and be rewarded in a manner consistent with these values" (Jones et al., 2008). However, in reality, action to confirm or correct medication errors or prevent future medication errors is often undermined by the person who is questioned or by others. This practice discourages health care workers from sharing valuable or concerning information with others to build a "Culture of Safety." Jenkins and Vaida (2007) stress promoting an "Equal Team Member" concept in practice settings in which all physicians and staff are encouraged to be responsible to detect and constructively act on potential or actual medical errors, and to prevent further medical errors or damage. The process can include debriefing cases involving medical errors, sharing information to improve practice safety, and supporting staff through education, resources, and/or system improvement. To establish a *Culture of Safety* and to promote quality of care and patient safety related to medical errors, an anonymous reporting system should be in place, allowing open collection and sharing of data within a system (Lindenberg, 2010).

STRATEGIES TO IMPROVE MEDICATIONS SAFETY

Guidelines for Patients/Caregivers

In many cases, older patients cannot easily recall what they wanted to ask when they see their physician and recognize that they forgot to ask important questions. The following guidelines are drawn from several research and review articles (Matz, 2011; Pfizer, 2008). These guidelines can be utilized for older patients to improve their confidence with regard to medication use and adherence and to encourage them to communicate with the physicians. Ultimately, these guidelines are designed to increase the effectiveness of disease management while improving medication safety. Older patients are considered a "high-risk group" for medication safety when the older patient lives alone, takes three or more medications, has memory problems or experiences decreased memory and mental function, and/or gets prescriptions from more than one doctor (Pfizer, 2008). Seniors should consider asking for help from a family member, caregiver, doctor, or pharmacist to support the safe use of medication.

Here are some recommendations for older patients to follow to ensure medication safety.

At Home

- Read the information packaged with your medicine for important information
- Keep your medical history and medication lists up to date
- Keep your medicine schedule straight by using reminders or an organizer
  - Set an alarm on your watch or cellphone
  - Ask help from family to keep medication schedule or appointment schedule
  - Use a pill organizer to track whether you have taken your pills
  - Link your medication routine to something you do every day (such as brush your teeth) OR use checklists
  - Refill a pill organizer daily or weekly
  - Update a new pill checklist each day
- Keep a daily log for measures requested by a doctor such as blood pressure, blood glucose level, or trends of symptoms.

At Doctor's Office

- Make a list of questions you want to ask about your health or medication.
- Always carry and bring with you a complete list of your prescribed or non-prescribed medication as well as an updated list of your medical history and allergies.
- Request a "brown-bag" review of your doctor's advice at least once a year. In the brown-bag, include all the medications prescribed and non-prescribed that you are taking routinely and intermittently.

- Ask three major questions, utilizing the "Ask Me 3" questionnaire (NPSF, n.d.):
  - **What is my main problem?**
  - **What do I need to do?**
  - **Why is it important for me to do this?**
- Ask about medication: the purpose, side effects, required lab monitoring, how long you will be taking medication.
- Ask your doctor or nurse to spell out any terminology or medication name for you.
- Be honest about any concerns related to having trouble managing current medication routines: increased forgetfulness, experiencing side effects, trouble affording your medication, or medication dependency.
  - There are several options of medications to treat the same disease. Your doctor may prescribe generic, low-cost medicines, or give samples to support your financial concerns, or refer to your social worker if necessary. Similarly, doctors can prescribe other medicines with no or fewer dependencies or side effects.
- Ask whether your doctor can simplify your medication routine (e.g., reduce the number of medicines by replacing it with combination medication, or reduce the frequency of doses of medicinve).

Guidelines for Clinicians/Practitioners for Safe Prescribing Practice

To promote patient safety related to medication for older adults, it is important for each health provider to build a safe prescribing practice considering the pharmacological action of each drug and patient factors such as age, weight, and family history. First, the clinician should be familiar with, and develop strategies to access, updated medication information at the time of prescribing in order to check adverse drug effects, drug–drug interactions, or drug–food interactions: the clinic or hospital itself may have an electronic medical chart system that supports a link to a core set of drug information references. The prescriber should also consider using personal digital devices with frequently updated information software such as *Epocrates*. Second, when prescribing a medication, the clinician should take into account individual differences in age, gender, functional or cognitive level, social life, finances, and their value to expand life at the end-of-life, as these variations in patient attributes may impact adherence to medication and disease management and to maintenance or improvement in quality of life (Clark, 2010; Huang, 2008; Jenkins & Vaida, 2007; Lindenberg, 2010; Pollock et al., 2007; Rochon, 2012).

The following are some factors that clinicians should consider when they prescribe medications for older adults:

- To control **acute moderate pain**, start with nonsteroidal medications. Medications like muscle relaxants and narcotics can increase the risk of falling and cause or worsen constipation.
- For patients on *Lasix who have difficulty walking*, prescribe the medication during the day and make sure that there is a commode nearby or that there is a caregiver available to help.
- **Narcotics** can cause constipation in older patients who already have decreased gastrointestinal motility. When narcotics are given, add lactulose or sorbitol and a stimulant laxative. Colace is not sufficient in most instances.
- **Steroids:** Long-term use of steroids can trigger or worsen osteoporosis or diabetes. When prescribing steroids for long-term treatment, it is important to think about osteoporosis prevention and glucose monitoring and control.

The following strategies/guidelines are provided to help clinicians to communicate effectively with patients and among health care workers and to promote safe prescribing practices, while taking into account an individual patient's differences and preferences. These approaches are supported by several studies (Huang, 2008; Jenkins & Vaida, 2007; Lindenberg, 2010; Pollock et al., 2007; Rochon, 2012).

Patient–Provider Communication Skills/Patient Engagement

- Evaluate the health literacy level of patient
  - Weiss and colleagues (2005) defined a patient's health literacy level as the "newest vital sign," affecting patient health outcomes, including medication adherence and self-management of chronic diseases and providing a quick tool for assessment of health literacy in primary care.
- Assess compliance with medication regimens and patient monitoring of therapeutic effects such as BP monitoring and blood glucose checks. In addition, evaluate major contributors to low medication adherence, including adverse drug effects, forgetfulness, financial constraints, and lack of transportation.
- Identify high-risk groups for medication problems, and discuss with patients concerns related to medication safety.
- Use plain language when providing patient education.
- Provide clear and simple instructions on medication or medical device use, including therapeutic purpose of the drugs, possible side effects, and when to report, especially when a new drug is started or there is a change in dose in previously prescribed drugs.
- Spend sufficient time on medication counseling.
- Support patients and empower them to be confident about medication use and management of their own disease (e.g., insulin injection, inhaler use, BP monitoring, glucose monitoring, etc.).

Communication Skills among Health Staff

- Improve handwriting skills. Print letters correctly in prescriptions.
- Avoid the use of abbreviations on allergy lists.
- Avoid the use of unauthorized/problematic abbreviations (e.g., q.d. → write out as "every day," h.s. → write out as "at bed time").
- Be aware of similar drug names.
  - Studies have shown that 25% of medication errors are the result of drugs' names that look alike or sound alike (Health Research and Educational Trust [HRET], ISMP, & Medical Group Management Association [MGMA], 2006).
- Indicate use of medication along with prescription, or use prescription pad containing checkbox for common indications.
- Require that orders be read back.
- Consider using electronic charting/prescription systems.

Safe Prescribing Practice

- Identify patient using two patient-specific identifiers.
- Verify allergies and reactions. Update at each visit.
- Check complete medication list and update current medications at each visit to a clinic or a hospital.

- Highlight critical diagnoses and conditions.
- Maintain updated drug references.
- Identify High-Alert *Medications List.*
  - For ISMP's High-Alert Medications List and High-Alert Meds in Community/Ambulatory Healthcare, see resources.
  - When prescribing and administering the "High-Alert Medications," provide mandatory patient education, employ automated or independent double checks when necessary, and standardize the prescribing, dispensing, and administering process of these products if possible.
- Avoid the use of medication in *Beers Medication Lists* for older adults aged 65 or older; use alternatives (For details of Beers List and Alternatives, refer to Therapeutic Research Center, 2007, see resources).
- Establish medication guidelines.
- If possible and manageable, start to treat a disease or symptom with non-pharmacological therapy, then pharmacological therapy if necessary.
- Always start with low doses and titrate slowly.
- Minimize the number of medications, if at all possible.
- Minimize the frequency of doses, if possible.
- Adjust dosage regimen to accommodate changes in physiology; start with doses smaller than adult doses.
- Provide detailed monitoring and periodic reevaluation of drug therapy.
- Provide clear information as to when patient should be seen for follow-up visit.

Guidelines for Administrators/Clinical Leaders/Organizations for Safe Prescribing Practice

The following are strategies/guidelines that health care agencies or administrator/clinical leaders can adopt to improve medication safety in their organizations.

Develop Evidence-Based Medication Guidelines

Administrators can establish and apply evidence-based, written standard medication guidelines in their practice, outlining frequently used drugs, correct dosages, maximum doses, contraindications, and precautions to promote medication safety. Standard practice guidelines are available on National Guidelines Clearinghouse Website, supported by AHRQ or specialized organizations such as the American Association of Family Practice or American Heart Association.

Adopt Electronic Prescribing Systems

E-prescribing system includes the generation and transmission of electronic prescriptions or prescription-related information between the prescriber, dispenser, pharmacy manager, or other health providers directly (Center for Medicare & Medicaid Services [CMS], 2009). The use of E-prescribing (e.g., iScribe, MEDeMORPHUS, TouchScript) has several advantages in that it can eliminate medication errors caused by illegible handwriting, allow automated screening, and trigger an alarm function for drug allergy lists, drug–drug interactions, and duplication of therapy. It also improves the communication of prescription information between prescribers and pharmacists by enhancing accuracy and reducing delayed transmission of prescription-related information.

The IOM recommended that all prescriptions be electronic by 2010. E-prescribing was adopted by Congress with the passage of the Medicare Improvements for Patients and Providers Act of 2008. The Act allows Medicare to provide incentives to providers who successfully adopt E-prescribing and improve health outcomes. Further, Medicare has reduced payment to providers who have not successfully adopted E-prescribing, starting in 2012 (Curtis, 2008; Lindenberg, 2010).

Create Culture of Safety

- Ensure that a system for reporting errors is in place, supported by a culture that allows medical staff to make it easy to share information and learn from errors.
- Assess regularly your practice performance and your office culture for patient safety using a formal assessment tool. The following tools can be used to evaluate and improve the culture of patient safety and staff performance:
    - The *Physician Practice Patient Safety Assessment* (PPPSA) is a self-assessment tool to help physician practices evaluate their patient-safety processes and detect areas for improvement. It was developed in 2006 by the HRET, the ISMP, and the MGMA.
    - The same partners also released *Pathways for Patient Safety*, a series of Web-based modules. These modules aim to increase awareness of patient safety as well as knowledge and implementation of best practices to reduce the risk of patient harm in both physician practices and organizational culture in 2009 (MGMA-American College of Medical Practice Executives [ACMPE], n.d.) (see resources).

CONCLUSION

Since the release of the IOM report (1999), efforts have been made to improve patient safety and quality of care through leadership, organization activities, development of error reporting systems, professional regulation, and standardization of education, training, and practice. However, the number of medical errors in hospitals and in the community is still high, ranking as the sixth leading cause of death, following heart disease, cancer, chronic lower respiratory disease, stroke, and accidents. In older adults, adverse drug events in older adults are a serious problem, along with polypharmacy and prescribing cascade. In a government study of Medicare patients in 2008, the Department of Health and Human Service reported that about 15,000 patients die each month partly on account of medical errors in the hospital (*USA Today*, 2010). Several studies have shown that approximately 50% to 88% of adverse drug events in older adults are preventable. Establishment of a consistent regulation system such as error reporting in institutions as well as among states, implementation of proven patient-safety interventions such as safe prescribing guidelines, involving patients in their care through education, and empowerment of patients for their own health management will improve the quality of care and patient safety.

REFERENCES

Adams M. P., Holland L. N., & Urban C. Q. (2011). *Pharmacology for nurses: A pathophysiologic approach* (3rd ed.). Upper Saddle River, NJ: Pearson.

Administration on Aging. (2013). Aging statistics. Department of Health and Human Services. Retrieved on Oct 13, 2013 from http://www.aoa.gov/AoARoot/Aging_Statistics/index.aspx

Agency for Healthcare Research and Quality. (2001, March). *Reducing and preventing adverse drug events to decrease hospital costs: Research in action, Issue 1* (AHRQ Publication No. 01-0020.). Rockville, MD: Author. Retrieved from http://www.ahrq.gov/qual/aderia/aderia.htm

Agency for Healthcare Research and Quality. (2004). *Literacy and health outcomes* (HCRQ reports). Retrieved from http://archive.ahrq.gov/clinic/epcsums/litsum.htm

Agency for Health Research and Quality. (2011). *Health Literacy Interventions and Outcomes:* An Updated Systematic Review. Executive Summary. Evidence Report/Technology Assessment. Number 199. Retrieved from http://www.ahrq.gov/research/findings/evidence-based-reports/litupsum.html

American Geriatrics Society. (2011). *AGS announces open public comment period on the draft AGS updated 2011 Beers criteria for potentially inappropriate medication use in older adults.* Retrieved from http://www.americangeriatrics.org/press/listservs/november_11_2011/id:2604

American Geriatrics Society 2012 Beers Criteria Update Expert Panel. (2012). American Geriatrics Society updated Beers Criteria for potentially inappropriate medication use in older adults. *Journal of the American Geriatrics Society, 60*(4), 616–631. doi:10.1111/j.1532-5415.2012.03923.x

American Society of Consultant Pharmacists. (n.d.). *The prescribing cascade.* Retrieved on Oct 13, 2013 from https://www.ascp.com/articles/prescribing-cascade

Anonymous. (1979). A study of physicians' handwriting as a time waster. *JAMA: The Journal of the American Medical Association, 242*(22), 2429–2430.

Avorn J., Gurwitz J. H., Bohn R. L., Mogun H., Monane M., & Walker A. (1995). Increased incidence of levodopa therapy following metoclopramide use. *JAMA: The Journal of the American Medical Association, 274*, 1780–1782.

Baker D. W., Gazmararian J. A., Williams M. V., Scott T., Parker R. M., Green D., . . . Peel J. (2002). Functional health literacy and the risk of hospital admission among Medicare managed care enrollees. *American Journal of Public Health, 92*(8), 1278–1283.

Baker D. W., Parker R. M., Williams M. V., & Clark W. S. (1998). Health literacy and the risk of hospital admission. *Journal of General Internal Medicine, 13*(12), 791–798.

Baker D. W., Wolf M. S., Feinglass J., Thompson J. A., Gazmararian J. A., & Huang J. (2007). Health literacy and mortality among elderly persons. *Archives of Internal Medicine, 167*(14), 1503–1509.

Barclay, L. (2007). Poor health literacy in the elderly predicts all-cause and cardiovascular mortality. Mescape Medical News. Retrieved from http://www.medscape.org/viewarticle/560695

Beach M. C., Keruly J., & Moore R. D. (2006). Is the quality of the patient-provider relationship associated with better adherence and health outcomes for patients with HIV? *Journal of General Internal Medicine, 21*(6), 661–665.

Beijer H. J., & de Blaey C. J. (2002). Hospitalizations caused by adverse drug reactions (ADR): A meta-analysis of observational studies. *Pharmacy World & Science: PWS, 24*, 46–54.

Benner J. S., Glynn R. J., Mogun H., Neumann P. J., Weinstein M. C., & Avorn J. (2002). Long-term persistence in use of statin therapy in elderly patients. *JAMA: The Journal of the American Medical Association, 288*(4), 455–461.

Bennet C. L., Ferreira M. R., Davis T. C., Kaplan J., Weinberger M., Kuzel T., . . . Sartor O. (1998). Relation between literacy, race, and stage of presentation among low-income patients with prostate cancer. *Journal of Clinical Oncology: Official Journal of the American Society of Clinical Oncology, 16*(9), 3101–3104.

Berkman N. D., Sheridan S. L., Donahue K. E., Halpern D. J., Viera A., Crotty K., . . . Viswanathan M. (2011). *Health literacy interventions and outcomes: An updated systematic review: Evidence reports/technology assessment,* No. 199 (AHRQ Publication No. 11-E006-1). Retrieved from http://www.ahrq.gov/research/findings/evidence-based-reports/litupsum.html

Bradley J. G., & Davis K. A. (2003). Orthostatic hypotension. *American Family Physician, 68*(12), 2393–2399. Retrieved from http://www.aafp.org/afp/2003/1215/p2393.html

Buchholz S. (2012). *Henke's Med-Math: Dosage calculation, preparation, & administration* (7th ed., chap. 9, p. 343). Philadelphia, PA: Lippincott Williams & Wilkins.

Budnitz D. S., Shehab N., Kegler S. R., & Richards C. L. (2007). Medication use leading to emergency department visits for adverse drug events in older adults. *Annals of Internal Medicine, 147*, 755.

Burley, P. (2007). 10 barriers to compliance-and how to overcome them. *Mondern Medicine.* Advanstar Communication. Retrieved from http://www.modernmedicine.com/modern-medicine/news/10-barriers-compliance%E2%80%94and-how-overcome-them assessed on Oct, 13, 2013

Carrière, I., Fourrier-Reglat, A., Dartigues, J.-F., Rouaud, O., Pasquier, F., Ritchie, K., & Ancelin, M.-L. (2009). Drugs with anticholinergic properties, cognitive decline, and dementia in an elderly general population: The 3-city study. *Archives of Internal Medicine, 169*, 1317.

Centers for Disease Control and Prevention. (2006). Medication safety basics. Retrieved from http://www.cdc.gov/MedicationSafety/basics.html

Centers for Disease Control and Prevention. (2010). Medication safety program: Adverse drug events in children/adverse events in older adults. Retrieved from http://www.cdc.gov/MedicationSafety/program_focus_activities.html

Centers for Disease Control and Prevention. (2011). Deaths/mortality in the United States, 2009, National Center for Health Care Statistics at the Centers for Disease Control and Prevention. Retrieved from http://www.cdc.gov/nchs/fastats/deaths.htm

Centers for Medicare & Medicaid Services. (2009). 2009 Electronic prescribing incentive program made simple. Retrieved from www.cms.hhs.gov/EPrescribing

Chew M. L., Mulsant B. H., Pollock B. G., Lehman M. E., Greenspan A., Mahmoud R. A., . . . Gharabawi G. (2008). Anticholinergic activity of 107 medications commonly used by older adults. *Journal of the American Geriatrics Society, 56*, 1333.

Clark, TR. (2010). Tough decisions about medications. *Aging Well magazine.* Winter.

Curtis, J. (2008). E-prescribing offers a carrot and a stick. *Journal for Nurse Practitioners. 4*(10).

Davis K., Schoenbaum S. C., & Audet A. M. (2005). A 2020 vision of patient-centered primary care. *Journal of General Internal Medicine, 20*(10), 953.

Dennis S. M., Williams A., Taggart J., Newall A., Denney-Wilson E., Zwar N., . . . Harris M. F. (2012). Which providers can bridge the health literacy gap in lifestyle risk factor modification education: A systematic review and narrative synthesis. *BMC Family Practice, 13*(1), 44.

Drugs.com. (n.d.-a). *Drug interactions between phenytoin and Vitamin D2.* Retrieved from http://www.drugs.com/drug-interactions/phenytoin-with-vitamin-d-1863-0-1003-5789.html

Drugs.com. (n.d.-b). *Drug Interactions Checker.* Retrieved from http://www.drugs.com/drug_interactions.html

Dwyer L. L., Han B., Woodwell D. A., & Rechtsteiner E. A. (2010). Polypharmacy in nursing home residents in the United States: Results of the 2004 National Nursing Home Survey. *American Journal of Geriatric Pharmacotherapy, 8*(1), 63–72.

ElDesoky E. S. (2007). Pharmacokinetic-pharmacodynamic crisis in the elderly. *American Journal of Therapeutics, 14*, 488–498.

Ferner R. E., & Aronson J. K. (2006). Communicating information about drug safety. *British Medical Journal, 333*, 143.

Fernstrom, M. (2006, October 26). Foods to avoid when you're taking meds. *Today Health.* Retrieved from http://today.msnbc.msn.com/id/14785552/ns/today-today_health/t/foods-avoid-when-youre-taking-meds/

Fick D. M., Cooper J. W., Wade W. E., Waller J. L., Maclean J. R., & Beers M. H. (2003). Updating the Beers criteria for potentially inappropriate medication use in older adults: Results of a US consensus panel of experts. *Archives of Internal Medicine, 163*(22), 2716–2724. doi:10.1001/archinte.163.22.2716

Field T. S., Gilman B. H., Subramanian S., Fuller J. C., Bates D. W., & Gurwitz J. H. (2005). The costs associated with adverse drug events among older adults in the ambulatory setting. *Medical Care, 43*(12), 1171–1176.

Field T. S., Gurwitz J. H., Avorn J., McCormick D., Jain S., Eckler M., . . . Bates D. W. (2001). Risk factors for adverse drug events among nursing home residents. *Archives of Internal Medicine, 161*(13), 1629.

Flach S. D., McCoy K. D., Vaughn T. E., Ward M. M., Bootsmiller B. J., & Doebbeling B. N. (2004). Does patient-centered care improve provision of preventive services? *Journal of General Internal Medicine, 19*(10), 1019–1026.

Flocke S. A., Miller W. L., & Crabtree B. F. (2002). Relationships between physician practice style, patient satisfaction, and attributes of primary care. *Journal of Family Practice, 51*(10), 835–840.

Flockhart D. A. (2007). *Drug Interactions: Cytochrome P450 Drug Interaction Table.* Indianapolis: Indiana University School of Medicine. Retrieved from http://medicine.iupui.edu/clinpharm/ddis/table.aspx

Fugh-Berman A. (2000). Herb–drug interactions. *Lancet, 355*, 134.

Fujita K. (2004). Food–drug interactions via human cytochrome P450 3A (CYP3A). *Drug Metabolism and Drug Interaction, 20*(4), 195–217.

Gerety, M.B., Cornell, J.E., et al. (1993). Adverse events related to drugs and drug withdrawal in nursing home residents. *JAGS,* 41:1326–32.

Gill S. S., Mamdani M., Naglie G., Streiner D. L., Bronskill S. E., Kopp A., . . . Rochon P. A. (2005). A prescribing cascade involving cholinesterase inhibitors and anticholinergic drugs. *Archives of Internal Medicine, 165*, 808–813.

Gurwitz J. H., Avorn J., Bohn R. L., Glynn R. J., Monane M., & Mogun H. (1994). Initiation of antihypertensive treatment during nonsteroidal anti-inflammatory drug therapy. *JAMA: The Journal of the American Medical Association, 272*, 781–786

Gurwitz J. H., Field T. S., Harrold L. R., Rothschild J., Debellis K., Seger A. C., . . . Bates D. W. (2003). Incidence and preventability of adverse drug events among older adults in the ambulatory setting. *JAMA: The Journal of the American Medical Association, 289*(9), 1107–1116.

Gurwitz J. H., Field T. S., Judge J., Rochon P., Harrold L. R., Cadoret C., . . . Bates D. W. (2005). The incidence of adverse drug events in two large academic long-term care facilities. *American Journal of Medicine, 118*, 251–258.

Gurwitz J. H., Field T. S., Rochon P., Judge J., Harrold L. R., Bell C. M., . . . Bates D. W. (2008). Effect of computerized provider order entry with clinical decision support on adverse drug events in the long-term care setting. *Journal of the American Geriatrics Society, 56*(12), 2225–2233.

Hakkarainen K. M., Hedna K., Petzold M., & Hägg S. (2012). Percentage of patients with preventable adverse drug reactions and preventability of adverse drug reactions—A meta-analysis. *PLoS ONE, 7*(3), e33236. Retrieved from http://www.plosone.org/article/info%3Adoi%2F10.1371%2Fjournal.pone.0033236

Health Research & Educational Trust, the Institute for Safe Medication Practices, & the Medical Group Management Association. (2006). *The physician practice patient safety assessment.* Retrieved from www.pathwaysforpatientsafety.org

Heerdink E. R., Leufkens H. G., Herings R. M., Ottervanger J. P., Stricker B. H., & Bakker A. (1998). NSAIDs associated with increased risk of congestive heart failure in elderly patients taking diuretics. *Archives of Internal Medicine, 158,* 1108–1112.

Heitterachi E., Lord S. R., Meyerkort P., McCloskey I., & Fitzpatrick R. (2002). Blood pressure changes on upright tilting predict falls in older people. *Age and Ageing, 31,* 181–186.

Hilmer S. N., Mager D. E., Simonsick E. M., Cao Y., Ling S. M., Windham B. G., . . . Abernethy D. R. (2007). A drug burden index to define the functional burden of medications in older people. *Archives of Internal Medicine, 167,* 781.

Hilmer S. N., Mager D. E., Simonsick E. M., Ling S. M., Windham B. G., Harris T. B., . . . Health ABC Study. (2009). Drug burden index score and functional decline in older people. *American Journal of Medicine, 122,* 1142.

Ho P. M., Rumsfeld J. S., Masoudi F. A., McClure D. L., Plomondon M. E., Steiner J. F., & Magid D. J. (2006). Effect of medication nonadherence on hospitalization and mortality among patients with diabetes mellitus. *Archives of Internal Medicine, 166,* 1836–1841.

Huang, A. (2008, November/December). *Optimizing prescribing among older adults* (Report of the 28th Canadian Geriatric Society Annual Meeting: Academic Career day, Vol. 11, No. 10, pp. 7–8). Retrieved from http://www.healthplexus.net/files/content/2008/CGS/CGSprescribing.pdf

Institute for Safe Medication Practices. (2011a). *ISMP list of high-alert medications in community/ambulatory healthcare.* Retrieved from http://www.ismp.org/communityRx/tools/ambulatoryhighalert.asp

Institute for Safe Medication Practices. (2011b). *ISMP's list of confused drug names.* Retrieved from http://www.ismp.org/tools/confuseddrugnames.pdf

Institute for Safe Medication Practices. (2012). *ISMP's list of high-alert medications.* Retrieved from http://www.ismp.org/Tools/institutionalhighAlert.asp

Institute for Safe Medication Practices. (2013). *ISMP's list of error-prone abbreviations, symbols, and dose designations.* Retrieved from http://www.ismp.org/tools/errorproneabbreviations.pdf

Institute of Medicine. (1999). *To err is human: Building a safer health system* (IOM Report, Shaping the Future for Health). Retrieved from http://iom.edu/~/media/Files/Report%20Files/1999/To-Err-is-Human/To%20Err%20is%20Human%201999%20report%20brief.pdf

Institute of Medicine. (2004). *Health literacy: A prescription to end confusion.* Washington, DC: National Academies Press.

Institute of Medicine. (2007). *Preventing medication errors: Quality chasm series.* Washington, DC: National Academies Press.

Jackevicius C. A., Mamdani M., & Tu J. V. (2002). Adherence with statin therapy in elderly patients with and without acute coronarysyndromes. *Journal of American Medical Association, 288*(4), 462–467.

Jenkins R. H., & Vaida A. J. (2007). Simple strategies to avoid medication errors. *Family Practice Management, 14*(2), 41–47. Retrieved from www.aafp.org/fpm/2007/0200/p41.html

Johnston C. B. (2001). UCSF Division of Geriatric Primary Care Lecture Series: Drugs and the elderly: Practical considerations. Retrieved from http://www.docstoc.com/docs/444572/Drugs-and-the-Elderly—Practical-Considerations

Joint Commission. (2010). *Fact about the official "do not use" list.* Retrieved from http://www.jointcommission.org/assets/1/18/Do_Not_Use_List.pdf

Jones, K. (2008). Challenges to improving safety at the point of care. Retrieved on Oct 13, 2013, from http://www.ahrq.gov/news/events/conference/2008/Jones.html

Kaiser Family Foundation. (2008). *Reducing medical errors.* Retrieved from http://www.kaiseredu.org/Issue-Modules/Reducing-Medical-Errors/Background-Brief.aspx

Kancelbaum B. (2011). *Medications in the older adult: Drugs to avoid and safer alternatives. Advances for nurses.* Pennsylvania, PA: Merion Matter.

Kane R. L., Ouslander J. G., Abrass I. B., & Resnick B. (2009). *Essentials of clinical geriatrics* (6th ed., chap. 14). New York, NY: McGraw-Hill.

Kaufman D. W., Kelly J. P., Rosenberg L., Anderson T. E., & Mitchell A. A. (2002). Recent patterns of medication use in the ambulatory adult population of the United States: The Slone survey. *JAMA: The Journal of the American Medical Association, 287*(3), 337.

Kirsch I. S., Jungeblut A., Jenkins L., & Kolstad A. (1993). *Adult literacy in America: A first look at the results of the National Adult Literacy Survey (NALS)*. Washington, DC: National Center for Education Statistics, U. S. Department of Education.

Kocurek B. (2009). Promoting medication adherence in older adults . . . and the rest of us. *Diabetes Spectrum, 22*(2), 80–84.

Kohn L., Corrigan J., & Donaldson M. (Eds.). (2000). *To err is human: Building a safer health care system*. Washington, DC: National Academies Press.

Lai S. W., Liao K. F., Liao C. C., Muo C. H., Liu C. S., & Sung F. C. (2010). Polypharmacy correlates with increased risk for hip fracture in the elderly: A population-based study. *Medicine (Baltimore), 89*, 295–299.

Leipzig R. M., Cumming R. G., & Tinetti M. E. (1999). Drugs and falls in older people: A systematic review and meta-analysis: I. Psychotropic drugs. *Journal of the American Geriatrics Society, 47*, 30–39.

Lindenberg J. A. (2010). Medication safety in the elderly: Translating research into practice. *Clinical Scholars Review, 3*(1), 43–48.

Liu B. A., Topper A. K., Reeves R. A., Gryfe C., & Maki B. E. (1995). Falls among older people: Relationship to medication use and orthostatic hypotension. *Journal of the American Geriatrics Society, 43*, 1141–1145.

Matz J. (2011). Why taking your meds as prescribed is important. *MyOptumHealth*. Retrieved from http://www.myoptumhealth.com/portal/Information/item/Medication+Safety+for+the+Elderly?archiveChannel=Home%2FArticle&clicked=true

McLean A. J., & Le Couteur D. G. (2004). Aging, biology, and geriatric clinical pharmacology. *Pharmacological Reviews, 56*, 163–184.

Medical Group Management Association & American College of Medical Practice Executives. (n.d.). *Patient safety tools for physician practices*. Retrieved from http://www.mgma.com/pppsahome/

Nahin R. L., Pecha M., Welmerink D. B., Sink K., DeKosky S. T., Fitzpatrick A. L., & Ginkgo Evaluation of Memory Study Investigators. (2009). Concomitant use of prescription drugs and dietary supplements in ambulatory elderly people. *Journal of the American Geriatrics Society, 57*, 1197.

National Center for Complementary and Alternative Medicine. (n.d.). *Herbs at a glance: A quick guide to herbal supplements*. Bethesda, MD: U.S. Department of Health and Human Services, National Institutes of Health. Retrieved from http://nccam.nih.gov/sites/nccam.nih.gov/files/herbs/NIH_Herbs_at_a_Glance.pdf

National Center for Education Statistics. (2006). *The health literacy of America's adults: Results from the 2003 National Assessment of Adult Literacy*. Washington, DC: U.S. Department of Education. Retrieved from http://nces.ed.gov/pubsearch/pubsinfo.asp?pubid=2006483

National Network of Libraries of Medicine. (2011). *Health literacy*. Retrieved from http://nnlm.gov/outreach/consumer/hlthlit.html

National Patient Safety Foundation. (2011). *Health literacy: Statistics at-a-glance*. Retrieved from http://www.npsf.org/wp-content/uploads/2011/12/AskMe3_Stats_English.pdf

National Patient Safety Foundation. (n.d.). *Ask Me 3*. Retrieved from http://www.npsf.org/for-healthcare-professionals/programs/ask-me-3/

New England Healthcare Institute. (2009). *Thinking outside the pillbox: A system-wide approach to improving patient medication adherence for chronic disease*. Retrieved from http://www.nehi.net/publications/44/thinking_outside_the_pillbox_a_systemwide_approach_to_improving_patient_medication_adherence_for_chronic_disease

Odegard P. S., & Gray S. L. (2008). Barriers to medication adherence in poorly controlled diabetes mellitus. *Diabetes Educator, 34*, 692–697.

Osterberg L., & Blaschke T. (2005). Adherence to medication. *New England Journal of Medicine, 353*(5), 487–497.

Parker R. M., & Kindig D. A. (2006). Beyond the Institute of Medicine Health Literacy Report: Are the recommendations being taken seriously? *Journal of General Internal Medicine, 21*, 891–892. doi:10.1111/j.1525-1497.2006.00541.x

Pfizer. (2008). Medication Safety for the Elderly: A guide for patients and caregivers. August.

Pollock M., Bazaldua O. V., & Dobbie A. E. (2007). Appropriate prescribing of medications: An eight-step approach. *American Family Physician, 75*(2), 231–236.

Psaty BM, Koepsell TD, Wagner EH, *et al.* The relative risk of incident coronary heart disease associated with recently stopping use of beta blockers. JAMA 1990;263:1653–7.

Qato D. M., Alexander G. C., Conti R. M., Johnson M., Schumm P., & Lindau S. T. (2008). Use of prescription and over-the-counter medications and dietary supplements among older adults in the United States. *JAMA: The Journal of the American Medical Association, 300*(24), 2867–2878.

Riefkohl E. Z., Bieber H. L., Burlingame M. B., & Lowenthal D. T. (2003). Medications and falls in the elderly: A review of the evidence and practical considerations. *Pharmacy and Therapeutics, 28*(11), 724–733.

Rochon P. A. (2012). Drug prescribing for older adults. *UpToDate.* Retrieved from http://www.uptodate.com/contents/drug-prescribing-for-older-adults/abstract/19

Rochon P. A., & Gurwitz J. H. (1997). Optimising drug treatment for elderly people: The prescribing cascade. *British Medical Journal, 315*, 1096.

Rochon P. A., Stukel T. A., Sykora K., Gill S., Garfinkel S., Anderson G. M., . . . Gurwitz J. H. (2005). Atypical antipsychotics and parkinsonism. *Archives of Internal Medicine, 165*, 1882–1888.

Romero, K., Vargo, D. L., & Woosley, R. L. (n.d.). *Clinical Pharmacology Education Module 1—Preventable adverse drug reactions: A focus on drug interactions* (Funded by AHRQ). Centers for Education & Research on Therapeutics. Retrieved from http://www.azcert.org/medical-pros/education/CERT%20Lecture%20Guide.pdf

Schillinger D., Grumbach K., Piette J., Wang F., Osmond D., Daher C., . . . Bindman A. B. (2002). Association of health literacy with diabetes outcomes. *JAMA: The Journal of the American Medical Association, 288*(4), 475–482.

Schillinger D., Piette J., Grumbach K., Wang F., Wilson C., Daher C., . . . Bindman A. B. (2003). Closing the loop: Physician communication with diabetic patients who have low health literacy. *Archives of Internal Medicine, 163*(1), 83–90.

Scott T. L., Gazmararian J. A., Williams M. V., & Baker D. W. (2002). Health literacy and preventive health care use among Medicare enrollees in a managed care organization. *Medical Care, 40*(5), 395–404.

Slone Epidemiology Center at Boston University. (n.d.-b). *Patterns of medication use in the United States 2006: A report from the Slone survey.* Boston, MA: Author. Retrieved from http://www.bu.edu/slone/files/2012/11/SloneSurveyReport2006.pdf

Soumerai S. B., Pierre-Jacques M., Zhang F., Ross-Degnan D., Adams A. S., Gurwitz J., . . . Safran D. G. (2006). Cost-related medication nonadherence among elderly and disabled Medicare beneficiaries: A national survey 1 year before the Medicare drug benefit. *Archives of Internal Medicine, 166*(17), 1829–1835.

Therapeutic Research Center. (2007). Potentially harmful drugs in the elderly: Beers list and more. *Pharmacist's Letter/Prescriber's Letter, 23*, Doc. No. 230907. Retrieved from http://www.fmda.org/beers.pdf

Tinetti M. E., Bogardus S. T., Jr., & Agostini J. V. (2004). Potential pitfalls of disease-specific guidelines for patients with multiple conditions. *New England Journal of Medicine, 351*(27), 2870.

University of Rochester Medical Center. (2005, January 26). Grapefruit juice and medication can be a dangerous mix. *ScienceDaily.* Retrieved from http://www.sciencedaily.com/releases/2005/01/050124010803.htm

USA Today. (2010). Hospital care fatal for some Medicare patients. Retrieved from http://www.usatoday.com/yourlife/health/healthcare/2010-11-16-medicare_N.htm?csp=34news#uslPageReturn

U.S. Department of Health and Human Services/ Office of Disease Prevention and Health Promotion. Office of Quick guide to health literacy. Fact Sheet: Health literacy and Health Outcomes. Retrieved from http://www.health.gov/communication/literacy/quickguide/factsliteracy.htm

Weisbart E. S. (2006). Safer prescribing for older adults: Clinical and business imperatives aligned. *Clinical Geriatrics: A Clinical Journal of the American Geriatrics Society, 14*(11), 18–24. Retrieved from http://www.sbggpr.org.br/artigos/Prescricao%20para%20idosos.pdf

Weiss B. D., Mays M. Z., Martz W., Castro K. M., DeWalt D. A., Pignone M. P., . . . Hale F. A. (2005). Quick assessment of literacy in primary care: The newest vital sign. *Annals of Family Medicine, 3*(6), 514–522.

Williams M. V., Baker D. W., Honig E. G., Lee T. M., & Nowlan A. (1998). Inadequate literacy is a barrier to asthma knowledge and self-care. *Chest, 114*(4), 1008–1015.

Williams M. V., Parker R. M., Baker D. W., Parikh N. S., Pitkin K., Coates W. C., & Nurss J. R. (1995). Inadequate functional health literacy among patients at two public hospitals. *JAMA: The Journal of the American Medical Association, 274*(21), 1677–1682.

Wilson N. M., Hilmer S. N., March L. M., Cameron I. D., Lord S. R., Seibel M. J., . . . Sambrook P. N. (2011). Associations between drug burden index and falls in older people in residential aged care. *Journal of the American Geriatrics Society, 59*, 875.

Wold R. S., Lopez S. T., Yau C. L., Butler L. M., Pareo-Tubbeh S. L., Waters D. L., . . . Baumgartner R. N. (2005). Increasing trends in elderly persons' use of nonvitamin, nonmineral dietary supplements and concurrent use of medications. *Journal of the American Dietetic Association, 105*, 54.

Zhan C., Arispe I., Kelley E., Ding T., Burt C. W., Shinogle J., & Stryer D. (2005). Ambulatory care visits for treating adverse drug effects in the United States, 1995–2001. *Joint Commission Journal on Quality and Patient Safety/Joint Commission Resources, 31*, 372–378.

CHAPTER 18: IT RESOURCES

Websites

Agency for Healthcare Research and Quality
www.ahrq.gov

AHRQ—National Guidelines Clearinghouse (standard practice guidelines)
http://www.guideline.gov

National Council on Aging—Medication Safety
http://www.ncoa.org/calendar-of-events/medication-management.html

Women's Health—Medication Safety
http://www.womenshealth.gov/aging/drugs-alternative-medicine/medication-safety.cfm

ConsultGerin—Nursing Standard of Practice Protocol: Reducing Adverse Drug Events
http://consultgerirn.org/topics/medication/want_to_know_more

American Society of Consultant Pharmacists
www.ascp.com

American Society of Health System Pharmacists (ASHP)
http://www.ashp.org/

CDC—Medication Safety Program: Adults and Older Adult Adverse Drug Events
http://www.cdc.gov/medicationsafety/adult_adversedrugevents.html

Healthcare Quality Strategies, Inc., Project in a Box: Medication Safety in Older Adults
http://hqsi.org/index/providers/Adverse-Drug-Events/Medication-Safety-in-Older-Adults
.html

Geriatric Pharmacotherapy Practice Resource Center
https://www.ascp.com/articles/geriatric-pharmacotherapy

Health Literacy Program, American Medical Association Foundation
http://www.ama-assn.org/ama/pub/about-ama/ama-foundation/our-programs/public-health/
health-literacy-program.page

Health Literacy Resources, American Medical Association Foundation
http://www.ama-assn.org//ama/pub/about-ama/ama-foundation/our-programs/public-
health/health-literacy-program/health-literacy-kit.page

Institute of Medicine
http://www.iom.edu/

Institute for Safe Medication Practice
http://www.ismp.org/default.asp

National Council on Patient Information and Education (NCPIE)—Educate Before You Medicate
www.talkaboutrx.org

National Patient Safety Institute
http://www.npsf.org/

Center for Medication Safety of the South Carolina College of Pharmacology
http://medsafety.org/

Institute for Safe Medication Practices
http://www.ismp.org/Tools/MSK.asp

Patient Safety and Medical Errors Information—Agency for Healthcare Research and Quality
(AHRQ)
http://www.ahrq.gov/qual/patientsafetyix.htm

Patient Safety Tools: Improving Safety at the Point of Care. Toolkit by Patient Safety Issue/Area (AHRQ)
  http://www.ahrq.gov/qual/pips/issues.htm
American Society of Health System Pharmacists (ASHP)—Medication Safety
  http://www.ashp.org/menu/Advocacy/FederalIssues/MedicationSafety
American Society of Health System Pharmacists (ASHP)—Implementing a Bar-Coded Medication Safety Program
  http://www.ashpfoundation.org/MainMenuCategories/PracticeTools/BarCodeGuide
Drug Interactions Checker
  http://www.drugs.com/drug_interactions.html
Patient Safety Tools for Physician Practices from the Health Research and Education Trust (HRET), Institute for Safe Medication Practices (ISMP), and the Medical Group Management Association (MGMA)
  http://www.mgma.com/pppsahome/
Institute for Safe Medication Practice (ISMP)—Medication Safety Tools and Resources
  http://www.ismp.org/tools/default.asp
ISMP List of High-Alert Medications in Community/Ambulatory Healthcare
  http://www.ismp.org/communityRx/tools/ambulatoryhighalert.asp
The National Committee on Quality Assurance (NCQA)'s 2011 High-Risk Medication Lists
  http://www.ncqa.org/tabid/1274/Default.aspx
WHO Patient Safety Curriculum Guide for Medical Schools
  http://www.who.int/patientsafety/activities/technical/medical_curriculum_slides/en/index.html
Health Literacy Intervention Program: Ask Me 3 (Sponsored by the Partnership for Clear Health Communication at the National Patient Safety Foundation)
  http://www.npsf.org/askme3
HealthCoach4Me Virtual Health Library
  www.takingmeds.com
FDA—Index to Drug-Specific Information
  http://www.fda.gov/Drugs/DrugSafety/PostmarketDrugSafetyInformationforPatientsandProviders/UCM111085
AHRQ—Check Your Medicines: Tips for Using Medicines Safely
  http://www.ahrq.gov/consumer/checkmeds.htm
Medication Use Safety Training for Seniors (MUST)
  www.mustforseniors.org
National Patient Safety Foundation—Ask Me 3 Health Literacy Reference Resources
  http://www.npsf.org/for-healthcare-professionals/programs/ask-me-3/ask-me-3-resources/
AHRQ—Your Medicine: Be Smart. Be Safe
  http://www.ahrq.gov/patients-consumers/diagnosis-treatment/treatments/safemeds/yourmeds.html

PDF Documents

American Geriatrics Society Updated Beers Criteria for Potentially Inappropriate Medication Use in Older Adults
  http://www.americangeriatrics.org/files/documents/beers/2012BeersCriteria_JAGS.pdf

American Geriatrics Society Beers Criteria for Potentially Inappropriate Medication Use in
  Older Adults—Pocket Card
    http://www.americangeriatrics.org/files/documents/beers/PrintableBeersPocketCard.pdf
Potentially Harmful Drugs in the Elderly: Beers List and More
    http://www.fmda.org/beers.pdf
Institute for Safe Medication Practices' List of High-Alert Medications
    http://www.ismp.org/Tools/highalertmedications.pdf
ISMP's Lists of Confused Drug Names
    http://www.ismp.org/tools/confuseddrugnames.pdf
ISMP's List of Error-Prone Abbreviations, Symbols, and Dose Designations
    http://www.ismp.org/tools/errorproneabbreviations.pdf
The Health Literacy of America's Adults—Institute of Education Sciences
    http://nces.ed.gov/pubs2006/2006483.pdf
Medications and the Older Adult (MetLife Mature Market Institute)
https://www.metlife.com/assets/cao/mmi/publications/since-you-care-guides/
    mmi-medications-older-adult.pdf
Medication Safety for the Elderly: A Guide for Patients and Caregivers
    http://www.pfizer.com/files/health/medicine_safety/4-6_Med_Safety_for_Elderly.pdf

Videos

Health IT Success: Multimedia Intervention &; Medication Management for Older Adults
  (2013)
    The development of DVD segments on topics such as insomnia, depression, heart failure, and
    diabetes shows promise as a way to help older adults address medication health care chal-
    lenges. (10:28 minutes)
    http://youtu.be/Njahg5irzbc
An Update on Medication Safety
    SmarterMeds pharmacist Aaron Emmel discusses the findings in a recent *New England Jour-
    nal of Medicine* study examining adverse drug events in older adults. (4:11 minutes)
    http://youtu.be/v7JvXN_vFHQ
Prevention of Medication-Related Complications with Older Adults (2012) (6:20 minutes)
    http://youtu.be/eySJ-NDm1fA
Beers Criteria Updated—Meds Not Good for Seniors (2012)
    The Beers Criteria (or Beers List) is a list of specific medications that are generally considered
    inappropriate when given to elderly people. For a wide variety of individual reasons, the med-
    ications listed tend to cause side effects in the elderly because of the physiologic changes of
    aging. The list was originally created by geriatrician Mark H. Beers. The criteria were created
    through consensus of a panel of experts and originally published in the Archives of Internal
    Medicine. It has now been updated.
    http://youtu.be/3Z6aF90FcNA
NCOA Offer Medication Mgt Tips (2013)
    Every year, one in three adults older than 65 has one or more harmful reactions to a medica-
    tion, according to the American Geriatrics Society. Here are six tips to keep in mind to man-
    age medication wisely to stay healthy and safe. (1:01 minutes)
    http://youtu.be/DFvE0kQWyPY

Medication Use in Older Adults (2011)
Lynsey E. Brandt, MD, a geriatric medicine doctor at Penn Medicine, discusses medication use in older adults. (28:50 minutes)
http://youtu.be/QfbCP-Y6v1M
Medication Adherence in the Elderly Population (2013). (4:28 minutes)
http://youtu.be/MEfPIUeLwu0

Images

Google images for Medication Safety and Older Adults
http://www.google.com/search?q=medication+safety+and+older+adult&;safe=active&;source=lnms&;tbm=isch&;sa=X&;ei=mwGuUaPzN8uu0AGejYCgBw&;ved=0CAcQ_AUoAQ&;biw=988&;bih=178

Psychiatric Assessment and Diagnostic Evaluation

Rizwan Ali, MD, DFAPA
Kye Y. Kim, MD

INTRODUCTION AND BACKGROUND

Healthy aging as defined by Erik Erikson is the time of "integrity," and not a time of "despair." Aging is a developmental stage and is not a disease (Kaplan & Sadock, 2007). Erickson was one of the first developmental theorists to identify aging as a developmental stage. Older age is theorized by ego integrity versus despair. Ego integrity begins in later adulthood when the individual begins to experience a sense of mortality, though not in a negative way. It is a productive introspection that leads to the person viewing his or her life as a harmonious and contented one. Conversely, despair occurs when the individual comes to a negative resolution of life. They fear death, have a sense that life is short, and are frequently depressed (Melillo & Houde, 2011).

At the same time that the clinician assesses for daily functioning, special senses, and mobility, special attention must be given to older adults when assessing their emotional health and their cognitive abilities (Melillo & Houde, 2011).

> The meaning that people attach to life events and their emotional, physical, and social sequelae often constitute a major influence on one's healthy or unhealthy response to life's hardships, challenges of role transition, and recovery from traumatic experiences. (Melillo & Houde, 2011, p.53)

The present population of those over 65 will increase from 35 million in 2000 to 72 million in 2030, with the oldest old, those over 85, projected to grow from 5.8 million in 2010 to 8.7 million in 2030 (US Census Bureau, 2010). Studies have shown that formalized comprehensive geriatric assessments can result in improved survival, reduced hospital and nursing home stays, decreased medical costs, and improved functional status (Applegate et al., 1990; Quinn et al., 2008). Lewis and Bottomley (2007) have written a text, *Geriatric Rehabilitation: A Clinical Approach*, on the subject. Owing to the multiple comorbid medical conditions and intake of several medications, older adults are at risk for accelerated deterioration not only in functional ability but also in cognitive and emotional ability.

There is little difference in the psychiatric examination of older patients and younger patients; however, because of the cognitive decline in older adults, it is essential to pay special attention to comprehension and understanding in the diagnostic process. In one study, 176 homebound older adults (mean age 77 years) referred for psychiatric evaluation were assessed in the home by a geriatric psychiatrist (Levy, 1985). The comprehensive neuropsychiatric assessment can decrease the number of medical specialist visits and the overall health care costs, and increase patient satisfaction and quality of life. It is often used to determine the current and future health care and psychosocial needs of older patients. The comprehensive neuropsychiatric assessment provides useful diagnostic and prognostic information and serves as a baseline for better understanding immediate and long-term patient and family needs and wishes. A comprehensive geriatric assessment often requires the involvement of a trained interdisciplinary team who will allow sufficient time for a thorough patient workup (see Chapter 3). Standard and potentially complicated testing may be involved. Members of the "core team" generally include the geriatrician (internist or family medicine physician with fellowship training in geriatric medicine), a social worker, and a nurse, academically and/or experientially trained in gerontological nursing. Other health care disciplines are often involved in initial or subsequent assessment visits, such as the medicine specialties of neurology and psychiatry and other staff such as a dietitian, pharmacist, physical therapist, occupational therapist, and clinical psychologists.

Performing a comprehensive assessment is an ambitious undertaking. A team of geriatric providers may choose to assess current symptoms and illnesses and their functional impact, current medications, their indications and effects, relevant past illnesses, recent and impending life changes, and objective measure of overall personal and social functionality. Current and future living environment and its appropriateness to function and prognosis, family situation and availability, current caregiver network, including its deficiencies and potential, are all part of comprehensive geriatric evaluation. Objective measure of cognitive status, assessment of mobility/balance, rehabilitative status/prognosis, and current emotional health, including history of substance abuse, are also included in initial evaluation. Nutritional status and needs, disease risk factors, screening status, health promotion activities, and services required and received will all give a better idea about the overall status of an older patient and will help assess the needs in a more realistic and compassionate way (see Chapter 3).

PSYCHIATRIC ASSESSMENT

Source of Referral and Review of Records

Once the patient is referred for comprehensive psychiatric assessment, source of referral is of prime importance. If the patient is referred by a primary care physician, a reason for referral and review of comprehensive physical examination and laboratory results is a common place to start. A face-to-face or a telephone consult with the referring physician is very helpful. Often the patient himself or herself is not aware of the need for a psychiatric assessment, and a discussion with the primary care physician, caregivers, and family members is critical to develop a clear picture about the current situation and to verify the need for referral. If the patient is self-referred or referred by a family member, it becomes more critical to communicate with the primary care physician to ascertain the general physical health of the patient and to learn what baseline blood tests have already been done, including a detailed neurological examination with computed tomography (CT) or magnetic resonance imaging (MRI) scans of the head and other parts of the body. There are very many medical conditions, and there is a list of medications that can interfere with patient's cognition, mood, and overall mental status. A good knowledge of the older patient's medical condition is generally a safe place to start a comprehensive psychiatric assessment (Meeks et al., 2009).

Identifying Data

A comprehensive understanding and knowledge of the older patient's age, sex, marital status, employment, finances, and living situation cannot be emphasized more. Is the patient living independently or is totally dependent on a family member or a caregiver for his activities of daily living (ADLs)? Is he living in an assisted living facility (ALF) or a skilled nursing facility (SNF)? Is he divorced, single, or widowed or had he recently lost a close family member or a spouse? Who brought the patient for the assessment and who has the main concern (the patient or the family member)? Who has the power of attorney and is authorized to make decisions for the patient if the patient lacks the capacity to decide for himself? All these questions have huge implications for psychiatric evaluation, treatment, and overall prognosis of an older patient.

Chief Complaints

The primary reason for the assessment, preferably in the patient's own words, and the duration of these symptoms is captured under this heading. Chronic, painful conditions are very common in older patients. Arthritis generally leads the list. Multiple medical problems and organ pathology make the presenting complaint confusing. Both dementia and delirium may present with altered mental status and deterioration in memory, orientation, and behavior. Communication barriers due to hearing impairment, cognitive decline, and overall frailty in older patients may impose further challenges in gathering accurate information. Sometimes patients may downplay or deny otherwise serious problems, and the role of caregivers becomes crucial in getting the exact nature, duration, and severity of current symptoms. Sometimes, depression may be present, further complicating the chief complaint, and may be present along with dementia and/or delirium (Meeks et al., 2009).

History of Present Illness

Details related to chief complaints are documented next. When did the problem start? Was the onset sudden, as in the case of delirium, or slowly developing, as in the case of dementia? What are the other symptoms associated with the chief complaints? How is the patient sleeping? Has there been any weight loss associated with the current problem? Duration of the symptoms helps identify if the condition is acute or chronic. Most of the conditions in older patients are chronic, and the chief complaint may be an acute exacerbation of a chronic illness. Special attention is given to medical history and the list of medications, with careful consideration to any recent changes in medication or overall medical status of the patient. How are these chief complaints and present illness affecting other people involved in the patient's care? Has the patient been aggressive or violent, and are there any legal charges pending? A detailed history of present illness helps formulate the case and points toward the possible differential diagnoses and treatments. Examples of other variables compounding the picture is the presence of infection such as urinary tract infection or upper respiratory infection.

Past Psychiatric History

Central to comprehensive psychiatric assessment is the past psychiatric history. The main difference from evaluating a younger patient is that the data in an older patient are more extensive, generated by more providers, and the source is potentially more distant. Patients and caregivers alike may not know or recall important details from medical, surgical, or psychiatric events taking place 30, 40, or 50 years ago. In their effort to be comprehensive and accurate, therefore, geriatric practitioners need to frequently locate and obtain medical records from multiple sources existing long ago and far away. Prior psychiatric hospitalizations and treatments are always helpful to know the baseline of an older patient. History of suicide attempts and psychiatric inpatient treatments for depressive or psychotic disorders are going to determine the current choice of medications to help with the recent presentation. A history of bipolar disorder is very important in assessing a patient with current depressive or manic symptoms (see Chapter 24). Use of psychiatric medications in the past is a good indicator to tell which medication may or may not work this time and what side effects should be expected from these medications. Multiple psychiatric hospitalizations in the past generally indicate that the condition is chronic and treatment may be longer to stabilize the patient. Patients with delirium and dementia may show severe behavioral problems, and with a history of aggressive behavior in the past, one can be better prepared for the safety measures for the staff and the patient (Meeks et al., 2009).

Medical History and List of Medications

A patient's medical history should note all major illnesses, especially seizure disorders, loss of consciousness, headaches, visual problems, and hearing loss. Stroke and a recent cardiovascular event are known to result in depression. Older individuals are very susceptible to the adverse effects of drugs, which may present as behavioral and cognitive disturbances. A detailed list of all medications, including the ones that are taken on an as-needed basis and over-the-counter (OTC) drugs, is very important for psychiatric assessment of an older patient. Use of herbal and dietary supplements is an additional source of information that is essential to obtain as many patients do not tell their health care providers about these supplements that can interact with prescribed agents. Because of the chronic nature of most of the problems, like sleep disturbances or painful arthritis, older patients tend to take OTC or herbal remedies that may not show on their regular list of medications being prescribed by their family physicians. Therefore, specifically asking for OTC and herbal medicines is a good idea. Many sleeping aids and OTC analgesics interfere with cognition, can affect balance and coordination, and can increase the risk of falls. Benzodiazepines can cause sedation, behavioral disinhibition, depression, and memory impairment as side effects (Kaplan & Sadock, 2007). Many antidepressant drugs cause nervousness and insomnia. Several medications used to treat general medical conditions, including cardiovascular, pulmonary, and endocrine disorders, are also known to cause psychiatric side effects (Posner et al., 2007).

Major depression has been found in approximately 12% of hospitalized patients and other depressive syndromes in 23%. Among patients with Alzheimer disease, it is estimated that 23% to 54% have major depression (HelpGuide.org, 2013; Parmelee et al., 1989). Since the risk of suicide is significantly higher in older white men and older persons tend to underuse psychiatric services, geriatricians should look for signs of depression and cognitive impairment in older patients with physical illnesses, including recent stroke, coronary artery bypass grafting, or myocardial infarct (Choi et al., 2013; Levy, 1985). In a past study on older adults who were homebound for various causes, the most common discrete psychiatric diagnoses were dementia, with or without secondary symptoms, major depression, and paranoid states without dementia (Brody, 2002).

History of Substance Abuse

The prevalence of alcoholism is 1% to 5% in community dwelling older persons and 5% to 10% among those who seek medical care (Brody, 2002). Because of the pharmacokinetic changes, older patients retain higher circulating levels of alcohol and thus have more severe and more prolonged toxic effects. Alcohol abuse is a major contributing factor in 10% to 20% of psychiatric, nursing home, and hospital admissions (Brody, 2002). Use of alcohol in older patients is associated with depression, anxiety, sleep disturbances, incontinence, falls, and malnutrition. Interaction of alcohol with other medications may also result in complications. Delirium and dementia may become severe if alcohol is on board. The most useful tool in assessing alcohol use is a four-item questionnaire, called CAGE (Have you ever felt you should cut down on your drinking? Have people annoyed you by criticizing your drinking? Have you ever felt bad or guilty about your drinking? Have you ever had a drink first thing in the morning to steady your nerves or get rid of a hangover?) The positive predictive value with two or more affirmative answers exceeds 75% in older patients (see Chapters 21 and 22).

Use of other illicit drugs is also increasing in older patients as their population is growing. On the basis of the definition of substance abuse and substance dependence in DSM IV (American Hospital Association, 2013), a study found that among older adults (50+) who met the criteria for substance abuse and dependence, 10.2% were dependent on or abusing illicit drugs only, 85.8% were dependent on or abusing alcohol only, and 4.0% were dependent on or abusing both illicit drugs and alcohol. Among the older adults dependent on or abusing illicit drugs, the most common drugs of abuse were marijuana (42%), cocaine (36%), pain relievers (25%), stimulants (18%), and sedatives (17%) (Gfroerer et al., 2003). Whereas older adults constitute 13% of the U.S. population, they account for 30% of prescription drugs and 40% of OTC medications sold in this country (Delafuente, 2003). OTC analgesics are used by 35% of older persons and 30% use laxatives. Careful inquiry about alcohol use, illicit drug use, and the use of OTC medications should always be part of comprehensive geriatric assessment (Cummings & Mega, 2003). A recent conference call (2012) conducted by the American Psychiatric Association's section on substance abuse discussed reducing psychiatric readmissions to cut costs.

Family, Social, Developmental, and Work History

It is important to assess the past. Many times it may not be possible to extract all of the necessary information from the patient owing to cognitive decline, and this is where the role of caregivers, other family members, providers, and clinicians becomes extremely important.

A patient's childhood, place of birth, persons involved with their care—parents or others—attitude of parents, hardship or trauma in early years of life, all play a major role in shaping the personality and future interactions in the person's entire life. The provider should also ask about patient's schooling, highest education, employment history and retirement age, and circumstances in which retirement was decided (if applicable). A history of learning disability in school and difficulties in finding and maintaining a job are good indicators of early psychiatric problems. Inquiry should also be made about hobbies, friends, sports, social and leisure activities, and overall satisfaction with life (Meeks et al., 2009).

Family history includes number of siblings, relationship of family members with each other, and history of any psychiatric or physical illness in the family. Several psychiatric conditions, including Alzheimer disease, run in families. Previous exposure of a family member to psychiatric medications helps the clinician choose a medication that may be helpful to the patient. Family history of suicide is very important, especially when assessing a patient with depression (National Institute of Mental Health [NIMH], 2013b). Marital status is generally also part of the family history, which includes health and presence of the spouse and number, availability, and involvement of children. In a patient who is a widow or a widower, grief related to that loss should be evaluated, and coping strategies must be explored in detail. Patients with a recent loss of their spouse are at a high risk for an adverse physical and psychological event (Kaplan & Sadock, 2007). Sexual history should not be neglected in older patients. Problems related to sexual activity may be a major concern in older persons. Sexual orientation, frequency, and desire for sexual activity, and any difficulty around sexuality should be explored further.

Mental Status Examination

Appearance, Grooming, and Level of Cooperation

The neuropsychiatric assessment starts with the first observation of the patient's general appearance. Drowsiness or sedation may interfere with every aspect of psychiatric evaluation. It is important to make sure that sedation is not related to drug or alcohol intoxication or a medication side effect. Patients' emotional status is displayed in the way they are dressed and interact with the environment. A poorly groomed, disheveled appearance with poor hygiene reflects lack of self-care and inability to perform basic activities of cleaning and dressing appropriately. This may be a sign of frontal lobe syndromes, including stroke, dementia, severe depression, or schizophrenia. Unilateral left-sided neglect in dressing or grooming (hemispatial neglect) is evident in right parietal lesions. Unilateral right-sided neglect does sometimes occur in patients with left hemisphere damage; however, it is fairly uncommon. Right-sided neglect occurs in approximately 20% of patients with left hemisphere damage. It is also less severe and usually of shorter duration than left-sided neglect. Inappropriate dressing, for instance, dressing in multiple layers or wearing warm clothes in hot, sizzling weather may be seen in patients with schizophrenia or dementia. Bright and loud makeup, with flashy and colorful clothes, is inappropriately worn by patients with manic symptoms, schizophrenia, or frontal lobe lesions (Morris et al., 2000).

Patient's attitude about the interview process, in general, and particularly toward the interviewer, speaks volumes about his/her state of mind. Cooperative and engaged attitude should be differentiated from detached, uncooperative, and hostile or guarded attitude. Every behavior points toward a different diagnosis and is important to notice in the assessment process. Anxious and paranoid patients may be very guarded. A manic patient may be gregarious, disinhibited, loud, and sometimes belligerent. Some patients with dementia or dependency traits may turn to their spouses for answers during the interview. On the other hand, some spouses may interject answers before the patient can speak. Depression may result in psychomotor retardation and paucity of speech. Movements and responses of depressed patients are slow, and they avoid eye contact with a downward gaze and stooped posture. Paranoid patients may have difficulty with trusting the interviewer and may be suspicious. Special attention must be paid to abnormalities of gait, posture, and spontaneous movements, as each abnormality in these areas is characteristic of certain types of neuropsychiatric disorder. Medications used in psychiatry may result in certain side effects that resemble Parkinson disease, including tremors, akathisia (restlessness and inability to sit still; driven like a motor inside), body stiffness (rigidity), and dystonia (NIMH, 2013a).

Orientation

Awareness of one's surroundings and having knowledge of the correct year, month, day, date, and time of the day as well as one's current location will reveal important information about the learning process and recent memory. Impairment in orientation to time, place, and person is associated with cognitive disorders. Disorientation may be seen in depressive disorders, anxiety disorders, and personality disorders, especially under severe stress. Orientation to person can be tested by asking the patient's name or by asking names of the other people involved in his/her care. Also important is to know how the patient knows about these facts. In terms of degree of deterioration, disorientation to person signifies a higher degree of impairment, then the place and then time (Kaplan & Sadock, 2007).

Attention and Concentration

As mentioned earlier, a sedated or drowsy patient will have difficulty in every exam of neuropsychiatric assessment. Therefore, attention and concentration should be tested in every patient with utmost care. Several degrees of reduced arousal are recognized, including clouding (mildly reduced wakefulness or awareness), obtundation (mildly to moderately reduced alertness with lessened interest in the environment, drowsiness while awake, and increased sleep), stupor (deep sleep or similar unresponsiveness state from which the patient can be aroused only with vigorous and repeated stimuli), and coma (unarousable unresponsiveness) (Cummings & Mega, 2003). A disturbance in attention and concentration is usually seen in patients with frontal lobe dysfunction or toxic-metabolic encephalopathy.

Digit Span measures short-term auditory memory and attention. The digits have no logical relationship to each other and are presented in random order by the examiner. The patient must then recite the digits correctly by recalling them in the same order. On the second part of this subtest, the patient must remember the order in which digits are presented, but recite them in reverse order. Digit Span is an untimed core working memory subtest. For Digit Span forward, the examiner reads numbers such as "2, 3, 9, 1," and the patient responds with the same numbers. For Digit Span backward, the examiner reads numbers such as "24, 3, 7, 12," and the patient responds "12, 7, 3, 24." The "A" test is used to assess the ability to sustain the concentration. The patient is asked to raise his hand whenever the letter "A" is heard in a list of letters read aloud by the examiner (Strub & Black, 2000). See http://www.learninginfo.org/digit-span.htm for additional information.

Serial 7 test is a very useful test for educated patients with average mathematical skills. This test not only assesses attention and concentration but also requires recent memory and intact executive functions. The examiner asks the patient to subtract 7s from 100 or subtract 3s from 10, depending on the patient's ability to tolerate the complexity of the task. Spelling "world" backward and saying the month of the year in reverse order are other tests to assess mental control and sustained attention. See http://attentionmmse.com/ for additional information.

Memory—Immediate, Recent, and Remote

Immediate retention and recall are tested by giving the patient six digits to repeat forward and backward. Patients with normal immediate memory and those without anxiety are able to repeat all six digits forward and five to six digits backward. Remote memory can be tested by asking the patient about his/her place and date of birth or names and birthdays of the family members. Impairment in recent memory is the most important cognitive decline seen in psychiatry and is generally tested by a test called "object recall." The examiner gives the patient names of three objects to remember and asks for a recall after 3 to 5 minutes. Asking the patient to recall what he/she ate for breakfast or his/her current address and details of other recent events may also be used to test the recent memory. Loss of memory before the event is called retrograde amnesia, and loss of memory after the event is known as anterograde amnesia.

Speech and Language Output

Problems with language output that are manifested in the impairment of speech are called aphasia. Some examples of common aphasias are non-fluent or Broca aphasia, fluent or Wernicke aphasia, andglobal aphasia, a combination of fluent and non-fluent aphasias. Non-fluent aphasias are characterized by decreased verbal output, effortful speech, dysarthria, decreased phrase length, dysprosody (loss of speech rhythm), and agrammatism (omission of the small relational words). The patient's understanding remains intact, but the ability to speak is impaired. Non-fluent aphasia generally reflects damage to the left frontal lobe. Fluent aphasias have a normal or increased verbal output, normal articulation, normal phrase length, preserved prosody, empty speech, circumlocution, and paraphasia. A simple test for Wernicke aphasia is to show the patient common objects, such as a pen, watch, paper, and doorknob—and ask the patient to name them. The patient does not understand the use of these objects either and thus is unable to name them correctly. Fluent aphasias are generally the result of lesions at the posterior temporal, inferior parietal, or temporo parietooccipital junction region (Kirshner & Hoffmann, 2012).

Mood and Affect

Mood refers to emotion as experienced and expressed by the patient, whereas affect refers to emotion manifested by the patient in speech, facial expression, and behavior (Cummings & Mega, 2003). Congruency between mood and affect is noted as a normal aspect of normal mental status examination. Incongruent mood and affect is seen in conditions such as pseudobulbar palsy, in which the patient may laugh while feeling depressed or may cry when reporting happiness. Euphoria with silly gestures and facial expressions may be noted in frontal lobe diseases. Elevated mood with euphoria and grandiose sense of self is seen in hypomania and mania and is a hallmark symptom of bipolar illness. Depressed mood is characterized by slow movement, paucity of speech, and psychomotor retardation in general. Other emotions reported by the patient may include anxiety, anger, rage, irritability, apathy, emotions blunting, and so on, and they should be matched with affective congruency. Sometimes, the mood may be labile, fluctuating quickly from tears to laughter to anger.

Perceptual Abnormalities

Hallucination (wrong perception of a stimulus when nothing is present) and illusion (misperception of a stimulus when something is present) are commonly seen in older patients in confusional states and organic conditions. These perceptual abnormalities may manifest in any of the five perceptual modalities (senses), including visual, auditory, touch, olfactory, and gustatory. Organic brain diseases can also cause impaired perceptual phenomena called agnosia (the inability to recognize and interpret the significance of sensory impressions). It is important to note the type of agnosia—anosognosia (denial of illness), atopognosia (the denial of a body part), simultanagnosia (inability to perceive two objects at once), or visual agnosia (the inability to recognize objects) or prosopagnosia (the inability to recognize faces) (The Merck Manual, 2013).

Thought Processes and Contents

A disturbed thought form is referred to abnormal relationships between ideas in the flow of conversation. Some examples of formal thought disorders include loose associations, flight of ideas, perseveration, tangentiality, derailment and circumstantiality, word salad, and neologism. Paucity of thoughts is noticed in depression and Parkinsonism, while flight of ideas with rhyming, punning, or assonance in seen in mania. Loosening of association with word salad or neologism is very common in severe schizophrenia. Perseveration is seen in dementia and other frontal lobe syndromes.

Disturbance of thought content is manifested as delusions in which the patient is unable to assess the reality correctly. Delusion of paranoia is the most common delusion when the patient becomes preoccupied with the idea that someone is trying to harm him or his family. Delusions may be centered toward one's health and well-being (somatic delusion), infidelity of spouse or significant other (delusion of jealousy), idea that someone famous or of higher status is in love with the patient (erotomania), or belief that the person has acquired unbelievable education, wealth, or power (delusion of grandiosity). In some patients, there are two or more delusions at one time (mixed), and sometimes it is not possible to name a delusion (unspecified). When delusions are plausible and are possible in real day-to-day life, they are called non-bizarre delusions, but when they are incomprehensible and are totally based on unrealistic possibilities, as for example, "there is a chip in my brain and someone from Mars is controlling me," they are called bizarre delusions. Less severe disturbances of thought content include obsessions, overvalued ideas, magical thinking, phobias, and hypochondriasis (see Chapters 24 and 25).

Intelligence

Simple questions related to day-to-day life can be useful ("How many nickels and dimes are in $ 1.35?"). Decline in intelligence should be compared with the previous highest level of functioning. Intelligence may reflect in every aspect of psychiatric evaluation. Patients with lower levels of education or intelligence may not be able to perform simple tests such as serial 7s or serial 3s, despite intact attention and concentration, as noted above. Socioeconomic status and general life experiences also affect patient's intellectual abilities and should be taken into account. The patient's general knowledge, which is indirectly reflective of his or her intelligence, may be assessed by asking the names of the last five presidents of the country, famous landmarks in different cities, population of the United States, and so on.

Judgment and Insight

Judgment is the capacity of the person to act appropriately in different situations, and insight is the ability to see what is wrong with self and what needs to be done to correct it. Common questions that a patient may be asked to test for appropriate judgment are "What would you do if you found a stamped, sealed envelope in the street?" or "What would you do if you saw and smelled smoke in a crowded place?" Insight is examined by inquiring about what the patient understands of his or her illness, intends to do after leaving the hospital, or perceives about current personal medical and psychological needs.

NEUROPSYCHOLOGICAL EVALUATIONS

Clinicians may consider neuropsychological evaluations for their intended purposes and patient factors. They are generally useful tools to assist in the diagnosis of and the prognosis of disease progression, especially in cognitive disorders. Individual tests are selected depending on the general and specific goals of the evaluation such as evaluations involving differential diagnosis, or memory function, or language function. When the patient is referred for a neuropsychological evaluation, it is more efficient and cost-effective to ask specific questions rather than vague referrals. In addition, the clinician may need to decide on requesting a screening test or a comprehensive neuropsychological evaluation. The objective of a screening test is to detect a problem and determine whether or not a function is abnormal. By contrast, the goal of a comprehensive evaluation is to describe function, determine the nature and extent of deficits, provide information relevant to everyday functioning, and assist in differential diagnosis. There are brief or quick screening tests available to the clinicians that can be practical and valuable in their daily clinical work (Koss & Attix, 2006).

- Mini-Mental Status Examination is the most commonly used test of cognitive functioning, which assesses orientation, attention, calculation, immediate and short-term recall, language, and the ability to follow simple commands. The maximum score on MMSE is 30. It is used widely to monitor the treatment response and the progress in the course of time. This test is now under stricter copyright in terms of availability for all to use (Folstein et al., 1975).
- Clock Drawing Test is commonly used as a screening instrument for dementia and neuropsychiatric disorders. A mix of visuospatial abilities and executive function abilities makes this test very useful while it has challenges as to an appropriate scoring system. The Clock Drawing Test is particularly useful as a monitoring instrument since it can provide an easily recognizable change over time (Shulman, 2000).
- Mini-Cog is a cognitive screening test that consists of a test of delayed recall and the Clock Drawing Test (Borson et al., 2000).
- The Montreal Cognitive Assessment is a screening tool to assist clinicians in detection of mild cognitive impairment (Nasreddine, 2005).
- The Geriatric Depression Scale is useful in assessing depression in older individuals because it excludes somatic complaints from its list of items (Yesavage et al., 1983).

LABORATORY TESTS AND NEUROIMAGING

Laboratory tests, including electrocardiogram, comprehensive metabolic panel, rapid plasma reagin, vitamin B_{12} levels, endocrinological tests, toxicology panels, and other relevant or specific tests, are indicated according to the unique presenting problem and should be ordered to assess the patients. Typically, the role of imaging studies is to exclude treatable etiologies of dementia, but only 5% of dementia patients have structural abnormalities. However, in practice, the incidence of significant treatable abnormalities is much smaller (Kantarci & Jack, 2003; Murray, 2007). Neuroimaging, including high-resolution MRI and CT, is helpful in assessing the degree and place of structural damage to the brain. In many cases, the specific pattern of cortical and subcortical abnormalities on MRI has diagnostic utilities, such as early diagnosis and detection of subcortical vascular changes (Vitali et al., 2008). Functional studies, including positron emission tomography (PET) or single-photon emission computed tomography (SPECT), are not routinely used in clinics, but are helpful research tools. Even though these neuroimaging techniques are becoming sophisticated every day, for psychiatric assessment of an older patient, emphasis is still laid heavily on the detailed history and thorough clinical examination, as outlined above.

REFERENCES

American Psychiatric Association. (2012). *Position statement on substance use disorders.* Retrieved from http://www.psy chiatry.org/advocacy—newsroom/position-statements.

American Hospital Association. (2013). *Section for psychiatric and substance abuse services.* Retrieved from http://www .aha.org/about/membership/constituency/psych/index.shtml.

Applegate, W. B., Miller, S. T., Graney, M. J., Elam, J. T., Burns, R., & Akins, D. E. (1990). A randomized, controlled trial of a geriatric assessment unit in a community rehabilitation hospital. *New England Journal of Medicine, 322,* 1572–1578.

Borson, S., Scanlan, J., Brush, M., Vitaliano, P., & Dokmak, A. (2000). The mini-cog: A cognitive 'vital signs' measure for dementia screening in multi-lingual elderly. *International Journal of Geriatric Psychiatry, 15,* 1021–1027.

Brody, J. A. (2002, April 2). Hidden plague of alcohol abuse by the elderly. *New York Times.* Retrieved from http://www .nytimes.com/2002/04/02/health/personal-health-hidden-plague-of-alcohol-abuse-by-the-elderly.html?src=pm.

Choi, N. G., Sirey, J. A., & Bruce, M. L. (2013). Depression in homebound older adults: Recent advances in screening and psychosocial interventions. *Current Translational Geriatrics and Experimental Gerontology Reports, 2*(1), 16–23.

Cummings, J., & Mega, M. (2003). Neuropsychiatric assessment. In *Neuropsychiatry and behavioral neuroscience* (pp. 24–42). New York, NY: Oxford University Press.

Delafuente, J. C. (2003). Understanding and preventing drug interactions in elderly patients. *Critical Reviews in Oncology/ Hematology, 48*(2), 133–143.

Folstein, M. F., Folstein, S. E., & McHugh, P. R. (1975). Mini-mental state: A practical method for grading the cognitive state of patients for the clinicians. *Journal of Psychiatric Research, 12,* 189–198.

Gfroerer, J., Penne, M., Pemberton, M., & Folsom, R. (2003). Substance abuse treatment need among older adults in 2020: The impact of the aging baby-boom cohort. *Drug and Alcohol Dependence, 69,* 127–135.

HelpGuide.org. (2013). *Depression in older adults and the elderly: Recognize the signs and find treatment that works.* Retrieved from http://www.helpguide.org/mental/depression_elderly.htm.

Kantarci, K., & Jack, C. R., Jr. (2003). Neuroimaging in Alzheimer's disease: An evidence-based review. *Neuroimaging Clinics of North America, 13,* 197–209.

Kaplan, H. I., & Sadock, B. J. (2007). Geriatric psychiatry. In B. J. Sadock & V. A. Sadock (Eds.), *Synopsis of psychiatry: Behavioral sciences/clinical psychiatry* (10th ed., pp. 1348–1358). Baltimore, MD: Williams & Wilkins.

Kirshner, H. S., & Hoffmann, M. (2012). *Aphasia.* Retrieved from http://emedicine.medscape.com/article/1135 944-overview.

Koss, E., & Attix, D. K. (2006). Neuropsychological assessment. In M. E. Argonin & G. L. Maletta (Eds.), *Principles and practice of geriatric psychiatry* (pp. 119–136). Philadelphia, PA: Lippincott, Williams & Wilkins.

Levy, M. T. (1985). Psychiatric assessment of elderly patients in the home: A survey of 176 cases. *Journal of the American Geriatrics Society, 33,* 9–12.

Lewis, C. B., & Bottomley, J. (2007). *Geriatric rehabilitation: A clinical approach* (3rd ed.). Upper Saddle River, NJ: Prentice Hall.

Meeks, T. W., Lanouette, N., Vahia, I., Dawes, S., Jeste, D. V., & Lebowitz, B. (2009). Psychiatric assessment and diagnosis in older adults. *FOCUS, 7*(1), 3–14.

Melillo, K. D., & Houde, S. C. (2011). *Geropsychiatric and mental health nursing* (2nd ed., pp. 37–38). Sudbury, MA: Jones & Bartlett Learning.

Morris, R. G., Worsley, C., & Matthews, D. (2000). Neuropsychological assessment in older people: Old principles and new directions. *Advances in Psychiatric Treatment, 6,* 362–370.

Murray, A. D. (2007). Imaging in dementia. *Imaging, 19,* 133–141.

Nasreddine, Z. S., Phillips, N. A., Bédirian, V., Charbonneau, S., Whitehead, V., Collin, I., Cumming, J., Chertkow, H. (2005). The Montreal Cognitive Assessment, MoCA: A brief tool for mild cognitive impairment. *Journal of the American Geriatrics Society, 53,* 695–699.

National Institute of Mental Health. (2013a). *Mental health medications: Which groups have special needs when taking psychiatric medications?* Retrieved from http://www.nimh.nih.gov/health/publications/mental-health-medications/complete-index.shtml#pub9.

National Institute of Mental Health. (2013b). *Older adults: Depression and suicide facts (Fact Sheet).* Retrieved from http://www.nimh.nih.gov/health/publications/older-adults-depression-and-suicide-facts-fact-sheet/index.shtml.

Parmelee, P. A., Katz, I. R., & Lawton, M. P. (1989). Depression among institutionalized aged: Assessment and prevalence estimation. *Journal of Gerontology, 44*(1), M22–M29.

Posner, J. B., Saper, C. B., Schiff, N., & Plum, F. (2007). *Plum and Posner's diagnosis of stupor and coma* (4th ed.). New York, NY: Oxford University Press.

Quinn, C. C., Port, C. L., Zimmerman, S., Gruber-Baldini, A. L., Kasper, J. D., Fleshner, I., . . . Magaziner, J. (2008). Short-stay nursing home rehabilitation patients: Transitional care problems pose research challenges. *Journal of the American Geriatrics Society, 56*(10), 1940–1945.

Shulman, K. I. (2000). Clock-drawing: Is it the ideal cognitive screening test? *International Journal of Geriatric Psychiatry, 15*, 548–561.

Strub, R. L., & Black, F. W. (2000). *The mental status examination in neurology* (4th ed.). Philadelphia, PA: F. A. Davis.

The Merck Manual. (2013). *Routine psychiatric assessment.* Retrieved from http://www.merckmanuals.com/professional/psychiatric_disorders/approach_to_the_patient_with_mental_symptoms/routine_psychiatric_assessment.html.

U. S. Census Bureau. (2010). Retrieved from https://www.census.gov/newsroom/releases/archives/facts_for_features_special_editions/cb10-ff06.html.

Vitali, P., Migliaccio, R., Agosta, F., Rosen, H., & Geschwind, M. (2008). Neuroimaging in dementia. *Seminars in Neurology, 28*, 467–483.

Yesavage, J. A., Brink, T. L., Rose, T. L., Lum, O., Huang, V., Adey, M., & Leirer, V. O. (1983). Development and validation of a geriatric depression screening scale: A preliminary report. *Journal of Psychiatric Research, 17*, 37–49.

CHAPTER 19: IT RESOURCES

Websites

Psychiatric Assessment and Diagnosis in Older Adults
http://focus.psychiatryonline.org/article.aspx?articleID=52781

Neuropsychological Assessment in Older People: Old Principles and New Directions
http://apt.rcpsych.org/content/6/5/362.full

Assessment of Older Adults
http://www.bmj.com/bmj-series/assessment-older-adults

Digit Span Test
http://www.anselm.edu/internet/compsci/faculty_staff/mmalita/HOMEPAGE/ProjectPsych-WEB/lmendez/Project/index.html

The use of the Digit Span Test in screening for cognitive impairment in acute medical inpatients
http://www.ncbi.nlm.nih.gov/pubmed/21729426

What is Digit Span?
http://www.learninginfo.org/digit-span.htm

Attention Testing in Mental State Examination
http://attentionmmse.com/

PDF Documents

Assessment of Older Adults with Diminished Capacity: A Handbook for Lawyers
http://www.apa.org/pi/aging/resources/guides/diminished-capacity.pdf

The Mental Status Examination
http://www.testandcalc.com/richard/resources/Teaching_Resource_Mental_Status_Examination.pdf

AGS Beers Criteria for Potentially Inappropriate Medication Use in Older Adults
http://www.americangeriatrics.org/files/documents/beers/PrintableBeersPocketCard.pdf

American Geriatrics Society Updated Beers Criteria for Potentially Inappropriate Medication Use in Older Adults—The American Geriatrics Society 2012 Beers Criteria Update Expert Panel
http://www.americangeriatrics.org/files/documents/beers/2012BeersCriteria_JAGS.pdf

What Practitioners Should Know about Working with Older Adults
http://www.nova.edu/gec/forms/practitioners_older_adults.pdf

Mental Status Assessment in Older Adults: MoCA Version 7.1
http://consultgerirn.org/uploads/File/trythis/try_this_3_2.pdf

Videos

Montreal Cognitive Assessment (MoCA) (2012) (7:29 minutes)
http://youtu.be/3e3oKmtRfgM

Images

Google Images for Digit Span Test
http://www.google.com/search?q=digit+span+test&hl=en&rls=com.microsoft:en-us:
IE-Address&tbm=isch&tbo=u&source=univ&sa=X&ei=-suTUdvmKePB0AGPp4DwAw&
sqi=2&ved=0CEwQsAQ&biw=1280&bih=705

Psychosocial Challenges

Victoria Bierman, PhD, LCSW, FNP-BC

INTRODUCTION

Successful aging, healthy aging, and *productive aging* are several terms used to describe a positive approach to growing old. Old age, unfortunately, has negative connotations, such as inevitable decline, disability, and loss of independence. These negative perceptions are pervasive in society and especially among health care providers (Blazer, 2006; Hill, 2005).

The prevalence of chronic disease management and bias toward older adults increases the complexity of providing health care (Ryan & Coughlan, 2011). Approximately 80% of older adults have one chronic disease and 50% have at least two (Administration on Aging [AOA, 2009]). Biased attitudes, also known as ageism, play a significant role in the negative opinion toward treating the older population.

Within the last 50 years, the perception of aging in the United States has improved. The view of getting older has changed from one of decline in vitality to a more positive state of health and well-being. Research studies have been influential in dispelling the myth that all older adults are a burden to society. Many researchers and theorists have described successful aging using different criteria (Baltes & Baltes, 1990; Crowther et al., 2002; Depp & Jeste, 2006; Koenig, 2001; Phelan et al., 2004; Pruchno et al., 2010; Rowe & Kahn, 1987, 1997; Strawbridge et al., 2002), but, unfortunately, the ambiguity and lack of consensus on defining healthy aging has resulted in differences of opinion to the influential predictors of health.

Some of the most significant studies on aging include the Duke Longitudinal Studies of Normal Aging (Busse & Maddox, 1986), the Baltimore Longitudinal Study of Aging (Shock et al., 1984), Veterans Affairs Normative Aging Study (Bosse et al., 1991), the Study of Adult Development (Vaillant & Mukamal, 2001), Swedish Twin Study (Ljundquist et al., 1998), and particularly the MacArthur Studies of Successful Aging (Rowe & Kahn, 1987). They have all contributed valuable information to understanding the process of growing older. However, none of these studies provide strong evidence for specific predictor variables that can increase the likelihood of successful aging (Vaillant & Mukamal, 2001).

The fountain of youth has not been found; but in this chapter, we will examine the many factors, both risk and protective, that can facilitate successful aging. Health care providers will be encouraged to consider using a person-centered holistic approach and the biopsychosocial framework to identify these many factors.

HEALTHY AGING PERSPECTIVES

In the previous chapters, healthy aging was presented from a biomedical perspective focusing primarily on the disease. From a biopsychosocial approach, the focus is on assessing biological as well as psychological and social factors that impact an individual's health and well-being. This paradigm has a person-centered holistic approach that encourages patients' active participation in determining impacting factors on their illness and the meaning of the illness.

In the 1970s, Drs. George Engle and John Romano introduced the biopsychosocial approach to medicine to promote a greater understanding of health, illness, and health care delivery (Engel, 1977). This approach included both a philosophy of clinical care and a practical guideline for patient care. This paradigm has been around for a number of years and continues to be promoted by many health care professions; however, the biomedical model is the most prevalent used by the US medical health care system. The biomedical model promotes a reductionist view and encourages paternalism (Knickman & Kovner, 2008; Wade & Halligan, 2004). This model also negates the complex interaction of the multidimensional influences of biological, psychological, and social factors on health and wellness.

Most illness, whether physical or psychiatric, is influenced and determined by the combination of biopsychosocial and cultural phenomena. Many factors can influence the predisposition, onset, course, and disease outcomes (Cole et al., 1998); therefore, it is important to consider all the variables (past and present) contributing to the disease states, interfering with one's sense of well-being, and impacting social functioning.

Older adults face a number of different challenges to maintaining their health than younger adults. These challenges are a combination of factors, and include attitudes and beliefs of older adults and their health care providers (Kane et al., 2009). Currently, 13.1% of the US population is considered older (Centers for Disease Control and Prevention [CDC], 2010), and it is projected that over the next 20 years 20% of the population of the United States will be old. With the aging of America, health care services have increased demands and readjustments to meet changing needs of the aging population. One adjustment would be to change from the traditional biomedical model and embrace the biopsychosocial paradigm.

A biopsychosocial approach has been shown to improve diagnostic accuracy, promote functional and mental status, decrease medication use, reduce out-of-home placement, prolong survival rate, and decrease health care costs (Butler & Lewis, 1982; Cole et al., 1998; Engel, 1977). Others have suggested that this integrative method will improve accuracy in diagnosing and promote time-saving interventions (Kane et al., 2009). The following example explains the problems of a focused assessment. A 70-year-old, recently widowed male, presents to his primary care provider with symptoms for 3 days of persistent chest pain, shortness of breath, cough, and low grade fever. His chest x-rays were unremarkable, and his CBC was slightly elevated. He was diagnosed with bronchitis, prescribed azithromycin and an albuterol inhaler. The patient goes home alone and does not obtain his medications. In the past, his wife had managed the family finances and completing all the shopping. This patient did not obtain his medication because he lacked the knowledge of the medication's purpose, he was not familiar with the pharmacy, and he was anxious about shopping alone. His pride prevented him from asking for help; in addition, his underlying grief and limited literacy level resulted in nonadherence to treatment. The health care provider's problem focus orientation to assessing and treating only his respiratory symptoms resulted in compromised and suboptimal care.

Geriatric clinicians are notably the most skilled in providing biopsychosocial assessments; however, the number of providers trained and practicing as geriatricians is inadequate (AOA, 2009; Kane et al., 2009). The Institute of Medicine Report (Institute of Medicine of the National Academies, Committee on the Future Health Care Workforce for Older Americans, Board on Health Care Services, 2008) has recommended that all providers be educated and skilled in caring for older adults to address the projected growth of this population. This will require health care providers, as described previously, trained in providing holistic assessments to address the complexity of care (Melillo & Houde, 2011).

DEFINING THE OLDER ADULT

The term older adult reflects the chronological age of individuals 65 years and older because the United States Census Bureau (2010) unfortunately continues to categorize old age at age 65. The age of 65 is a historically socially constructed number arbitrarily selected by Chancellor Bismarck of Germany in 1880. He used age 65 as a benchmark to facilitate social policy development for older adults (Butler & Lewis, 1982). Although the United States continues to define old age beginning at age 65, this number is both an unreliable and inaccurate indicator of a person's physical and mental status (Ryan et al., 2011). Fortunately, there is a growing acknowledgment that despite chronological age, individuals age at different rates and in different ways. According to Seeman and associates (1994), individuals who appear to age optimally often display specific characteristics, activities, and lifestyle choices that appear to facilitate aging. Exercise is one of the most modifiable protective factors to promote aging (Singh et al., 2001), along with social support (Depp & Jeste, 2006) and optimistic view of life (Vaillant, 2002). By examining the demographic profile using the United States Census Bureau data (2010), this population of older adults can be better defined. The following data were obtained from the AOA (2009) and the United States Census Bureau (2010) website.

The majority of older adults live in their own homes, and only 2% reside in assisted living facilities, and 4% reside in nursing homes. Among community dwellers, 29% live alone and 47% of them, older than 75, live alone. Universally, older adults prefer to live at home and receive health care from their primary care provider and necessary in-home assistance rather than from an institutional setting. For those with functional disabilities, most in-home assistance is provided by family or friends (80%), and many spouse caregivers are as frail as their spouses. Women are primarily the caregivers (72%), and often they have to leave the workforce as a result of caregiving activities. Approximately 25% of family caregivers remain employed.

The demands of providing care for an older cognitively or physically impaired family member increases the risk of abuse or neglect (Greenberg et al., 1999). Elder mistreatment, both physical abuse and neglect, psychological abuse and neglect, financial abuse and neglect, and the violation of personal rights has become a public health issue with between 1.5 and 2 million older adults annually reporting mistreatment (National Center on Elder Abuse, Administration on Aging, 2008).

When older adults decide to leave their home, it is usually related to concerns for safety associated with a deteriorated neighborhood, limited mobility due to structural barriers, inadequate resources to maintain their home, limited accessibility to public transportation, and limited support systems (Center for Civic Partnerships, 2010). The most active elders choose to move into a retirement community for the available amenities and social activities.

Despite the choice some have to live near family for added support, others have limited options. The increase in mobility among many younger adults does not support parental caregiving and inhibits relationship building among grandparents and grandchildren. The limited opportunities to experience the vitality of healthy aging parents and the necessity to intervene when health issues arise can alter perceptions and contribute to ageism. Research has shown children who are more familiar with older adults, such as grandparents, develop more positive attitudes toward the older adult (Bales et al., 2000). In addition, families can benefit from the nurturance and guidance provided by grandparents.

This generation of older adults experience higher rates of divorce and marital separation (12.4%) than previous generations. The educational level has increased, with 22.5% having obtained at least a bachelor's degree, and the number of older women (65 to 69) continuing to work has steadily increased. Women continue to outlive men by 23%, and 40% of older women are widowed.

According to the Administration on Aging (2009), Social Security provides 87% of income for older people, and 26% continued to earn income from employment. Nine percent live below the poverty level, and another 5.8% are classified as near poor (income between the poverty level). Those with the highest poverty rates are women (10.7%) and those living alone (16%). The number of women living to a very old age has increased with many unique and difficult late-life issues associated with widowhood. Women are three times more likely to have stressful transitions and greater negative socioeconomic consequences than men. Many women did not establish careers and are therefore dependent upon widow pensions or assistance programs. Among the women who were employed outside the home, they retired with less income due to receiving less salary than men doing the same job.

Older Americans spent 13.2% of their total expenses on health, which is greater than twice the amount spent by all consumers. The cost of insurance is 65% of all expenditures; additionally, 18% of expenses are for medical services and 17% for medications. Fortunately, less than 1% lack insurance coverage, and 93.1% receive supplemental Medicare (AOA, U.S. Department of Health and Human Services [HHS], 2011).

Racial diversity among the older adults has increased in the United States, with documented disparities in income, health insurance, and health care (Laditka et al., 2009). The highest poverty rates are among older Hispanics and African Americans (CDC, 2010). Ethnic minorities also face other barriers, such as limited access to all types of services and lower health literacy (AOA, HHS, 2011).

BIOPSYCHOSOCIAL CHALLENGES

Older adults, as discussed, are a diverse group exposed to a wide range of physical, psychological, social, environmental, cultural, and historical factors that contribute to both vulnerability and resilience (Greene & Adelman, 1996; Ryan et al., 2011). What makes one individual more vulnerable and another resilient to life's stressors remains theoretical. We can only speculate as to the causes, but many suggest that the longer one lives, the more likely they are exposed to experiences and stressors requiring adaptation (Kahana et al., 2012; Kasen et al., 2010).

Successful aging is associated with many risk and protective factors, and from a home health perspective, assessing these factors requires a holistic approach, considering the environmental, cultural, spiritual, nutritional, and physical assessments (Barry, 1998). The study of successful aging and identifying modifiable factors will be even more essential as the number of older adults increases and their impact on health care delivery is extensive.

A comprehensive review of quantitative studies by Depp and Jeste (2006) identified 28 studies on successful aging. Most of the definitions associated with healthy aging focused on an absence of disease or physical impairment, a biological perspective, and very few considered psychosocial factors in their definition. The strongest predictors for successful aging included the absence of arthritis, absence of hearing problems, not smoking, being chronologically younger, and better performance at activities of daily living. The moderate influential predictors of successful aging were ability to perform higher physical activities, better self-rated health, lower systolic blood pressures, fewer chronic diseases, higher cognitive function, and the absence of depression. Those predictors of less importance were higher income levels, higher education level, being currently married, and being white. The use of socioeconomic variables in the definitions was so limited that their strength in predicting successful aging could not be measured. Despite the lack of consensus on defining successful aging, one third of the subjects were classified as aging successfully. Even though the predictors for successful aging varied, several modifiable variables were suggested.

Rowe and Kahn's (1997) prevailing model described successful aging as a multidimensional concept. The characteristics most attributed to successful aging were freedom from disease and disability, greater cognitive, physical, and social functioning. Yet another multidimensional perspective by Baltes and Baltes (1990) emphasized that success at aging included the ability to respond and adapt to changes in life. The biological, psychological, and social constructs of Rowe and Kahn's model were expanded by Crowther and colleagues (2002) to include the concept of positive spirituality. Positive spirituality incorporated both religion and spirituality and explained the importance of religious beliefs to aging successfully. Their cognitive framework proposes that religious beliefs result in decreased stress and add an increase in purpose and meaning to life.

A subjective dimension to successful aging was proposed by Strawbridge et al. (2002). They promote defining successful aging from older persons' rating their own success at aging, independent of disease and disability. Pruchno et al. (2010) added both objective and subjective criteria to define successful aging.

Although individual variability with aging is explained by multiple theoretical models, and many account for social and contextual factors that impact healthy adjustment, psychosocial theories focus on how people cope with health challenges.

Physiological Challenges and Successful Aging

Multiple biopsychosocial factors impact health and aging, and these factors, although outlined under separate headings in the following sections, are inseparable. From a physiological perspective, disease processes and functional limitations have the greatest impact on successful aging (Hill, 2005). Themes of loss, deterioration of health and function, and the decline in functional reserves are persistent challenges associated with age-related decline. Functional impairments with limitations in activity are common, with over 50% of older adults reporting having at least one type of disability: physical, mental, or sensory (AOA, 2010). The presence of any disability has a major impact on aging successfully. The increased risk of chronic disease is an additional burden related to the general decline in body processes (Aiken, 1999; Hill, 2005). When co-morbid conditions are added, such as acute or chronic illness, nutrition and hydration deficits, delirium, dementia, decline in economic resources, environmental stressors, additional medica-tions, psychological and social stressors, the challenges can be overwhelming (Barry, 1998). The loss of independence that occurs because of decline in health puts an additional burden on the older population (Callahan et al., 2005).

Despite the significant increase in life expectancy in the last 100 years, from age to 49.2 to 83.8 (CDC, 2010), the prospects of aging appear bleak when we focus on the prevalence of chronic diseases and functional impairment. Unfortunately, 37% of older persons reported some type of disability (CDC, 2010). These disabilities included hearing, vision, and ambulation difficulty, or a decline in cognition or self-care. The risk of disability increases with age. Fifty-six percent report a severe disability and a need for assistance with activities of daily living or instrumental activities of daily living. The presence of severe disabilities has been associated with lower-income levels and educational attainment (AOA, 2010).

Conversely, many older adults experience a sense of well-being despite disabilities and func-tional decline. Positive responses to change, diseases, and disabilities shape how one interprets events and experiences of life (Vaillant, 2002). When the focus is on the positive, and not the problems and difficulties with growing old, actions to enhance health and promote optimal func-tioning can occur. A decline in health can motivate the older adult to modify risk factors and adopt protective factors. These behavioral changes can include increasing physical activity, cessa-tion of smoking, accessing resources to make physical modifications to the environment, and re-framing thoughts to positively interpret life events (Hill, 2005). The perception of positive aging can generate an affirmative sense of well-being and cultivate flexibility to cope with additional life experiences (Greve & Staudinger, 2006).

Psychological Challenges and Healthy Aging

Psychological aging focuses on the ability to respond and adapt to changing environments (Baltes & Baltes, 1990; Ryan et al., 2011). This involves engaging cognitive processes with learn-ing, memory, intelligence, motivation, emotions, feelings, and assigning meaning to life (Birren & Schaie, 1977; Depp & Jeste, 2006; Meis, 2005). As previously asserted, psychological adjustments are a frequent reality for older adults.

One of the most common emotional experiences encountered by the older adult is loss, and, unfortunately, loss is an inevitable consequence of aging. Losses impact many aspects of life, and much physical and emotional energy is expended in dealing with grief. This can include adapting to change associated with losses and resolving grief (Ryan et al., 2011). Multiple losses can occur simultaneously, such as the death of a significant other, a change in living standards, a decline in health and loss of independence, and the loss of prestige and status with retirement. A wide range of experiences can be interpreted as loss. Some of these include loss of health, function, mobility, independence, and loss of sensory function (hearing and vision). Some psychological losses as-sociated with physiological changes include cognitive, libido, and body image (Kane et al., 2009). Other psychological losses can include self-esteem, loss of influence and power, a purpose to life, willingness to live, and spiritual beliefs. Social losses can include financial security, home, friend-ships, church associations, and affiliation with groups. Considering the individuals' perception and meaning of the loss is vital to their well-being (Vaillant & Mukamal, 2001).

Coping with loss is complex and takes place on multiple levels. Personal factors influence the reaction to loss; such factors include age, prior losses, gender, race/ethnicity, relationship with the deceased, and type of death (expected or unexpected). Losses can threaten the psychology reserves and well-being of those who grieve and result in lower levels of functioning. The experiences of loss and grief have been identified as risk factors for mental health issues; however, other studies reveal that losses in later life can both facilitate and hinder adjustment (Zisook et al., 1997).

The existence of a spiritual belief system is a strength that facilitates resolving grief and contributes to the subjective sense of successful aging (Pruchno et al., 2010). Worldwide, religious beliefs influence an individual's perception of the world and provide meaning to the circumstances and experiences with living (Hill, 2005). The concept of religion is pervasive in the US culture, and 82% of the population acknowledges a personal need for spiritual growth (Gallup & Jones, 2000). A body of research suggests that perceptions based on religious beliefs are positively associated with health; one's personal belief system can be a protective factor for the prevention of diseases (Miller & Thoresen, 2003). Diseases can be prevented by an enhanced sense of well-being associated with services to others, attending church services, socializing with other believers, and engaging in church activities. According to Hill (2005), older adults are the most likely group to consider religious beliefs as an important resource in coping with life's challenges.

Other factors that contribute most to resilience and ability to cope with losses include personal and social competence, family and social support systems, and physical and emotional resources (Greve & Staudinger, 2006; Hill, 2005; Nilsson et al., 2000). Evidence exists that older adults can manage the experiences of loss well and progress through the normal reactions and stages of grief (Hansson & Stroebe, 2007; Ryan et al., 2011), but the experience of coping with grief is complex, and bereavement is highly variable.

Frequent experiences with losses have also been associated with a significant threat to the subjective quality of life and increase in distress. Symptoms of anxiety and depression early in the course of bereavement have been linked with subsequent medical and psychological illness (Chen et al., 1999), and it becomes more difficult to assess and differentiate between symptoms of anxiety and depression in later life (Beckman et al., 2000). The prevalence of anxiety symptoms ranges from 15% to 52.3% in the community of older adults (Mental Health America [MHA], 2012). The fear of one's own mortality and nature of death contributes to anxiety (Field, 2000) as well as past regrets and the associated meaning of loss (Tomer, 2000). The increase in death anxiety is associated with greater psychological and physical health problems (Fortner & Neimeyer, 1999). Experiences of loss and unresolved grief issues are one of the most serious risk factors for suicide (De Leo et al., 2002).

Suicide of our older adults has a significant impact on society. The CDC (2010) reports that 13% of all deaths are attributed to suicide, while 20% of older adults die from suicide. Those at most risk are older men who are three times as likely to commit suicide, and 81% of them use a firearm (CDC, 2010). Risk factors for suicide also include untreated depression, feelings of desperation, chronic illness, social isolation, and the use of alcohol and substance abuse, which increases disinhibition and fosters impulsive acts (American Foundation for Suicide Prevention, 2013). Older adults with untreated mental illness are the most vulnerable.

In the United States, mental health care needs have been viewed as secondary and disconnected from physical needs (Sivis et al., 2005). Prior to the mid-20th century, mental illness in the older adult was assumed to be part of the aging process (Gerontological Society of America, 2008). When symptoms of mental illness appeared in later life, it was commonly attributed to age-related changes. This is a common perception that results in untreated symptoms and neglect by the medical community (Collier & Sorrell, 2011). Neglected mental health care needs, such as depression, exacerbate physical health and lead to greater consequences with increased self-neglect, premature institutionalization, hospitalization, and increasing greater costs to society (O'Donoghue & Ryan, 2011).

Depression also coincides with other medical issues, and the symptoms of depression are often overlooked and untreated as people age (MHA, 2012). This may be due to the continued assumption that depression is a normal consequence of aging, but depression is not a normal response. Over 34 million older adults suffer with depression, and it is a leading cause of disability, morbidity, and risk of suicide (Blazer, 2006). The MHA Survey (2012) revealed that 68% of older adults know very little about depression, 58% believe it is normal for people to get depressed as they grow older, and 38% believe depression is a health problem. It is important for providers to assess for anxiety and depression because it can be triggered by chronic illnesses and older adults with depression increase health care costs by 50% (MHA, 2012).

The number of older adults with mental illness is expected to double in the next 20 years (Cohen et al., 2008), and as the number of older adults increases, the number of those who experience mental health issues and serious psychiatric illnesses will also increase. Those who experience mental disorders, such as depression, dementia, anxiety, unresolved grief issues, or even schizophrenia, are more vulnerable to the lack of continuity of care and less likely to receive a comprehensive biopsychosocial assessment. Stigma is a very powerful obstacle to seeking care for mental health issues and is especially strong among the older population. Studies have shown that medical providers lack uniformity in evaluating older adults with mental health issues, such as not gathering routine information or failing to provide treatment (Butler & Lewis, 1982; Shawler, 2010). Only 50% of older adults receive mental health treatment from primary care providers, and primary care providers accurately recognize less than 50% of patients with depression (Segal et al., 2005). Older adults with a history of mental illness have increased mortality, which may be due to attitudes of health care providers, patient characteristics from nonadherence to treatment, unhealthy lifestyles, lack of financial resources, and health care system dynamics limiting service availability (Collier & Sorrell, 2011).

The decline in cognition has a significant impact on successful aging. Dementia is the general term for cognitive decline that is both progressive and devastating. This neurodegenerative disorder impairs memory, thinking, and behaviors and is the most prevalent mental illness experienced by older adults (Alzheimer's Association, 2012). Dementia has the greatest impact on the older adult's emotional, social, and physical functioning; it is not a normal aging process, but as one ages, the risk of dementia increases (O'Reilly et al., 2011). The number of those experiencing dementia will double by 2030 and more than triple by 2050; dementia is described as a "public health priority" by the World Health Organization (WHO, 2013), and the ramifications of dementia are devastating. With the lack of awareness and understanding of dementia and the resulting stigmatization and barriers to the diagnosis of dementia, the Alzheimer's Association (2012) has published recommendations to help providers detect cognitive impairment. Society must address the physical, psychological, and economic impact of dementia.

Emotional adjustments are a frequent reality for older adults. Those who are most successful with psychological aging have a more optimistic appraisal of life and develop a positive sense of well-being. Protective factors contributing to healthy aging are a sense of spirituality, optimistic life view, increased self-identity, and self-confidence. Strawbridge and colleagues (2002) suggest emotional experiences improve with aging, as evidenced by a greater regulation of emotions and a less negative effect from life experiences.

Social Challenges and Healthy Aging

Most changes and difficulties associated with growing older have social implications (Ryan et al., 2011; Segerstrom et al., 2012). Generally, older adults experience a decline in financial resources, reduced social support, increase in chronic diseases and functional decline.

Social factors with the greatest health impact include level of independence, financial security, family role, support network, and social relationships (Hill, 2005). The meaning attributed to a decline in any of these social factors can have a significant impact on the success of aging.

Social influences inducing positive aging are identified as being currently married, being employed or volunteering, practicing healthy behaviors, having adequate support systems, and practicing religious beliefs (Pruchno et al., 2010; Rowe & Kahn, 1997). Many have suggested that the quality of our support systems has a direct positive effect on health and buffers some of the health-related effects of aging (Eysenck, 2000; Thanakwang, 2009; Wienclaw, 2009; Yoon, 2006).

Having caregiver support is a lifeline for many older adults unable to care for themselves. Close friends and family members have historically been providers of care for the older adult and are considered the backbone of the health care systems worldwide (IOM, 2008). With the projected growth of this population and increase in chronic illnesses, the need for and demands on caregivers is even greater. Many have projected caregiving as a public health crisis due to the number of family members having to provide care, hours spent with caregiving, and the overwhelming tasks they perform (Gitlin & Schultz, 2012). Despite its rewards, the role of a caregiver is challenging, and many suffer from negative health effects and higher rates of anxiety and depression than non-caregivers (Pinquart & Sorensen, 2003). The act of caregiving does not end once a family member is placed in long-term care; many provide frequent, if not daily, onsite monitoring and hands-on personal care. Caregiving is also episodic, with accompanying the older adult to medical appointments, or intermittent, providing limited care during recuperation from surgery. It is estimated that caregiving is equivalent to $257 billion in free care annually (AOA, 2004). In 2000, the National Family Caregiver Support Act was signed into law by President George W. Bush. This act mandated support and education to assist family caregivers with resources administered through the National Family Caregiver Support Program (AOA, 2004). With the provision of support and resources to caregivers, the long-term impact will be to diminish caregiver burden, prevent and delay the costly out-of-home placements, and improve care for the older adult.

In the United States, the average life expectancy favors those with greater social and economic resources (Hill, 2005; United States Census Bureau, 2010). This group tends to have greater access to medical care, fewer exposures to environmental hazards and stressors, improved diet, advanced education to navigate the health care system, greater participation in health promotion activities, resources for recreational outlets, participation in more social activities, and resources to modify their environment to allow for greater mobility (Pinquart & Sorensen, 2000). When older adults participate in civic and service activities, the meaning and purpose to their lives is enhanced (Segerstrom et al., 2012).

The lower socioeconomic groups have fewer economic resources and have more difficulty achieving healthy aging owing to limited access to health care (Cloutterbuck, 2011; Gallo et al., 2005; Marmot, 1999). Poverty and illness together increase vulnerabilities for the older adult. The poor are more likely to become ill and die at younger ages; they have a higher prevalence of disabilities and chronic diseases than those at higher economic levels. Those of lower-income status tend to reside in poor environmental situations and have limited health care resources. The relationship among poverty and health is complex. Those in poverty have lower educational levels, decreased awareness of needed medical care, financial barriers to access health services, and lack of resources to maintain good health status (Matthews et al., 2010). A limited budget results in more processed, fatty, and less nutritious food choices. Access to care can be poor owing to a limited number of providers in lower-income areas, transportation issues, provider discrimination, inability to pay for care and medications (Marmot, 1999). Public programs play a vital role in decreasing health disparities, but provide only for the most basic needs (Ryan & Wroblewska, 2011).

All older adults living on fixed incomes are especially vulnerable to local economic hardships. The reductions in public services related to declines in property and sales tax revenues, the decline in housing markets, rising unemployment, and reduced consumer spending have resulted in cuts to public services and welfare programs (Center for Civic Partnerships, 2010).

Environmental challenges for older adults include affordable housing and mobility concerns. Older adults may have difficulty finding adequate housing at a reasonable cost, and physical barriers may limit access. Buildings are often designed both inside and out, which make them unsuitable for people with a limited range of physical ability. The existence of uneven sidewalks multiple-level floor plans requiring maneuvering of staircases, narrow halls and bathroom doorways are some of the features that can be challenging to older adults. Some apartments discriminate against the older adult and restrict the sharing of housing. The loss of driving privileges, lack of available transportation, and unaffordable transit fees are often barriers to independence. This can reduce access to grocery stores, pharmacies, medical clinics and dental offices, as well as to community centers for social activities (Center for Civic Partnerships, 2010).

Thankfully, the protective factors of healthy aging are primarily modifiable factors independent of economic status or education and include subjective well-being, perceived health, good social relationships, and an active lifestyle (Nilsson et al., 2000). A change in the older adult's perspective from one of being materialistic and self-centered to a more introspective discernment can promote adaptation to their experience with multiple losses (Brown & Lowis, 2003).

Retired persons are valuable assets to any community with more time to volunteer their skills and experiences to promote service and civic affairs. Volunteering in turn enhances their health and well-being and reduces feelings of isolation and loneliness.

Cultural Perspectives and Successful Aging

Racism and poverty are tied to health outcomes. Racial and ethnic groups are generally poorer and face significant health disparities with more illness and more complications (Cloutterbuck, 2011). Differences in poverty rates exist among minorities, Blacks and Latinos experiencing greater poverty rates and poorer health outcomes. Heart disease rates are 40% greater in Blacks than Whites, Latinos are twice as likely to die from diabetes, and the rate of diabetes among American Indians and Alaska Natives is twice that of Whites (CDC, 2010). These disparities have been associated with the complex interaction of genetics, environmental factors, and specific health behaviors (Marmot, 1999). Racism has been shown to impact lives with increased prejudicial stressors. Being of a minority race results in greater exploitation due to insecurities, and a sense of self-hatred was found in victims of discrimination (Cloutterbuck, 2011).

Other victims of discrimination are those with mental illness. Mental illness is both a cause and a consequence of poverty (O'Connell-Kehoe & Coughlan, 2011). Mental health issues compromise education, increase vulnerabilities, and present with greater difficulties accessing housing, health care, employment, and health promotion interventions. Those who suffer the most from mental health disparities are racial minorities, those with low incomes, and residents of rural areas. Less than half of the people diagnosed with mental illness, particularly Blacks, do not receive treatment. Stigma and the failure to seek treatment are only two of the associated causes (O'Connell-Kehoe & Coughlan, 2011).

Older adults are multiracial and multicultural with unique cultural values, beliefs, and perceptions that impact their lives (Butler & Lewis, 1982; Ryan & Wroblewska, 2011). Care and respect for the older population is influenced by different beliefs and values. Some ethnic groups demonstrate care and respect better than others. Asian cultures express a fundamental belief in and ascribe value to parental caregiving, under the influence of Confucianism associated with the concept of care (Fan, 2002). Koreans believe families live together to provide support and care for parents, and the neglect of this role results in shame to the family (Park & Cho, 1995; Yang & Rosenblatt, 2001). In Latin America, the cultural norm is for women to be the primary caregivers of aging parents, and they are expected to provide care as long as possible (Phillips et al., 2000). In the United States, care and respect toward older adults can be lacking, and a discriminatory attitude toward the older population as burdens to society can persist (Tataru & Dicker, 2009).

Now that diversity makes up 20% of the US older adult population and in the next 50 years, diversity will increase to 64% of the population (CDC, 2010), ageism can improve. Because ageism plays a significant role in the negative opinion about older adults and influences delivery of care (Lalor & Ryan, 2011), providers are in a position to modify this issue. They need to acknowledge and eliminate their own discriminatory practices and serve as models for others. As community leaders, providers can gain knowledge in cultural competence and respect for ethnic older adults' cultural values and beliefs.

In summary, successful aging is multidimensional and is impacted by a combination of biological, psychological, and sociocultural factors and ageism. Despite the lack of an agreement on the definition of successful aging, many of the identified risk and protective factors are modifiable. When we place an emphasis on modifying risk factors and a greater focus on the assets and not the deficits of older adults, we can adjust the distorted societal view of the older adult.

CONCLUSION

The prevalent image of older adults includes physical frailty, poverty, social isolation, loneliness, depression, and imminent death. This perception can change, and the reader is encouraged to examine the individual's uniqueness and focus on the contributions and resilience of this population.

With the growing aging population and the associated costs of care, the necessity to provide quality health care cannot be ignored. A patient-centered holistic approach with a biopsychosocial framework enhances the well-being of individuals, families, and communities. This begins with addressing ageism on the part of provider and patient, recognizing the importance of relationships in health delivery, eliciting the patient's history and perspective of the illness, allowing adequate time to process questions, determining what aspects of the biological, psychological, and social factors are most important in promoting health, and providing multidimensional treatment with services and referrals (Kane et al., 2009). Interventions are available to address many of the psychological and social factors if needs are identified; therefore a focus of health care would include both reducing factors that increase risks and strengthening factors that protect health.

Older adults are living longer, enjoying better health, and experiencing the benefits of activities more than any past generation. Although chronic disease and functional decline are a part of age-related decline, health promotion and disease prevention have reduced this burden. As the increase in diversity continues in the United States, cultural influences can improve the concept of care for the older population. The perception of older adults as a burden on society and consumer of most economic resources can change by focusing education on communities, providers, and policy makers. This emphasis would be on promoting a better understanding of the interrelationship among all the biopsychosocial and cultural factors that contribute to health and a sense of well-being and reducing barriers, and providing access to available resources.

REFERENCES

Administration on Aging. (2004). *Compassion in action.* Retrieved from http://www.aoa.gov/aoaroot/program_results/docs/Program_Eval/FINAL%20NFCSP%20Report%20July22,%202004.pdf

Administration on Aging. (2009). *A profile of older Americans: 2009.* Washington, DC: Author. Retrieved from http://www.aoa.gov/AoARoot/Aging_Statistics/Profile/2009/2.aspx

Administration on Aging, U.S. Department of Health and Human Services. (2011). *A profile of older Americans: 2011.* Retrieved from http://www.aarp.org/content/dam/aarp/livable-communities/learn/demographics/a-profile-of-older-americans-2011-aarp.pdf

Aiken, L. (1999). *Human differences.* Mahwah, NJ: Lawrence Erlbaum Associates.

Alzheimer's Association. (2012). *Alzheimer's disease: facts & figures.* Retrieved from http://www.alz.org/documents_custom/report_alzfactsfigures2010.pdf

American Foundation for Suicide Prevention. (2013). Risk factors for suicide. Retrieved from http://www.afsp.org/preventing-suicide/risk-factors-and-warning-signs

Bales, S., Eklund, S., & Siffin, C. (2000). Children's perceptions of elders before and after a school-based intergenerational program. *Educational Gerontology, 26*(7), 667–689.

Baltes, P. B., & Baltes, M. M. (1990). Psychological perspectives on successful aging: The model of selective optimization with compensation. In P. B. Baltes & M. M. Baltes (Eds.), *Successful aging: Perspectives from the behavioral sciences* (pp. 1–34). Cambridge, MA: Cambridge University Press. doi:10.1017/CBO9780511665684.003

Barry, C. B. (1998). Assessing the older adult in the home. *Home Healthcare Nurse, 16*(8), 519–529.

Beckman, A. T., de Beurs, E., van Balkom, A., Deeg, D., van Dyck, R., & van Tilburg, W. (2000). Anxiety and depression in later life: Co-occurrence and communality of risk factors. *American Journal of Psychiatry, 157*, 89–95.

Birren, J., & Schaie, K. (1977). *Handbook of the psychology of aging.* San Diego, CA: Academic Press.

Blazer, D. G. (2006). Successful aging [Editorial]. *American Journal of Geriatric Psychiatry, 14*(1), 2–5.

Bosse, R., Aldwin, C. M., Levenson, M. R., & Workman-Daniels, K. (1991). How stressful is retirement? Findings from the Normative Aging Study. *Journal of Gerontology, Psychology, and Science, 46*, 9–14.

Brown, C., & Lowis, M. J. (2003). Psychosocial development in the elderly: An investigation into Erikson's ninth stage. *Journal of Aging Studies, 17*, 415–426.

Busse, E. W., & Maddox, G. L. (1986). *The Duke longitudinal studies of normal aging: 1955–1980.* New York, NY: Springer.

Butler, R. N., & Lewis, M. L. (1982). *Aging and mental health: Positive, psychological and biomedical approaches* (3rd ed.). St. Louis, MO: C. V. Mosby.

Callahan, C., Kroenke, K., Counsell, S., Hendrie, H., Perkins, A., Katon, W., . . . Unützer, J. (2005). Treatment of depression improves physical functioning in older adults. *Journal of the American Geriatrics Society, 53*, 367–373.

Center for Civic Partnerships. (2010). *Aging well in communities: A toolkit for planning, engagement and action.* Retrieved from http://www.civicpartnerships.org/docs/services/CHCC/aging-well.htm

Centers for Disease Control and Prevention. (2010). *Behavioral risk factor surveillance system survey data.* Atlanta, GA: U.S. Department of Health and Human Services, Centers for Disease Control and Prevention. Retrieved from http://cdc.gov/brfss/

Chen, J., Bierhals, A., Prigerson, H., Kasl, S., Mazure, C., & Jacobs, S. (1999). Gender differences in the effects of bereavement-related psychological distress in health outcomes. *Psychological Medicine, 29*, 367–380.

Cloutterbuck, J. (2011). Ethnic elders. In K. D. Melillo & S. C. Houde (Eds.), *Geropsychiatric and mental health nursing* (2nd ed.). Sudbury, MA: Jones & Bartlett Learning.

Cohen, C., Vahia, I., Reyes, P., Diwan, S., Bankole, A.O., Palekar, N., Kehn, M., Ramirez, P. (2008). Focus on geriatric psychiatry: Schizophrenia in later life: Clinical symptoms and social well-being. *Psychiatric Services, 59*(3): 232–234.

Cole, S. A., Saravay, S. M., & Levinson, R. M. (1998). The biopsychosocial model in medical practice. In A. Stoudemire (Ed.), *Human behavior: An introduction for medical students* (3rd ed., pp. 36–84). Philadelphia, PA: Lippincott, Williams & Wilkins.

Collier, E., & Sorrell, J. M. (2011). Schizophrenia in older adults. *Journal of Psychosocial Nursing and Mental Health Services, 49*(11), 17–21. doi:10.3928/02793695-20111004-04

Crowther, M. R., Parker, M. W., Achenbaum, W. A., Larimore, W. L., & Koenig, H. G. (2002). Rowe and Kahn's model of successful aging revisited: Positive spirituality—The forgotten factor. *Gerontologist, 42*(5), 613–620. doi:10.1093/geront/42.5.613

De Leo, D., Buono, M., & Dwyer, J. (2002). Suicide among the elderly: The long-term impact of a telephone support and assessment intervention in northern Italy. *British Journal of Psychiatry, 181*, 226–229.

Depp, C. A., & Jeste, D. V. (2006). Definitions and predictors of successful aging: A comprehensive review of larger quantitative studies. *American Journal of Geriatric Psychiatry, 14*, 6–20.

Engel, G. (1977). The need for a new medical model: A challenge for biomedicine. *Science, 196*, 129–136.

Eysenck, M. W. (2000). *Psychology—A student's handbook*. Hove, England: Psychology Press.

Fan, R. (2002). Reconstructionist Confucianism and health care: An Asian moral account of health care resource allocation. *Journal of Medicine and Philosophy, 27*(6), 675–682.

Field, D. (2000). Older people's attitudes toward death in England. *Mortality: Promoting the Interdisciplinary Study of Death and Dying, 5*(3), 277–297.

Fortner, B., & Neimeyer, R. (1999). Death anxiety in older adults: A quantitative review. *Death Studies, 23*(5), 387–411.

Gallo, L. C., Bogart, L. M., Vranceanu, A. M., & Matthews, K. A. (2005). Socioeconomic status, resources, psychological experiences, and emotional responses: A test of the reserve capacity model. *Journal of Personality and Social Psychology, 88*(2), 386–399.

Gallup, G., Jr., & Jones, T. (2000). *The next American spirituality: Finding God in the twenty-first century*. Colorado Springs, CO: Cook Communications.

Gerontological Society of America. (2008). Fact sheet. Retrieved from http://www.geron.org/About%20Us/Fact%20 Sheet

Gitlin, L., & Schultz, R. (2012). Family caregiving of the older adult. In T. R. Prohaska, L. A. Anderson, & R. Binstock (Eds.), *Public health for an aging society* (pp. 181–204). Baltimore, MD: John Hopkins University Press.

Greenberg, S., Ramsey, G., Mitty, E., & Fulmer, T. (1999). Elder mistreatment: Case law and ethical issues in assessment, reporting and management. *Journal of Nursing Law, 6*(3), 7–20.

Greene, M., & Adelman, R. (1996). Psychosocial factors in older patients' medical encounters. *Research on Aging, 18*(1), 84–102.

Greve, W., & Staudinger, U. (2006). Resilience in later adulthood and old age: Resources and potentials for successful aging. In D. Cicchetti & D. J. Cohen (Eds.), *Developmental psychopathology: Risk, disorder, and adaptation* (2nd ed., Vol. 3). Hoboken, NJ: John Wiley & Sons.

Hansson, R. O., & Stroebe, M. S. (2007). *Bereavement in late life: Coping, adaptation, and developmental influences*. Washington, DC: American Psychological Association.

Hill, R. D. (2005). *Positive aging: A guide for mental health professionals and consumers*. New York, NY: W. W. Norton.

Institute of Medicine of the National Academies, Committee on the Future Health Care Workforce for Older Americans, Board on Health Care Services. (2008). *Retooling for an aging America: Building the health care workforce*. Washington, DC: National Academies Press.

Kahana, E., Kelley-Moore, J., & Kahana, B. (2012). Proactive aging: A longitudinal study of stress, resources, agency, and well-being in late life. *Aging & Mental Health, 16*(4), 438–451.

Kane, R. L., Ouslander, J. G., Abrass, I. B., & Resnick, B. (2009). *Essentials of clinical geriatrics* (6th ed.). New York, NY: McGraw Hill.

Kasen, S., Chen, H., Sneed, J. R., & Cohen, P. (2010). Earlier stress exposure and subsequent major depression in aging women. *International Journal of Geriatric Psychiatry, 25*(1), 91–99. doi:10.1002/gps.2304

Knickman, J. R., & Kovner, A. R. (2008). Overview: The state of health care delivery in the United States. In A. R. Kovner & J. R. Knickman (Eds.), *Jonas & Kovner's health care delivery in the United States* (9th ed.). New York, NY: Springer.

Koenig, H. G. (2001). Religion and medicine III: Developing a theoretical model. *International Journal of Psychiatry in Medicine, 31*, 199–216.

Laditka, S., Corwin, S., Laditka, J., Liu, R., Tseng, W., Wu, B., . . . Ivey, S. (2009). Attitudes about aging well among a diverse group of older Americans: Implications for promoting cognitive health. *Gerontologist, 49*(Suppl. 1), S30–S39. doi:10.1093/geront/gnp084

Lalor, J., & Ryan, P. (2011). Ageism: Myth or fact? In P. Ryan & J. Coughlan (Eds.), *Ageing and older adult mental health: Issues and implications for practice* (pp. 36–49). New York, NY: Routledge.

Ljundquist, B., Berg, S., Lanke, J., McClearn, G. E., & Pedersen, N. L. (1998). The effect of genetic factors for longevity: A comparison of identical and fraternal twins in the Swedish Twin Registry. *Journal of Gerontology, Series A: Biological Sciences and Medical Sciences, 53A*(6), M441–M446.

Marmot, M. (1999). Acting on the evidence to reduce inequalities in health. *Health Affairs, 18*(3), 42–44.

Matthews, K. A., Gallo, L. C., & Taylor, S. E. (2010). Are psychosocial factors mediators of socioeconomic status and health connections? A progress report and blueprint for the future. *Annals of the New York Academy of Sciences, 1186*, 146–173. doi:10.1111/j.1749-6632.2009.05332.x

Meis, M. (2005). Geriatric orphans: A study of severe isolation in an elderly population. *Dissertation Abstracts International Section A,* 65.

Melillo, K. D., & Houde, S. C. (2011). *Geropsychiatric and mental health nursing* (2nd ed.). Sudbury, MA: Jones & Bartlett Learning.

Mental Health America. (2012). Social determinants of health. Retrieved from http://www.mentalhealthamerica.net/go/socialdeterminants

Miller, W. R., & Thoresen, C. E. (2003). Spirituality, religion, and health: An emerging research field. *American Psychologist, 58*(1), 24–35.

National Center on Elder Abuse, Administration on Aging. (2008). Retrieved from http://ncea.aoa.gov/FAQ/Type_Abuse/

Nilsson, M., Sarvimäki, A., & Ekman, S. (2000). Feeling old: Being in a phase of transition in later life. *Nursing Inquiry, 7*(1), 41–49.

O'Connell-Kehoe, D., & Coughlan, B. (2011). Assessment of mental health issues: Approaches and frameworks. In P. Ryan & B. Coughlan (Eds.), *Ageing and older adult mental health: Issues and implications for practice* (pp. 50–65). New York, NY: Routledge.

O'Donoghue, M., & Ryan, P. (2011). Depression and aging: Assessment and intervention. In P. Ryan & J. Coughlan (Eds.), *Ageing and older adult mental health: Issues and implications for practice* (pp. 127–142). New York, NY: Routledge.

O'Reilly, O., Lavin, D., & Coughlan, B. (2011). Ageing and dementia: Assessment and intervention. In P. Ryan & B. Coughlan (Eds.), *Ageing and older adult mental health: Issues and implications for practice* (pp. 89–108). New York, NY: Routledge.

Park, I. H., & Cho, L. J. (1995). Confucianism and the Korean framework for Asian family study. *Journal of Comparative Family Studies, 26*, 117–125.

Phelan, E. A., Anderson, L. A., LaCroix, A. Z., & Larson, E. B. (2004). Older adults' views of "successful aging"—How do they compare with researchers' definitions? *Journal of the American Geriatrics Society, 52*, 211–216.

Phillips, L. R., Torres de Ardon, R., Kommenich, P., Killen, M., & Rusinak, R. (2000). The Mexican American caregiving experience. *Hispanic Journal of Behavioral Sciences, 22*, 296–313.

Pinquart, M., & Sorensen, S. (2000). Influences of socioeconomic status, social network, and competence on subjective well-being in later life: A meta-analysis. *Psychology and Aging, 15*(2), 187–224.

Pinquart, M., & Sorensen, S. (2003). Differences between caregivers and non-caregivers in psychological health and physical health: A meta-analysis. *Psychology and Aging, 18*, 250–267.

Pruchno, R. A., Wilson-Genderson, M., Rose, M., & Cartwright, F. (2010). Successful aging: Early influences and contemporary characteristics. *Gerontologists, 50*(6), 821–833.

Rowe, J. W., & Kahn, R. L. (1987). Human aging: Usual and successful. *Science, 237*, 143–149.

Rowe, J. W., & Kahn, R. L. (1997). Successful aging. *Gerontologist, 37*(4), 433–440.

Ryan, P. & Coughlan, B. Introduction. In P. Ryan & B. Coughlan (Eds.). Ageing and older adult mental health: Issues and implications for practice (pp.1-2). New York, NY: Routledge.

Ryan, P., Coughlan, B., Shahid, Z., & Aherne, C. (2011). Older adults' experience of loss, bereavement and grief. In P. Ryan & B. Coughlan (Eds.), *Ageing and older adult mental health: Issues and implications for practice* (pp. 109–126). New York, NY: Routledge.

Ryan, P., O'Rourke, L., Ward, M., & Aherne, C. (2011). Ageing: Historical and current perspectives. In P. Ryan & J. Coughlan (Eds.), *Ageing and older adult mental health: Issues and implications for practice* (pp. 3–23). New York, NY: Routledge.

Ryan, P., & Wroblewska, A. (2011). Caring for older adults: Who cares and who does not? In P. Ryan & J. Coughlan (Eds.), *Ageing and older adult mental health: Issues and implications for practice* (pp. 214–229). New York, NY: Routledge.

Seeman, T. E., Charpentier, P. A., Berkman, L. F., Tinetti, M. E., Guralnik, J. M., Albert, M., . . . Rowe, J. W. (1994). Predicting change in physical performance in a high functioning elderly cohort: MacArthur studies of successful aging. *Journal of Gerontology, 49*(3), 97–108.

Segal, D. L., Coolidge, F. L., Mincic, M. S., & O'Riley, A. (2005). Beliefs about mental illness and willingness to seek help: A cross-sectional study. *Aging & Mental Health, 9*(4), 363–367. doi:10.1080/13607860500131047

Segerstrom, S. C., Al-Attar, A., & Lutz, C. T. (2012). Psychosocial resources, aging, and natural killer cell terminal maturity. *Psychology and Aging, 27*(4), 892–902. doi:10.1037/a0029093

Shawler, C. (2010). Assessing and maintaining mental health in elderly individuals. *Nursing Clinics of North America, 45,* 635–650.

Shock, N. W., Greulich, R. C., Andres, R., Arenberg, D., Costa, P., Lakatta, E., & Tobin, J. D. (1984). *Normal human aging: The Baltimore longitudinal study of aging* (NIH Publication No. 84-2450). Washington, DC: National Institutes of Health.

Singh, N., Clements, K. M., & Fiatarone Singh, M. (2001). The efficacy of exercise as a long-term antidepressant in elderly subjects: A randomized, controlled trial. *Journal of Gerontology Series A: Biological Sciences and Medical Sciences, 56A*(8), M497–M504.

Sivis, R., McCrae, C. S., & Demir, A. (2005). Availability of mental health services for older adults: A cross-cultural comparison of the United States and Turkey. *Aging and Mental Health, 9*(3), 223–234.

Strawbridge, W. J., Wallhagen, M. I., & Cohen, R. D. (2002). Successful aging and well-being: Self-rated compared with Rowe and Kahn. *Gerontologist, 42*(6), 727–733.

Tataru, N., & Dicker, A. (2009). Ageing-ethical issues and stigma. *European Psychiatry, 24,* S204.

Thanakwang, K. (2009). Social relationships influencing positive perceived health among Thai older persons: A secondary data analysis using the National Elderly Survey. *Nursing & Health Sciences, 11*(2), 144–149.

Tomer, A. (2000). Death related attitudes: Conceptual distinctions. In *Death attitudes and the older adult: Theories, concepts, and applications* (pp. 183–225). New York, NY: Brunner-Routledge.

United States Census Bureau. (2010). American fact finder. Retrieved from http://factfinder2.census.gov/

Vaillant, G. E. (2002). *Aging well: Surprising guideposts to a happier life.* Boston, MA: Little, Brown.

Vaillant, G. E., & Mukamal, K. (2001). Successful aging. *American Journal of Psychiatry, 158,* 839–847.

Wade, D. T., & Halligan, P. W. (2004). Do biomedical models of illness make for good healthcare systems? *British Medical Journal, 329*(7479), 1398–1401. doi:10.1136/bmj.329.7479.1398

Wienclaw, R. (2009). Growing old: Social aging. *Research Starters Sociology, 1,* 1–6.

World Health Organization. (2013). Mental health: Suicide prevention (SUPRE). Retrieved from http://www.who.int/mental_health/prevention/suicide/suicideprevent/en/

Yang, S., & Rosenblatt, P. C. (2001). Shame in Korean families. *Journal of Comparative Family Studies, 32,* 361–375.

Yoon, D. P. (2006). Factors affecting subjective well-being for rural elderly individuals: The importance of spirituality, religiousness, and social support. *Journal of Religion & Spirituality in Social Work, 25*(2), 59–75.

Zisook, D., Paulus, M., Shuchter, S. R., & Judd, L. L. (1997). The many faces of depression following spousal bereavement. *Journal of Affective Disorders, 45,* 85–95.

CHAPTER 20: IT RESOURCES

Websites

American Osteopathic Association website
http://www.osteopathic.org/Pages/default.aspx
National Center on Elder Abuse
http://www.ncea.aoa.gov/
Social Security Administration
http://www.ssa.gov/
United States Census Bureau
http://www.census.gov/
The Center for Successful Aging
http://hhd.fullerton.edu/csa/

American Psychological Association: Successful Aging—The Second 50
   http://www.apa.org/monitor/jan00/cs.aspx
Promoting Successful Aging
   http://gero.usc.edu/AgeWorks/core_courses/gero500_core/successful_lect/
The Facts on Successful Aging
   http://www.egyptianaaa.org/healthsuccessfulaging2.htm
Grief Counseling in the Elderly
   http://www.livestrong.com/article/157605-what-are-the-stages-of-grief-counseling-in-the-elderly/
Grief Issues of the Aged
   http://revlady.hubpages.com/hub/Grief-Issues-of-the-Aged
Grief and the Elderly
   http://www.after55blog.com/?p=843
Elder Grief: The Hidden Burden of Advanced Age
   http://www.psychologytoday.com/blog/beautiful-grief/201205/elder-grief-the-hidden-burden-advanced-age
Mental Health America Surveys
   http://www.mentalhealthamerica.net/go/surveys
Center for Civic Partnerships
   http://www.civicpartnerships.org/
Biomedical Model
   http://www.wisegeek.org/what-is-the-biomedical-model.htm
What Is the Biomedical Model of Healthcare?
   http://wiki.answers.com/Q/What_is_biomedical_model_of_health_care
Paradigms of Psychiatry: Eclecticism and Its Discontents: The Biopsychosocial Model: Anything Goes?
   http://www.medscape.com/viewarticle/547497_2
Positive Aging
   http://s404764450.initial-website.com/
The TAOS Institute—Positive Aging
   http://www.taosinstitute.net/positive-aging-newsletter
Positive Aging Resource Center
   http://www.positiveaging.org/
Positive Aging Act
   http://www.apa.org/about/gr/issues/aging/positive-aging-facts.aspx
National Family Caregiver Support Program
   http://www.aoa.gov/aoa_programs/hcltc/caregiver/index.aspx
The National Alliance for Caregiving
   http://www.caregiving.org/

PDF Documents

Successful Aging: Myth or Reality
   http://deepblue.lib.umich.edu/bitstream/handle/2027.42/49494/2004%20Winkelman%20Lecture%20Kahn.pdf;jsessionid=4A4A43A089653090E514DCDF74C1334F?sequence=3

Videos

Successful Aging Research (2011)
  People who feel a purpose in life and who can cope with change are poised to age successfully. That is what Valerie McCarthy, RN, PhD, found through her theory-based research. The assistant nursing professor said that successful aging is not the absence of disease or physical difficulty, but the ability to choose and accomplish goals that are personally important. (2:20 minutes)
  http://youtu.be/cLRrm0knVyk

Jessie Jones, PhD, Lectures on 'Successful Aging' at the United Nations (2008)
  Dr. Jessie Jones gave a vibrant lecture at the Brain Education conference at the United Nations in New York, NY, on June 20, 2008. From her many years of research and clinical experience at the Center for Successful Aging at CalState, Fullerton, she shares her tips and philosophy on aging well for the rest of our lives. Dr. Jones has also coauthored a book on the subject with Ilchi Lee called "In Full Bloom: A Brain Education Guide for Successful Aging." (8:40 minutes)
  http://youtu.be/q1cbfBJVJ0o

Successful Cognitive and Emotional Aging—Research on Aging (2008)
  The next 25 years will witness the largest-ever increase in our elderly population, especially those living an active life. Yet research on successful aging has lagged behind that on age-related diseases. Although successful aging involves both mental and physical health, new research suggests that the critical component of successful aging is related to brain and mind. Dr. Dilip Jeste shares the latest research and reviews some evidence-based strategies for successful aging. (1 hour)
  http://youtu.be/QXvAZsC_UmA

Successful Aging (2011) (36:33 minutes)
  http://youtu.be/ddWSfticYeM

Images

Google images for Successful Aging
  http://www.google.com/search?q=successful+aging&hl=en&tbm=isch&tbo=u&source=univ&sa=X&ei=uuBZUZfVJKzB4AO5yIHoBA&sqi=2&ved=0CHYQsAQ&biw=1280&bih=705

Google images for Positive Aging
  http://www.google.com/search?q=positive+aging&hl=en&source=lnms&tbm=isch&sa=X&ei=kUuZUdSmHejD4AOsqIHADw&sqi=2&ved=0CAcQ_AUoAQ&biw=1024&bih=564

Alcohol Use Disorders

Nancy Brossoie, PhD

INTRODUCTION

For thousands of years, people have fermented fruits, grains, and vegetables to produce alcoholic beverages. Variations of those early versions of beer, wine, and spirits continue to be produced today for religious ceremonies, social celebrations, and as beverages to complement the foods we eat. Anheuser-Busch, the world's largest brewer of beer, has capitalized on the connection people make between alcohol and socialization and is proud to claim they have "been creating social networks since 1366" (AB InBev, 2012). Public thirst for alcohol has remained robust throughout the history of the United States, even during Prohibition (1920 to 1933) when production, sales, and possession of alcohol were illegal. Its sustaining appeal continues to be its relaxing and disinhibiting effects, which help the drinker unwind and feel euphoric, if only for a short time.

Older adults, like their younger counterparts, consume alcohol at social gatherings and as part of their own daily routines. While many people believe that adults "mature out" of engaging in heavy drinking as they age, focus on their careers, raise families, and take on more responsibilities (O'Malley, 2004/2005; Winick, 1962), there is increasing evidence that many older adults have either never stopped drinking or are resuming the drinking behaviors of their youth as a way to cope with stress in later life (Duncan et al., 2010; Glantz, 1981). For chronic heavy drinkers (i.e., persons with recurring drinking patterns that exceed recommended limits), the toll of alcohol on the body is evidenced by adverse health and social consequences, including liver damage (Carithers & McCLain, 2010), cardiovascular problems (Lucas et al., 2005), gastrointestinal issues (Bode & Bode, 1997), memory loss (White, 2004), poor cognition (Kim et al., 2012), and fractured personal relationships (Klingemann, 2001; Roberts & McCrady, 2003).

Alcohol can even have serious health consequences for older adults who limit their drinking to small amounts on a regular basis (e.g., a glass of wine every night). Older bodies undergo physiological changes that make it difficult to metabolize alcohol as efficiently as in younger years. Moreover, alcohol can exacerbate existing health conditions and reduce the effectiveness of medications taken for those problems (National Institute on Alcohol Abuse and Alcoholism [NIAAA], 2007a). Unfortunately, health care providers often neglect to think about alcohol use as a potential problem behavior in the lives of their older patients and frequently overlook it when addressing other health problems (Fink et al., 1996; National Institute on Aging [NIA], 2012; Stewart & Oslin, 2001). With increasing numbers of adults living longer and aging in place in their communities, increased awareness of alcohol use and misuse is critical for health care providers to provide effective care, support their patients' independence, and contain medical costs.

BACKGROUND AND STATISTICS

The impact of alcohol misuse on public health is arguably extensive. The World Health Organization reports that alcohol (i.e., ethyl alcohol or ethanol) is the world's third largest risk factor for disease burden (Rehm, 2011). More than 60 different preventable medical conditions are attributable to alcohol, and 4% of all disease can be attributed to alcohol. Alcohol-induced health problems account for as much death and disability as tobacco and hypertension worldwide (Room et al., 2005). In the United States,

- Liver cirrhosis is the 12th leading cause of death and the 7th leading cause among adults aged 45 to 64 (Murphy et al., 2012).
- Alcoholic dementia accounts for 10% of all cases of dementia (Weyerer et al., 2011).
- Approximately one out of every three persons dependent on alcohol displays alcoholic cardiomyopathy of varying severity (Zhang & Ren, 2011).
- Over 50% of adults aged 50 to 64 years and 40.3% of adults aged 65+ used alcohol in the past month (Substance Abuse and Mental Health Services Administration [SAMHSA], 2012).
- Older people with alcohol dependence have more binge drinking episodes per month than do their younger counterparts (Ginzer & Richardson, 2009).
- About 8.4% of adults aged 55 to 59 years, 7.8% of adults aged 60 to 64 years, and 3.2% of adults aged 65+ reported driving while intoxicated during the past year (SAMHSA, 2012).

The economic impact of alcohol on society is also formidable. While major beer manufacturers like Anheuser-Busch and MillerCoors may enjoy a healthy bottom line (AB InBev, 2012), their US profits pale in comparison with the $223.5 billion (or $1.90 per drink) that excessive drinking cost the United States economy in 2006 in lost worker productivity (missed hours and reduced output—72.2%), increased health care costs (11%), and additional criminal justice costs (9.4%). Crime-related costs for government alone exceeded $94 billion (or $0.80 per drink) (Bouchery et al., 2011). However, no dollar amount can be placed on the intangible costs of pain and suffering resulting from incidents involving excessive drinking.

Determining the prevalence of drinking among older adults remains a challenge for epidemiologists. The first challenge to collecting accurate information is identifying older adults willing to talk. In general, older adults tend not to participate in surveys (Quinn, 2010), and if they do, they are not apt to divulge personal habits that may be considered socially inappropriate, like drinking (Rice et al., 1993). Secondly, survey items used to capture drinking habits and patterns of the adult population are often ill-suited to uncovering the drinking habits of older adults

(Blow et al., 1992). Lastly, secondary data sources like medical codes (i.e., ICD 9) used to track incidences of alcohol-related health problems cannot fully capture the spectrum of alcohol use found among patients (Rehm, 2011). Despite facing such challenges, researchers concur that alcohol use in the second half of life is a growing hidden public health problem (Blow et al., 2002; Merrick et al., 2008; National Institute on Alcohol Abuse and Alcoholism, 2005a). Recent statistics indicate:

- Up to 4% of community dwelling older adults may suffer from full-blown alcohol dependence (Oslin, 2005).
- Nurse aides estimate that 69% of residents in assisted living facilities drink alcohol, and for 19% of them, alcohol has impacted their health (Castle et al., 2012).
- Up to 50% of nursing home residents suffer from alcohol problems (Klein & Jess, 2002).
- Nearly 1 in 10 Medicare beneficiaries report exceeding recommended drinking limits (Merrick et al., 2008).
- Approximately 7% to 22% of hospital inpatients and 10% to 15% of older persons treated in the emergency room have a problem abusing alcohol (SAMHSA, Center for Behavioral Health Statistics and Quality, 2011).
- Although 87% of older adults see a physician regularly (Bartels et al., 2005), 40% do not self-identify or seek treatment (Center for Substance Abuse Treatment [CSAT], 1998).

HEALTHY PEOPLE 2020 OBJECTIVES

Public health problems associated with alcohol misuse can be reduced if health care providers can identify patients with potential health problems and provide them with treatment options. The Healthy People 2020 (U.S. Department of Health and Human Services, Office of Disease Prevention and Health Promotion, 2010) objectives developed to reduce chronic heavy drinking, and the effects of alcohol on patient health include:

A. Screening and treatment
  - SA-8—Increase proportion of persons who need alcohol treatment in past year
  - SA-9—Increase proportion of persons referred for follow-up care from ER
B. Epidemiology and surveillance
  - SA-11—Reduce cirrhosis deaths
  - SA-14—Reduce proportion of persons engaged in binge drinking
  - SA-15—Reduce proportion of adults who drank excessively in the previous 30 days
  - SA-20—Decrease number of deaths attributable to alcohol

PATHOPHYSIOLOGY

The process in which the body excretes, absorbs, and metabolizes alcohol is the same for everyone. Yet there are differences in how quickly or efficiently each person can process alcohol. Differences are associated with age, sex, body composition, health status, and genetics. Perhaps not surprisingly, a young healthy adult can consume more alcohol before feeling its effects than older less fit adults experiencing health problems. In the following sections, associations between individual characteristics and the body's ability to process alcohol are highlighted when applicable.

Unmetabolized Alcohol

After alcohol is ingested, up to 10% is excreted unmetabolized through body fluids like perspiration, urine, and the moisture in breath. For a period of time following consumption, traces of unmetabolized alcohol remain in the breath and on the body, even if only a small amount of alcohol has been consumed. Research on detecting and measuring the alcohol left behind is generally aligned with public safety efforts to reduce incidences of drunk driving. For example, breathalyzer tools like those used by police officers to screen potential drunk drivers measure the unmetabolized alcohol found in breath and translate it into a blood alcohol concentration (BAC) metric that estimates the percentage of alcohol in the bloodstream (Jones & Andersson, 2003). A BAC of 0.08 is equivalent to 0.08% (eight tenths of 1%) of a person's blood (by volume) containing alcohol. A BAC of 0.08 surpasses the blood alcohol limit of less than 0.08 g alcohol per 100 ml blood allowed by US state laws when driving a personal vehicle (Insurance Institute for Highway Safety, 2013).

Absorption

Any remaining alcohol that has not been excreted through body fluids is absorbed through the gastrointestinal tract (i.e., stomach, small intestines, and colon) into the bloodstream, where it passes throughout the body for processing. Because alcohol is water and lipid soluble, it can pass through cell walls easily and no energy or catalyst is required for diffusion. Consequently, individuals with more muscle and fat absorb more alcohol than their thinner and lighter drinking companions, which can slow down the absorption of alcohol into their bloodstreams. This explains why males (who are more likely to have more muscle and fat than females) can generally consume more alcohol than females before showing signs of intoxication and why females should be discouraged from matching their male drinking companions drink for drink (Graham et al., 1998). Having food in the stomach before drinking or while drinking can slow down absorption of alcohol into the blood, but will not prevent it. While absorption rates may differ among individuals owing to varying body types and patterns of alcohol consumption, the rate at which alcohol is metabolized remains constant. As a general rule, the body can only produce enough enzymes to metabolize alcohol at the rate of approximately 14 g of alcohol per hour—or one standard drink (e.g., a 5-oz [141.7 g] glass of wine or a 12-oz [340.2 g] beer) (NIAAA, 2007c).

Metabolization

Once alcohol is ingested, it is either metabolized in the stomach or passed through the digestive tract and circulated in the bloodstream (NIAAA, 2007c). Although most alcohol is processed in the liver, other tissues in the body (including the brain and pancreas) can metabolize it if the appropriate alcohol dehydrogenase (ADH) enzymes are present. Simply stated, metabolization involves several oxidation processes initiated by ADH enzymes. During the first step, ADH enzymes interact with alcohol and convert it into acetaldehyde—a toxic substance to the body. If acetaldehyde is not broken down and allowed to remain in the system in its toxic form, it can produce vomiting, headaches, heart palpitations, and permanent tissue damage. The body reacts to the presence of acetaldehyde by initiating a second oxidation process using an acetaldehyde dehydrogenase (ALDH2) enzyme to eliminate it. When acetaldehyde combines with ALDH2, it loses toxicity and transforms into acetic acid. The acetic acid is then further oxygenated and reduced to carbon dioxide and water, which is eventually expelled through the lungs and urine. Unfortunately, ADH and ALDH2 enzymes needed for metabolization are not stored in the body. Enzyme production is stimulated by demand and takes time to produce—evidence that metabolism occurs at a constant rate.

Low levels of ADH enzymes are normally present in the gastric mucosa (mucus layer of the stomach lining), although the concentration is not enough to metabolize large quantities of alcohol at any given time. Males generally have higher concentrations of ADH enzymes stored than females, which allows them to metabolize as much as 20% of alcohol present in their stomachs—another reason why females show signs of intoxication sooner than males when drinking similar quantities (Graham et al., 1998).

PHYSIOLOGICAL RESPONSES

Flushing

Nearly 8% of the world population possesses an inherited deficiency that affects the structure of their ALDH2 enzymes, which compromise their ability to metabolize alcohol. Persons with this genetic variation may experience facial flushing, nausea, and tachycardia as acetaldehyde accumulates in their body (NIAAA, 2003). Approximately 36% of East Asians (i.e., Japanese, Chinese, and Korean) possess this characteristic and will appear flushed after drinking alcohol; a response often referred to as "Asian flush" or "Asian glow" (Edenberg, 2003; Nurnberger & Bierut, 2007). Understandably, most individuals with this genetic expression abstain from drinking altogether to avoid the undesirable side effects.

Dehydration and Kidney Functioning

The diuretic effects of alcohol prompt frequent urination and disrupt normal kidney functioning. Drinking can cause a person to expel up to four times the amount of water as alcohol consumed, depending on the alcoholic content and type of beverage consumed (i.e., beer, whisky, wine). The ongoing need to eliminate water can explain why some individuals drinking a great deal experience episodes of incontinence while they sleep.

When alcohol enters the body, it signals the pituitary gland to stop distributing vasopressin, an antidiuretic hormone. The resulting drop in vasopressin triggers the kidneys to stop reabsorbing water and reroute it directly to the bladder for elimination. By circumventing the kidneys, metabolic functioning is disrupted. As concentrations of metabolic waste, glucose, and salts rise in the blood, ionic imbalances are created.

Brain Response

The simple molecular structure of alcohol (i.e., ethanol) enables it to pass easily through the "blood–brain barrier," which normally protects brain tissue from toxins in the blood (NIAAA, 2007c). When alcohol reaches the brain, chemical changes begin. Alcohol affects brain functioning largely by interfering with the activities of neurotransmitters responsible for brain communication (NIAAA, 2004). Two neurotransmitters—gamma-aminobutyric acid (GABA) and glutamate—are especially sensitive to alcohol. GABA is an inhibitory neurotransmitter that reduces or depresses neuronal activity. Glutamate is an excitatory neurotransmitter that increases activity in neurons. Together, these two amino acids maintain balance in synaptic transmissions and control excitability within neurons. When alcohol is consumed, it disrupts their neuronal balance by suppressing the excitatory actions of the glutamate and boosting the inhibitory effects of GABA. The resulting chemical interaction produces a depressive effect, which is why alcohol is referred to as a central nervous system (CNS) depressant.

As the level of alcohol consumed rises and continues to depress the CNS, the brain responds by producing more and more glutamate to achieve equilibrium. When individuals drinking small amounts of alcohol stop drinking, glutamate levels fall back to normal and neural excitement subsides. However, when chronic heavy drinkers withdraw from alcohol, high levels of glutamate remain in the brain owing to past overproduction. The remaining high levels of glutamate continue to excite the CNS—a prolonged brain hyperactivity that leads to symptoms of withdrawal, including hallucinations, delirium tremens, and seizures.

Many people drink alcohol for its relaxed and euphoric effects. However, as the amount of alcohol ingested increases and the CNS becomes more depressed, those desirable effects fade. Brain activity becomes increasingly sluggish and impaired as more alcohol is consumed. Regions of the brain affected by alcohol are illustrated in Figure 21.1, and the associated losses in functioning for each region are described below.

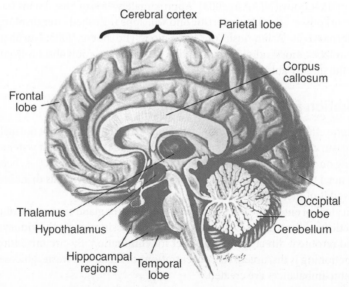

FIGURE 21.1. Areas of the brain affected by alcohol: frontal lobe—loss of reason, caution, and inhibitions; parietal lobe—loss of fine motor skills, slower reaction time, and shaking; temporal lobe—slurred speech and impaired hearing; occipital lobe—blurred vision and poor distance judgment; cerebellum—lack of muscle coordination and balance; brain stem—loss of vital functions. (From National Institute on Alcohol Abuse and Alcoholism. [2004]. Alcohol's damaging effect on the brain. *Alcohol Alert, 63*. Retrieved from http://pubs.niaaa.nih.gov/publications/aa63/aa63.htm. All material contained in the Alcohol Alert is in the public domain and may be used or reproduced without permission from NIAAA.)

TOLERANCE

The brain can become tolerant or insensitive to the effects of alcohol over time. As alcohol consumption increases, the persons need to consume more to experience its relaxing and euphoric effects. Persons who allow their alcohol consumption patterns to increase are at risk for a number of health problems, including alcohol dependence—a condition in which an individual physically needs alcohol and focuses on obtaining and consuming it at the expense of all other personal responsibilities, including work, family, finances, and personal relationships (NIAAA, 2009).

REINFORCEMENT

The neurobiology underlying alcohol dependence is not yet completely understood. However, through the use of human and animal models, scientists have learned that the pleasurable effects that reward a drinker also reinforce drinking. The reinforcement process occurs in the brain's mesolimbic system—a specialized neural network that serves as a reward pathway for activities like drinking, eating, and sex. When alcohol is consumed, it triggers the release of neurotransmitters (e.g., dopamine and opioid) that produce heightened feelings of euphoria (di Chiara, 1997; Goodman, 2008).

The pleasurable feelings or rewards associated with alcohol are difficult for chronic heavy drinkers to ignore and resist. They have built up so much tolerance to alcohol that even if they want to quit drinking, they need to continue to drink just to feel normal. If they do stop drinking, the craving for a pleasurable reward is often stronger than their will to withstand the unpleasant side effects of withdrawal. This explains why so many individuals relapse repeatedly in their attempts to remain sober (NIAAA, 2001).

PRESENTATION

Many health problems that lead older adults to seek medical assistance are influenced by personal habits, including the use of alcohol. Yet, self-disclosure of alcohol use is quite limited between patients and health care providers (CSAT, 1998; Hanson & Gutheil, 2004). Personal drinking habits are not revealed for several reasons. Some older adults tend to think that a long-standing routine like drinking a glass of wine every night before bed is not worth mentioning; especially when it has never led to a problem in the past. Other older adults may be hesitant to reveal their alcohol use because they are embarrassed and fear being labeled as having a drinking problem. Social stereotypes of older adults still abound. Old women are often assumed to be teetotalers, and old men who drink too much are often viewed as town drunks and derelicts. In reality, older adults are a heterogeneous population, and their drinking patterns range from abstinence to chronic heavy drinking (SAMHSA, 2012). When health care providers and other community service professionals refrain from asking older adults about their alcohol use at each appointment because they believe that asking would be irrelevant or inappropriate, they perpetuate the false belief that drinking in late life does not exist or indicates some type of personal defect if revealed (Sharp & Vacha-Haase, 2010).

Even though older adults metabolize alcohol in the same manner as they did when they were young, they develop an increased sensitivity to it, which does not allow them to safely consume the same amounts as they once did (CSAT, 1998). Older bodies are often dehydrated (from lack of fluids or medications), which leaves less water circulating in the body to dilute the alcohol. Older bodies also carry a higher proportion of body fat to lean muscle, which increases levels of alcohol absorption and circulation in the body. Moreover, the aged liver is less efficient in processing alcohol than in younger years. Thus, older adults consuming alcoholic beverages become intoxicated quicker and remain intoxicated longer than younger similarly sized adults drinking the same quantities.

The effects of alcohol on brain functioning, movement, coordination, and sleep are easy to overlook among older adults because the same or similar impairments are attributable to other health problems associated with normal aging (e.g., slowed or impaired speech, thinking, judgment, and memory). When those same conditions coexist with alcohol misuse and dependency, identifying the cause of a problem or illness becomes more challenging. Moreover, many medications taken by older adults have side effects similar to intoxication (e.g., drowsiness, unsteady gait, impaired attention or memory, and sleep problems) and can mask detection of alcohol-related health problems. Some common signs and symptoms of alcohol misuse that can mimic health problems experienced by older adults are shown in Table 21.1.

Risk of falling is especially high for older adults drinking alcohol—even at low levels and rates of consumption. Loss of coordination, slowed reaction time, and poor judgment become amplified with intoxication and challenge persons already experiencing balance and coordination problems. Older chronic heavy drinkers are at the most risk of falling because of their increased neuromuscular impairments caused by long-term alcohol use compounded by other health problems. The risk of falling is further heightened when alcohol is consumed with medications contraindicated with alcohol.

Bone health is also impacted by chronic heavy drinking. Alcohol interferes with the healthy development and proliferation of osteoblasts (bone building cells). During middle age, the production of osteoblasts naturally begins to decline. Heavy alcohol consumption further compromises bone structure and places chronic heavy drinkers at risk of fractures.

TABLE 21.1 • Signs and Symptoms of Potential Alcohol Problems

Physical Health	Mental Health	Emotional and Social Health
Dizziness	Anxiety	Bereavement and sadness
Disorientation	Depression	Lack of hope
Headaches	Mood swings	Poor self-esteem
Memory loss	Increased alcohol use	Relationship problems
Insomnia		Changes in social status
Falls, scrapes, and bruises		Social isolation
Incontinence		Increased legal or financial troubles
Physical distress		

IMMEDIATE OR SHORT-TERM EFFECTS

Intoxication

Intoxication is a physiological state induced by the presence of a toxin (e.g., alcohol) resulting in abnormal behavior and thinking not associated with any other medical condition. As the level of alcohol in the body increases, physical and mental functioning become progressively impaired because the body cannot process it as quickly as it is consumed. General signs of intoxication or inebriation include slurred speech, uncoordination, unsteady gait, nystagmus, impaired attention or memory, and stupor or coma.

There are four general methods for determining intoxication: self-report, observation, breathalyzer, and laboratory tests. Self-report is the first step to uncovering alcohol use problems, although it is not foolproof. Report accuracy is influenced by the respondents' comfort level with the person asking for information, the questions asked, assurance of confidentiality, and being alcohol-free during questioning (Sobell & Sobell, 2003). While observation may provide general clues, it cannot be relied upon because each individual can vary in how he or she processes alcohol and exhibits signs of intoxication. In emergency situations, health care professionals often receive breathalyzer scores when members of law enforcement are involved. Even though the breathalyzer reading is an accurate estimator, health providers may wish to verify the amount of alcohol in the system using a blood test. The progressive effects of alcohol and the associated blood alcohol values can be found in Table 21.2.

Effects of Intoxication

Drinking alcohol can produce numerous undesirable health outcomes that do not necessarily involve chronic heavy drinking (Virginia Tech Campus Alcohol Abuse Prevention Center, n.d.). Memory blackouts are episodes of amnesia generally experienced by individuals at risk of becoming chronic heavy drinkers. "Blacking out" is caused by a rapid rise of alcohol in the bloodstream owing to the consumption of a large volume of alcohol within a short period. When blackouts occur, memory formation processes are interrupted, and the brain is unable to form long-term memories. Even though a blacked-out person may be actively engaged in his or her surroundings and may be able to recount events within a few minutes of their occurrence, he or she will not have the ability to store those events in long-term memory. Additionally, he or she will have no memory of events or interactions that occurred during the blackout. Only after the body is able to reduce the level of alcohol in the bloodstream will the blacked-out person's brain begin to form long-term memories again (White, 2004).

Alcohol poisoning can occur when the amount of alcohol circulating in the blood is dangerously high. Brain functioning becomes seriously impaired, and the drinker exhibits signs of slurred speech, ataxia, and stupor. Alcohol poisoning causes the brain to become partially anesthetized and interferes with neurotransmissions. The drinker's heartbeat and breathing can also become irregular and even stop. Even though the media is more likely to report incidents of alcohol poisoning among persons inexperienced with how alcohol might affect them, death from alcohol poisoning is more common among chronic heavy drinkers because their blood alcohol content is more likely to reach a lethal level (Yoon et al., 2003).

Alcoholic ketoacidosis (AKA) is an acute form of metabolic acidosis characterized by a buildup of ketones in the blood. Alcoholic ketoacidosis is caused by drinking excessive amounts of alcohol while dehydrated and fasting. Without water and food, the body lacks the fluid and

TABLE 21.2 • Progressive Effects of Alcohol

Intake (mg/dl)	BAC (% by vol.)	Behavior	Impairment
10–29	0.010–0.029	Average individual appears normal	Subtle effects that can be detected with special tests
30–59	0.030–0.059	Mild euphoria Relaxation Joyousness Talkativeness Decreased inhibition	Concentration
60–90	0.06–0.09	Blunted feelings Disinhibition Extraversion	Reasoning Depth perception Peripheral vision Glare recovery
100–190	0.10–0.19	Overexpression Emotional swings Anger or sadness Boisterousness Decreased libido	Reflexes Reaction time Gross motor control Staggering Slurred speech Temporary erectile dysfunction
200–290	0.20–0.29	Stupor Loss of understanding Impaired sensations	Severe motor impairment Loss of consciousness Memory blackout
300–390	0.30–0.39	Severe CNS depression Unconsciousness Possibility of death	Bladder function Breathing Heart rate
400–500	0.40–0.50	General lack of behavior Unconsciousness Possibility of death	Breathing Heart rate
500+	>0.50	Death	

Adapted from Center for Substance Abuse Treatment. (1999). *Enhancing motivation for change in substance abuse treatment. Treatment Improvement Protocol (TIP) series, No. 35* (HHS Publication No. [SMA] 12-4212). Rockville, MD: Substance Abuse and Mental Health Services Administration. Contents are in public domain and may be freely reproduced.

glucose needed for organ functioning and reduces the excretion of keto acids from the kidneys and impairs the liver's ability to metabolize the alcohol.

"Holiday heart syndrome" is a condition most often seen around holidays when excessive drinking is likely to occur. Increased levels of alcohol in the blood create arrhythmias by disrupting the movement of sodium, calcium, and potassium ions across myocyte membranes—a condition that reverts to normal after alcohol levels are reduced (Sterner & Keough, 2003; Zakhari, 1997).

Dehydration can become a problem for individuals while they drink, because signs of dehydration—dizziness, confusion, and tiredness—can be readily attributed to other causes. After drinking, the effects of dehydration become more pronounced and recognizable as nausea, headache, and dry mouth—commonly associated with hangovers (Prat et al., 2009). Replacing a drink of water for every other drink consumed will not only combat dehydration but will help slow absorption and dilute toxins building up in the body (NIAAA, 2010b).

Vasodilation causes some individuals to feel warm after drinking because alcohol dilates blood vessels. Even though the enlarged vessels increase blood flow and produce sensations of warmth, the body actually loses heat while drinking. Thus, vasodilation may lead to potentially serious consequences when an individual is exposed to low temperatures. In situations where high levels of alcohol are consumed, blood vessels will start to constrict and increase blood pressure, which can exacerbate some health problems such as migraine headaches (Prat et al., 2009).

Sleep is often interrupted after drinking, causing a person to feel quite fatigued. Alcohol stops the body's normal production of glutamine—a natural stimulant and neural transmitter. Once drinking stops, glutamine production resumes at a high rate to compensate for lost production. The sudden increase of glutamine stimulates brain activity and can prevent a drinker from sleeping soundly or reaching deep sleep. Thus, individuals may feel tired up to 2 days after heavy drinking due to the rebounding levels of glutamine that are keeping them awake. Among chronic heavy drinkers, increased production of glutamine can be more serious and lead to feelings of anxiety and restlessness, high blood pressure, and tremors (Brower, 2003).

A hangover is a nonmedical term to describe the ill feelings experienced after a bout of heavy drinking. The discomforts associated with a hangover have been recorded for centuries, yet there is little consensus on its definition or understanding of why every person who consumes alcohol does not end up with a hangover (Wiese et al., 2000). Common symptoms reported include headache, diarrhea, fatigue, dry mouth, stomach irritation, and general feelings of poor health. A review of scientific evidence (Prat et al., 2009; Verster, 2008) reveals that a hangover may be a side effect from acetaldehyde and glutamine lingering in the body, although those actions are not yet fully understood. There is also evidence that suggests that hangovers are caused by congeners found in alcoholic beverages (Verster, 2008; Wiese et al., 2000). Congeners are the chemical byproducts produced during fermentation, which contribute to the flavor, look, and aroma of alcohol. Clear alcohol has fewer congeners than alcohol with dark coloring. Even though there have been a limited number of studies conducted on the effects of congeners on individuals who drink, there is evidence that congeners can be toxic to the body and frequently contribute to unwanted side effects. Similarly, histamine compounds are often found in foods (e.g., grape skins) included in the fermentation process. Persons who lack sufficient quantities of the enzyme needed to break down histamines in the small intestine often experience headaches after drinking. Because drinking alcohol suppresses production of these enzymes, those individuals with limited ability to process histamines are more likely to experience headaches than others.

LONG-TERM EFFECTS

Chronic heavy drinking can cause significant and often irreversible damage to the body. Early signs of alcohol-induced health problems often manifest in the gastrointestinal tract and often start with acute gastritis (Bode & Bode, 1997).

Gastrointestinal Functioning

The consumption of large quantities of alcohol during a single drinking session or consistently over an extended period breaks down or inflames the stomach's protective lining (gastric mucosa) and overstimulates production of hydrochloric acid, a digestive aid in the stomach. With the stomach lining exposed, the buildup of acids and toxins can cause additional irritation and bleeding. For some individuals, the increased levels of hydrochloric acid will induce vomiting, which can be helpful in ridding the body of alcohol and other toxins causing irritation. Vomiting can be especially helpful for females because they have a thinner gastric mucosa and increased susceptibility to gastrointestinal irritation than males. Chronic symptoms of acute gastritis are often described as a pain or dull ache, nausea, gas, loss of appetite, and burning sensation in the mouth. The treatment for alcoholic acute gastritis is abstinence, and prognosis for healing is excellent if there is treatment adherence.

Pancreatitis

Pancreatitis develops when pancreatic enzymes produced for digesting food in the small intestine activate within the pancreas and digest pancreatic tissue (parenchyma). Most incidences of pancreatitis (acute and chronic) are attributed to alcohol, and the first acute attack typically appears after 5 to 10 years of chronic heavy drinking. As alcohol is metabolized by the pancreas, it stimulates production of digestive enzymes. In persons with pancreatitis, the enzymes activated within the pancreas begin to autodigest the gland. Signs of acute pancreatitis include pain, edema, and hemorrhaging. Persons with chronic pancreatitis also have signs of fibrosis and calcification in their pancreas, which reduce its ability to produce digestive enzymes and beta cells needed for insulin production. Thus, pancreatitis can contribute to other serious health conditions, including maldigestion, diabetes, and pancreatic cancer (Ammann, 2001; NIAAA, 2010a).

The liver is the primary organ responsible for metabolizing and eliminating alcohol from the body. Alcohol that is absorbed into the bloodstream through the stomach and small intestine first passes through the liver for processing—exposing it to high concentrations of alcohol. Additional stress is placed on the liver when large quantities of alcohol are passed through it over a short period or when medications (e.g., acetaminophen) and alcohol are simultaneously processed. The additive stress that alcohol places on the liver can lead to alcoholic liver disease (ALD), which can manifest as one of three physical conditions: steatosis, alcoholic hepatitis, and cirrhosis (NIAAA, 2005b).

Steatosis or "fatty liver" is the most common ALD in which fat deposits build up within liver cells and impair liver functioning. Individuals may be unaware that they have steatosis because there are no known symptoms to indicate that a problem exists. The condition can be reversed through abstinence.

Alcoholic hepatitis is an inflammation of the liver caused by chronic heavy drinking that can lead to liver failure and death. Individuals can experience mild-to-severe symptoms of nausea, vomiting, fever, abdominal pain and bleeding, jaundice, and mental confusion. Nearly 70% of persons with alcoholic hepatitis will ultimately develop cirrhosis if they do not stop drinking. Those persons who commit to abstaining from alcohol can reduce inflammation and reverse some damage to the liver.

Cirrhosis

Cirrhosis is an irreversible condition in which normal liver tissue is replaced by scar tissue. As healthy liver cells die and are replaced with scar tissue, the blood flow through the liver becomes increasingly restricted. As liver functioning and efficiency decrease, the risk of liver failure increases. In the early stages of cirrhosis, signs of the condition may not be evident. However, as the amount of scar tissue increases, symptoms similar to alcoholic hepatitis slowly emerge followed by symptoms of ascites (fluid in the space between the membranes lining the abdomen and abdominal organs), limb and truncal ataxia (lack of coordination of muscles), myoclonus of the limbs (involuntary twitching and jerking), and areflexia (absence of reflex). Approximately 15%

of persons dependent on alcohol develop cirrhosis, and 12.5% of them receive a liver transplant (Anantharaju & Van Thiel, 2003).

Diagnosing ALD is challenging because symptoms are not always present or recognizable, chronic heavy drinkers are likely to deny or minimize their drinking patterns and behaviors, and laboratory tests are not conclusive for alcohol-related conditions. For example, blood can be tested for three key liver enzymes to determine whether liver damage has occurred. Yet, even though approximately 75% of chronic heavy drinkers have elevated levels of gamma-glutamyltransferase (GGT), other conditions like congestive heart failure can cause GCT levels to rise too. Similarly, aspartate aminotransferase (AST) and alanine aminotransferase (ALT) levels are also elevated in persons who drink, but their ratio is relatively low. Only among persons with ALD is the ratio between AST and ALT high. However, the larger ratio can also be seen after a heart attack. Thus, knowledge of drinking patterns is invaluable in connecting liver problems with alcohol.

A related alcohol-induced health problem caused by scarred liver tissue is portal hypertension. Damaged liver tissue inhibits blood flow and subsequently creates increased pressure in the portal vein entering the liver from the digestive organs. Large veins or varices begin to develop across the esophagus and stomach in an effort to bypass the blockages. As a result, even though pressure may be reduced, the varices are fragile and can tear and bleed. The condition, Mallory–Weiss syndrome is characterized by esophageal bleeding from torn varices precipitated by forceful vomiting following binge drinking (i.e., drinking large quantities during a short period).

CARDIOVASCULAR FUNCTIONING

Alcoholic cardiomyopathy is a condition precipitated by chronic heavy drinking in which the heart becomes enlarged and loses its ability to contract. Unlike other nonischemic cardiomyopathies, the damage caused by alcohol can be reversed or significantly reduced through abstinence. Heavy drinking can also disturb the heart's ability to beat normally. Two types of arrhythmias that can be attributed to heavy drinking include atrial fibrillation (rapid, irregular beats in the arterial heart chambers) and ventricular tachycardia (rapid beating in the ventricular heart chambers). Among "holiday drinkers" with heart disease, an episode of heavy drinking can also produce angina (Sterner & Keough, 2003).

Sudden death from ventricular arrhythmias is a major cause of death for chronic heavy drinkers, with or without other preexisting health conditions. For many, death occurs during times of detoxification or abstinence when alcohol levels in the blood are relatively low. However, elevated levels of adrenaline and noradrenaline sometimes remain and increase the heart's sensitivity to arrhythmias. In addition, the lack of magnesium and potassium (brought on by heavy drinking) further increases chances of arrhythmias.

Other cardiovascular conditions that can be exacerbated by alcohol include mild-to-moderate hypertension and mitral regurgitation. The red flushed look of some chronic heavy drinkers is the result of peripheral vasodilation, in which alcohol causes capillaries to rise to the surface of the skin.

BRAIN FUNCTIONING

Chronic heavy drinkers risk developing serious and persistent changes in the brain caused directly by alcohol or indirectly by factors such as an unbalanced diet (e.g., missed meals and high fat diet), nutritional deficiencies (e.g., thiamine), or co-occurring health conditions. Moreover, sleep apnea and head injuries, which are common health problems for chronic heavy drinkers, can also contribute to limited brain functioning (Cook et al., 1998; Meyerhoff et al., 2005).

For over 50 years, scientists have found that toxins, like alcohol, can permanently damage the "hard wiring" of the brain, cause brain shrinkage, and disrupt brain cell regeneration. More recently, brain imaging studies have shown that abstinence from alcohol can actually improve brain health. If chronic heavy drinkers abstain from alcohol for at least a year, some brain cells begin to regenerate, brain mass increases, and brain functioning starts to improve. Still, years of abstinence cannot reverse all the damage caused by alcohol in the brain (NIAAA, 2004; Rosenbloom et al., 2003).

Dementia

Alcohol-induced dementia is an irreversible condition caused by chronic heavy drinking. Brain cell damage associated with alcohol-induced dementia is generally nonspecific but located primarily in the frontal lobes and cerebellum. Subsequently, persons with alcohol-induced dementia often experience behavior changes related to those regions, which can make supporting them challenging. They can be apathetic, irritable, and resistive to help. Fortunately, long-term sobriety can help reverse some cell damage and improve cognition.

Delirium

Before the diagnosis of alcohol-induced dementia is made, delirium caused by alcohol must be ruled out or a separate diagnosis made. Delirium is a disturbance in consciousness and cognition occurring within a short time frame (American Psychological Association, 1994). It is generally precipitated by a combination of multiple risk factors (some modifiable), including advanced age, cognitive impairment, severe illness, surgery, diabetes, metabolic abnormalities, pharmacological interactions, and substance abuse. Failure to recognize delirium and treat its cause can result in a downward spiral in health and functioning (Fong et al., 2009).

Psychoses

Alcohol-induced psychoses can occur even after short periods of exposure to alcohol. That is, persons who drink in moderation or drink heavily on occasion are potentially at risk of psychotic episodes brought on by alcohol. Psychotic episodes can emerge while intoxicated or within a month of withdrawing from alcohol, and commonly include delusions and hallucinations. For most individuals, alcohol-induced psychoses subside after extended periods of abstinence, but may require additional treatment with medications.

Delusions are fixed false beliefs that an individual believes to be true, despite evidence to the contrary. For example, a delusional person may believe that he or she is married to the President of the United States, even though that is obviously not true. Hallucinations are false perceptions involving the five senses—sight, sound, smell, taste, and touch. Hallucinations induced by alcohol are generally auditory (e.g., voices telling an individual what to do) or tactile (e.g., bugs crawling up a person's arm).

Korsakoff psychosis is a form of irreversible short-term memory loss caused by alcohol exposure and often confused with alcohol-induced dementia. Persons with the condition maintain long-term memory, but do not have short-term recall. Like other persons with extensive short-term memory loss, patients with Korsakoff psychosis may be conscious of their inability to recall and resort to confabulating stories when confused.

NEUROLOGICAL SYSTEM

Chronic heavy drinking can permanently damage the nervous system by diminishing sense of touch, muscle coordination, and movement. Complex motor skills like dressing become difficult and place a person at risk for falling.

Unbalanced diets and nutritional deficiencies associated with heavy alcohol use are major contributors to neurological impairments. The food choices and eating patterns of chronic heavy drinkers often deteriorate in quality and quantity as alcohol consumption increases. Participation in meal time activities such as food preparation and socialization, which can deter drinking, are reduced or eliminated. Meals are often missed or substituted with alcoholic beverages. The resulting carbohydrate- and fat-based diets have limited nutritional value and lack essential nutrients needed for healthy body functions. Consequently, deficits in essential nutrients (vitamins A, C, B, and B_1 [thiamine], calcium, and iron) increase and can lead to alcohol-induced neurological conditions, including Wernicke syndrome, polyneuropathy, cerebellar degeneration, and amblyopia (Heuberger, 2009).

Wernicke Syndrome

This is caused by thiamine deficiency (NIAAA, 2004). Symptoms include ophthalmoplegia (wandering eye), ataxia (staggering gait), and confusion. Generally, patients with the Wernicke syndrome are also diagnosed with Korsakoff psychosis. While a therapy regime of thiamine can reverse some of the neurological damage, it will not reverse short-term memory loss.

Nutritional deficiencies also contribute to alcoholic polyneuropathy. Onset of the often painful condition is gradual and may emerge years after damage from alcohol is done. Early symptoms of peripheral neuropathy include tingling (i.e., "pins and needles") or burning sensations in the toes as axonal degeneration begins at distal ends of nerve fibers. Pain may be constant or intermittent and include sharp piercing pain or dull aches. Over time, increased sensory and motor losses affect the body in a symmetrical pattern (e.g., one side first, then the other). Moreover, signs of impairment usually start in the legs followed by the arms. Hands generally become impaired only after impairment is noticed above the ankle. Patients report muscle cramping and weakness, muscle atrophy, gait unsteadiness due to ataxia, and falls. The debilitating effects of impairment vary as do degrees of impairment. As the condition progresses, some patients may have difficulty swallowing (dysphagia), speech impairments (dysarthria), increased muscle spasms, and muscle atrophy. The unsteady gait often associated with alcoholic polyneuropathy may also be associated with cerebellar degeneration also induced by alcohol.

Alcoholic Cerebellar Degeneration

Alcoholic cerebellar degeneration (ACD) is caused by long-term alcohol use and nutritional deficits. Scientists suspect that the interference of alcohol on glutamate (the excitatory neurotransmitter that increases activity in neurons) is involved with the irreversible degeneration of Purkinje cells responsible for motor movements. Patients with ACD exhibit similar clinical symptoms, including truncal ataxia and impaired gait. Symptoms can appear suddenly and will eventually stabilize. Even though patients with ACD may abstain from alcohol and correct their nutritional deficiencies, damage to the Purkinje cells is permanent and motor activity will not improve over time.

Alcohol Amblyopia

This is another condition linked to thiamine deficiency and unique to chronic heavy drinkers. Individuals with alcohol amblyopia experience decreased vision and visual acuity within the center of their visual field. The condition is caused by damage and swelling of the optic nerve by alcohol and exacerbated by a lack of thiamine. If treatment begins early, symptoms can be reversed with improved diet and thiamine supplements.

NUTRITIONAL DEFICIENCIES

Poor nutrition among chronic heavy drinkers can also lead to other health problems such as pellagra or exacerbate health conditions like diabetes. Pellagra is a nutritional condition resulting from niacin deficiency. It is generally found among impoverished populations and chronic heavy drinkers. Niacin is obtained through diet and used by the body to metabolize alcohol. Symptoms of pellagra include the eruption of a photosensitive rash on the face, hands, neck, arms, and feet; gastrointestinal problems, including vomiting, diarrhea, and abdominal pain; and general irritability and fatigue. Eruption of the rash is pivotal to diagnosis. As the condition progresses, the rash resembles a blistering sunburn and with a chronic scaly rash. Pellagra can be easily treated with niacin supplements, but can turn fatal if left unattended.

Alcohol also interferes with the body's ability to regulate blood sugar and can cause serious health problems for individuals with diabetes. When alcohol is consumed, insulin is released to lower the resulting blood sugar, but the body focuses on metabolizing the alcohol rather than producing the much-needed glucose. Diabetics taking insulin or other oral diabetes medications that work to lower blood glucose levels are at risk of developing hypoglycemia (low blood sugar) when drinking, especially when drinking on an empty stomach or when glucose levels are already low. Symptoms of hypoglycemia mimic signs of intoxication such as dizziness, disorientation, and sleepiness. Thus, a diabetic is often assumed to be intoxicated when, in fact, they are exhibiting signs of hypoglycemia.

The effect of chronic heavy drinking on the effectiveness of insulin produced by the body is also dramatic. Insulin can become less effective over time and lead to hyperglycemia (high blood sugar). Most persons with liver disease, including those with ALD, are diabetic or glucose intolerant (Blendea et al., 2010).

IMMUNE SYSTEM

Chronic heavy drinking can lead to immune deficiencies by increasing susceptibility to infections and diseases. Although the exact mechanisms are not completely understood, the prevalence of alcohol and urinary tract infections, septicemia, and bacterial peritonitis has long been noted (Szabo & Mandrekar, 2009). Higher incidence of bacterial pneumonia, pulmonary tuberculosis, and hepatitis C are also found more among persons who drink heavily than among nondrinkers. Even though HIV infection is associated with heavy drinking, scientists have yet to confirm that alcohol increases susceptibility and facilitates progression to full-blown AIDS.

CANCERS

The causal relationship between alcohol and cancer remains unclear, although mounting scientific evidence suggests that chronic heavy drinking may contribute to development of cancers of the neck and head, stomach, pancreas, colon, breast, and prostate (NIAAA, 2010a). The combination of heavy drinking with other substances, medications, or health conditions also appears to increase the risk of developing cancers. For example, when alcohol and tobacco use co-occur, the risk of developing cancers of the mouth, throat, and colon increases (NIAAA, 2007b). Adults with chronic inflammation of the pancreas appear to be more likely to develop pancreatic cancer if they are chronic heavy drinkers (NIAAA, 2010a). Among women, the combination of hormone replacement therapy and heavy alcohol use may also increase the risk of breast cancer (NIAAA, 2008b). However, additional studies need to be completed to identify the underlying mechanisms, before a clear connection between alcohol and cancer can be stated.

CO-OCCURRING DISORDERS

The co-occurrence of alcohol misuse and other types of substance abuse (e.g., tobacco, medications, and recreational drugs) or mental health disorders (e.g., depression, anxiety, and bipolar disorder) has been well documented. While the relationships and underlying biological mechanisms are not completely understood, several explanations exist that underscore the connections.

Tobacco Use

Alcohol and tobacco use go hand in hand (NIAAA, 2007b). Smokers dependent on nicotine are four times more likely to drink than nonsmokers, and persons dependent on alcohol are more likely to smoke than nondrinkers. Even though the risk factors associated with the two substances vary, both substances act on the brain's mesolimbic system to deliver pleasurable rewards to the user. When alcohol and tobacco are consumed together, the combined pleasurable effect is even greater than either drug alone, explaining, in part, the high rates of co-occurrence.

Drug Use

The co-occurrence of alcohol and drug (i.e., prescription or recreational drug) dependence is frequently noted (NIAAA, 2008a), although people dependent on drugs are more likely to be dependent on alcohol than people with alcohol dependence are dependent on drugs. Gender differences arise in use of alcohol and drugs with men more likely than women to be dependent on both drugs either separately or combined. Still, persons using alcohol and drugs share many of the same risk factors that may place them at risk for dependence, including genetics, social environment, and psychological disorders.

Psychiatric Disorders

It is not clearly understood whether alcohol abuse is a consequence of psychiatric disorders or contributes to their emergence. Either way, the co-occurrence of alcohol abuse and psychiatric disorders is high, especially among persons diagnosed with depression, anxiety, and bipolar disorder. In persons with these disorders, chemical imbalances are suspected to trigger the use of alcohol. The rewarding effects achieved through alcohol not only provide the desired rewards but also alleviate psychiatric symptoms (NIAAA, 2007b). However, recurring alcohol use unbalances brain chemistry and can subsequently mask or exacerbate psychiatric problems. Treatment for co-occurring alcohol and psychiatric disorders can be complex and should include withdrawal from alcohol. Psychiatric problems induced by alcohol can potentially be eradicated through abstinence.

Withdrawal

When drinking ceases, neurons in the brain become hyperexcited, and the body begins to exhibit signs of withdrawal. While the exact mechanisms underlying withdrawal are not yet completely understood, the inhibition of GABA neurotransmitters (as described in the section on the brain's response to alcohol) is believed to be largely responsible. Imbalances in neurochemical and metabolic functioning caused by chronic heavy alcohol use are also suspected to exacerbate withdrawal symptoms by causing seizure activity and delirium. Moreover, the phenomenon of "kindling," a neuronal response associated with how individuals are sensitized to alcohol through repeated exposure, is also linked to increasingly severe alcohol-induced seizures each time a person attempts to withdraw from alcohol, brain damage, and cognitive impairment (Hartsell et al., 2007).

Initial symptoms of alcohol withdrawal generally appear 48 to 72 hours after the last drink (Hartsell et al., 2007) and begin with mild autonomic hyperactivity, including tremulousness and changes in mental functioning (e.g., agitation, confusion, fear, anxiety, and excitement), tachycardia, hypertension, vomiting, sweating, insomnia, and vivid dreams. Symptoms of withdrawal fall along a spectrum of intensity, can worsen quickly, and generally peak in intensity between days 4 and 6. When only mild symptoms are present, withdrawal can last from 1 to 2 days. However, symptoms can last 10 to 14 days for chronic heavy drinkers.

Major symptoms of alcohol withdrawal include seizures, hallucinations, and delirium tremens (DTs). Five to ten percent of persons withdrawing from alcohol experience generalized tonic–clonic seizures during the first 12 to 48 hours after the last drink (Compton, 2002; Hartsell et al., 2007). The likelihood of experiencing seizures increases with the number of withdrawal episodes. For example, individuals who have withdrawn five or more times have a 42% chance of experiencing seizures during withdrawal. Up to 25% of hospitalized persons withdrawing from alcohol will also experience alcohol-induced visual and persecutory hallucinations (Compton, 2002; Hartsell et al., 2007). Moreover, nearly 5% of persons in withdrawal will experience DTs and require medical intervention. Symptoms accompanying DTs include seizures, irregular heartbeat, tachycardia, muscle tremors, heavy sweating, increased startle reflex, and nystagmus.

The mortality rate associated with withdrawal is between 2% and 10%. Underlying poor health conditions are often the primary contributors to death during withdrawal (Hartsell et al., 2007). Even though the withdrawal process can be a humbling and debilitating experience, living through it does not automatically deter a person dependent on alcohol from relapsing. Despite having good intentions, many individuals are lured back to drinking by a craving for its relaxing and euphoric effects or the need to feel "normal" as they struggle to remain sober (NIAAA, 2007b).

PROTECTIVE EFFECTS

Amidst the scientific literature evidencing the detrimental effects of alcohol, there is evidence that drinking low-to-moderate amounts of alcohol every day can protect individuals from health problems, including cardiovascular disease, breast cancer, diabetes, and obesity (NIAAA, 2000). Statistically speaking, persons consuming low-to-moderate amounts of alcohol appear to have a lower risk of developing those conditions than persons consuming high amounts or abstainers. One might assume that abstinence would also be a protective factor. However, epidemiologists have yet to clearly determine its influence on health outcomes because nationally representative surveys of abstainers include two groups of individuals: people who can drink but choose not to and people who no longer drink because of poor health. The health status of the second group complicates complete understanding of the effects of drinking or not drinking and challenges our interpretation of the role of abstinence in health outcomes. Regardless, scientists agree that no one should be advised to start drinking in an attempt to benefit from the protective effects of alcohol, and people who drink more than moderate amounts should consider cutting back their consumption to benefit from alcohol's protective effects.

Alcohol also shares a protective role in promoting personal well-being and social relationships (NIAAA, 2000). Socialization opportunities that often accompany drinking can improve a participant's satisfaction and happiness with life. Moreover, when older adults join together to share a meal, they tend to eat a better balanced diet, which helps them maintain good health and process the alcohol they consume.

TERMINOLOGY, RISK FACTORS, AND SCREENING

Terminology

Before screening patients for potential alcohol problems, health care professionals need to be aware of the terminology associated with drinking and knowledgeable of drinking guidelines promulgated by the NIAAA, one of the National Institutes of Health.

The myriad of social terms often used to describe a person who drinks heavily or is dependent on alcohol (e.g., boozer, drunkard, and lush) and their drinking patterns (e.g., on a bender, social drinker) have subjective meanings, and their use by professionals can hinder understanding of alcohol-related behaviors and working with persons with drinking problems. Terms that label individuals as "alcoholics" or "drunks" are stigmatizing and judgmental. Use of such terms with persons in denial of their drinking problems will only impede efforts to help them confront their alcohol use.

Successful interactions with persons who are dependent on alcohol are based on an understanding that alcohol dependency involves a complex set of interactions influenced by biological, psychological, social, and environmental factors and that drinking behaviors occur on a continuum spanning from abstinence to dependence. The World Health Organization (2012) has adopted an approach to conceptualize drinking behaviors and has recommended categorizing and thinking about drinking habits using three categories: nonhazardous (no risks involved), hazardous (alcohol use associated with risks of complications), or harmful (alcohol use causes complications such as dependence). This broader conceptualization of alcohol use helps place intervention efforts in perspective and helps professionals focus on the specific needs of a person as they travel on the road to recovery.

Until broader definitions of alcohol use are fully adopted in the United States, criteria for diagnosing alcohol misuse, specifically alcohol abuse and alcohol dependence, are outlined in the

American Psychological Association's *DSM-IV: Diagnostic and Statistical Manual of Mental Disorders* (1994). Alcohol abuse is defined as patterns of alcohol use that lead to significant impairment in functioning during a 12-month period measured by meeting at least one of the following criteria:

- Failure to fulfill major obligations at work, school, or home due to recurring alcohol use
- Recurrent alcohol use in situations that are physically hazardous (e.g., driving while intoxicated or operating machinery)
- Legal problems related to alcohol use
- Significant social or interpersonal problems caused by alcohol use.

Alcohol dependence is an extension of alcohol abuse that requires meeting three or more of the following criteria in a 12-month period:

- Increased tolerance of alcohol (more needed to achieve rewarding effect)
- Characteristic withdrawal symptoms and alcohol consumed to relieve symptoms
- Alcohol consumed in larger amounts and for longer periods than intended
- Persistent desire or repeated unsuccessful attempts to stop drinking
- Time and energy spent on obtaining, consuming, and recovering from alcohol
- Reduced social, occupational, or recreational activities due to alcohol use.

The terms "alcoholic" and "alcoholism" are no longer linked to medical diagnostic criteria, although they continue to imply alcohol dependency.

Standard Unit of Drink

Discussions with older adults about their alcohol use must be based on a mutual understanding of what constitutes a standard unit of drink. According to the NIAAA (2010b), a standard unit of drink contains about 14 g of alcohol. Figure 21.2 illustrates different types of alcoholic

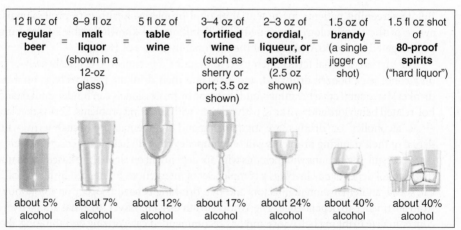

FIGURE 21.2. Standard unit of drinks. (Adapted from National Institute on Alcohol Abuse and Alcoholism. [2010]. *Rethinking drinking* [NIH Publication No. 10-3770]. Rockville, MD: Author. Retrieved from http://rethinkingdrinking.niaaa.nih.gov/WhatCountsDrink/WhatsAstandardDrink.asp. Information available on the NIAAA Web site is within the public domain, and unless otherwise noted, may be freely downloaded and reproduced.)

beverages and their volume equivalents in relation to a standard unit of drink. Use of a standard unit of drink helps patients recognize how much alcohol they are consuming and helps health care providers facilitate discussion for reducing intake without infringing on alcoholic preferences.

DRINKING GUIDELINE RECOMMENDATIONS

Guidelines for daily and weekly alcohol consumption for older adults are consistent with studies on the effects of alcohol on functional impairments. Older adults drinking seven or more alcoholic drinks per week experience functional impairments in completing their instrumental activities of daily living (IADL) (e.g., driving, housekeeping, and managing finances). Similarly, consuming more than three drinks on one occasion also results in impairments with IADLs. Thus, the NIAAA used those findings to establish drinking guidelines for adults aged 65+ to promote successful functioning and reduce health risks (see Table 21.3). Individuals who exceed the recommended drinking guideline per occasion are referred to as binge drinkers.

Risk Factors

Risk factors for problems with alcohol include biological, social, and environmental factors. As covered in previous sections, the physiology of the older body is sensitive to alcohol, and it becomes more difficult for older adults to manage the effects of alcohol as they age and cope with other health problems.

Genetic makeup can also be a risk factor for alcohol use (NIAAA, 2003). Geneticists studying associations between alcohol dependency and genes estimate that 40% to 60% of the population has genetic tendencies toward alcohol dependency. However, no single gene is responsible for alcohol use. Rather, a combination of several genes and variations within those genes are more likely responsible for placing some individuals at higher risk for alcohol dependency. Scientists continue to explore those genetic associations—especially ones that connect alcohol dependency with depression and nicotine dependency.

Social and environmental changes that accompany lifestyle changes and transitions can also increase the risk of alcohol problems in late life (Rigler, 2000). Retirement, death of a spouse or loved one, increasing caregiving responsibilities, declining health, financial insecurity, and social isolation are often accompanied by periods of stress. Retirees, especially women, are at risk for becoming binge drinkers. Individuals with physical disabilities, persons with limited mobility,

TABLE 21.3 • Drinking Guidelines for Older Adults

Women	Men
<1 drink per day	Up to 2 drinks per day
Up to 7 drinks per week	Up to 14 drinks per week
No more than 2 drinks per occasion	No more than 3 drinks per occasion

and other older socially isolated adults are at risk for increasing their dependence on alcohol as a means to cope (Menninger, 2002).

How well older adults cope when distressed, depends, in part, on their history of alcohol use (i.e., early onset, late onset, or returning drinkers—see Screening Tools for additional information) and how they use alcohol to cope (Liberto & Oslin, 1995). Certain groups of individuals—men, smokers, unmarried persons, depressed individuals, and the bereaved— have been shown to be at risk for alcohol use problems, even after a history of abstention (Karlamangla et al., 2006; Sacco et al., 2009; Stevenson, 2005). Thus, when health care professionals can keep track of the life events of patients, potential problems with alcohol can be recognized sooner than later.

Medications

Many classifications of medications (i.e., prescription and over-the-counter) taken by older adults are contraindicated when used in combination with alcohol. Health care professionals need to ask older patients about their medication use at each visit so that potential alcohol and medication interaction problems can be quickly identified and treatments can be better managed. The NIAAA (2007a) produces a list of common medications contraindicated by alcohol and their possible reactions with alcohol (reproduced in Table 21.4). As shown in the table, many of the reactions mimic intoxication and withdrawal (e.g., drowsiness, impaired motor control, memory problems, and nausea), which confirms the importance of understanding the role of alcohol use in the lives of older patients and being able to recognize when it is or is not a contributing factor to reported health concerns.

Screening Tools

A number of screening tools for alcohol problems have been developed and standardized, but do not have high validity with older adults. That is, questions asked about alcohol use are not sensitive to the lifestyles and behaviors of older adults. For example, asking a socially isolated older adult whether relatives or friends have expressed concerns over their drinking habit is not meaningful. The 10-item Short Michigan Alcoholism Screening Test–Geriatric Version (S-MAST-G) (Blow et al., 1992) has been shown to be valid and sensitive to older respondents and recommended for inclusion as part of the health care screening process. The questions can be asked as written or incorporated into conversation with an older patient (see Table 21.5). If respondents answer "yes" to two or more questions, they likely have a problem managing their drinking, and further discussion is warranted.

Often, the manner in which a person presents to a health care provider provides clues as to whether alcohol use might be problematic. Despite evidence to the contrary, it is possible that an individual may not perceive a problem with alcohol when the health care professional does. The most successful approach to talking with older adults about sensitive topics such as alcohol use is to incorporate questions into conversations about other health concerns (e.g., exercise and smoking) and social activities. By routinely incorporating questions at each health visit, conversations about alcohol use become normalized and patients can become more comfortable talking about their drinking. Moreover, conditions that mimic intoxication and withdrawal can be more effectively uncovered (Compton, 2002; Donnelly et al., 2012; Puz & Stokes, 2005).

TABLE 21.4 · Effects of Alcohol on Medications

Symptoms/Disorders	Medication		Possible Reactions with Alcohol
	Brand Name	Generic Name	
Allergies/colds/flu	Alavert	Loratadine	Drowsiness, dizziness; increased risk of overdose
	Allegra	Fexofenadine	
	Benadryl	Diphenhydramine	
	Clarinex	Desloratadine	
	Claritin	Loratadine	
	Dimetapp Cold & Allergy	Brompheniramine	
	Sudafed Sinus & Allergy	Chlorpheniramine	
	Triaminic Cold & Allergy		
	Tylenol Allergy Sinus		
	Tylenol Cold & Flu		
	Zyrtec	Cetirizine	
Angina/chest pain	Isordil	Isosorbide	Rapid heartbeat, sudden changes in blood pressure, dizziness, fainting
Anxiety and epilepsy	Ativan	Lorazepam	Drowsiness, dizziness; increased risk of overdose; slowed or difficulty breathing; impaired motor control; unusual behavior; and memory problems
	Klonopin	Clonazepam	
	Librium	Chlordiazepoxide	
	Paxil	Paroxetine	
	Valium	Diazepam	
	Xanax	Alprazolam	
	Herbal Preparations (Kava Kava)		Liver damage, drowsiness
Arthritis	Celebrex	Celecoxib	Ulcers, stomach bleeding, liver problems
	Naprosyn	Naproxen	
	Voltaren	Diclofenac	
Blood clots	Coumadin	Warfarin	Occasional drinking may lead to internal bleeding; heavier drinking also may cause bleeding or may have the opposite effect, resulting in possible blood clots, strokes, or heart attacks
Cough	Delsym Robitussin Cough	Dextromethorphan	Drowsiness, dizziness; increased risk of overdose
	Robitussin A-C	Guaifenesin & codeine	
Depression	Anafranil	Clomipramine	Drowsiness, dizziness, increased risk of overdose; increased feelings of depression
	Celexa	Citalopram	
	Desyrel	Trazodone	
	Effexor	Venlafaxine	
	Elavil	Amitriptyline	
	Lexapro	Escitalopram	
	Luvox	Fluvoxamine	
	Norpramin	Desipramine	
	Paxil	Paroxetine	
	Prozac	Fluoxetine	
	Serzone	Nefazodone	
	Wellbutrin	Bupropion	
	Zoloft	Sertraline	
	Herbal preparations		

(Continued)

TABLE 21.4 • Effects of Alcohol on Medications *(Continued)*

| Symptoms/Disorders | Medication | | Possible Reactions with Alcohol |
	Brand Name	Generic Name	
Diabetes	Glucophage	Metformin	Abnormally low blood sugar levels, flushing reaction (nausea, vomiting, headache, rapid heartbeat, sudden changes in blood pressure)
	Micronase	Glyburide	
	Orinase	Tolbutamide	
Enlarged prostate	Cardura	Doxazosin	Dizziness, light headedness, fainting
	Flomax	Tamsulosin	
	Hytrin	Terazosin	
	Minipress	Prazosin	
Heartburn, indigestion, sour stomach	Axid	Nizatidine	Rapid heartbeat, sudden changes in blood pressure (metoclopramide); increased alcohol effect
	Reglan	Metoclopramide	
	Tagamet	Cimetidine	
	Zantac	Ranitidine	
High blood pressure	Accupril	Quinapril	Dizziness, fainting, drowsiness; heart problems such as changes in the heart's regular heartbeat (arrhythmia)
	Capozide	Hydrochlorothiazide	
	Cardura	Doxazosin	
	Catapres	Clonidine	
	Cozaar	Losartan	
	Hytrin	Terazosin	
	Lopressor HCT	Hydrochlorothiazide	
	Lotensin	Benazepril	
	Minipress	Prazosin	
	Vaseretic	Enalapril	
High cholesterol	Advicor	Lovastatin and niacin	Liver damage (all medications); increased flushing and itching (niacin), increased stomach bleeding (pravastatin and aspirin)
	Altocor	Lovastatin	
	Crestor	Rosuvastatin	
	Lipitor	Atorvastatin	
	Mevacor	Lovastatin	
	Niaspan	Niacin	
	Pravachol	Pravastatin	
	Pravigard	Pravastatin and aspirin	
	Vytorin	Ezetimibe and simvastatin	
	Zocor	Simvastatin	
Infections	Macrodantin*	Nitrofurantoin	Fast heartbeat, sudden changes in blood pressure; stomach pain, upset stomach, vomiting, headache, or flushing or redness of the face; liver damage (isoniazid, ketoconazole)
	Flagyl	Metronidazole	
	Grisactin	Griseofulvin	
	Nizoral	Ketoconazole	
	Nydrazid	Isoniazid	
	Seromycin	Cycloserine	
	Tindamax	Tinidazole	
Muscle pain	Flexeril	Cyclobenzaprine	Drowsiness, dizziness; increased risk of seizures; increased risk of overdose; slowed or difficulty breathing; impaired motor control; unusual behavior; memory problems
	Soma	Carisoprodol	

TABLE 21.4 · Effects of Alcohol on Medications *(Continued)*

Symptoms/Disorders	Medication		Possible Reactions with Alcohol
	Brand Name	Generic Name	
Nausea, motion sickness	Antivert	Meclizine	Drowsiness, dizziness; increased risk of overdose
	Atarax	Hydroxyzine	
	Dramamine	Dimenhydrinate	
	Phenergan	Promethazine	
Pain (such as headache, muscle ache, minor arthritis pain), fever, inflammation	Advil	Ibuprofen	Stomach upset, bleeding, and ulcers; liver damage (acetaminophen); rapid heartbeat
	Aleve	Naproxen	
	Excedrin	Aspirin, Acetaminophen	
	Motrin	Ibuprofen	
	Tylenol	Acetaminophen	
Seizures	Dilantin	Phenytoin	Drowsiness, dizziness; increased risk of seizures
	Klonopin	Clonazepam phenobarbital	
Severe pain from injury. Postsurgical care, oral surgery, migraines	Darvocet-N	Propoxyphene	Drowsiness, dizziness; increased risk of overdose; slowed or difficulty breathing; impaired motor control; unusual behavior; memory problems
	Demerol	Meperidine	
	Fiorinal w/codeine	Butalbital w/codeine	
	Percocet	Oxycodone	
	Vicodin	Hydrocodone	
Sleep problems	Ambien	Zolpidem	Drowsiness, sleepiness, dizziness; slowed or difficulty breathing; impaired motor control; unusual behavior; memory problems
	Lunesta	Eszopiclone	
	ProSom	Estazolam	
	Restoril	Temazepam	
	Sominex	Diphenhydramine	
	Unisom	Doxylamine	
	Herbal preparations (chamomile, valerian, lavender)		Increased drowsiness

Adapted from National Institute on Alcohol Abuse and Alcoholism. (2007). *Harmful interactions: Mixing medications and alcohol.* Rockville, MD: Author. Content is in public domain and may be reproduced freely.

Even though gathering information about alcohol use in the recent past is invaluable, learning about the drinking history of an older adult can also help uncover and predict drinking behaviors. Older persons dependent on alcohol or suspected of having a drinking problem are generally categorized as early onset, late onset, or returning drinkers (Liberto & Oslin, 1995). Early onset drinkers are established drinkers. They have been drinking alcohol throughout their lives and have likely relied on alcohol as a coping mechanism in the past. Late onset drinkers begin drinking in late life—usually when faced with a stressful situation (e.g., retirement, caregiving responsibilities, death of a spouse). Returning drinkers are older adults who return to drinking after many years of abstinence. Their decision to drink can also be motivated by many factors, including lifestyle changes, poor health, relationship loss, financial trouble, and caregiving burdens.

TABLE 21.5 • Short Michigan Alcoholism Screening Test–Geriatric Version (S-MAST-G)

S. No.	Item	Yes	No
1	When talking with others, do you ever underestimate how much you actually drink?		
2	After a few drinks, have you sometimes not eaten or been able to skip a meal because you didn't feel hungry?		
3	Does having a few drinks help decrease your shakiness or tremors?		
4	Does alcohol sometimes make it hard for you to remember parts of the day or night?		
5	Do you usually take a drink to relax or calm your nerves?		
6	Do you drink to take your mind off your problems?		
7	Have you ever increased your drinking after experiencing a loss in your life?		
8	Has a doctor or nurse ever said they were worried or concerned about your drinking?		
9	Have you ever made rules to manage your drinking?		
10	When you feel lonely, does having a drink help?		

From Blow, F. C., Brower, K. J., Schulenberg, J. E., Demo-Dananberg, L. M., Young, J. P., & Beresford, T. P. (1992). The Michigan Alcoholism Screening Test–Geriatric Version (MAST-G): A new elderly-specific screening instrument. *Alcoholism: Clinical and Experimental Research, 16,* 372, with permission. ©The Regents of the University of Michigan, 1991.

TREATMENT

Treatment strategies for alcohol problems vary according to the presenting status of the individual, level of alcohol use, willingness to change alcohol use, and the availability of family and friends to provide support on the road to recovery. Thus, treatment options can include multiple approaches, including short- and long-term options. Any approach chosen needs to reflect each person's individual needs (Tucker and Simpson, 2011).

Brief Intervention

Older adults who consume enough alcohol on a regular basis to place them at risk for problems with alcohol (i.e., at or above the recommended guidelines) respond well to brief interventions during routine health care visits. Brief interventions are designed to take place in a clinic or home setting and can last 5 to 30 minutes. The intervention focus is placed on how current level of alcohol use and drinking behaviors affect the individual's health, well-being, and quality of life. During the conversation, the patient is invited to help identify strategies for change that are consistent with their personal goals, values, and lifestyle. Studies have shown that older patients who receive a brief intervention will change their drinking habits and remain compliant up to 12 months after the intervention (Fleming et al., 1999). Moreover, brief interventions also appear to reduce alcohol-related hospitalizations and health care utilization in the year following intervention (Fleming et al., 2002).

Because the purpose of the intervention is to help the older adult move past ambivalence about their drinking habits and negotiate successful lifestyle changes, the use of a motivational interviewing (MI) approach (Miller & Rollnick, 2002) has been shown to be effective. Motivational interviewing requires more than just being a good listener and dispensing sage advice. Motivational interviewing elicits talk about change from the individual by using nonjudgmental encouraging language and reflective listening techniques. Resistance on the part of the individual is met with reflection to stimulate their involvement and acceptance of change. Through the use of MI strategies, the health care provider and the patient gain a mutual understanding of the patient's perceptions of current alcohol use and how he or she wants the future to look.

The FRAMES approach (Miller & Sanchez, 1994) is a framework for guiding conversation in a brief intervention and complements MI strategies. FRAMES is an acronym for key concepts (Feedback, Responsibility, Advice, Menu of options, Empathy, and Self-efficacy) used to facilitate a brief intervention. Because no two conversations are alike, no standard scripts exist on what participants should say. Still, the FRAMES approach can be used to guide each conversation. Elements of the FRAMES approach are presented in Table 21.6 with sample statements to illustrate the types of statements that might be made by an interventionist.

If in the process of conducting a brief intervention it becomes clear to the health care professional that the patient has an alcohol dependence problem and could benefit from an intervention with a specialized treatment program, referral to appropriate treatment should be discussed and integrated into the brief intervention.

Readiness for Change

The biggest barrier to treatment is the patient. Many individuals continue to deny they have a problem with alcohol even after the people closest to them begin to express concerns. Early onset drinkers are inherently poised to deny a drinking problem because they have used alcohol throughout their lives—and generally without any major impact on their daily activities (Liberto & Oslin, 1995). Late onset drinkers are most likely to accept treatment once they participate in a brief intervention and become aware of the effects of alcohol on their life. Still, regardless of the

TABLE 21.6 • FRAMES Approach to a Brief Intervention

Element	Element Description	Sample Statement
Feedback	Provide feedback on personal risk due to drinking	Your drinking may be increasing the anxiety you feel
Responsibility	Emphasize personal responsibility for change	No one can make you change. It is up to you
Advice	Advise the person to make changes in their behavior	If you limit yourself to only two drinks per evening, you will be putting less stress on your body
Menu	Offer a menu of options that can facilitate change	A daily diary can help you monitor your drinking
Empathy	Use empathy while engaged in conversation	This must be difficult for you to hear
Self-efficacy	Promote self-efficacy and optimism that change is possible	You have the strength to make this change in your life

Adapted from Center for Substance Abuse Treatment. (1999). *Enhancing motivation for change in substance abuse treatment. Treatment Improvement Protocol (TIP) series, No. 35* (HHS Publication No. [SMA] 12-4212). Rockville, MD: Substance Abuse and Mental Health Services Administration. Content is in public domain and may be reproduced freely.

levels of consumption and drinking history, each individual must be willing to make a change in how they use alcohol before treatment interventions are effective.

Unfortunately, the positive rewards associated with drinking often override a person's best intentions. The Transtheoretical Model (TTM) (Prochaska et al., 2008) is used to explain a person's readiness to change and the steps he or she goes through on the road to recovery. Persons relapsing in their efforts to stop drinking are assumed to reenter the model at the stage at which they are prepared to succeed.

Within each stage of change, certain key activities or processes need to be completed or addressed so that the individual can be successful in achieving sobriety. These catalysts for change and corresponding steps for an interventionist to pursue are provided in Table 21.7.

Pharmacological Interventions

Medications are often prescribed in conjunction with other intervention strategies to help individuals dependent on alcohol manage their withdrawal symptoms or refrain from drinking. As noted in Table 21.8, one generic medication (disulfam) affects the body's metabolism and three other generic medications (i.e., benzodiazepines, naltrexone, and acamprosate) interact with neurotransmissions in the brain (NIAAA, 2008a, 2009).

Disulfam is prescribed for individuals wanting to abstain from drinking. It works by increasing levels of acetaldehyde in the body, which will cause users to feel violently ill if they consume alcohol. However, this aversive approach is only effective if the patient adheres to the prescribed medication regime.

Benzodiazepines are the first line of pharmacologic therapy prescribed to alleviate withdrawal symptoms (Hartsell et al., 2007). The underlying mechanism of the drug enhances the depressive effect of GABA while delivering the effects of alcohol to the patient. Different forms of the drug can be short- or long-acting, and their prescribed use is dependent on the patient's health and withdrawal symptoms. Because benzodiazepines are highly addictive, patients should not be discharged with a prescription unless closely monitored.

Older adults medicated with benzodiazepine generally receive short-acting dosages (Compton, 2002; McKay et al., 2004; Myrick & Anton, 1998). This helps health care professionals effectively manage withdrawal symptoms and identify other health conditions unmasked by the benzodiazepine. Because older patients are at risk for poor health and multiple health problems, they are monitored closely (during and after withdrawal) as benzodiazepine levels are tapered to ensure their health is not further compromised.

Regardless of the medication prescribed or the use of short- or long-acting dosages, successful treatment relies on medication adherence and permanent lifestyle changes, which include abstinence from drinking.

Detoxification and Inpatient Treatment

The health care professional's role in the withdrawal process is to provide a supportive environment, alleviate symptoms, prevent progression of withdrawal to DTs, manage co-occurring health conditions, and provide information about treatment options after discharge (Hartsell et al., 2007; Myrick & Anton, 1998).

Supportive care is provided by ensuring a quiet, safe, and comfortable environment with supervision. Unnecessary stimulation and noise (e.g., television, movies, or loud conversations)

TABLE 21.7 • Stages of Change, Catalysts for Change, and Interventionist Steps

TTM Stage	Catalysts for Change	Interventionist Steps

Precontemplation The older adult (OA) is not yet considering change or is unwilling or unable to change	**Consciousness raising**—possessing information about problem
	Environmental reevaluation—assessing how problem affects personal and physical environment
	Emotional arousal and dramatic relief—experiencing and expressing personal feelings about problem
		■ Establish a rapport, ask permission, build trust
		■ Raise doubts or concerns in the OA about alcohol use by:
		  ■ Exploring the meaning of the events that brought the OA to treatment or the results of previous treatments
		  ■ Eliciting the OA's perceptions of the problem
		  ■ Offering factual information about the risks of alcohol use
		  ■ Providing personalized feedback about assessment findings
		  ■ Exploring the pros and cons of alcohol abuse
		  ■ Examining discrepancies between the OA's and others' perceptions of the problem behavior
		■ Express concern and keep the door open

Contemplation The OA acknowledges concerns and is considering the possibility of change, but is ambivalent and uncertain	**Self-evaluation**—assessing how one thinks about one's problems
	Environmental reevaluation—assessing how problem affects personal and physical environment
	Emotional arousal and dramatic relief—experiencing and expressing personal feelings about problem
		■ Normalize ambivalence
		■ Help the OA tip the decisional balances scale toward change by:
		  ■ Eliciting and weighing pros and cons of alcohol abuse and change
		  ■ Changing extrinsic to intrinsic motivation
		  ■ Examining the OA's personal values in relation to change
		  ■ Emphasizing the OA's free choice, responsibility, and self-efficacy for change
		■ Elicit self-motivational statements of intent and commitment
		■ Elicit ideas of the OA's perceived self-efficacy and expectation regarding treatment
		■ Summarize self-motivational statements

Preparation The OA is committed to and planning to make a change in the near future, but is still considering what to do	**Self-liberation**—choosing and committing to change **Counterconditioning**—substituting alternative coping strategies **Helping relationships**—working with others who care	■ Clarify the OA's own goals and strategies for change ■ Offer a menu of options for change or treatment ■ With permission, offer expertise and advice ■ Negotiate a change or treatment plan and behavior contract ■ Consider and lower barriers to change ■ Help the OA enlist social support ■ Explore treatment expectancies and the OA's role ■ Elicit from the OA what has worked in the past ■ Assist the OA to negotiate finances, transportation, or other potential barriers ■ Have the OA publicly announce plans to change

(Continued)

TABLE 21.7 · Stages of Change, Catalysts for Change, and Interventionist Steps (*Continued*)

TTM Stage	Catalysts for Change	Interventionist Steps
Action The OA is actively taking steps to change, but has not yet reached a stable state	**Counterconditioning**—substituting alternative coping strategies **Helping relationships**—working with others who care **Stimulus control**—avoiding stimuli that elicit problem behaviors **Reinforcement management**—rewarding oneself for making changes	▪ Engage the OA in treatment and reinforce importance of recovery ▪ Support a realistic view of change through small steps ▪ Acknowledge difficulties in early stages of change ▪ Help the OA identify high-risk situations and develop appropriate coping strategies to overcome ▪ Assist the OA in finding new reinforcers of positive change ▪ Help the OA assess whether he or she has family and social support
Maintenance The OA has achieved initial goals such as abstinence and is now working toward maintaining gains	**Environmental reevaluation**—assessing how problem affects personal and physical environment **Self-liberation**—choosing and committing to change **Helping relationships**—working with others who care **Reinforcement management**—rewarding oneself for making changes	▪ Help the OA identify and sample new reinforcers ▪ Support lifestyle changes ▪ Affirm the OA's resolve and self-efficacy ▪ Help the OA practice and use new coping strategies to avoid relapse ▪ Maintain supportive contact ▪ Develop a plan if OA were to resume alcohol use ▪ Review long-term goal with OA
Recurrence The OA has experienced a recurrence of symptoms and must cope with consequences and what to do next	Use catalysts associated with at point of reentry	▪ Help the OA reenter the change cycle and commend any willingness to reconsider positive change ▪ Explore the meaning and reality of the recurrence as a learning experience ▪ Assist the OA in finding alternative coping strategies ▪ Maintain supportive contact

Adapted from Center for Substance Abuse Treatment. (1999). *Enhancing motivation for change in substance abuse treatment. Treatment Improvement Protocol (TIP) series, No. 35* (HHS Publication No. [SMA] 12-4212). Rockville, MD: Substance Abuse and Mental Health Services Administration. Content is in public domain and may be reproduced freely.

TABLE 21.8 · Medications for Treating Alcohol Abuse

Medications		Treatment Use	Effect
Generic Name	Brand Name		
Benzodiazepines	Valium Xanax	Treating alcohol withdrawal	Increases GABA activity, curbing the brain's "excitability" during its withdrawal from alcohol, allowing the brain to restore its natural balance
Disulfiram	Antabuse	Main effect on alcohol metabolism rather than on the brain	Increases the concentration of acetaldehyde, causing unpleasant symptoms such as nausea and flushing of the skin if alcohol is consumed
Naltrexone	ReVia Vivitrol Naltrel	Reducing/stopping drinking	Blocks opioid receptors involved in the pleasant sensations associated with drinking
Acamprosate	Campral	Enhancing abstinence	Thought to dampen glutamate activity, may reduce some of the hyperexcitability associated with alcohol withdrawal

Adapted from National Institute on Alcohol Abuse and Alcoholism. (2009). Neuroscience: Pathways to alcohol dependence. *Alcohol Alert, 77*. Retrieved from http://pubs.niaaa.nih.gov/publications/AA77/AA77.htm. All material contained in the *Alcohol Alert* is in the public domain and may be used or reproduced without permission from NIAAA.

can exacerbate confusion and excitability—especially during hallucinogenic states—and should be avoided. Patient electrolyte levels should be monitored and kept in balance through intravenous fluids. Thiamine supplements (100 mg) should also be offered for prophylaxis against or for Wernicke–Korsakoff syndrome.

Symptom management can be achieved through fixed-dose or symptom-triggered regimes of medication therapy (Hartsell et al., 2007). A fixed-dose approach is based on dosing at regularly scheduled intervals regardless of manifested symptoms. While the approach is effective, patients can become oversedated, and health care professionals often find it difficult to respond effectively to a patient's challenging behaviors as they erupt. With symptom-triggered therapy, benzodiazepines are administered in response to patient symptoms and only at levels necessary to alleviate discomfort. The patient's withdrawal status is assessed frequently using a tool like the Clinical Institute Withdrawal Assessment for Alcohol Scale (CIWA-Ar) (Sullivan et al., 1989) (see Table 21.9). The CIWA-Ar not only helps health care professionals identify the severity and progress of withdrawal symptoms, it helps guide medication dosages. When compared, fixed-dose and symptom-triggered regimes result in comparable outcomes with similar complications. However, the time spent with symptom-triggered therapy is shorter (20 vs. 63 hours) and relies on less medication (37 vs. 231 mg), a potential benefit for both patient and health care facility.

After withdrawal and prior to discharge, health care professionals need to have a frank discussion with each patient about drinking and the effects of alcohol on the body. A brief intervention (as previously outlined) accompanied by basic information about alcohol dependence and resources in the community is an essential step in helping a patient become successful on the road to recovery.

TABLE 21.9 · Clinical Institute Withdrawal Assessment for Alcohol Scale (CIWA-Ar)

Nausea and vomiting	**Tactile disturbances**
Ask "Do you feel sick to your stomach? Have you vomited?"	Ask "Have you any itching, pins and needles sensations, any burning, any numbness, or do you feel bugs crawling on or under your skin?"
Observation	*Observation*
0 no nausea and no vomiting	0 none
1 mild nausea with no vomiting	1 very mild itching, pins and needles, burning, or numbness
2	2 mild itching, pins and needles, burning, or numbness
3	3 moderate itching, pins and needles, burning, or numbness
4 intermittent nausea with dry heaves	4 moderately severe hallucinations
5	5 severe hallucinations
6	6 extremely severe hallucinations
7 constant nausea, frequent dry heaves and vomiting	7 continuous hallucinations
Tremor	**Auditory disturbances**
Arms extended and fingers spread apart.	Ask "Are you more aware of sounds around you? Are they harsh? Do they frighten you? Are you hearing anything that is disturbing to you? Are you hearing things you know are not there?"
Observation	
0 no tremor	
1 not visible, but can be felt fingertip to fingertip	*Observation*
2	0 not present
3	1 very mild harshness or ability to frighten
4 moderate, with patient's arms extended	2 mild harshness or ability to frighten
5	3 moderate harshness or ability to frighten
6	4 moderately severe hallucinations
7 severe, even with arms not extended	5 severe hallucinations
	6 extremely severe hallucinations
	7 continuous hallucination
Paroxysmal sweats	**Visual disturbances**
Observation	Ask "Does the light appear to be too bright? Is its color different? Does it hurt your eyes? Are you seeing anything that is disturbing to you? Are you seeing things you know are not there?"
0 no sweat visible	
1 barely perceptible sweating, palms moist	
2	*Observation*
3	0 not present
4 beads of sweat obvious on forehead	1 very mild sensitivity
5	2 mild sensitivity
6	3 moderate sensitivity
7 drenching sweats	4 moderately severe hallucinations
	5 severe hallucinations
	6 extremely severe hallucinations
	7 continuous hallucinations
Anxiety	**Headache, fullness in head**
Ask "Do you feel nervous?"	Ask "Does your head feel different? Does it feel like there is a band around your head?" Do not rate for dizziness or lightheadedness. Otherwise, rate severity.
Observation	
0 no anxiety, at ease	
1 mildly anxious	*Observation*
2	0 not present
3	1 very mild

TABLE 21.9 • Clinical Institute Withdrawal Assessment for Alcohol Scale (CIWA-Ar) (Continued)

4 moderately anxious, or guarded, so anxiety is inferred	2 mild
5	3 moderate
6	4 moderately severe
7 equivalent to acute panic states as seen in severe delirium or acute schizophrenic reactions	5 severe
	6 very severe
	7 extremely severe
Agitation	**Orientation and clouding of sensorium**
Observation	Ask "What day is this? Where are you? Who am I?"
0 normal activity	*Observation*
1 somewhat more than normal activity	0 oriented and can do serial additions
2	1 cannot do serial additions or is uncertain about date
3	2 disoriented for date by no more than 2 calendar days
4 moderately fidgety and restless	3 disoriented for date by more than 2 calendar days
5	4 disoriented for place/or person
6	Total **CIWA-Ar** Score _____
7 paces back and forth during most of the interview, or constantly thrashes about	Rater's Initials _____
	Maximum Possible Score 67

The CIWA-Ar is not copyrighted and may be reproduced freely. Patients scoring less than 10 do not usually need additional medication for withdrawal.
Adapted from Sullivan, J. T., Sykora, K., Schneiderman, J., Naranjo, C. A., & Sellers, E. M. (1989). Assessment of alcohol withdrawal: The revised Clinical Institute Withdrawal Assessment for Alcohol scale (CIWA-Ar). *British Journal of Addiction, 84,* 1353–1357, with permission.

Long-Term or Outpatient Treatment

Outpatient interventions take place in a variety of home and community settings. The type of intervention delivered is initially based on the individual's level of alcohol consumption (i.e., above or below recommended limits) and associated level of risk. Because drinking problems and the factors that contribute to drinking vary by individual, long-term interventions need to be tailored to meet the medical and social needs of each participant (McKay & Hiller-Sturmhofel, 2011).

A barrier to outpatient treatments is the lack of therapeutic options designed specifically for older individuals and offered at accessible locations and times (White et al., 2011). While some group treatment options may serve older adults, they tend to be based on processes developed with younger adults in mind. Until older adults demand treatments that specifically address their needs and lifestyles, treatment options are likely to remain limited.

Specialized Formal Interventions or Treatment Approaches

Specialized intensive treatment programs for alcohol dependency are now available in most communities. Two scientifically valid and popular therapeutic intervention models include cognitive behavioral therapy (CBT) and motivational enhancement therapy (MET) (CSAT, 1999; NIAAA, 2008a). Sessions are led by licensed clinical therapists trained in conducting each approach and are offered as individual and group formats. CBT strategies are well-suited to individuals agreeable to working on their alcohol dependence. Participants learn to identify situations that place them at risk and develop alternative responses that can support their efforts to abstain from drinking. CBT is personalized and focused on changing behaviors as well as thinking.

MET is most effective with individuals resistant to change. The MET process uses a client-centered nonconfrontational approach to effect change. It incorporates MI strategies such as those used in the brief intervention process to facilitate personal recognition and acceptance of alcohol-related problems. MET is particularly effective in helping participants resolve their ambivalence toward drinking and commit to change.

Another community-based treatment option includes 12-step programs like Alcoholics Anonymous (AA). The AA organization literature describes itself as *a fellowship of men and women who share their experience, strength, and hope with each other that they may solve their common problem and help others to recover from alcoholism. The only requirement for membership is a desire to stop drinking. There are no dues or fees for AA membership; we are self-supporting through our own contributions. AA is not allied with any sect, denomination, politics, organization, or institution; does not wish to engage in any controversy; neither endorses nor opposes any causes. Our primary purpose is to stay sober and help other alcoholics to achieve sobriety* (AA Grapevine, Inc., 2011).

Twelve-step programs, like AA, are guided by common principles, which participants accept and work through to regain control of their lives. The 12-step process includes:

- Admitting that one cannot control one's addiction
- Recognizing a higher power that can give strength
- Examining past errors with the help of a sponsor—a more experienced member
- Making amends for errors
- Learning to live a new life with a code of behavior
- Helping others who suffer from the same problems of addiction.

While there is limited scientific evidence that indicates programs such as AA significantly increase abstinence, the 63,845 groups in the United States and Canada, supported by over 1.3 million members, suggest it has an important role in helping individuals succeed on the road to recovery. The unconditional acceptance of new members and lack of stigmatization among them no doubt facilitates the powerful fellowship that helps them move toward their goals.

CULTURAL AND RELIGIOUS CONSIDERATIONS

How individuals view alcohol use varies by culture. In some regions (e.g., Mediterranean and some South American cultures), drinking is regarded as a peaceful communal activity, whereas in other parts of the world (e.g., United States, United Kingdom, Scandinavia, and Australia), drinking is primarily a singular activity often associated with violence and disruptive behaviors (Social Issues Research Centre, 1998).

In the United States and United Kingdom, whites tend to drink more and abstain less than the minority ethnic groups living in the same regions (Hurcombe et al., 2010). For minority immigrants, the acculturation process (i.e., identifying with the traits of another culture while retaining one's own ethnic identity) can be challenging when drinking alcoholic beverages is an expectation in the new culture. Those immigrants who retain strong ties to their ethnic heritage, home country, and religion appear to have less difficulty managing their alcohol consumption (Hurcombe et al., 2010).

Many immigrants choosing to drink often place themselves in a moral dilemma if they have cultural ties to regions in which alcohol use is low or not tolerated (e.g., Arab countries) or their religion prohibits its use (e.g., Buddhism, Islam, Bahá'í). Ultimately, those immigrants who choose to drink are likely to increase their alcohol consumption as they achieve greater socioeconomic status and become more socially integrated (Hurcombe et al., 2010). Among older Hispanic and Asian immigrants, as the acculturation process proceeds, alcohol consumption increases as the frequency of binge drinking episodes decreases (Bryant & Kim, 2013). Immigrants struggling with alcohol problems are often too ashamed or hesitant to seek help because acknowledging the problem would suggest a betrayal of their cultural and religious roots to their families and ethnic communities (Holt et al., 2006; Hurcombe et al., 2010). Thus, more work needs to be done on identifying immigrants with alcohol-related problems and encouraging them to seek help.

Religious affiliation is a strong predictor of alcohol use among all races and ethnicities worldwide. In the United States, followers of Judaism and most of the 139 denominations of Christianity permit their members to drink. Yet, as in other areas of the world, members of Islam, Seventh Day Adventist, and The Church of Jesus Christ of Latter-day Saints do not sanction the use of alcohol in food or drink (Holt et al., 2006).

Within the United States, drinking patterns are notably different between Hispanics and non-Hispanics (NIAAA, 2011) and between Native and non-Native Americans (Centers for Disease Control and Prevention [CDC], 2008; Chartier & Caetano, 2010). Hispanic adults have high rates of abstinence and are less likely to drink than non-Hispanic Whites. However, among Hispanics who do drink, the frequency of binge drinking episodes is higher than among non-Hispanics. Within the Hispanic community, Mexican Americans and Puerto Ricans share a more relaxed attitude toward drinking than Cuban Americans. As a group, Hispanic men who are Catholic have a more relaxed attitude about drinking, tend to drink heavily, and have more problems with alcohol than Protestants. When Hispanic women drink, they tend to drink only among family and close friends. Yet, as acculturation progresses, their drinking habits become more public. Similarly, as the population of Hispanics increases and Hispanic immigrants acculturate into US society, their consumption of alcohol is expected to increase and mirror that of the larger society.

The high rates of alcohol abuse and dependency among Native American and Alaska Native populations are legendary and their relationship to native culture has still not been fully understood (Mail & Johnson, 1992). The CDC (2008) reports that between 2001 and 2005, 11.7% of deaths among Native Americans and Alaska Natives were alcohol-related compared with 3.3% for the entire United States. Theories used to explain usage range from biological differences (e.g., genetic variations), psychological weaknesses (e.g., anxiety, depression, and low self-esteem), and social problems (e.g., peer pressure, persistent poverty) to environment (e.g., isolation) and government paternalism. Regardless, alcohol abuse and dependency continue to be a serious problem even though intervention activities within Native American communities have increased and alcohol-related deaths have dropped since the 1960s.

Although there is scant information on the influences of culture, ethnicity, or religion on alcohol use in late life, conversations with older adults about their alcohol use should be initiated with respect for the cultural and religious norms and values that guide their use. The best way to identify cultural and religious influences on an individual's drinking behavior is to simply ask, and then work with each person to identify resolutions that are consistent with cultural and religious beliefs.

PREVENTION

Older adults who abstain from drinking and those who drink under the recommended guidelines are considered to be at low risk for alcohol problems. However, they can still benefit from prevention and education resources that highlight the relationship between alcohol use and health problems or the importance of responsible drinking in late life. As with any literature distributed among older adults, materials should incorporate design formats that are easy to read, use words that are easily understood, and cover content that accurately depicts the drinking habits and lifestyles of older adults; pamphlets on college binge drinking will not effectively convey the intended message.

In discussions with older adults about alcohol use, MI techniques (used in brief interventions) can be implemented to motivate listeners to think about how alcohol affects their current lifestyle. Moreover, health care professionals can utilize teach-back strategies (Schillinger et al., 2003) to ensure that older adults understand important information like standard drink size and recommended drinking guidelines.

Prevention efforts to raise awareness of the effects of alcohol on older adults are not extensive and are generally limited to the health care field. Some consumer-oriented materials have been developed for older adults and designed to raise awareness. Increased interest in the interactions between alcohol and medications has prompted development of additional brochures on the topic. Links to brochures developed specifically for older adults are provided in the electronic resource section at the end of the chapter.

PATIENT EDUCATION COMPONENTS FOR PROVIDERS

Continuing education on alcohol use among older adults is limited, although available through professional organizations offering continuing education opportunities. In 2007, a group of community professionals started the Aging and Alcohol Awareness Group (AAAG) with support from the Commonwealth of Virginia's Alcoholic Beverage Control Division to provide community presentations, health professional trainings, and professional conferences on the effects of alcohol on older adults. The AAAG sponsors annual Screening and Brief Intervention Trainings (SBIRT) (Babor et al., 2007) covering alcohol use in older adults. The SBIRT training is a continuing education opportunity developed by the Florida BRITE project (Schonfeld et al., 2010) and shown to be an effective way to train health professionals in how to conduct screenings and brief interventions. Opportunities to participate in SBIRT trainings are regularly scheduled across the United States through onsite and Web-based instruction.

REFERENCES

AA Grapevine, Inc. (2011). *Alcoholics Anonymous Preamble*. New York, NY: A. A. World Services.

AB InBev. (2012). *Annual report 2011: Financial report 2011*. Retrieved from http://www.ab-inbev.com/pdf/Financial_Report_2011.pdf

American Psychological Association. (1994). *DSM-IV: Diagnostic and statistical manual of mental disorders* (4th ed., pp. 176–204). Washington, DC: Author.

Ammann, R. W. (2001). The natural history of alcoholic chronic pancreatitis. *Internal Medicine, 40*, 368–375.

Anantharaju, A., & Van Thiel, D. H. (2003). Liver transplantation for alcoholic liver disease. *Alcohol Research & Health: The Journal of the National Institute on Alcohol Abuse and Alcoholism, 27*, 257–268. Retrieved from http://pubs.niaaa.nih.gov/publications/arh27-3/257-269.pdf

Babor, T., McRee, B., Kassebaum, P., Grimaldi, P., Ahmed, K., & Bray, J. (2007). Screening, Brief Intervention, and Referral to Treatment (SBIRT): Toward a public health approach to the management of substance abuse. *Substance Abuse: Official Publication of the Association for Medical Education and Research in Substance Abuse, 28*, 7–30. doi:10.1300/J465v28n03_03

Bartels, S. J., Blow, F. C., Brockmann, L. M., & Van Citters, A. D. (2005). *Substance abuse and mental health among older Americans: The state of the knowledge and future directions*. Rockville, MD: Westat.

Blendea, M. C., Thompson, M. J., & Malkani, S. (2010). Diabetes and chronic liver disease: Etiology and pitfalls in monitoring. *Clinical Diabetes, 28*, 139–144. doi:10.2337/diaclin.28.4.139

Blow, F. C., Brower, K. J., Schulenberg, J. E., Demo-Dananberg, L. M., Young, J. P., & Beresford, T. P. (1992). The Michigan Alcoholism Screening Test–Geriatric Version (MAST-G): A new elderly-specific screening instrument. *Alcoholism: Clinical and Experimental Research, 16*, 372.

Blow, F. C., Oslin, D. W., & Barry, K. L. (2002). Misuse and abuse of alcohol, illicit drugs, and psychoactive medication among older people. *Generations, 26*, 50–54.

Bode, C., & Bode, J. C. (1997). Alcohol's role in gastrointestinal tract disorders. *Alcohol Health & Research World, 21*, 76–83. Retrieved from http://pubs.niaaa.nih.gov/publications/arh21-1/76.pdf

Bouchery, E. E., Harwood, H. J., Sacks, J. J., Simon, C. J., & Brewer, R. D. (2011). Economic costs of excessive alcohol consumption in the U.S., 2006. *American Journal of Preventive Medicine, 41*, 516–524. Retrieved from http://download .journals.elsevierhealth.com/pdfs/journals/0749-3797/PIIS0749379711005381.pdf

Brower, K. J. (2003). Insomnia, alcoholism, and relapse. *Sleep Medicine Reviews, 7*, 523–539. doi:10.1016/S1087-0792 (03)90005-0

Bryant, A. N., & Kim, G. (2013). The relation between acculturation and alcohol consumption patterns among older Asian and Hispanic immigrants. *Aging & Mental Health, 17*(2), 147–156. doi:10.1080/13607863.2012.727382

Carithers, R. L., Jr., & McClain, C. J. (2010). Alcoholic liver disease. In M. Feldman, L. S. Friedman, & L. J. Brandt (Eds.), *Sleisenger & Fordtran's gastrointestinal and liver disease* (pp. 1383–1400). Philadelphia, PA: Saunders Elsevier.

Castle, N. G., Wagner, L. M., Ferguson-Rome, J. C., Smith, M. L., & Handler, S. M. (2012). Alcohol misuse and abuse reported by nurse aides in assisted living. *Research on Aging, 43*, 321–336. doi:10.1177/0164027511423929

Center for Substance Abuse Treatment. (1998). *Treatment improvement protocol (TIP) #26. Substance abuse among older adults.* Rockville, MD: SAMHSA.

Center for Substance Abuse Treatment. (1999). *Treatment improvement protocol (TIP) #35. Enhancing motivation for change in substance abuse treatment.* Rockville, MD: SAMHSA.

Centers for Disease Control and Prevention. (2008). Alcohol-attributable deaths and years of potential life lost among American Indians and Alaska Natives—United States, 2001–2005. *MMWR, Morbidity and Mortality Weekly Reports.* Retrieved from http://www.cdc.gov/mmwr/preview/mmwrhtml/mm5734a3.htm

Chartier, K., & Caetano, R. (2010). Ethnicity and health disparities in alcohol research. *Alcohol Research & Health: The Journal of the National Institute on Alcohol Abuse and Alcoholism, 33*, 152–160. Retrieved from http://pubs.niaaa.nih .gov/publications/arh40/152-160.htm

Compton, P. (2002). Caring for an alcohol-dependent patient. *Nursing, 32*, 58–63.

Cook, C., Hallwood, P., & Thompson, A. (1998). B vitamin deficiency and neuropsychiatric syndromes in alcohol misuse. *Alcohol and Alcoholism, 33*, 317–336.

Di Chiara, G. (1997). Alcohol and dopamine. *Alcohol Health & Research World, 21*, 108–114.

Donnelly, G., Kent-Wilkinson, A., & Rush, A. (2012). The alcohol-dependent patient in hospital: challenges for nursing. *Medsurg Nursing: Official Journal of the Academy of Medical-Surgical Nurses, 21*, 9–14.

Duncan, D. F., Nicholson, T., White, J. B., Bradley, D. B., & Bonaguro, J. (2010). The baby boomer effect: Changing patterns of substance abuse among adults ages 55 and older. *Journal of Aging & Social Policy, 22*, 237–248. doi:10.1080/ 08959420.2010.485511

Edenberg, H. J. (2003). *The collaborative study on the genetics of alcoholism: An update.* Rockville, MD: NIAAA.

Fink, A., Hays, R. D., Moore, A. A., & Beck, J. C. (1996). Alcohol-related problems in older persons: Determinants, consequences, and screening. *Archives of Internal Medicine, 156*, 1150–1156. doi:10.1001/archinte.1996.00440100038006

Fleming, M. F., Manwell, L. B., Barry, K. L., Adams, W., & Stauffacher, E. A. (1999). Brief physician advice for alcohol problems in older adults: A randomized community-based trial. *Journal of Family Practice, 48*, 378–384.

Fleming, M. F., Mundt, M. P., French, M. T., Manwell, L. B., Stauffacher, E. A., & Barry, K. L. (2002). Brief physician advice for problem drinkers: Long-term efficacy and benefit-cost analysis. *Alcoholism: Clinical and Experimental Research, 26*, 36–43. doi:10.1111/j.1530-0277.2002.tb02429.x

Fong, T. G., Tulebaev, S. R., & Inouye, S. K. (2009). Delirium in elderly adults: Diagnosis, prevention, and treatment. *Nature Reviews Neurology, 5*, 210–220. doi:10.1038/nrneurol.2009.24

Ginzer, L., & Richardson, V. E. (2009). *How much are people drinking, anyway: Findings from NESARC.* Paper presented at the annual meeting of the Gerontological Society of America, Atlanta, GA.

Glantz, M. (1981). Predictions of elderly drug abuse. *Journal of Psychoactive Drugs, 13*, 7–16.

Goodman, A. (2008). Neurobiology of addiction: An integrative review. *Biochemical Pharmacology, 75*, 266–322. doi:10.1016/j.bcp.2007.07.030

Graham, K., Wilsnack, R., Dawson, D., & Vogeltanz, N. (1998). Should alcohol consumption measures by adjusted for gender differences? *Addiction, 93*, 1137–1147.

Hanson, M., & Gutheil, I. A. (2004). Motivational strategies with alcohol-involved older adults: Implications for social work practice. *Social Work, 49*, 364–372.

Hartsell, Z., Drost, J., Wilkens, J. A., & Budavari, A. I. (2007). Managing alcohol withdrawal in hospitalized patients. *JAAPA: Journal of the American Academy of Physician Assistants, 20*, 20–25. Retrieved from http://media.haymarket-media.com/documents/2/alcohol0907_1601.pdf

Heuberger, R. A. (2009). Alcohol and older adult: A comprehensive review. *Journal of Nutrition for the Elderly, 28*, 203–235. doi:10.1080/01639360903140106

Holt, J. B., Miller, J. W., Naimi, T. S., & Sui, D. Z. (2006). Religious affiliation and alcohol consumption in the United States. *Geographical Review, 96*, 523–542. doi:10.1111/j.1931-0846.2006.tb00515.x

Hurcombe, R., Bayley, M., & Goodman, A. (2010). *Ethnicity and alcohol: A review of the UK literature.* York, England: Joseph Roundtree Foundation. Retrieved from www.jrf.org.uk

Insurance Institute for Highway Safety. (2013). *DUI/DWI laws.* Arlington, VA: Highway Loss Data Institute. Retrieved from http://www.iihs.org/laws/dui.aspx

Jones, A. W., & Andersson, L. (2003). Comparison of ethanol concentrations in venous blood and end-expired breath during a controlled drinking study. *Forensic Science International, 132*, 18–25.

Karlamangla, A., Zhou, K., Reuben, D., Greendale, G., & Moore, A. (2006). Longitudinal trajectories of heavy drinking in adults in the United States of America. *Addiction (Abingdon, England), 101*, 91–99. doi:10.1111/j.1360-0443.2005.01299.x

Kim, J. W., Lee, D. Y., Lee, B. C., Jung, M. H., Kim, H., Choi, Y. S., & Choi, I. G. (2012). Alcohol and cognition in the elderly: A review. *Korean Neuropsychiatric Review, 9*, 8–16. doi:10.4306/pi.2012.9.1.8

Klein, W. C., & Jess, C. (2002). One last pleasure? Alcohol use among elderly people in nursing homes. *Health & Social Work, 27*, 193–203. doi:10.1093/hsw/27.3.193

Klingemann, H. (2001). *Alcohol and its social consequences—The forgotten dimension.* Geneva, Switzerland: World Health Organization. Retrieved from www.ias.org.uk/btg/policyeu/pdfs/2001-klingermann.pdf

Liberto, J. G., & Oslin, D. W. (1995). Early versus late onset of alcoholism in the elderly. *International Journal of the Addictions, 30*, 1799–1818.

Lucas, D. L., Brown, R. A., Wassef, M., & Giles, T. D. (2005). Alcohol and the cardiovascular system: Research challenges and opportunities. *Journal of the American College of Cardiology, 45*, 1916–1924. doi:10.1016/j.jacc.2005.02.

Mail, P. D., & Johnson, S. (1992). Boozing, sniffing, and toking: An overview of the past, present, and future substance use by American Indians. *American Indian and Alaska Native Mental Health Research, 5*, 1–33.

McKay, A, Kornada, A., & Axen, D. (2004). Using a symptom-triggered approach to manage patients in acute alcohol withdrawal. *Medsurg Nursing: Official Journal of the Academy of Medical-Surgical Nurses, 13*, 15–20.

McKay, J. R., & Hiller-Sturmhofel, S. (2011). Treating alcoholism as a chronic disease: Approaches to long-term continuing care. *Alcohol Research & Health: The Journal of the National Institute on Alcohol Abuse and Alcoholism, 33*, 356–370.

Menninger, J. A. (2002). Assessment and treatment of alcoholism and substance-related disorders in the elderly. *Bulletin of the Menninger Clinic, 66*, 166–183.

Merrick, E. L., Horgan, C. M., Hodgkin, D., Garnick, D. W., Houghton, S. F., Panas, L., . . . Blow, F. C. (2008). Unhealthy drinking among older adults: Prevalence and associated factors. *Journal of the American Geriatrics Society, 56*, 214–223. doi:10.1111/j.1532-5415.2007.01539.x

Meyerhoff, D. J., Bode, C., Nixon, S. J., de Bruin, E. A., Bode, C., & Seitz, H. K. (2005). Health risks of chronic moderate and heavy alcohol consumption: How much is too much? *Alcoholism: Clinical and Experimental Research, 29*, 1334–1340.

Miller, W. R., & Rollnick, S. (2002). *Motivational interviewing: Preparing people to change addictive behavior.* New York, NY: Guilford Press.

Miller, W. R., & Sanchez, V. C. (1994). Motivating young adults for treatment and lifestyle change. In G. S. Howard & P. E. Nathan (Eds.), *Alcohol use and misuse by young adult* (pp. 55–81). South Bend, IN: University of Notre Dame Press.

Murphy, S. L., Xu, J. Q., & Kochanek, K. D. (2012). *Deaths: Preliminary data for 2010* (National Vital Statistics Reports, Vol. 60, No. 4). Hyattsville, MD: National Center for Health Statistics. 2012.

Myrick, H., & Anton, R. (1998). Treatment of alcohol withdrawal. *Alcohol Health & Research World, 22*, 38–43.

National Institute on Aging. (2012). *Alcohol use in older people* (AgePage). Gaithersburg, MD: Author.

National Institute on Alcohol Abuse and Alcoholism. (2000). Health risks and benefits of alcohol consumption. *Alcohol Research & Health: The Journal of the National Institute on Alcohol Abuse and Alcoholism, 24*, 5–11. Retrieved from http://pubs.niaaa.nih.gov/publications/arh24-1/05-11.pdf

National Institute on Alcohol Abuse and Alcoholism. (2001). Craving research: Implications for treatment research. *Alcohol Alert, 54*. Retrieved from http://pubs.niaaa.nih.gov/publications/aa54.htm

National Institute on Alcohol Abuse and Alcoholism. (2003). *Concepts and terms in genetic research—A primer*. Rockville, MD: Author.

National Institute on Alcohol Abuse and Alcoholism. (2004). Alcohol's damaging effect on the brain. *Alcohol Alert, 63*. Retrieved from http://pubs.niaaa.nih.gov/publications/aa63/aa63.htm

National Institute on Alcohol Abuse and Alcoholism. (2005a). Module 10C: Older adults and alcohol problems. In *NIAAA: Social work education for the prevention and treatment of alcohol use disorders*. Retrieved from http://pubs.niaaa.nih.gov/publications/Social/ContentsList.html

National Institute on Alcohol Abuse and Alcoholism. (2005b). Alcoholic liver disease. *Alcohol Alert, 64*. Retrieved from http://www.niaaa.nih.gov/publications/journals-and-reports/alcohol-alert

National Institute on Alcohol Abuse and Alcoholism. (2007a). *Harmful interactions: Mixing alcohol with medicines*. Retrieved from http://pubs.niaaa.nih.gov/publications/Medicine/medicine.htm

National Institute on Alcohol Abuse and Alcoholism. (2007b). Alcohol and tobacco. *Alcohol Alert, 71*. Retrieved from http://www.niaaa.nih.gov/publications/journals-and-reports/alcohol-alert

National Institute on Alcohol Abuse and Alcoholism. (2007c). Alcohol metabolism: An update. *Alcohol Alert, 72*. Retrieved from http://www.niaaa.nih.gov/publications/journals-and-reports/alcohol-alert

National Institute on Alcohol Abuse and Alcoholism. (2008a). Alcohol and other drugs. *Alcohol Alert, 76*. Retrieved from http://www.niaaa.nih.gov/publications/journals-and-reports/alcohol-alert

National Institute on Alcohol Abuse and Alcoholism. (2008b). *Alcohol: A women's health issue* (NIH Publication No. 03-4956). Rockville, MD: Author.

National Institute on Alcohol Abuse and Alcoholism. (2009). Neuroscience: Pathways to alcohol dependence. *Alcohol Alert, 77*. Retrieved from http://www.niaaa.nih.gov/publications/journals-and-reports/alcohol-alert

National Institute on Alcohol Abuse and Alcoholism. (2010a). *Beyond hangovers: Understanding alcohol's effect on your health* (NIH Publication No. 10-7604). Rockville, MD: Author.

National Institute on Alcohol Abuse and Alcoholism. (2010b). *Rethinking drinking* (NIH Publication No. 10-3770). Rockville, MD: Author.

National Institute on Alcohol Abuse and Alcoholism. (2011). *Alcohol and the Hispanic community*. Rockville, MD: Author.

Nurnberger, J. I., Jr., & Bierut, L. J. (2007). Seeking the connections: Alcoholism and our genes. *Scientific American, 296*, 46–53.

O'Malley, P. M. (2004/2005). Maturing out of problematic alcohol use. *Alcohol Research & Health: The Journal of the National Institute on Alcohol Abuse and Alcoholism, 28*, 202–204. Retrieved from http://pubs.niaaa.nih.gov/publications/arh284/202-204.pdf?pagewanted=all

Oslin, D. W. (2005). Evidence-based treatment of geriatric substance abuse. *Psychiatric Clinics of North America, 18*, 897–911.

Prat, G., Adan, A., & Sanchez-Turet, M. (2009). Alcohol hangover: A critical review of explanatory factors. *Human Psychopharmacology: Clinical and Experimental, 24*, 259–267. doi:10.1002/hup.1023

Prochaska, J. O., Butterworth, S., Redding, C. A., Burden, V., Perrin, N., Leo, M., . . . Prochaska, J. M. (2008). Initial efficacy of MI, TTM tailoring and HRI's with multiple behaviors for employee health promotion. *Preventive Medicine, 46*, 226–231. doi:10.1016/j.ypmed.2007.11.007

Puz, C. A., & Stokes, S. J. (2005). Alcohol withdrawal syndrome: Assessment and treatment with the use of the Clinical Institute Withdrawal Assessment for Alcohol-revised. *Critical Care Nursing Clinics of North America, 17*, 297–304. doi:10.1016/j.ccell.2005.04.01

Quinn, K. (2010). Methodological consideration in surveys of older adults: Technology matters. *International Journal of Emerging Technologies and Society, 8*, 114–133.

Rehm, J. (2011). The risks associated with alcohol use and alcoholism. *Alcohol Research & Health: The Journal of the National Institute on Alcohol Abuse and Alcoholism, 34*, 135–143.

Rice, C., Longabaugh, R., Beattie, M., & Noel, N. (1993). Age group differences in response to treatment for problematic alcohol use. *Addiction (Abingdon, England), 88*, 1369–1375.

Rigler, S. K. (2000). Alcoholism in the elderly. *American Family Physician, 61*, 1710–1716.

Roberts, L. J., & McCrady, B. S. (2003). *Alcohol problems in intimate relationships: Identification and intervention* (NIH Publication No. 03-5284). Rockville, MD: NIAAA.

Room, R., Babor, T., & Rehm, J. (2005). Alcohol and public health. *Lancet, 365*, 519–530. doi:10.1016/S0140-6736(05)17870-2

Rosenbloom, M., Sullivan, E. V., & Pfefferbaum, A. (2003). Using magnetic resonance imaging and diffusion tensor imaging to assess brain damage in alcoholics. *Alcohol Research & Health: The Journal of the National Institute on Alcohol Abuse and Alcoholism, 27*, 146–152. Retrieved from http://pubs.niaaa.nih.gov/publications/arh27-2/toc27-2.htm

Sacco, P., Bucholz, K. K., & Spitznagel, E. L. (2009). Alcohol use among older adults in the National Epidemiologic Survey on Alcohol and Related Conditions: A latent class analysis. *Journal of Studies on Alcohol and Drugs, 70,* 829–838.

Schillinger, D., Piette, J., Grumbach, K., Wang, F., Wilson, C., Daher, C., . . . Bindman, A. B. (2003). Closing the loop: Physician communication with diabetic patients who have low health literacy. *Archives of Internal Medicine, 163,* 83–90.

Schonfeld, L., King-Kallimanis, B. L., Duchene, D. M., Etheridge, R. L., Herrera, J. R., Barry, K. L., & Lynn, N. (2010). Screening and brief intervention for substance misuse among older adults: The Florida BRITE project. *American Journal of Public Health, 100,* 108–114. Retrieved from http://ajph.aphapublications.org/doi/pdf/10.2105/AJPH.2008.149534

Sharp, L., & Vacha-Haase, T. (2010). Physician attitudes regarding alcohol use screening in older adult patients. *Journal of Applied Gerontology, 30,* 226–240. doi:0.1177/0733464810361345

Sobell, L. C., & Sobell, M. B. (2003). Alcohol consumption measures. In J. P. Allen & V. B. Wilson (Eds.), *Assessing alcohol problems: A guide for clinicians and researchers* (pp. 75–99). Retrieved from http://pubs.niaaa.nih.gov/publications/AssessingAlcohol/sobell.pdf

Social Issues Research Centre. (1998). *Social and cultural aspects of drinking: A report to the European Commission.* Oxford, England: Author. Retrieved from http://www.sirc.org/publik/social_drinking.pdf

Sterner, K. L., & Keough, V. A. (2003). Holiday heart syndrome: A case of cardiac irritability after increased alcohol consumption. *Journal of Emergency Nursing: JEN: official publication of the Emergency Department Nurses Association, 29,* 570–573.

Stevenson, J. S. (2005). Alcohol use, misuse, abuse, and dependence in later adulthood. *Annual Review of Nursing Research, 23,* 245–280.

Stewart, D., & Oslin, D. (2001). Recognition and treatment of late-life addictions in medical settings. *Journal of Clinical Geropsychology, 7,* 145–158. doi:10.1023/A:1009589706810

Substance Abuse and Mental Health Services Administration, Center for Behavioral Health Statistics and Quality. (2011). *The TEDS report: Older adult admissions reporting alcohol as a substance of abuse: 1992 and 2009.* Rockville, MD: Author. Retrieved from http://www.samhsa.gov/data/2k11/WEB_TEDS_021/021OlderAlcUse.htm

Substance Abuse and Mental Health Services Administration. (2012). *Results from the 2011 National Survey on Drug Use and Health: Summary of national findings* (NSDUH Series H-44, HHS Publication No. [SMA] 12-4713). Rockville, MD: Author. Retrieved from http://www.samhsa.gov/data/NSDUH/2011SummNatFindDetTables/Index.aspx

Sullivan, J. T., Sykora, K., Schneiderman, J., Naranjo, C. A., & Sellers, E. M. (1989). Assessment of alcohol withdrawal: The revised Clinical Institute Withdrawal Assessment for Alcohol scale (CIWA-Ar). *British Journal of Addiction, 84,* 1353–1357.

Szabo, G., & Mandrekar, P. (2009). A recent perspective on alcohol, immunity, and host defense. *Alcoholism: Clinical and Experimental Research, 33,* 220–232.

Tucker, J. A., & Simpson, C. A. (2011). The recovery spectrum: From self-change to seeking treatment. *Alcohol Research & Health: The Journal of the National Institute on Alcohol Abuse and Alcoholism, 33,* 371–379.

U.S. Department of Health and Human Services, Office of Disease Prevention and Health Promotion. (2010). *Healthy people 2020.* Washington, DC: Author. Retrieved from http://www.healthypeople.gov/2020/topicsobjectives2020/objectiveslist.aspx?topicId=40

Verster, J. C. (2008). The alcohol hangover—A puzzling phenomenon. *Alcohol and Alcoholism, 43,* 124–126. doi:10.1093/alcalc/agm163

Virginia Tech Campus Alcohol Abuse Prevention Center. (n.d.). *Alcohol's effects.* Retrieved from http://www.alcohol.vt.edu/Students/Alcohol_effects/index.html

Weyerer, S., Schaufele, M., Wiese, B., Maier, W., Tebarth, F., van den Bussche, H., . . . Riedel-Heller, S. G. (2011). Current alcohol consumption and its relationship to incident dementia: Results from a 3-year follow-up study among primary care attenders aged 75 years and older. *Age and Ageing, 40,* 456–463.doi:10.1093/ageing/afr007

White, A. M. (2004). *What happened? Alcohol, memory blackouts, and the brain.* Rockville, MD: NIAAA.

White, J. B., Duncan, D. F., Nicholson, T., Bradley, D., & Bonaguro, J. (2011). Generational shift and drug abuse in older Americans. *Journal of Social, Behavioral, and Health Sciences, 5,* 58–66. doi:10.5590/JSBHS.2011.05.1.06

Wiese, J., Shilpak, M. G., & Browner, W. S. (2000). The alcohol hangover. *Annals of Internal Medicine, 132,* 897–902.

Winick, C. (1962). Maturing out of narcotic addiction. *Bulletin of Narcotics, 14,* 1–7.

World Health Organization. (2012). *Global status report on alcohol and health 2011.* Retrieved from http://www.who.int/substance_abuse/publications/global_alcohol_report/en/index.html

Yoon, Y.-H., Stinson, F. S., Yi, H., & Dufour, M. C. (2003). Accidental alcohol poisoning mortality in the United States, 1996–1998. *Alcohol Research & Health: The Journal of the National Institute on Alcohol Abuse and Alcoholism, 27,* 110–118.

Zakhari, S. (1997). Alcohol and the cardiovascular system: Molecular mechanisms for beneficial and harmful action. *Alcohol Health & Research World, 21,* 21–29.

Zhang, Y., & Ren, J. (2011). ALDH2 in alcoholic heart diseases: Molecular mechanism and cellular implications. *Pharmacology & Therapeutics, 132,* 86–95. doi:10.1016/j.pharmthera.2011.05.008

CHAPTER 21: IT RESOURCES

Websites

National Institute on Alcohol Abuse and Alcoholism
  www.niaaa.nih.gov
Alcoholics Anonymous
  http://www.aa.org/?Media=PlayFlash
World Health Organization
  http://www.who.int/topics/alcohol_drinking/en/
Alcohol Alerts
  http://www.niaaa.nih.gov/Publications/AlcoholAlerts/Pages/default.aspx
Alcohol Research and Health
  http://www.niaaa.nih.gov/Publications/AlcoholResearch/Pages/default.aspx
About.com Alcoholism
  http://alcoholism.about.com/od/elder/Elderly_and_Alcohol.htm
The Alcoholism Guide
  http://www.the-alcoholism-guide.org/alcoholism-and-the-elderly.html
Substance Abuse Treatment Facility Locator
  http://findtreatment.samhsa.gov/
Blood Alcohol Content table
  http://www.brad21.org/bac_charts.html
Blood Alcohol Content Calculator
  http://www.ou.edu/oupd/bac.htm
Responsible Drinking: What Is a "Standard Drink?" from Prevention Lane Web site
  http://preventionlane.org/responsible-drinking.htm
Aging and Alcohol Awareness Group, Virginia Alcohol and Beverage Control Department
  http://www.abc.virginia.gov/Education/olderadults/aaagroup.html
Short Michigan Alcoholism Screening Test–Geriatric Version (S-MAST-G)
  http://www.nursingcenter.com/pdf.asp?AID=823032
Alcohol Use and Older Adults
  http://nihseniorhealth.gov/videolist.html#alcoholuse
The Best Is Yet to Come
  www.abc.virginia.gov/Education/brochures_and_other_resources.htm#alcaging
Harmful Interactions: Mixing Medications and Alcohol
  http://pubs.niaaa.nih.gov/publications/Medicine/medicine.htm
Florida BRITE Project: Brief Intervention and Treatment for Elders
  http://brite.fmhi.usf.edu/BRITE.htm
Substance Abuse and Mental Health Services Administration (SAMHSA)
  http://www.samhsa.gov/
The following publications on the SAMHSA website are aimed at alcohol abuse and the elderly:
  As You Age: Ask, Guard, Educate
    http://store.samhsa.gov/product/As-You-Age-Ask-Guard-Educate/AVD188 (to order)
    http://store.samhsa.gov/shin/content//AVD188/AVD188.pdf (downloadable, digital copy)
This free PSA from the SAMHSA website raises awareness among the elderly about the dangers
  of prescription drug and over-the-counter drug interactions and misuse as well as the mix of
  alcohol and medicines

As You Age: A Guide to Aging, Medicines, and Alcohol
http://store.samhsa.gov/product/As-You-Age-A-Guide-to-Aging-Medicines-and-Alcohol/SMA04-3940 (to order)
http://store.samhsa.gov/shin/content//SMA04-3940/SMA04-3940.pdf (downloadable, digital copy)
This free brochure from the SAMHSA website warns about the dangers of the elderly misusing alcohol, prescription drugs, and over-the-counter drugs. It describes the signs of misuse and steps that older adults can take to prevent problems. It also includes a chart for listing all medicines and dietary supplements.

As You Age: There's No Better Time to Learn More about How to Take Medications the Right Way
http://store.samhsa.gov/product/As-You-Age/AVD189 (to order)
http://store.samhsa.gov/shin/content//AVD189/AVD189.pdf (downloadable, digital copy)
This free PSA encourages the elderly to ask about the prescription drugs and over-the-counter drugs they use, learn about the dangers of mixing alcohol with medications, and guard against harmful interactions and misuse.

Aging, Medicines and Alcohol
http://store.samhsa.gov/product/Aging-Medicines-and-Alcohol/SMA08-3619 (to order)
http://kap.samhsa.gov/products/brochures/pdfs/Agingmed.pdf (downloadable, digital copy)
This brochure from the SAMHSA website is designed to increase awareness among older adult consumers about possible problems related to the misuse of alcohol, prescription drugs, or over-the-counter drugs. Lists signs of misuse and suggests actions the elderly can take to avoid or deal with problems.

Screening, Brief Intervention, and referral to Treatment (SBIRT)
http://www.samhsa.gov/samhsanewsletter/Volume_17_Number_6/SBIRT.aspx

TIP 26: Substance Abuse Among Older Adults
http://store.samhsa.gov/product/TIP-26-Substance-Abuse-Among-Older-Adults/SMA08-3918

Quick Guide for Clinicians: Based on TIP 26 Substance Abuse Among Older Adults
http://kap.samhsa.gov/products/tools/cl-guides/pdfs/QGC_26.pdf

PDF Documents

10th Special Report to the U.S. Congress on Alcohol and Health
http://pubs.niaaa.nih.gov/publications/10report/intro.pdf
Harmful Interactions: Mixing Alcohol with Medicines from the National Institute on Alcohol Abuse and Alcoholism
http://pubs.niaaa.nih.gov/publications/Medicine/Harmful_Interactions.pdf
Alcoholics Anonymous—as a Resource for the Health Professional
http://www.aa.org/pdf/products/p-23_aaasaresourceforhcp1.pdf
Older Adults and Alcohol, You Can Get Help
http://www.nia.nih.gov/sites/default/files/older_adults_and_alcohol.pdf
Clinical Institute Withdrawal Assessment for Alcohol Scale (CIWA-Ar)
http://umem.org/files/uploads/1104212257_CIWA-Ar.pdf

Videos

Alcoholics Anonymous—Videos and Audios
http://www.aa.org/subpage.cfm?page=421
Lists videos and audios on the Alcoholics Anonymous website, including Public Service Announcements, Videos for Professionals, Young People's Videos, and Audio PSAs
Ask the Geriatrician—Alcoholism and Depression in Elders (2010)
Ask the Geriatrician was developed to address the shortage of geriatricians available to meet with older adults and their caregivers in the United States. Geriatricians specialize in preventing and treating health issues in adults aged 65 plus, yet many people never have the opportunity to speak with one. (8:41 minutes)
http://youtu.be/0PjM0oJrY9U
Alcoholism and the Older Adult (2011)
Discussion with Dr. Andrew Carroll, Family Medicine Specialist, regarding the problem of alcoholism among older adults. This is a big problem that is greatly unrecognized. (4:02 minutes)
http://youtu.be/hyB0lgVBQg0
Alcohol Abuse among Seniors (2010)
Sherman Huff discusses alcohol abuse among older adults. (2:23 minutes)
http://youtu.be/OGE6HxncgvI
AA Video for Health Professionals
http://www.videostreamingservices.com/aa/cpc/health/index.php?lang=en

Images

Google images for Alcoholism and Older Adults
http://www.google.com/search?q=alcoholism+and+older+adults&source=lnms&tbm=isch&sa=X&ei=gs2nUZfXGqfi0gHO1YGwDA&ved=0CAcQ_AUoAQ&biw=1024&bih=564

Substance Abuse

Susan Russell, MSN, FNP-BC
David W. Hartman, MD

INTRODUCTION

In 2009, Olshansky et al. published forecast models with projections on aging trends in America using the US Census results from 2008 and Vital Statistics death rate records from 2000. Their results indicated that the population of Americans aged 65 years and older would rise from 38.7 million in 2008 to between 99 and 108 million by 2050. The study looked at the extension of life expectancy, advances in health care measures, and the aging of the baby boom generation. These "boomers" were born during the years 1946 to 1964. This period of population growth added 400 million people to humanity (Olshansky et al., 2009). These people came of age during an explosion of substance abuse in North America. In many areas of the country, this explosion of illegal drug abuse appeared less taboo and more as a coming-of-age tradition. The report posits the tremendous pressure this population will present to current health care resources designed to provide care for older adults.

The "boomers" are a large population group that has a well-documented substance use history. The 2009 study by Han et al. projected that this cohort will increase the number of average older adults with substance abuse issues from 2.8 to 5.7 million by 2020. This doubles the current number of older adults with substance abuse issues even after accounting for the higher mortality rate seen among substance abusers (Han et al., 2009). Generally, treatment programs are focused on younger patients and separated from primary care facilities. Now is the time to incorporate a more inclusive, interdisciplinary course of action in substance abuse treatment in which the scope of assessment for older adult patients separates symptoms of chronic medical issues and psychopathology and expands on possible substance abuse issues.

Subjects of abuse and addiction have been studied and written about for many years. "Voices From the Past" reported that as early as 1910, treatment for drug addiction was available (Fee,

2011). From 1910 to 1917, Dr. Charles Terry worked tirelessly as a city health officer in Jacksonville, Florida. He established the first "maintenance program" for addicts in the United States as part of his campaign against drug addiction.

What do we know about addiction? The *Diagnostic and Statistical Manual of Mental Disorders, fourth edition, text revision (DSM-IV TR)*, describes many types of addiction, each related to a specific substance or activity. In general, an addiction is a repeated and compulsive seeking of or use of a substance or activity despite adverse social, psychological, or physical consequences. According to *DSM-IV TR* (American Psychiatric Association [APA], 2000), to diagnose substance dependence or addiction, the patient must present with three of the following symptoms in a 12-month period:

- Tolerance as evidenced by increased amount needed to achieve desired effect
- Evidence of withdrawal symptoms when not using
- Using substance for a longer time than intended
- Unsuccessful attempts to cut down on use
- A great deal of time spent in getting it, using it, and recovering from the use
- Reducing social obligations because of use
- Continued use despite negative effects.

The *DSM-IV TR* also defines an individual having substance abuse disorder as needing to meet one of the following criteria in a 12-month period:

- The substance use interferes with one's ability to meet major responsibilities
- The substance use occurs in situations in which the individual or others are put in danger, such as driving under the influence
- Recurrent substance use–related legal problems such as arrest for driving when intoxicated
- Continued use of the substance in spite of adverse social, psychological, or physical consequences

The proposed *DSM-V* combines abuse and addiction into the diagnosis of substance use disorder. This diagnosis uses 11 criteria, including 3 of abuse, 7 of dependence, and the additional criterion of craving.

Use and misuse of alcohol and other substances may present differently in the older adult patient than it does in the younger adult patient. The symptoms may not fully meet the requirements of substance use disorder as defined in the *DSM-IV TR* or *DSM-V*. Screening of older patients should include changes in life pattern such as retirement or loss of life partner, chronic medical problems, sleep issues, chronic pain issues, and skin changes (Boyle & Davis, 2006). Persons retired or living alone may have just recently begun misuse of alcohol or substances as a coping strategy or sleep aid.

PATHOPHYSIOLOGY

In the brain, pleasure is registered during the release of the neurotransmitter dopamine. Abusive drugs cause a powerful surge of dopamine to be released into the brain, specifically the pleasure center in the nucleus accumbens. The interaction of the prefrontal cortex with the nucleus accumbens remodels the brain chemistry and changes the person's perception. Remodeling such as this can actually change how a person thinks and looks at the future. The hippocampus and amygdala store memories of the pleasure and cues associated with it. These memories help create the conditioned response or craving that makes addicts want to repeat the desired effect. This conditioned response contributes not only to the addiction itself, but also to relapse. The brain then becomes reprogrammed to desire a higher stimulation of pleasure. This new circuitry established with addiction then reinforces the use. Over time and with repeated abusive drug use, the brain receptors become overwhelmed and produce less dopamine, which reduces the impact of dopamine on the brain's reward center, thus reducing the pleasure. This effect is known as tolerance. When tolerance occurs, a higher quantity of the drug must be taken to experience the original level of pleasure or "high."

Changes in physiologic systems with aging affect pharmacokinetics and pharmacodynamics of an administered drug. Pharmacokinetics refers to what the body does to the medicines taken. Pharmacodynamics refers to the effect the medicine has on the body. The older adult patient can have many age-related physical changes that interfere with the processing of medicines. With normal aging, many changes can occur, including the rate of absorption, rate of distribution, rate of elimination, and rate of metabolism of medicine (Jesson, 2011). The rate of absorption changes owing to decreased gastrointestinal motility seen in a normal aging patient, thus interfering with transport of medicine into the body. The rate of distribution problems occur owing to lower total body water and the increase in body fat stores. An example of decreased distribution is a fat-soluble drug like benzodiazepine that may accumulate in the increased body fat of an older patient, thus prolonging and intensifying the effect (Jesson, 2011). The rate of elimination changes are seen on account of decreased kidney function seen in a normal aging patient. The rate of metabolism is decreased because of decreased mass of liver also seen in a normal aging patient. With decreased rate of absorption, medicine may not be as effective, causing the patient to overdose themselves to gain pain relief. Anticholinergic medicines have many adverse reactions, including incontinence, urinary retention, postural hypotension, and confusion, to name but a few adverse reactions (Jesson, 2011). Effects of normal aging lead to a lower rate of metabolism that puts older patients at risk for overuse and overdose.

Prescribing medicine for older adults has many challenges. Recent clinical trials often use younger subjects who have few, if any, chronic health problems. Older subjects are usually excluded from research trials because of increased risk of adverse side effects due to age, and they may not be available for follow-up because of death or simple transportation problems and also because many older subjects could have multiple chronic illnesses that automatically increase prescribing risks (Fialova & Onder, 2009).

In many older adult care settings, the resident assessment instrument (RAI) has been used to collate diagnosis, medicines used, and outcomes, helping to reduce treatment errors and improve standards of care (Fialova & Onder, 2009). Another tool found helpful when prescribing to older adults is the Beers Criteria. The Beers Criteria was established in 1991 by Dr. Mark Beers and associates. These criteria reference commonly used medicines and the possible interactions when used by older adults. Medicines are divided into categories of "high" and "low" potential for harm through inappropriate use in older adults. The list is updated every few years to stay current with changes in medicine and treatment options.

Three major areas of function important to remember when prescribing to older patients are mobility, continence, and mental functioning. These three items have a direct effect on patients maintaining their independence. Providers should begin dosing the older patient at a lower amount while closely monitoring the effects of the medicines. The rule of thumb to follow when prescribing to older patients is "start low and go slow."

PRESENTATION OF DISEASE

Functional Changes Seen with Alcohol Abuse

Alcohol is legal and socially accepted in most regions. Occasions when people gather often include alcohol such as weddings, birthdays, holidays, graduations, retirements, and happy hour celebrations to name a few. Alcohol abuse in younger adults may be associated with social problems, legal problems, or problems at work. The older adults may not be involved in those situations and are left with fewer ways to monitor alcohol use (St. John et al., 2009), thus receiving little, if any, attention. Older adults are quite vulnerable to effects of alcohol, considering their potential risk factors of physical changes, social isolation, and bereavement issues (Weyerer et al., 2009). Using the National Epidemiologic Survey on Alcohol and Related Conditions (NESARC) reports, alcohol use has been divided into three levels—light, moderate, and heavy (Moore et al., 2009)—with the following criteria:

- Light drinkers—3 or fewer drinks a week for men and women
- Moderate drinkers—4 to 14 drinks a week for men, 4 to 7 drinks a week for women
- Heavy drinkers—more than 14 drinks a week for men, more than 7 drinks a week for women

The NESARC guidelines are directed to younger and middle-aged adult alcohol use and may not sufficiently address alcohol use in older adults.

Guidelines for alcohol use in older adults establish lower parimeters, taking into consideration normal aging metabolism changes, possible chronic medical conditions, and sensitivity changes in the central nervous system (Johnson, 2010). The four categories are separated as follows:

- Light to none—one to two drinks in the past year
- Moderate to regular—no more than one drink daily
- Risky drinkers—more than one drink daily with minimal or no substance use–related health or social problems
- Problem drinkers—alcohol use has been related to health or social problems

The problem drinkers have dependence and abuse issues. The risky drinkers are the people on the edge. Intervention and education can be productive to reduce alcohol use in this group. They are the most likely to change behavior.

According to the results of a national survey of drug use and health in 2005 and 2006, factors associated with at-risk drinking in men include being 50 to 64 years of age, having a family income of more than $75,000, and tobacco smoking (Blazer & Wu, 2009a). For women, the associated factors for at-risk drinking are having an education greater than high school and a family income of more than $40,000.

The Primary Care Research in Substance Abuse and Mental Health for Elderly or PRISM-E study compared two treatment modalities for at-risk drinkers. They are the 12-step abstinence model and the harm reduction model (Lee et al., 2009). The harm reduction model was found more useful with older adults who may not see drinking as an addiction. Harm reduction supports safe drinking, eliminating binge drinking, thereby improving the situation for at-risk drinkers. The treatment is based on motivational interviewing and discusses the results of alcohol use on general health and possible interference with continued independence.

The Healthy Living as You Age study or HLAYA was conducted in a primary care setting to screen for at-risk older drinkers (Lin et al., 2010). The Comorbidity Alcohol Risk Evaluation tool was used to assess risk. This tool is helpful to delineate at-risk drinkers, placing them into appropriate groups according to drinking habits. The results found that those who received written and oral information as well as advice from the provider were more apt to reduce alcohol use (Lin et al., 2010), validating the importance of advice of providers.

Even brief interventions directed toward reduction of alcohol use have been effective. The use of telephone calls at regular intervals has been useful for at-risk drinkers (Lin et al., 2009). The time crunch at the primary care visit does not allow for in-depth discussion. But a reminder call from a health educator a week later solidifies the importance and the support of the health care staff.

Unhealthy drinking patterns were identified in Medicare beneficiaries in a 2003 study looking at community dwelling older adults (Merrick et al., 2008). Adult drinking limits are higher than older adult limits. Older adults may require education about appropriate limits for their current age and situation (Merrick et al., 2008). If adults continue the drinking pattern of younger aged adults, it may be because they do not understand the relevance of reducing the amount of alcohol, and may not be aware of the age-related risks.

Adults aged 65 and older are estimated to be 19.6% of the US population by 2030, and more than seven drinks per week for them is considered heavy drinking (Moore et al., 2009). Many of these adults will be the baby boomers generation who are likely to bring with them an increased rate of substance use for nonmedical purposes. Generally speaking, a safe limit of alcohol intake for adults aged 65 and older is one drink per day. This light level of drinking has been associated with a lower risk of death, cognitive impairment, and heart disease. However, considering that comorbidities such as dementia, diabetes, or hypertension may be present, even one or two drinks per day may be hazardous. Functional changes seen with alcohol abuse can include executive memory functioning, confusion, unsteady gait, hostility, and sequencing (Briggs et al., 2011). Abuse and excessive use can be associated with liver disease, poor nutrition, insomnia, injuries, heart disease, stroke, increased risk of cancer, and peripheral neuropathy.

Although alcohol consumption tends to decline with age, estimates show that 10% to 50% of older adults may continue to engage in heavy drinking (Moos et al., 2009). When men are compared with women, men more often exceed the recommendations and drink more rapidly, thereby consuming more alcohol at shorter intervals (Moos et al., 2009), resulting in increased harmful consequences.

Functional Changes Seen with Illegal Drug Use

Illicit drug use refers to street drugs such as marijuana, cocaine, heroin, hallucinogens, and prescription-type drugs used non-medically. Young adults who have an established addiction continue to need treatment as older adults. As baby boomers age, the incidence of abuse of illicit drugs is predicted to rise among the older population. Functional changes seen with illegal drug use include decreases in attention and verbal learning skills. Substance abuse is a chronic condition with periods of abstinence or remission as well as abuse or return of symptoms. Persons with a diagnosis of substance use disorder have a high mortality rate, averaging 22.5 less years of life than those without that diagnosis (Scott et al., 2011). Those same patients are likely to exhibit other high-risk behaviors such as tobacco and alcohol use, accidents, and chronic health problems. The Addiction Severity Index is a tool used for assessment of drug use that measures current usages as well as periods of abstinence (Scott et al., 2011). This tool includes questions regarding social and economic status, involvement with the legal system, and employment, as well as time and severity of substance abuse. Early intervention with intense initial treatment is associated with sustained abstinence and lower risk of mortality.

The misuse of prescription drugs is predicted to increase as the "baby boomers" age. Medications are often obtained from multiple providers, friends, and family members or by stockpiling or hoarding them (Culberson & Ziska, 2008). In this way, patients can dose themselves at higher levels than prescribed. Misuse is hard to determine in the older patient. Signs to watch for indicating misuse of medications include declining physical functioning, self-care, social isolation, or increased falls.

Functional Changes Seen with Over-the-Counter Drugs

Television commercials and store aisles are full of products advertising cures. Have a problem? There is a pill for that. Common uses for over-the-counter (OTC) medicines include fever, congestion, headache, body ache, indigestion, diarrhea, and constipation. These OTC medicines are easy to get, no appointment is necessary, and they can be obtained while shopping for food and paper products, requiring no extra money or time needed for a visit with their provider. This can save time and money, or does it?

In her 2011 review of alternative remedies, pharmacist Barbara Jesson discusses the difficulties providers have in assessment when patients use both prescription medicines and natural herbal remedies. The case study describes the combined use of Digoxin and St. John's Wort. The provider was unaware of the use of the herbal supplement St. John's Wort. The dose of Digoxin was increased due to ineffectiveness. The provider was unaware of the metabolic changes in the medicine that were caused by the use of St. John's Wort. This cascade of events resulted in Digoxin toxicity when the patient stopped using St. John's Wort, again not reported to the provider. The situation precipitated use of yet another medicine by this older patient for stabilization. The episode presented safety and independence issues for the patient.

Older adults consume more OTC medications than any other age group; the average older adult takes six to nine medications a day (Rolita & Freedman, 2008). Considering the normal physical changes occurring in older adults, adding more medications can put the patient at risk for adverse reactions and drug interactions. Using a combination of antidepressants, antipsychotics, benzodiazepines, and opioids can result in sedation (Tulner et al., 2008). A combination of nonsteroidal anti-inflammatory drugs (NSAIDs), salicylates, and selective serotonin reuptake inhibitors (SSRIs) can result in bleeding problems. Simply adding calcium and a vitamin D supplement to a thiazide diuretic can result in hypercalcemia.

Decongestants taken OTC interfere with blood pressure medicine and can cause arrhythmia (Rolita & Freedman, 2008). Cold remedies can have anticholinergic effects and the use of these can cause cognitive changes, unsteady gait, and urinary retention. The addition of NSAIDs for body aches and pain can increase the risk of GI bleeding and tinnitus, which are only a few of the possible adverse effects.

Cox-Curry et al. found in their 2010 study that the most common OTCs used are vitamins, minerals, and glucosamine chondroitin. This makes sense considering body aches and joint pain usually increase with aging. The Screening Tool of Older Persons' potentially inappropriate Prescriptions (STOPP) and the Screening Tool to Alert doctors to Right Treatment (START) may be helpful in evaluating the dearth of medications taken by older patients, both prescribed and OTC. These tools were originally designed by an expert academic panel with members from Ireland and the United Kingdom. Their study results, published in 2008, validated the screening tools for use in community dwelling older adults. These tools enable the provider to appraise current prescription use in relation to their current diagnoses (Gallagher et al., 2008).

The Brief Intervention and Treatment for Elders, or BRITE program, was a state-funded project used in Florida to provide screening and referrals to their underserved older adults with substance abuse issues. This program (Schonfeld et al., 2010) addressed retirees in their communities, at health fairs, and senior community centers. The screening tools focused on alcohol abuse, prescription medication misuse, as well as OTC misuse and illegal drug use. Common screening tools used (Schonfeld et al., 2010) included the 10-item Short Michigan Alcoholism Screening Test (SMAST-G) and the Short Geriatric Depression Scale (SGDS). The success of this program is reflected in obtaining a federal funding for expansion of the program and the continued care of many of Florida's seniors with substance abuse issues.

Functional Changes Seen with Pain Medicine Misuse

Chronic pain is very common in older adults. It is frequently underdiagnosed and therefore undertreated (Papaleontiou et al., 2010). The sequela associated with undertreatment of pain can include reduced quality of life (QOL) and changes in activities of daily living function. The American Geriatric Association recommends use of opioids for pain over nonsteroidal anti-inflammatory drugs, commonly referred to as NSAIDs (Campbell et al., 2010). Anti-inflammatory medicines or NSAIDs are often prescribed for chronic pain (Barkin et al., 2010). Different formulations are available, including oral, topical, intramuscular, and ophthalmic. Risks associated with the use of NSAIDs include GI bleeds, cardiac issues, peripheral edema, possible addiction, and overdose. Routine assessment should be in place for older patients placed on long-term NSAID therapy to quickly identify any adverse reactions of its use (Barkin et al., 2010).

The management of chronic pain in older adults is complex because of possible comorbidities and possible cognitive impairments. But older adults have a lower likelihood of abuse when using opioids than do their younger cohorts (Papaleontiou et al., 2010). Although opioid use for pain management may be more commonly seen in women, the potential for abuse is higher when used with male patients (Campbell et al., 2010). Older women are at risk for sedation, falls, accidental overdose, and constipation when using opioids (Campbell et al., 2010). Since many older women may take sleep aids, the risk of respiratory depression and cognitive impairment is a caution and must be considered as well when prescribing opioids.

When considering opioid treatment for pain management, many potential problems need to be addressed, including falls. Fall-related injuries are a leading cause of death in older adults (Buckeridge et al., 2010). The loss of coordination and sedation associated with the use of pain medicines could increase fall-related injuries and fractures. Using opioids for pain management has the potential for cumulative effects due to their long half-life. This can be a danger to older adults who have a reduced metabolism and clearance time. These normal changes of aging make it possible for higher levels of the drug to remain in their system, increasing the risk of overdose or poisoning.

Within the limited time of an office visit, assessment must be completed on a variety of systems. The presence or absence of pain must be one of them. The patient who is vague or inconsistent with previous pain medicine use may be hiding abuse (Dodrill et al., 2011). Use of UNCOPE, which is six questions regarding drug use, helps to quickly and effectively guide the interview (Dodrill et al., 2011). This tool was originally published by Zywiak et al. in 1999.

Several versions have been published with variations of the six basic questions. The mnemonic UNCOPE began with these words: (1) Used, (2) Neglected, (3) Cut down, (4) Objected, (5) Preoccupied, and (6) Emotional discomfort (Zywiak et al., 1999). Generally, the questions follow this line of thinking:

- Using more than intended; needing early refills
- Neglect of personal responsibilities
- Cutting down use considered
- Objection of medicine use from friends or family
- Preoccupation with having or getting the medicine
- Emotional state is relieved by the use.

Deaths in older patients from unintended drug poisoning are on the rise as more opioids are being prescribed. The most common problems associated with use of opioids including risk of injury from falls are dizziness, fatigue, and syncope. A survey by Blazer and Wu (2009b) on nonprescription use of prescription pain relievers showed interesting trends. Their results showed nonprescription use of prescription pain medicines in persons aged 65 and older low. However, a much higher use of these drugs was found in those aged 50 to 64. This reflects the idea that as baby boomers age, nonprescription use of prescription pain relievers will continue to increase.

Functional Changes Seen with Benzodiazepines

For many years, the use of benzodiazepines was commonplace. They have been prescribed for sleeping problems and anxiety issues. Current thinking recommends only short-term use of this type of medicine with older patients. Owing to changes in metabolism in the older patients, using short-acting benzodiazepines is recommended. Long-acting benzodiazepines could accumulate in the body and increase the risk of sedation.

The harmful effects of long-term use of benzodiazepines began to emerge in the 1990s (Smith & Tett, 2010), leading to a decrease in prescriptions. With long-term use, the effectiveness of the medicine can decline, and the risk of dependence increases. Side effects often seen with use in the older patient can include cognitive changes, dizziness, falls, and fractures. These findings open up educational opportunities for the provider and the patient. In one study, an assessment tool was tested to help providers to detect possible dependence in their older patients (Voyer et al., 2010). They interviewed the patients taking benzodiazepines and asked them two questions: "Have you tried to stop taking this medication?" "Over the past 12 months, have you noticed any decrease in the effect of this medication?" Yes answers to both questions were followed by further investigation and probable reduction of medicine. The results showed sensitivity of 97.1% and specificity of 94.9% regarding dependence, with sensitivity defined as the probability of being dependent and specificity defined as the probability of not being dependent (Voyer et al., 2010). These two questions prove to be an accurate simple tool.

Prescribing benzodiazepines places the patient at risk for falls, particularly due to the comorbidities that exist (Bartlett et al., 2009). Further incidence of long-term use of benzodiazepines was found when older patients had several different providers. The establishment of the prescription monitoring program nationwide gives providers Internet access to all prescriptions filled by their patients. This program can help to reduce "doctor shopping" and excessive medications.

Older adults are at a high risk for falls resulting from expected changes in vision, hearing, muscle tone, and proprioception (Al-Aama, 2011). Combined with chronic health issues and medication use, falling can be the main cause in disability or morbidity. Careful screening and assessment should be completed before beginning or continuing benzodiazepines. This class of medicine is associated with increased falls and cognitive changes in the older patient (Al-Aama, 2011). Patients who have fallen in the past years and those with abnormal gait or balance problems should be carefully assessed.

The risk of falls is greater in the older patient with higher levels of disability, poor cognitive function, previous falls, or fears of falling (Delbaere et al., 2010). Those with the highest risk are not usually involved in a regular exercise program focused on balance training. Simple daily walking on flat and uneven surfaces could reduce the risks of mobility problems and qualify as an exercise program. Basic fall prevention remains a concern for continuing independence in the older patient and should be assessed before beginning or maintaining treatment with a benzodiazepine.

Older patients are often diagnosed with anxiety and depression and may be taking benzodiazepines and undertreating the depression. Appropriate treatment for the depression may also control the anxiety (Culberson & Ziska, 2008). Again, the need for thoughtful evaluation, prescribing, and follow-up will assist providers with a more complete plan of care.

SCREENING AND RISK FACTORS

Older adults are not routinely screened for substance abuse (Briggs et al., 2011). Yet many are living alone, feeling lonely, dealing with physical challenges, and changing family dynamics, which can all put them at higher risk of substance abuse. Older adults respond better to treatment that is supportive, adaptive, creative, and less confrontational (Briggs et al., 2011). Owing to changes in metabolism and drug-to-drug interaction, tolerance in substance abuse may present differently in the older adult patient. The use of Screening, Brief Intervention, and Referral to Treatment (SBIRT) is useful to evaluate the need for services and provides a link to treatment in the community (Babor et al., 2007). The SBIRT model follows a line of screening from less risk to moderate or severe risk of alcohol or substance abuse. This model, directs a short-term plan for interventions that have been found useful for reduction of use.

What are the risk factors that contribute to substance abuse? Use of the P's formulation is helpful here. This is a group of questions providers may ask themselves while assessing the patient and formulating a plan of care. Contemplating these questions is a useful way to identify the patient's particular life path thus far. The provider looks for precipitating factors, perpetuating factors, predisposing factors, and possible protective factors as the patient explains or reviews their history or present illness.

- *What are precipitating factors*—economic forces/changes, what occurred that caused abuse—personal loss, retirement
- *What are perpetuating factors*—what environment supports "drinking," "smoking weed," perhaps a move into a retirement home with social events such as "happy hour," overuse of pain medicines for chronic pain, what things are ongoing to maintain and support abuses
- *What are predisposing factors*—genetics, grew up in environment of abuse
- *What is a protective factor*—what can decrease use of substance—going to live with family that avoids use of alcohol might prevent abuses, monitoring of medicines, monitoring use of assistive devices, that is, walker, safe alert jewelry. Patients with protective factors are more likely to respond to treatment.

There are multiple tools for screening substance abuse. The more common ones include Cage, QOL, the National Institute on Alcohol Abuse and Alcoholism guidelines (NIAAA), and Michigan Alcohol Screening Test (MAST). The Alcohol Use Disorder Identification Test (AUDIT) is another frequently used tool. This is a 10-question tool. The AUDIT C is a shorter version that is easier to use. It consists of only three questions focused on alcohol consumption (Dawson et al., 2005). A positive result from the AUDIT C suggests further investigation of alcohol abuse (Dawson et al., 2005). The SMAST-G or geriatric version was specifically developed for older adults and proves to be a more effective tool in identifying older adult alcohol abuse. The family interview is a very important screening tool. This gives the provider and the patient an objective look at the situation and establishes early involvement of the family in treatment planning and provides a social network for support in recovery and abstinence.

TREATMENT

How can we treat addictions? What is alcohol doing for the patient? What is the abusive behavior covering up; numbing? How can we promote increased independence in our older adult patient? How can we assist the older adult patient to move away from loneliness, grief, self-doubt, or chronic pain? What are options for treatment? A measure of pain relief may be found in physical therapy, occupational therapy, body mechanics training, and relaxation training. What is the QOL for the older adult patient? How can they resume or begin engagement in meaningful social activities? In his book *The Creative Age Awakening Human Potential in the Second Half of Life*, Dr. Gene Cohen states, "It is never too late to benefit from new opportunities and positive influences. We can more actively seek them out by taking special interest classes or meeting new people who affirm our sense of self-worth" (Cohen, 2000).

Evidence suggests that substance use treatment in the older patient has generally had results as good as or better than those with younger patients (Briggs et al., 2011). When it is determined that an individual has a substance use disorder, the provider could use motivational interviewing to help the patient come to grips with their problem. This type of interview utilizes questions to assist the individual to become aware of their substance use disorder. For example, the provider will ask the patient about their substance use and explore through questioning how their consumption of a substance might affect their life. "When you are drinking or using drugs, do you experience any problems with your balance and are you having an increased risk of falling? If so, what might happen to you should you fall and break a hip? Do you know of any of your older adult friends who have broken their hips and had to spend extensive time in a nursing home?" If the patient is able to acknowledge the relationship between their use of alcohol or drugs and their increased problem with balance, then one might ask: "Would you consider getting help to control your use of alcohol or drugs to reduce your risk of having a traumatic fall?"

Treatment begins by determining the stage of change the patient is currently in. One model of behavioral change has been offered by Norcross and his colleagues. The stages of change were studied through meta-analysis by Norcross et al. (2011). Their study looked at the interrelationship between the processes of change and the stages of change. The stage of change refers to what level of change the patient is in, and the process of change refers to how the change to another level occurs.

The first stage is labeled pre-contemplative. In this stage, the individual is in denial and has no insight into this or her behavior or how it affects others and puts them at risk. During this stage, the provider might utilize motivational interviewing to help the patient move past their denial and begin to consider the need for help. This could be accomplished by asking family members or friends to meet with the patient and the provider to better understand how the substance use is impairing their life. Another strategy is for the provider to challenge the patient to try stopping the substance use for several weeks, which might allow the person to appreciate their dependence on the substance and to experience the benefits of not using it.

The second stage is contemplative. The patient is beginning to show ambivalence toward their use of the substance. Again, using friends and family to help confront the patient may be helpful in moving them forward to further appreciate the extent of their problem with the substance. The provider should continue to ask the individual questions about how their use of the substance interferes with their personal goals and their dreams for the future. Older adults strive to be as independent as possible; their abuse of substances can put them at risk of losing their independence and ability to care for themselves.

Preparation is the third stage of behavioral change. The individual is now accepting the need for change and is ready to consider various options for treatment. The provider will now consider the severity of the problem. The action stage involves cessation of substance use. During this stage, regular treatment and support is essential.

If the patient is at risk for withdrawal or is unable to stop using the substance in their own home, residential treatment may be necessary. The treatment may require detoxification with medication such as a benzodiazepine, if the substance is alcohol. An opiate taper, such as suboxone would be considered if the substance is an opiate. If the patient has strong family support and great personal determination, home treatment may be sufficient. This might require frequent office visits to monitor their vital signs and to provide encouragement. Self-help groups such as Alcoholics Anonymous (AA) and Narcotics Anonymous (NA) are also often valuable, establishing another community of support and guidance.

The action stage or fourth stage is the time when the patient is receptive to getting treatment and support. During this stage, the provider will need to continue to give support and reinforce the patient's effort to get help and accept their treatment.

The maintenance stage is the final stage when behavior remains changed. No more substance use. This is the time when the provider works with the patient to avoid relapse and to help keep them focused on sobriety. The abusive behavior is replaced by healthy behavior, and the patient must now work continuously to avoid relapse.

A common pitfall occurs when a provider moves too quickly through the stages of change (Norcross et al., 2011). Often the patient will present at the clinic before they are ready to move into the action stage. Setting realistic goals will assure realistic change. As patients move through the stages of change, they often regress to previous stages, as they experience times of denial and struggle with their own personal resistance. Professionals need to be patient with the individual's progress, understanding the nature of addiction as a chronic, relapsing disease. During treatment, it is important for the practitioner to treat any comorbidities such as depression or anxiety disorders that present as the patient becomes sober. Antidepressants and nonaddictive antianxiety medications are often helpful.

Direct patient interview will guide the provider in pharmacologic management. Buspirone is an effective medication for the treatment of anxiety in the older adult, both since it is not addictive and since it is well tolerated by the aging patient. Selective serotonin reuptake inhibitors such as citalopram are well tolerated and have few drug-to-drug interactions. The Food and Drug Administration (FDA) guidelines note lower dosing limits for older patients owing to problems of possible Q-T lengthening.

Several medications may be considered in the treatment of alcohol use disorders. One such medicine is acamprosate. The precise action of this drug is still unclear; however, it seems to decrease the intensity of glutamate action in the brain. Studies have demonstrated the effectiveness of the drug in reducing the use of alcohol in middle-aged alcoholics. Its use in the older population, while as yet not fully studied, seems to indicate that it is safe and effective. Naltrexone, an opiate receptor blocker, has been shown to be effective in reducing the use of alcohol in a population of older Veterans (Johnson, 2010). Since the older adult population may be more prone to memory lapses, an injectable extended-release formulation of naltrexone might be considered. An antabuse, such as disulfiram, which inhibits aldehyde dehydrogenase, causes nausea, vomiting, and other unpleasant symptoms when alcohol is consumed. The use of this medicine in an aging population raises concerns that such symptoms might put older individuals at medical risk. Topiramate, a medicine that has been FDA approved for treatment of seizures, has been found to be helpful in the off-label treatment of patients with alcohol use disorder (Johnson, 2010). The drug decreases alcohol abuse. However, its effectiveness has yet to be demonstrated in the older patient. Topiramate has been known to produce problems with concentration and attention, psychomotor slowing and confusion; thus, its use in the older adult will need some caution, especially with an individual who may be experiencing some mild cognitive changes already. Older people who are addicted to opiates may benefit from detoxification with buprenorphine. Maintenance buprenorphine treatment might be considered with aging patients who suffer from chronic pain as well as dependence on pain medicine such as an opioid.

Pseudo-addiction can occur for older patients as they try to adjust pain medicines on their own. Buprenorphine can be useful in reducing opioid use while treating pain. This is office-based treatment requiring frequent follow-up visits (Dodrill et al., 2011). The treatment uses clearly defined protocols for dosing and maintenance stages. Buprenorphine is initiated during mild withdrawal in view of the medicine's affinity for the opioid receptors. This action would put the patient into an immediate withdrawal, but if it is started during mild symptoms of withdrawal, it will relieve them.

Detoxification and withdrawal may produce its own symptoms and needed treatments. When an older addicted patient either stops the abused chemical or significantly decreases the consumption, the individual is prone to experience withdrawal symptoms. Such symptoms may complicate the older person's medical situation. The withdrawal symptoms may be more severe and/or prolonged. The management of these symptoms often requires closer monitoring and more careful treatment. Alcohol withdrawal symptoms are manifested by nausea, vomiting diaphoresis, tremors, elevated pulse, blood pressure, agitation, anxiety, headaches, and insomnia. These symptoms can be effectively managed with benzodiazepine. The shorter acting benzodiazepine, lorazepam, can provide effective control of symptoms without prolonged sedation and instability for older adult patients. Anticonvulsants such as divalproex can provide medical protection against the possibility of a withdrawal seizure, which can occur 36 to 48 hours after the last drink. Should the patient experience symptoms consistent with delirium tremens such as confusion, agitation, marked elevation of blood pressure, heart rate, and temperature with hallucination and delusions, this is a medical emergency. That patient will need to be transferred to an intensive care unit where this medical emergency can be safely managed.

Motivational interviewing may be an effective way to guide older adult patients. This type of interviewing avoids confrontational questions and remains nonjudgmental. This communication style allows patients to arrive at their own conclusions about their problem with drinking or substance misuse, rather than having them feel controlled or manipulated by the professional. Sobriety can occur only when the individual is able to own the problem and accept the need for change.

PREVENTION/PATIENT EDUCATION

Providers underestimate the impact of their advice on patients. As educated, respected, health care providers, frank conversations are paramount when guiding patients regarding possible abusive behaviors such as alcohol use, OTC concoctions, pain medicines, and street drugs. Older adults often have several chronic medical issues, and providers need to be cautious when prescribing in order to eliminate or limit polypharmacy. Social events should downplay alcohol use, considering the changes older adults go through physically and mentally. What was normal for patients at age 30 may not be normal for them at age 65.

Twelve-step programs such as AA and NA may be helpful for the addicted older adult persons. These programs focus on one's identifying oneself as being powerless over the substance of abuse, accepting a higher power and identifying as well as asking forgiveness for past transgressions (Alcoholics Anonymous World Services, Inc., 2009). These self-help groups have the advantages of being free, less formal, and have meetings at various times and places in the community. This can accommodate the schedules of many participants. Since older adults may experience more problems with hearing, increased chronic medical illness, and increased difficulty with transportation, participation may be limited.

Questions remain regarding treatment and accurate assessment of marginalized aging adults such as Americans of different cultures, gay men, and lesbians. Estimates show 28% to 35% of gay men and lesbians have used recreational drugs, while the number of heterosexual users is 10% to 12% (Briggs et al., 2011). Little research has been done with these groups or other subgroups of the aging population to establish appropriate treatment or support needed.

The Healthy People initiative was started in 1979 by the U.S. Department of Health and Human Services. Every decade a new Healthy People plan is released with goals of health promotion and disease prevention in mind. With the establishment of the Healthy People 2020 protocols, the lower quality or complete lack of health care for minority older adults came into mainstream thinking (Byrd et al., 2007). Previously, this group of Americans that includes African Americans, Asians, Hispanics, Islanders, and Gays and Lesbians were found to receive less routine medical care or initial evaluations. The reasons vary but include the fact that fewer primary health care providers may be available near their home, which necessitates longer travel for health services and continued use of home remedies that are handed down for generations. Health care providers may need to gain the trust of these communities to be able to assist them. Patient compliance is part of the equation and the patient must seek out and value health care. An important way to partner with the patient is to engage the patient discussing their concerns and values. The LEARN plan of care can be a useful method for providers working with minority older adult patients (Byrd et al., 2007). The LEARN method was originally published in 1983 by Berlin and Fowkes outlining a framework for cross-cultural patient negotiation of care. This method consists of *Listening*, *Explaining*, *Acknowledging*, *Recommending*, and *Negotiating*. The patient and provider maintain a partnership moving forward. In other words, both sides bring ideas to the exam table to establish a mutual plan of care.

A study conducted in New York State compared three programs serving culturally diverse groups. These programs were community based and ambulatory patient–focused (Siegel et al., 2011). Often, a certain sense of mistrust can exist with patients of different cultures; there may be a stigma attached and shame about accessing the health care system. The importance of empowering and engaging the patient in their care and recovery cannot be overstated. Respect for their goals of treatment must be maintained. Be aware of differences. Take time to learn the values of the patient. What do they wish to take away from the treatment? Engage appropriate community and family member involvement to reduce stigma, build trust, and reduce possible communication or language barriers (Siegel et al., 2011).

Older adult patients should be encouraged to stay abreast of current thinking, use their talents for volunteering, stretch their brains, and stay involved in the world around them. Social media such as Internet email and Facebook are growing fast. These can be a great way for shut-ins to remain connected to family and friends. Other brain stimulation games can be found in books, crossword puzzles, Internet sites, video gaming, and reading. Accessing community services available can be another key resource for the older adult. Activities such as Senior Tai Chi or mall walking are often easy to find in communities and can help to maintain physical mobility and socialization opportunities.

Geriatrics and gerontology is often perceived as a nonglamorous profession with negative attitudes. A couple of issues that may contribute to those negative feelings are the difficulty of treatment for those patients with multiple comorbidities coupled with the poor reimbursement seen after all the extensive work and education time (Golden et al., 2010).

The cost of chronic care in America continues to rise. In an effort to find ways to improve efficiency and reduce current cost of health care, Boult et al. (2009) conducted a meta-analysis of current care models. Fifteen successful models were found for the older adult. The areas were in home acute care, long-term care, and work of interdisciplinary teams in comprehensive hospital care. These models can be used to improve the patient's QOL and extend functional independence. The Medicare program remains the facilitator of health care for the older adult. Research and negotiation must continue as the nation moves forward. Collaboration and change between health care providers and government agencies will be needed as the nation changes and ages.

Technology plays a significant role in health care reform and is designed to assist older people to maintain independence and remain in their private homes. Possible monitoring options include portable devices monitoring heart rate, blood pressure, and oxygen levels. Environmental ideas include motion sensors, door sensors, and electronic pillboxes (Kang et al., 2010). Although monitoring technologies may provide added safety, designers must be careful to create a balance between helpfulness and intruding on privacy (Kang et al., 2010).

Providers are strong advocates for continued physical and mental health. We need to keep the conversation open between patients, caregivers, and family members about ways to improve the QOL for our patients. Thorough assessment of older adults and access to educational materials are a beginning to a mutually beneficial relationship between providers, patients, and family members.

REFERENCES

Al-Aama T. (2011). Falls in the elderly: Spectrum and prevention. *Canadian Family Physician Médecin de Famille Canadien, 57,* 771–776.

Alcoholics Anonymous World Services, Inc. (2009). *Twelve steps & twelve tradition.* New York, NY: Author.

American Psychiatric Association. (2000). *Diagnostic and statistical manual of mental disorders* (4th ed., Text Rev.). Washington, DC: Author.

Babor T., McRee B., Kassebaum P., Grimaldi P., Ahmed K., & Bray J. (2007). Screening, Brief Intervention, and Referral to Treatment (SBIRT): Toward a public health approach to the management of substance abuse. *Substance Abuse: Official Publication of the Association for Medical Education and Research in Substance Abuse, 28*(3), 7–30.

Barkin R. L., Beckerman M., Blum S. L., Clark F. M., Koh E. K., & Wu D. S. (2010). Should nonsteroidal anti-inflammatory drugs (NSAIDs) be prescribed to the older adult? *Drugs & Aging, 27*(10), 775–789.

Bartlett G., Abrahamowicz M., Grad R., Sylvestre M. P., & Tamblyn R. (2009). Association between risk factors for injurious falls and new benzodiazepine prescribing in elderly persons. *BioMed Central Family Practice, 10*(1), 1–8.

Beers M. H., Ouslander J. G., Rollingher I., Reuben D. B., Brooks J., & Beck J. (1991). Explicit criteria for determining inappropriate medication use in nursing home residents. *Archives of Internal Medicine, 151*(9), 1825–1832.

Blazer, D. G., & Wu, L. T. (2009a). The epidemiology of at-risk and binge drinking among middle-aged and elderly community adults: National Survey on Drug Use and Health. *American Journal of Psychiatry, 166*, 1162–1169.

Blazer, D. G., & Wu, L. T. (2009b). Nonprescription use of pain relievers by middle-aged and elderly community-living adults: National Survey on Drug Use and Health. *Journal of the American Geriatrics Society, 57*, 1252–1257.

Boult C., Green A., Boult L. B., Pacala J., Snyder C., & Leff B. (2009). Successful models of comprehensive care for older adults with chronic conditions: Evidence for the institute of medicine's "retooling for an aging America" report. *Journal of the American Geriatrics Society, 57*, 2328–2337.

Boyle A. R., & Davis H. (2006). Early screening and assessment of alcohol and substance abuse in the elderly: Clinical implication. *Journal of Addictions Nursing, 17*(9), 95–103.

Briggs W. P., Magnus V. A., Lassiter P., Patterson A., & Smith L. (2011). Substance use, misuse, and abuse among older adults: Implications for clinical mental health counselors. *Journal of Mental Health Counseling, 33*(2), 112–127.

Buckeridge D., Huang A., Hanley J., Kelome A., Reidel K., Verma A., . . . Tamblyn R. (2010). Risk of injury associated with opioid use in older adults. *Journal of the American Geriatrics Society, 58*, 1664–1670.

Byrd L., Fletcher A., & Menifield C. (2007). Disparities in health care: Minority elders at risk. *ABNF Journal: Official Journal of the Association of Black Nursing Faculty in Higher Education, Inc., 18*, 51–55.

Campbell C. I., Weisner C., LeResche L., Ray T., Saunders K., Sullivan M. D., . . . VonKorff M. (2010). Age and gender trends in long-term opioid analgesic use for noncancer pain. *American Journal of Public Health, 100*(12), 2541–2547.

Cohen G. (2000). *The creative age: Awakening human potential in the second half of life* (p. 38). New York, NY: Avon Books.

Cox-Curry L., Walker C. A., & Hogstel M. (2010). Older adults' medication practices and risk. *Journal of Theory Construction and Testing, 13*(2), 69–74.

Culberson J. W., & Ziska M. (2008). Prescription drug misuse/abuse in the elderly. *Geriatrics, 63*(9), 22–31.

Dawson D. A., Grant B. F., Stinson F. S., & Zhou Y. (2005). Effectiveness of the derived alcohol use disorders identification test (AUDIT-C) in screening for alcohol use disorders and risk drinking in the US general population. *Alcoholism, Clinical and Experimental Research, 29*, 844–854.

Delbaere K., Close J. C. T., Heim J., Sachdev P. S., Brodaty H., Slavin M., . . . Lord S. R. (2010). A multifactorial approach to understanding fall risk in older people. *Journal of the American Geriatrics Society, 58*, 1679–1685.

Dodrill C. L., Helmer D. A., & Kosten T. R. (2011). Prescription pain medication dependence. *American Journal of Psychiatry, 168*(5), 466–471.

Fee E. (2011). Charles E. Terry (1878–1945): Early campaigner against drug addiction. *American Journal of Public Health, 101*(3), 451.

Fialova D., & Onder G. (2009). Medication errors in elderly people: Contributing factors and future perspectives. *British Journal of Clinical Pharmacology, 67*(6), 641–645.

Gallagher P., Ryan C., Byne S., Kennedy J., & O'Mahony D. (2008). STOPP (Screening Tool of Older Person's Prescriptions) and START (Screening Tool to Alert doctors to Right Treatment). Consensus validation. *International Journal of Clinical Pharmacology and Therapeutics, 46*(2), 72–83.

Golden A. G., Van Zuilen M. H., Mintzer M., Issenberg S. B., Silverman M. A., & Roos B. (2010). A fourth-year medical school clerkship that addressed negative attitudes toward geriatric medicine. *Journal of the American Geriatrics Society, 58*, 746–750.

Han B., Gfroerer J. C., Colliver J. D., & Penne M. A. (2009). Substance use disorder among older adults in the United States in 2020. *Addiction (Abingdon, England), 104*, 88–96.

Jesson B. (2011). Minimising the risk of polypharmacy. *Nursing Older People, 23*(4), 14–20.

Johnson B. (2010). Medication treatment of different types of alcoholism. *American Journal of Psychiatry, 167*, 630–639.

Kang H. G., Mahoney D. F., Hoenig H., Hirth V. A., Bonato P., Hajjar I., & Lipsitz L. A. (2010). In situ monitoring of health in older adults: Technologies and issues. *Journal of the American Geriatrics Society, 58*, 1579–1586.

Lee H. S., Mericle A. A., Ayalon L., & Arean P. A. (2009). Harm reduction among at-risk elderly drinkers: A site-specific analysis from the multi-site Primary Care Research in Substance Abuse and Mental Health for Elderly (PRISM-E) study. *International Journal of Geriatric Psychiatry, 24*, 54–60.

Lin J. C., Karno M. P., Barry K. L., Blow F. C., Davis J. W., Tang L., & Moore A. A. (2010). Determinants of early reductions in drinking in older at-risk drinkers participating in the intervention arm of a trial to reduce at-risk drinking in primary care. *Journal of the American Geriatrics Society, 58,* 227–233.

Lin J. C., Karno M. P., Tang L., Barry K. L., Blow F. C., Davis J. W., . . . Moore A. A. (2009). Do health educator telephone calls reduce at-risk drinking among older adults in primary care? *Journal of General Internal Medicine, 25*(4), 334–339.

Merrick E. L., Horgan C. M., Hodgkin D., Garnick D. W., Houghton S. F., Panas L., . . . Blow F. C. (2008). Unhealthy drinking patterns in older adults: Prevalence and associated characteristics. *Journal of the American Geriatrics Society, 56*(2), 214–223.

Moore A. A., Karno M. P., Grella C. E., Lin J. C., Warda U., Liao D. H., & Hu P. (2009). Alcohol, tobacco, and nonmedical drug use in older U.S. adults: Data from the 2001/02 national epidemiologic survey of alcohol and related conditions. *Journal of the American Geriatrics Society, 57*(12), 2275–2281.

Moos R. H., Schutte K. K., Brennan P. L., & Moos B. S. (2009). Older adults' alcohol consumption and late-life drinking problems: A 20-year perspective. *Addiction (Abingdon, England), 104,* 1293–1302.

Norcross J. C., Kreb P. M., & Prochaska J. O. (2011). Stages of change. *Journal of Clinical Psychology: In Session, 67*(2), 143–154.

Olshansky S. J., Goldman D. P., Zheng Y., & Rowe J. W. (2009). Aging in America in the twenty-first century: Demographic forecasts from the Macarthur Foundation Research Network on the Aging Society. *Milbank Quarterly, 87*(4), 842–862.

Papaleontiou M., Henderson C. R., Jr., Turner B. J., Moore A. A., Olkhovskaya Y., Amanfo L., & Reid M. C. (2010). Outcomes associated with opioid use in the treatment of chronic noncancer pain in older adults: A systematic review and meta-analysis. *Journal of the American Geriatrics Society, 58,* 1353–1369.

Rolita L., & Freedman M. (2008). Over-the-counter medication use in older adults. *Journal of Gerontological Nursing, 34*(4), 8–17.

Schonfeld L., King-Kallimanis B. L., Duchene D. W., Etheridge R. L., Herrera J. R., Barry K. L., & Lynn N. (2010). Screening and brief intervention for substance misuse among older adults: The Florida BRITE project. *American Journal of Public Health, 100*(1), 108–114.

Scott C. K., Dennis M. L., Laudet A., Funk R. R., & Simeone R. S. (2011). Surviving drug addiction: The effect of treatment and abstinence on mortality. *American Journal of Public Health, 101*(4), 737–744.

Siegel C., Haugland G., Reid-Rose L., & Hopper K. (2011). Components of cultural competence in three mental health programs. *Psychiatric Services (Washington, D. C.), 62*(6), 626–631.

Smith A. J., & Tett S. E. (2010). Improving the use of benzodiazepines—Is it possible? A non-systematic review of interventions tried in the last 20 years. *BMC Health Services Research, 10*(321), 1–12.

St. John, P. D., Montgomery, P. R., & Tyas, S. L. (2009). Alcohol misuse, gender and depressive symptoms in community-dwelling seniors. *International Journal of Geriatric Psychiatry, 24,* 369–375.

Tulner L. R., Frankfort S. V., Gijsen G. J. P. T., van Campen J. P. C. M., Koks C. H. W., & Beijnen J. H. (2008). Drug-drug interaction in a geriatric outpatient cohort. *Drugs & Aging, 25*(4), 343–355.

Voyer P., Roussel M. E., Berbiche D., & Preville M. (2010). Effectively detect dependence on benzodiazepines among community-dwelling seniors by asking only two questions. *Journal of Psychiatric and Mental Health Nursing, 17,* 328–334.

Weyerer S., Schaufele M., Eifflaender-Gorfer S., Kohler L., Maier W., Haller F., . . . Riedel-Heller S. G. (2009). At-risk alcohol drinking in primary care patients aged 75 years and older. *International Journal of Geriatric Psychiatry, 24,* 1376–1385.

Zywiak W. H., Hoffman N. G., & Floyd A. S. (1999). Enhancing alcohol treatment outcomes through aftercare and self-help group. *Medicine and Health, Rhode Island, 82*(3), 87–90.

CHAPTER 22: IT RESOURCES

Web sites

Alcoholics Anonymous
http://www.aa.org/?Media=PlayFlash

Narcotics Anonymous
http://www.na.org/

American Psychiatric Association
http://www.psych.org/

Society for the Study of Addiction
http://www.addiction-ssa.org/

National Institute on Alcohol Abuse and Alcoholism
http://www.niaaa.nih.gov/

Substance Abuse and Mental Health Services Administration
http://www.samhsa.gov/

Study finds high rates of at-risk drinking among elderly adults
http://newsroom.ucla.edu/portal/ucla/study-finds-high-rates-of-at-risk-156797.aspx

About.Com—Elderly and Alcohol. Website provides several articles on elderly and Alcoholism.
http://alcoholism.about.com/od/elder/Elderly_and_Alcohol.htm

Alcohol screening tools—includes information on the FAST Alcohol Screening Test, the
AUDIT test, the CAGE test. Includes links to the TWEAK Test, the MAST Test, the RAPS4
Test, Top 10 LSAT Test Tips
http://alcoholism.about.com/od/tests/a/fast.htm

Substance abuse among the elderly: a growing problem. Hazelden helps restore hope, healing,
and health to people affected by addiction to alcohol and other drugs. This Web site provides
resources to assist in substance abuse recovery.
http://www.hazelden.org/web/public/ade60220.page

A John Hopkins health alert on prescription drug abuse and the elderly.
http://www.johnshopkinshealthalerts.com/reports/prescription_drugs/3363-1.html

Effects of Drug Abuse on the Elderly
http://www.livestrong.com/article/194729-the-effects-of-drug-abuse-on-the-elderly/

The Impact of Substance Use and Abuse by the Elderly: The Next 20 to 30 Years
http://www.oas.samhsa.gov/aging/chap1.htm

Elderly Drug Abuse a Rising Problem
http://www.treatmentsolutions.com/elderly-drug-abuse-a-rising-problem/

FastStats from the CDC for Alcohol Use
http://www.cdc.gov/nchs/fastats/alcohol.htm

Identification and Treatment of Senior Citizens with Addiction Problems
http://www.kap.samhsa.gov/products/manuals/taps/17q.htm

PDF Documents

American Geriatrics Society Updated Beers Criteria for Potentially Inappropriate Medication
Use in Older Adults
http://www.americangeriatrics.org/files/documents/beers/2012BeersCriteria_JAGS.pdf

The Prevention of Substance Abuse and Misuse among the Elderly: Review of the Literature and Strategies for Prevention. Report includes: Reasons for Concern, Prevalence of Alcohol and Licit and Illicit Drugs among the Elderly, Demographic and Socioeconomic Relationships, Social and Psychological Factors, Considerations for Prevention, and Models for Prevention. (1994)
http://depts.washington.edu/adai/pubs/tr/elderly/elderly.pdf

Co-Occurring Disorders–Related Facts: Elderly—A brief summary of mental illness, substance use, and homelessness among the elderly taken from the SAMHSA website.
http://www.samhsa.gov/co-occurring/topics/data/elderly-quick-facts.aspx

Geriatric Substance Abuse
http://www.alzbrain.org/pdf/handouts/6000.%20GERIATRIC%20SUBSTANCE%20ABUSE%20IN%20THE%20ELDERLY.pdf

Substance Abuse among the Elderly Population—PowerPoint/PDF document
http://www.reachoflouisville.com/SIG/elderly%20substance%20abuse.pdf

The ICAP (International Center for Alcohol Policies) Blue Book: Practical Guidelines for Alcohol Policies and Prevention Approaches—this module is entitled *Alcohol and the Elderly*.
http://www.icap.org/LinkClick.aspx?fileticket=JrDTh3DzjMw%3d&tabid=181

Videos

Substance Abuse in the Elderly (4/10/12)
"Ask the Geriatrician" was developed to address the shortage of geriatricians available to meet with older adults and their caregivers in the United States. Geriatricians specialize in preventing and treating health issues in adults aged 65+, yet many people never have the opportunity to speak with one. (7:12 minutes)
http://youtu.be/wTCEMvU0Jtk

Alcohol Risks for Over 60s (11/27/08) (5:01 minutes)
http://youtu.be/If89PU2NjcY

Images

Google images for Substance Abuse and the Elderly
http://www.google.com/search?q=substance+abuse+and+elderly&hl=en&qscrl=1&nord=1&rlz=1T4ADFA_enUS417US433&tbm=isch&prmd=imvns&source=lnms&sa=X&ei=iT7bT7qSK-z26gHY_OyPCw&ved=0CCoQ_AUoAQ&biw=1152&bih=530

Dementia

Martha Smith Anderson, DNP, CNS-BC, FNGNA

INTRODUCTION AND BACKGROUND

Dementia is a progressive disease of the brain causing decline in intellect and daily functioning. It is often referred to as a syndrome that may be caused by many different neuropathologies with varied clinical symptoms. Typically, memory and abstract reasoning are affected, but the presenting signs and symptoms vary according to the specific cause of dementia. Alzheimer disease is the most frequent form of dementia. The first set of diagnostic criteria in 27 years were released in 2011. Previous criteria were developed by the National Institute of Neurological and Communicative Disorders and Stroke (NINCDS) and the Alzheimer's Disease and Related Disorders Association in 1984. The new criteria from the National Institute on Aging-Alzheimer's Association (NIA-AA) workgroup are a work in progress, addressing the neuropathology and the clinical symptomatology of the dementia syndrome as related to Alzheimer dementia (AD; Jack et al., 2011). Research has demonstrated that the neuropathologies exist in approximately 30% of cognitively normal older adults, often a decade before clinical symptoms present. The preclinical phase is important to identify for health promotion and possible prevention strategies, for research opportunities, and for patient and family education about treatment options. When cognitive impairment progresses and causes impaired daily function, the diagnosis of AD dementia is made (Albert et al., 2011).

AD, the most frequent dementia, affects over 5.2 million Americans over the age of 65. These prevalence data are based on 2010 census data and 2020 extrapolation data (Alzheimer's Association, 2011). AD was identified over 100 years ago in 1906 by Dr. Alois Alzheimer. However, research into causes, risk factors, treatment, and presenting symptoms has flourished only in the last 30 years. A focus on primary prevention in dementia is imperative with the increasing number of older adults effective with cognitive impairment. Revision of diagnostic criteria for clinical practice and additional research targeting the preclinical phase are important.

Age is one of the key risk factors in developing AD, with incidence increasing with longevity. Other dementias include vascular dementia (VaD), the second most frequent dementia, and mixed dementia—Alzheimer with another dementia. Also, dementia with Lewy bodies, Parkinson dementia, frontotemporal dementia (FTD), Creutzfeldt–Jakob, and normal pressure hydrocephalus cause other progressive dementia syndromes (Cardarelli et al., 2010; Schneider et al., 2007; Vanneste, 2000).

Mild cognitive impairment (MCI) is memory loss or cognitive changes more than aging, but is not dementia (Winblad et al., 2004). Initially, the syndrome was called benign senescent forgetfulness. Consensus criteria were developed in 2004 and are supported by the 2011 criteria. Efforts to better define MCI, looking at both clinical presentation and cognitive and functional assessment, are the focus of much research. The new criteria consider the MCI due to AD (Albert et al., 2011); however, there are persons with MCI who do not progress to dementia; thus early identification is important for health promotion, possible prevention, education, and planning. Since some with MCI convert to normal, early identification and targeted evaluation and treatment are essential.

Delirium is an acute and fluctuating sensorium due to medical illness. Increased morbidity, mortality, and institutionalization are associated with patients experiencing delirium (Witlox et al., 2010). However, the presence of beta amyloid and tau in the CSF were not associated with delirium (Witlox, J., Eurelings, L. S., de Jonghe, 2011). In patients undergoing aortic vascular surgery, delirium was present in 36% of patients after surgery and post operative cognitive dysfunction (POCD) was present in 66% at discharge. Three months after discharge, 6% of subjects continued to have POCD (Bryson et al., 2011). Persons may experience a delirium without an underlying dementia; however, those with dementia have an increased risk of delirium. The disturbances in consciousness and cognition occur over short periods, usually hours to days, and fluctuate within a 24-hour time frame (DSM-IV TR). Evaluation and treatment of the underlying medical condition is urgent, but prevention is the goal.

PATHOPHYSIOLOGY

Brain aging—and everything that it entails, from the annoying inconvenience of age-related memory loss to more serious conditions such as Alzheimer and dementia—was equated with neuron failure; however, it is now known that unless a specific disease that causes loss of nerve cells is diagnosed, most, if not all, of the neurons remain healthy until death. That's a big change, and it has only come about in the last decade (Khan et al., 2011, Mathias & Burke, 2009).

Different dementias have unique pathologies, definitively defined by brain autopsy at death. New research considers biomarkers that are either from cerebrospinal fluid or imaging, such as positron emission tomography (PET) scans. Biomarkers are objective measurable components of a process or disease (AAIC, 2012). One biomarker being studied to understand the dementia syndrome is C-PIB (C-labeled Pittsburg Compound B), studied in cerebrospinal fluid. AD is characterized by a neurodegenerative pathophysiological process and distinct clinical symptoms that are considered a continuum, but the course of development may not be concurrent (Sperling et al., 2011). It is thought that extracellular beta-amyloid protein plaques develop years before symptoms, accumulating along the synapses in the neocortex, appearing to inhibit neuronal communication. The hippocampus, which is central to memory, is first affected, and then the amygdala, part of the limbic system, impacting emotion and instincts. Neuronal loss spreads throughout the cerebral cortex, affecting the frontal, parietal, and temporal lobes as the disease progresses. Neurotransmitter decline results from this cell death; particularly, acetylcholine decline occurs, and it is essential in formation and then retrieval of memories (Petersen, 2002). As cell loss progresses, other neurotransmitters are affected, including dopamine, which impacts movement; glutamate, impacting learning and long-term memory; norepinephrine, which affects emotional responses; and serotonin, impacting mood and anxiety.

Whether this beta-amyloid accumulation is causative in the development of the dementia syndrome is not yet established, yet the damage may be present a decade before symptoms present. Intracellular neurofibrillary tangles are more closely correlated with the onset of clinical symptoms. High levels of the protein tau form tangles that inhibit transport of important nutrients within the cell throughout regions of the brain. The resultant cell death is attributed to the cerebral atrophy seen on head scans in advanced Alzheimer's; the brain's shrinkage due to neuronal death (National Institute of Aging, 2008). Early onset Alzheimer disease is no longer accepted as a different pathology from late onset ($\geq$65years). Heavier amyloid pathological burden may represent a more aggressive form of AD based on comparisons of early onset and late onset AD patients. Comparisons of living brain amyloid burden using C-PIB biomarkers were matched for dementia severity, illness duration, and genotype (Choo et al., 2011).

AD pathology of diffuse amyloid plaques may be present without any presenting clinical symptoms, and symptom presentation may vary greatly; thus, pathology and clinical presentation are distinguished in treatment and research criteria of the syndrome in the new NIA-AA workgroup consensus (Khachaturian, 2011). Jack et al. (2011) note that the non-AD dementias have more overlap than realized previously. Vascular dementia, Lewy body disease, and AD coexist much more often than understood a decade previously (Schneider et al., 2007). The presence of multiple pathologies is associated with greater decline (Viswanathan et al., 2009).

Vascular Dementia

The concept of VaD has been recognized for over a century. Its definition and diagnostic criteria remain unclear and generate confusion and debate, although several clinical criteria have been used for defining VaD. The term VaD substantially means a disease with a cognitive impairment often resulting from cerebrovascular disease and ischemic or hemorrhagic brain injury. Dementia represents only a portion of the burden of cognitive dysfunction associated with cerebrovascular disease. The older term "vascular dementia" is being replaced with a new one: "vascular cognitive impairment" (VCI) (Alzheimer's Association, n.d.).

Vascular dementia is the second most common form of dementia and is attributed to 20% of dementia in older adults (Wimo et al., 2006). Treatment of vascular risk factors in high-risk populations has been shown to influence the incidence of dementia (Schneider et al., 2007). Hypertension is a risk factor for cardiovascular disease, and stroke and can lead to cognitive impairment. Executive function is the most vulnerable cognitive domain to hypertension, impacting abstract reasoning, planning, and the ability to initiate, sequence, and monitor goal-directed behavior. The antihypertensives and vascular, endothelial, and cognitive function (AVEC) trial studied hypertensives with early cognitive impairment (Hajjar et al., 2009). There is strong evidence that white matter hyperintensities, even when found on brain imaging studies, incidentally, are associated with increased risk of stroke, dementia, and mortality (Debette & Markus, 2010). White matter hyperintensities are seen more in patients with cerebrovascular disease or cardiovascular risk factors and associated with small vessel disease changes impairing blood flow to the brain. Vascular dementia is most directly attributed to hemorrhagic and/or ischemic stroke leading to brain tissue necrosis. Atherosclerosis is often present and risk factors include hypertension, diabetes, smoking, hyperlipidemia, and cardiac disease (Viswanathan et al., 2009).

A meta-analysis of BMI and risk of dementia (Anstey et al., 2011) indicated that underweight, overweight, and obesity were correlated with increased incidence of dementia. However, authors report that further study is needed both with the risk of underweight subjects and in clarifying whether overweight subjects were barely overweight or almost obese. Longitudinal studies of older subjects are also needed.

Lewy Body Dementia

Lewy body pathology of alpha-synuclein protein is present in the cerebrum, brain stem, and/or autonomic nervous system in Lewy body dementia. Lewy bodies are also seen in dementia of Parkinson disease. The dementia with Lewy body (DLB) consortium (McKeith et al., 2004) defines diagnostic criteria based on presentation of dementia occurring before or with parkinsonism as DLB and Parkinson disease dementia (PDD) as dementia occurring after established Parkinson disease. To verify these diagnostic criteria, Fujishiro et al. (2008) evaluated clinically diagnosed DLB at autopsy by high, intermediate, or low probability finding diffuse cortical Lewy bodies with Braak NFT V at 90% of the high-probability cases and low Alzheimer pathology. Core clinical features of fluctuating attention, extrapyramidal signs, including tremor or muscle rigidity, and REM sleep behavior disorder were higher in the high-probability cases also—except for visual hallucinations that occurred across all levels of the DLB pathology (Fujishiro et al., 2008).

Mixed Dementia

Mixed dementia is most often AD pathology mixed with another pathology, usually VaD or Lewy body dementia. The incidence of mixed dementia is particularly high in persons of advanced age with dementia. Thus, the pathology of most dementia cases is mixed and will be more challenging to target treatments (Brodaty et al., 2011). Most community dwelling elders have neuropathological changes of dementia on autopsy. Most common diagnoses in the elders with dementia were mixed pathology, usually AD with vascular infarcts. Those with a greater than one neuropathology at autopsy had dementia three times more than those with only one pathology (Schneider et al., 2007). The incidence of pure AD and pure VaD are less than that of mixed dementias.

Frontotemporal Dementia

Frontotemporal dementias affect the frontal and temporal lobes and include Pick disease, progressive supranuclear palsy, and primary progressive aphasia (PPA) and variants. Behavioral presentation is most often impulsivity or early changes in social behavior. Disinhibition and embarrassing behavior are typical. Apathy and lack of motivation may also present. Recent reclassification (Gorno-Tempini et al., 2011) defines PPA as a clinical syndrome with varied neuropathology but with the most prominent initial clinical presentation of language difficulty. ADLs are preserved except in areas affected by the language impairment, and aphasia is the most significant presenting symptom in the early stages of the disease. On the basis of clinical presentation early in the disease, the 2011 workgroup identified three of the most common forms of PPA—nonfluent progressive aphasia, semantic dementia, and lopogenic PPA. Nonfluent progressive aphasia is the most frequent PPA with tau-positive pathology, semantic dementia is ubiquitin/TDP43-positive, and the newest classification, lopogenic, has AD pathology. Frontotemporal lobar degeneration varies according to neuroimaging findings along these three variants. Nonfluent progressive aphasia affects left posterior frontal and insular neuroanatomy, semantic dementia impacts the anterior temporal regions of the brain, and damage in the left temporal and parietal regions are found in lopogenic PPA. The reclassification workgroup defined presenting symptoms along the three variants also, developing tables of inclusion and exclusion criteria (Gorno-Tempini et al., 2011).

MCI is a state between normal aging that may be transitional toward dementia or indicative of high-risk or even very early mild dementia (Petersen, 2004; Pinals & Teresa, 2004; Plassman et al., 2008).

The prevalence of MCI was found to be 19% in patients less than 75 years and 29% in those greater than 85 years in the cardiovascular health study (Lopez et al., 2003). Researchers identified MCI as a heterogeneous syndrome. MCI patients had a higher conversion rate to dementia; rates of conversion varied greatly. Petersen et al. (2001) reported 10% to 15% and Marcos et al. (2006) found 46.3% conversion to dementia. Persons with MCI had 1.7 times higher death rates and developed Alzheimer disease 3.1 times more often than age-, education-, and sex-matched peers (Petersen et al., 2001). Plassman et al. (2008) found 22.2% greater than or equal to 71 years in the United States had mild cognitive or functional impairment without dementia with an annual conversion rate of 11.7% to dementia, but a 17% to 20% conversion in those with prodromal Alzheimer disease or stroke. Decline in episodic and semantic memory and perceptual speed was more significant in persons with MCI (Bennett et al., 2002). Functional parameters of MCI offer opportunities for helpful, individualized strategies for the MCI patient. The International Working Group on MCI (Winblad et al., 2004) reached consensus on a working diagnosis of MCI to include: (a) memory complaint, (b) essentially normal function, (c) decline supported by family or others as not normal for age, (d) no dementia, and (e) cognitive impairment on standardized tests. In 2004, Petersen et al. described subtypes of MCI. Amnestic MCI, nonamnestic MCI, and multiple-domain MCI (both amnestic and nonamnestic) were classified according to primary impact on extensive neuropsychological testing.

Diagnostic criteria of MCI reviewed as a Report of the Quality Standards Subcommittee of the American Academy of Neurology (Petersen et al., 2001) made the argument that MCI was a diagnostic entity. The need for research to develop sensitive functional and neuropsychological measures and monitor progression with cultural influences was identified.

The new criteria from the NIA-AA workgroup addressing the neuropathologies and the clinical symptomatology of the dementia syndrome emphasize the earliest presentations of symptoms, the MCI criteria (Jack et al., 2011). Albert et al. delineates the core clinical criteria in this workgroup (2011). "MCI due to AD" recommendations note that these cognitive changes are not normal for age, and thus AACD (age-associated cognitive decline) or AAMI (age-associated memory impairment) are different. MCI due to AD is one of many causes of cognitive impairment that is not dementia (CIND) such as metabolic abnormalities, substance abuse, or head injury. MCI is a syndrome with clinical, cognitive, and functional criteria; clinical judgment is essential to distinguish between normal cognition, MCI, and dementia. When the clinical assessment points to AD, but the patient is not demented, it is essential that other potential causes of decline be ruled out, including degenerative, depressive, traumatic, vascular, medical, or mixed brain disease (Albert et al., 2011).

PRESENTATION OF DISEASE: ACUTE AND CHRONIC

Dementia is always progressive. There is often a period of MCI, or a prodrome, to most dementias. However, MCI is not always due to the prodrome of AD and is thus not always progressive. The insidious nature of an AD makes it difficult for families to identify when they first noticed cognitive changes. Memory is the most typical complaint, but forgetting names beyond the level of same age peers, difficulty performing activities that were once part of normal functioning, such as managing finances, finding familiar locations while driving, and several episodes of forgetting appointments are clues that often bring patients and families in for assessment. All complaints should be addressed as very few memory complaints are verified as pertaining only to the worried well. Syndromes that should be assessed because symptoms mimic dementia include depression or delirium. Delirium has a high mortality if not identified and treated promptly. It is an acute illness that can become chronic and lead to dementia.

Delirium frequently affects older patients, particularly those with a preexisting cognitive dysfunction. The presentation of this acute confusional state differs from dementia because it is acute and fluctuating. It is extremely common in older hospitalized patients, affecting 14% to 56% of older hospitalized patients with mortality rates of 25% to 33% (Leslie & Inouye, 2011). Functional recovery rates decline with the longer the syndrome exists, creating increasing return to the functional state after 2 weeks. (Witlox et al., 2010). The complexity of the delirium syndrome is best addressed by the interprofessional team. Johns Hopkins Delirium Consortium (Neufeld et al., 2011) is a model for interdisciplinary collaboration to prevent and treat delirium. Successful strategies include reduced heavy sedation in ICU patients, particularly minimizing benzodiazepines and narcotic infusions, reduced bed rest and early mobilization and physical rehabilitation, and, more recently, modifying sleep deprivation. The team reports improvement in the ratio of medical ICU days without delirium (21% versus 53%) (Neufeld et al., 2011).

Delirium may be hypoactive or hyperactive (DSM-IV-RV). The hyperactive patient is known to pull out catheters and lines, climb out of bed, and experience frightening hallucinations, all with risks of falls and subsequent trauma. While causative factors for most delirium cases are not definitively identified, prompt and thorough clinical evaluation for infection, electrolyte imbalance, medication adverse events, and other geriatric syndromes are essential to reduce morbidity and mortality. The quiet or subdued patient may have a physiological crisis without forewarning or may be assumed to be depressed; the nuances of the geriatric syndromes require critical thinking in assessment, evaluation, and planning. Bedside assessments with standardized instruments such as the CAM-ICU to assess delirium and agitation–sedation assessments are reliable over time in the clinical setting and assist with prompt medical decisions (Vasilevskis et al., 2011).

Depression is associated with cognitive impairment, yet the relationship has been unclear. Reppermund et al. (2011) studied depression symptoms as defined by a Geriatric Depression Scale greater than or equal to 6 (GDS), past episodes of depression, and the use of antidepressant medications, and found that current or past reports of depression requiring medical interventions were associated with lower cognition but not with lower function on ADLs. In this sample of community dwelling older persons, memory was impacted more than executive function after controlling for anxiety. Potential effect of antidepressant use, cardiovascular risks, and life satisfaction was controlled showing no relationship to memory impairment in depressed older individuals living in the community and currently showing depressive symptoms. Other studies demonstrate subsequent cognitive decline in those with a history of depressive episodes, (Köhler et al., 2010). Community dwelling elders with depressive symptoms as demonstrated with a positive GDS are at risk for cognitive decline, similarly to elders with a history of major depression (Reppermund et al., 2011).

Comprehensive assessment is essential in diagnosing and treating cognitive concerns. Earlier identification allows time to address risk factors and comorbidities contributing to progression. Clinical evaluation must include standardized testing and a thorough history of early symptoms and impact on function. Depression must be considered and treated with counseling and antidepressants for optimal impact. Executive function is specifically affected in persons with previous or current depression (Reppermund et al., 2011) (see Chapter 26).

TREATMENT

Treatment involves assessment of the total patient. Lab work that can discern possible causes of cognitive dysfunction include B_{12} and thyroid and must be conducted. Vascular risk factors should be treated to optimal levels of management, including hypertension, diabetes, and elevated lipids. Depression should be ruled out and treated if suspected. Symptom presentation determines whether head imaging is needed.

As pointed out in the new recommendations (Albert et al., 2011), when the clinical assessment points to AD, but the patient is not demented, it is essential that other potential causes of decline be ruled out. These include other neurological degenerative disorders, depression, traumatic brain injury, vascular, medical or mixed brain disease.

While there are no effective treatments for dementia, there are FDA-approved medications aimed at decreasing the rate of decline and lengthening the time to dependency in persons with mild-to-moderate dementia. There are three cholinesterase inhibitors, donepezil (Aricept), galantamine (Razadyne), and rivastigmine (Exelon). The efficacy data are similar for each of these medications; decisions on which to choose come down to cost, convenience, and side effects.

In addition, there is one approved N-methyl-D-aspartate antagonist, Memantine (Namenda), approved for the treatment of dementia in the moderate-to-severe stages. This medication can be used alone or in combination with the cholinesterase inhibitors (Table 23.1).

TABLE 23.1 · Medications for Dementia

Brand Name	Generic Name	Dosage	Side Effects	Action
Aricept	donepezil	10 mg once daily After titration, 23 mg once daily is available.	Nausea, vomiting, diarrhea, anorexia, bradycardia, sleep changes, leg cramps	Acetylcholinesterase inhibitor
Exelon	rivastigmine	6 mg b.i.d. or 9.5 mg patch daily	Nausea, vomiting, diarrhea, sleep changes, headache, interactions with other drugs	Acetylcholinesterase inhibitor
Razadyne (initially Reminyl)	galantamine	24 mg once daily	Nausea, vomiting, diarrhea, anorexia, dizziness, headache, syncope	Acetylcholinesterase inhibitor
Namenda	memantine	10 mg b.i.d.	Cough, chest pain, confusion, hallucinations, sudden numbness or weakness, seizures, increased blood pressure	N-methyl-D-aspartate receptor antagonists

Additional information on medications for dementia should be reviewed in a pharmacology textbook. Web site information may be briefly referenced at drugs.com.

CULTURAL CONSIDERATIONS

Diagnosis of dementia varies geographically in the United States. Gillum and Obisesan (2011) analyzed data from the US multiple-cause-of-death files from 1999 to 2004. In the middle Atlantic and the United States, blacks were found to have nonspecified dementia diagnoses such as senility 66% more than AD (30%) as compared with whites (58% and 41%). Speculation as to the cause of this pattern of diagnosis variability along geography and race includes variability in accepted practice or custom for diagnosis and lack of access to technology and treatment centers.

PREVENTION

The role of hypertension and hyperlipidemia in prevention of dementia is currently under investigation. A meta-analysis of hypertension as a risk factor (Sharp et al., 2011) found that hypertension significantly increased risk for VaD. Hypertension has been shown to be a risk factor for AD also. There is no strong evidence that lowering blood pressure actually reduces the risk of VaD, but there have been few large, well-controlled studies with cognition as a key variable (Sharp et al., 2011). Thus, the importance of preventing hypertension and treating it aggressively are emphasized in prevention of VaD.

Use of statin medications has not been shown to be effective in established AD or VaD in a meta-analysis comparing randomized controlled trials where dementia patients received statins for at least 6 months (McGuinness et al., 2010). No effect was seen in cognition, function, or behavior as a treatment modality.

Genetic risk for AD is primarily for persons who carry APOE4 alleles. The apolipoproteins have increased risk of developing AD dementia, but do not always develop symptoms (Sperling et al., 2011). In a cross-sectional study of MCI subjects (He et al., 2009), all four MCI subtypes were compared and no difference was found in the APOE-4 genotype. However, persons with amnestic MCI demonstrated almost double the prevalence of the APOE-4 allele than the non-amnestic MCI subjects.

Other risk factors for development of MCI include men more than women. Petersen studied predominantly white Midwestern subjects and found 19% men and 14% women with MCI. The total of 16% included both amnestic MCI, more likely to progress to AD, and non-amnestic MCI. Amnestic MCI was seen twice as much in this study of almost 2,000 randomly selected 70- to 89-year-olds. Education was protective based on years in school: less than 9 years in school for 30% of the MCI subjects as compared with 11% in those with 16+ years of education. Subjects who were currently or previously married had less MCI than those who never married (Petersen, 2010).

Several meta-analyses have identified the benefit of physical activity in reducing the risk of AD (Hamer & Chida, 2009) and also VaD (Aarsland et al., 2010). Multiple small studies of impact on memory in MCI with dietary modifications include green tea (Park et al., 2011), grape juice (Krikorian et al., 2009) and low fat/low glycemic index (Bayer-Carter et al., 2011), all of which were encouraging, but larger studies are needed and quantities of dietary supplementations are understudied.

Although outside the realm of this work, there are numerous smaller studies looking at various non-pharmacologic or dietary methods of preventing or treating early mild memory loss. Regular physical exercise, including dance and Tai Chi, are often recommended. New learning and regular cognitive stimulation are often addressed, including involvement with music. Spirituality and faith and stress reduction are also considered. Larger, randomized controlled studies are needed to clarify what modifiable activities and intellectual pursuits are most beneficial.

PATIENT EDUCATION COMPONENTS FOR PROVIDERS

Memory complaints need to be addressed. Early memory complaints or cognitive concerns offer an opportunity to identify risk factors and treatment plans. Until research on biomarkers and new more effective medications are realized, Brodaty and colleagues argue, the best strategy currently is to postpone the clinical onset of dementia. A 1-year delay now will save the global economic and personal burden for almost 12 million persons by 2050 (Brookmeyer et al., 2007). To postpone the onset of dementia clinically, early diagnosis must be a priority.

The influence of age on four diagnostic measures of Alzheimer disease was studied in a sample of 55- to 90-year-olds (Schmand et al., 2011). Neuroimaging with structural magnetic resonance imaging (MRI) and neuropsychological testing did not diminish diagnostic value with age in those greater than 75 years. Cerebrospinal fluid evaluation for beta-amyloid and tau nor FDG-PET scan added diagnostic value to the older adults with MCI or AD. Thus hippocampal volume measured with by MRI and memory performance measured by neuropsychology assessment provided the most accurate diagnoses in the older subjects, as opposed to CSF fluid evaluation or FDG-PET scans. Ruling out reversible causes of dementia such as B_{12} deficiency and hypothyroidism are first steps. A computed tomography or MRI of the head is recommended in the revised standards (McKhann et al., 2011), but reimbursement by insurance has been a practical difficulty in some cases unless symptoms include nontypical AD progression (National Institute of Neurological Disorders and Stroke [NINDS], 2012). Future imaging studies that might be of value include PET, functional MRI (fMRI), and single photon emission computed tomography (SPECT). These studies are rarely used today outside the research environment.

Providers must be alert to concerns and complaints about memory or cognitive function. Memory clinics offer early assessment expertise, and neuropsychology availability is essential. If such clinics are unavailable, standardized assessment tools should be utilized in the primary care office.

SCREENING AND RISK FACTORS

Screening tools provide standardized methods of assessment and objective data in determining and monitoring levels of cognitive impairment. Nurse researchers studied the role of nurses in identifying MCI in older patients, based on the memory subtypes described by Petersen (2004) and Winblad et al. (2004). Floetke et al. (2008) studied amnestic MCI only, in a secondary analysis within their population of patients with pain. They were able to discriminate amnestic MCI with a cognitive test battery of the Dementia Rating Scale-2 and the Hopkins Verbal Learning Test, taking over 40 minutes. The GDS was used to assess depression. Floetke et al. suggest that APRNs are in a position to screen, but recognize that shorter screening batteries are needed for the primary care practice. They suggest that APRNs are certainly responsible for screening and referral, and encourage nurses to become involved with developing faster assessment methods.

Connor et al. (2005) used the animal fluency test in comparison with three clock drawing tests (CDT) and found the animal fluency test to be a better lone predictor of dementia than either of the CDT, which were only predictive of moderate-to-severe dementia in the two groups of pair-matched controls and dementia. Among the instruments used, the MMSE (Folstein et al., 1975) the MMSE (Folstein, Folstein, & McHugh, 1975) was found to be the best predictor of cognitive impairment, utilizing a cut-off of 26 on the MMSE. The MMSE is a brief screening instrument, typically taking 7-10 minutes to administer, and assessing cognitive function of orientation, word recall, attention and calculation, language, and visuospatial. Scores range from 0 to 30, with the cut-off of 24 or less indicating cognitive impairment. The MMSE is helpful in screening for dementia and in following change in persons with dementia. Scores are related to older age and education (Alzheimer's Society, Mitchell, 2009; Jacova, Kertesz, Blair, Fisk, & Feldman, 2007).

The MMSE was found to be a reliable and valid cognitive screen in a dementia group determined by Dementia Rating Scale (DRS) scores. The CDT was sensitive only in the more demented groups, when functional impairments would be more evident and formal testing less revealing. Loewenstein et al. (2006) determined which measures were of the most use or what was the optimal cut-off to determine impairment or MCI. Different memory measures were given to 80 normal subjects leading to eight different memory indices with co-normed data. The MCI study group of 23 had CDR of 0.5, MMSE greater than 23, and memory deficits. Researchers determined guidelines for specific tests, alone or combined, to classify MCI. They used the Fuld Object Memory Evaluation, which was three trials of recall of 10 objects with a distractor task and Wechsler subtests. More than two of any tests decreased accuracy of classification.

There was no consensus on which tests best described MCI and which cut-off values were most accurate (Loewenstein et al., 2006). Connor et al. (2005) used a cut-off score of 26 on the MMSE to define the study population of MCI. The typical cut-off for the MMSE was generally 24 for cognitive impairment at the dementia level (Folstein et al., 1975).

Researchers (Wood et al., 2006) found age, education, and racial differences with the MMSE. After adjustment for age and education, MMSE scores were still significantly lower in black older adults as compared with white older adults. The potential for the MMSE to produce bias among ethnic groups should be considered when using the MMSE to define practice or study groups (Wood et al. 2006). Age and education should be adjusted in community dwelling older adults. These scientists recommended further study of intervention acceptance or success after reclassification of groups by cognitive status using the adjusted MMSE scores.

The MMSE is recommended for the best stand-alone screen of early mild dementia (Connor et al., 2005). The Blessed or Mini-Cog is suggested if the MMSE, which takes about 7 minutes to administer, is considered too lengthy for practitioners to use. Animal fluency, with a cut-off of 12 animals named, had some merit as a lone cognitive screen, although it has bias of education and was inappropriate in speech abnormalities. The Mini-Cog combines the three-word recall of the MMSE with a distraction clock drawing. In a recent review of some dementia screening tools, the Mini-Cog was one of the recommendations for general practitioners, based on lack of educational bias, improved sensitivity and specificity over the MMSE and efficiency in time of administration (Brodaty et al., 2006). This study supported the use of the CLOX 1. Screens such as CDT, Mini-Cog, and category fluency tests are recommended for nurses to increase the frequency of screening persons with memory concerns or those with advanced age, probably greater than 75 years. Screening should be repeated in subsequent visits, with increased awareness of the clinician to seek further evaluation and assessment and particularly to develop interventions to maintain function in those with early memory deficits.

A web site maintained by the John A Hartford Foundation through the Hartford Institute for Geriatric Nursing (ConsultGeriRN.org) offers access to many of the screening and assessment tools discussed. This web site is a valuable resource for written and video demonstrations and explanations of tools such as the MMSE, Mini-Cog, GDS, executive dysfunction assessment using the Trails test, a verbal fluency test, and the Clox drawing tests. The APRN should develop expertise in a validated set of screening and assessment tools to guide recommendations and interventions over time.

Neuropsychology assessment offers expertise in differential diagnosis of the type of dementia, level of impairment, and assists in treatment plan and follow-up through evaluation of the unique characteristics of each patient's symptoms. Commonly used scales such as the MMSE or Blessed do not discern the patterns of deficit as in thorough neuropsychological evaluation. Deficits in dementia assessed by neuropsychology include memory—whether retention, retrieval, or organizational; language—such as aphasia, echolalia, or semantic disorders; perception—such as agnosia or spatial perception and motor function (Snowden, 1994). Memory clinics utilize standardized testing and most often involve the expertise of a neuropsychologist.

Geriatric assessment offers comprehensive assessment of older adults from several functional domains and most often with an interdisciplinary team. Assessments of functional parameters of memory, mood, environment, and social support are included alongside the medical evaluation. The comprehensive nature of the assessment can be beneficial across settings and has been demonstrated in hospitals, primary care offices, and in home care (Gudmundsson & Carnes, 1996). Expert education and training to caregivers and identification of resources and support services offer numerous benefits and reduced burden, including improving mood and delaying institutionalization.

REFERENCES

AAIC Press Release: New Research Reported at the Alzheimer's Association International conference advances validation of new diagnostic guidelines. (2012). Retrieved from http://www.alz.org/aaic/wed_130pmct_nia.asp

Aarsland, D., Sardahaee, F. S., Anderssen, S., Ballard, C., & the Alzheimer's Society Systematic Review group. (2010). Is physical activity a potential preventive factor for vascular dementia? A systematic review. *Aging & Mental Health, 14*(4), 386–395.

Albert, M. S., DeKosky, S. T., Dickson, D., Dubois, B., Feldman, H. H., Fox, N. C., . . . Phelps, C. H. (2011). The diagnosis of mild cognitive impairment due to Alzheimer's disease: Recommendations from the National Institute on Aging-Alzheimer's Association workgroups on diagnostic guidelines for Alzheimer's disease. *Alzheimer's & Dementia, 7*, 270–279.

Alzheimer's Association. (n.d.). *Vascular dementia.* Retrieved from http://www.alz.org/dementia/vascular-dementia-symptoms.asp

Alzheimer's Association. (2011). *Alzheimer's disease facts and figures.* Chicago, IL: Author.

Alzheimer's Society Mini-Mental State Exam. http://www.alzheimers.org.uk/site/scripts/documents_info.php?document ID=121

Bayer-Carter, J. L., Green, P. S., Montine, T. J., VanFossen, B., Baker, L. D., Watson, G. S., . . . Craft, S. (2011). Diet intervention and cerebrospinal fluid biomarkers in amnestic mild cognitive impairment. *Archives of Neurology, 68*(6), 743–752.

Bennett, D. A., Wilson, R. S., Schneider, J. A., Evans, D. A, Beckett, L. A., Aggarwal, N. T., (2002). Natural history of mild cognitive impairment in older persons. *Neurology, 61*, 1179–1184.

Brodaty, H., Breteler, M. M. B., DeKosky, S. T., Dorenlot, P, Fratiglioni, L., Hock, C., . . . De Strooper, B. (2011). The world of dementia beyond 2020. *Journal of the American Geriatrics Society, 59*, 923–927.

Brodaty, H., Low, L., Gibson, L., & Burns, K. (2006). What is the best dementia screening instrument for general practitioners to use? *American Journal of Geriatric Psychiatry, 14*(5), 391–400.

Brookmeyer, R., Johnson, E., Ziegler-Graham, K., & Arrighi, H. M. (2007). Forecasting the global burden of Alzheimer's disease. *Alzheimer's and Dementia, 3*, 186–191.

Cardarelli, R., Kertesz, A., & Knebl, J. A. (2010). Frontotemporal dementia: A review for primary care physicians. *American Family Physician, 82*(11), 1372–1377.

Choo, I. H., Lee, D. Y., Kim, J. W., Seo, E. H., Lee, D. S., Kim, Y. K., . . . Yoon, E. J. (2011). Relationship of amyloid-beta burden with age-at-onset in Alzheimer disease. *American Journal of Geriatric Psychiatry, 19*(7), 627–634.

Connor, D. J., Seward, J. D., Bauer, J. A., Golden, K. S., & Salmon, D. P. (2005). Performance of three clock scoring systems across different ranges of dementia severity. *Alzheimer Disease and Associated Disorders, 19*(3), 119–127.

Debette, S., & Markus, H. S. (2010). The clinical importance of white matter hyperintensities on brain magnetic resonance imaging: Systematic review and meta-analysis. *British Medical Journal*, doi:10.1136/bmj.c3666

Floetke, E. A., Horgas, A. L., & Marsiske, M. (2008). Nurses' role in identifying mild cognitive impairment in older adults. *Geriatric Nursing, 29*, 38–47.

Folstein, M. F., Folstein, S. E., & McHugh, P. R. (1975). "Mini-mental state": A practical method for grading the cognitive state of patients for the clinician. *Journal of Psychiatric Research, 12*, 189–198.

Fujishiro, H., Ferman, T. J., Boeve, B. F., Smith, G. E., Graff-Radford, N. R., . . . Dickson, D. W. (2008). Validation of the neuropathologic criteria of the third consortium for dementia with Lewy bodies for prospectively diagnosed cases. *Journal of Neuropathology & Experimental Neurology, 67*(7), 649–656. doi:10.1097/NEN.0b013e31817d7a1d.

Gillum, R. F., & Obisesan, T. O. (2011). Differences in mortality associated with dementia in U. S. blacks and whites. *Journal of the American Geriatrics Society, 59*, 1823–1828. doi:10.1111/j.1532-5415.2011.03598.x.

Gorno-Tempini, M. L., Hillis, A. E., Weintraub, S., Kertesz, A., Mendez, M., Cappa, S. F., . . . Grossman, M. (2011). Classification of primary progressive aphasia and its variants. *Neurology, 76*, 1006–1014.

Gudmundsson, A., & Carnes, M. (1996). Geriatric assessment: Making it work in primary care practice. *Geriatrics, 51*(3), 55–65.

Hajjar, I., Hart, M., Milberg, W., Novak, V., & Lipsitz, L. (2009). The rationale and design of the antihypertensives and vascular endothelial, and cognitive function (AVEC) trial in elderly hypertensives with early cognitive impairment: Role of the renin angiotensin system inhibition. *BMC Geriatrics, 9*, 48. doi:10.1186/1471-2318-9-48.

Hamer, M., & Chida, Y. (2009). Physical activity and risk of neurodegenerative disease: A systematic review of prospective evidence. *Psychological Medicine, 39*(1), 3–11.

He, J., Farias, S., Martinez, O., Reed, B., Mungas, D., & DeCarli, C. (2009). Differences in brain volume, hippocampal volume, cerebrovascular risk factors, and APOE4 among MCI subtypes. *Archives of Neurology, 66*(11), 1393–1399.

Jack, C. R., Jr, Albert, M. S., Knopman, D. S., McKhann, G. M., Sperling, R. A., Carrillo, M. C., . . . Phelps, C. H. (2011). Introduction to the recommendations from the National Institute on Aging-Alzheimer's Association workgroups on diagnostic guidelines for Alzheimer's disease. *Alzheimer's & Dementia, 7*, 257–262.

Jacova, C., Kertesz, A., Blair, M., Fisk, J.D., & Feldman, H. H. (2007). Neuropsychological testing and assessment for dementia, *Alzheimer's & Dementia, 3*(4), 299–317.

Khachaturian, Z. S. (2011). Revised criteria for diagnosis of Alzheimer's disease: National Institute on Aging-Alzheimer's Association diagnostic guidelines for Alzheimer's disease. *Alzheimer's & Dementia, 7*, 253–256.

Khan, B. A., Zawahiri, M., Campbell, N. L., & Boustani, M. A. (2009). Biomarkers for delirium—A review. *Journal of the American Geriatrics Society, 59*(Suppl. 2), S256–S261.

Köhler, S., Thomas, A. J., Barnett, N. A., & O'Brien, J. T. (2010). The pattern and course of cognitive impairment in late-life depression. *Psychological Medicine, 40*, 591–602. doi:10.1017/S0033291709990833.

Krikorian, R., Nash, T. A., Shidler, M. D., Shukitt-Hall, B., & Joseph, J. A. (2009). Concord grape juice supplementation improves memory function in older adults with mild cognitive impairment. *British Journal of Nutrition, 103*, 730–734.

Leslie, D. L., & Inouye, S. K. (2011). The importance of delirium: Economic and societal costs. *Journal of the American Geriatrics Society, 59*(Suppl. 2), S241–S243.

Loewenstein, D. A., Acevedo, A., Ownby, R., Agron, J., Barker, W. W., Isaacson, R., . . . Duara R. (2006). Using different memory cutoffs to assess mild cognitive impairment. *American Journal of Geriatric Psychiatry, 14*(11), 911–919.

Lopez, O. L., Jagust, W. J., DeKosky, S. T., Becker, J. T., Fitzpatrick, A., Dulberg, C., et al. (2003). Prevalence and classification of mild cognitive impairment in the cardiovascular health study cognition study. *Archives of Neurology, 60*, 1385–1389.

Marcos, A., Gil, P., Barabash, A., Rodriquez, R., Encinas, M., Fernandez, C., et al. (2006). Neuropsychological markers of progression from mild cognitive impairment to Alzheimer's Disease. *American Journal of Alzheimer's Disease & Other Dementias, 21*(3), 189–196.

Mathias, J. L., & Burke, J. (2009). Cognitive functioning in Alzheimer's and vascular dementia: A meta-analysis. *Neuropsychology, 23*(4), 411–423.

McGuinness, B., O'Hare, J., Craig, D., Bullock, R., Malouf, R., & Passmore, P. (2010). Statins for the treatment of dementia. *Cochrane Database of Systematic Reviews*, (8), CD007514.

McKeith, I., Mintzer, J., Aarsland, D., Burn, D., Chiu, H., Cohen-Mansfield, J., . . . Reid, W. (2004). Dementia with Lewy bodies. *Lancet Neurology, 3*, 19–28.

McKhann, G. M., Knopman, D. S., Chertkow, H., Hyman, B. T., Jack, C. R., Kawas, C. H., . . . Phelps, C. H. (2011). The diagnosis of dementia due to Alzheimer's disease: Recommendations from the National Institute on Aging-Alzheimer's Association workgroups on diagnostic guidelines for Alzheimer's disease. *Alzheimer's & Dementia, 7*, 263–269.

Mitchell, A. J. (2009). A meta-analysis of the accuracy of the mini-mental state examination in the detection of dementia and mild cognitive impairment. *Journal of Psychiatric Research, 43*(4), 411–431.

National Institute on Aging, (2008). Hallmarks of Alzheimer's Disease. http://www.nia.nih.gov/alzheimers/publication/part-2-what-happens-brain-ad/hallmarks-ad

National Institute of Neurological Disorders and Stroke. (2012). Department of Health and Human Services Director's overview. Retrieved from http://www.ninds.nih.gov/news_and_events/congressional_testimony/ninds_fy_2013_cj.pdf.

Neufeld, K. J., Bienvenu, O. J., Rosenberg, P. B., Mears, S. C., Lee, H. B., Kamdar, B. B., . . . Needham, D. M. (2011). The Johns Hopkins Delirium Consortium: A model for collaborating across disciplines and departments for delirium prevention and treatment. *Journal of the American Geriatrics Society, 59*(Suppl. 2), S244–S248.

Park, S-K., Jung, I-C., Lee, W. K., Lee, Y. S., Park, H. K., Go, H. J., . . . Rho, S. S. (2011). A combination of green tea extract and L-Theanine improves memory and attention in subjects with mild cognitive impairment: A double-blind placebo-controlled study. *Journal of Medicinal Food, 14*(4), 334–343.

Petersen, R. C. (Ed.). (2002). *Mayo Clinic on Alzheimer's disease*. Rochester, MN: Mayo Clinic.

Petersen, R. C. (2004). Mild cognitive impairment as a diagnostic entity. *Journal of Internal Medicine, 256*, 183–194.

Petersen, R. C. (2010). The Prevance of mild cognitive impairment is more common in men. *Neurology, 75*(10), 889–897. doi: HYPERLINK "http://dx.doi.org/10.1212%2FWNL.0b013e3181f11d85" \t "pmc_ext" 10.1212/WNL.0b013e3181f11d85

Petersen, R. C., Stevens, J. C., Ganguli, M., Tangalos, E. G., Cummings, J. L., & DeKosky, S. (2001). Practice parameter: Early detection of dementia: Mild cognitive impairment (an evidence-based review). Report of the Quality Standards Subcommittee of the American Academy of Neurology. *Neurology, 56*, 1133–1142.

Pinals, S. L., & Teresa, M. M. S. (2004). Early recognition, management, and treatment of mild cognitive impairment and its relationship to Alzheimer's disease. *Primary Psychiatry, 11*(1), 41–47.

Plassman, B. L., Langa, K. M., Fisher, G. G., Heeringa, S. G., Weir, D. R., Ofstedal, M. B., . . . Wallace, R. B. (2008). Prevalence of cognitive impairment without dementia in the United States. *Annals of Internal Medicine, 148*(6), 427–436.

Reppermund, S., Brodaty, H., Crawford, J. D., Kochan, N. A., Slavin, M. J., Trollor, J. N., . . . Sachdev, P. S. (2011). The relationship of current depressive symptoms and past depression with cognitive impairment and instrumental activities of daily living in an elderly population: The Sydney Memory and Ageing Study. *Journal of Psychiatric Research, 45*, 1600–1607.

Schmand, B., Eikelenboom, P., van Gool, W. A., & the Alzheimer's Disease Neuroimaging Initiative. (2011). Value of neuropsychological tests, neuroimaging, and biomarkers for diagnosing Alzheimer's disease in younger and older age cohorts. *Journal of the American Geriatrics Society, 59*, 1705–1710.

Schneider, J. A., Arvanitakis, Z., Bang, W., & Bennett, D. A. (2007). Mixed brain pathologies account for most dementia cases in community-dwelling older persons. *Neurology, 69*, 2197–2204.

Sharp, S. I., Aarsland, D., Day, S., Sønnesyn, H., Ballard, C., & Alzheimer's Society Vascular Dementia Systematic Review Group. (2011). Hypertension is a potential risk factor for vascular dementia: Systematic review. *International Journal of Geriatric Psychiatry, 26*(7), 661–669. doi:10.1002/gps.2572.

Snowden, J. S. (1994). Contribution to the differential diagnosis of dementias. 1: Neuropsychology. *Reviews in Clinical Gerontology, 4*, 227–234.

Sperling, R. A., Aisen, P. S., Beckett, L. A., Bennett, D. A., Craft, S., Fagan, A. M., . . . Phelps, C. H. (2011). Toward defining the preclinical stages of Alzheimer's disease: Recommendations from the National Institute on Aging-Alzheimer's Association workgroups on diagnostic guidelines for Alzheimer's disease. *Alzheimer's & Dementia, 7*, 280–292.

Vanneste, J. A. L. (2000). Diagnosis and management of normal-pressure hydrocephalus. *Journal of Neurology, 247*(1), 5–14.

Vasilevskis, E. E., Morandi, A., Boehm, L., Pandharipande, P. P., Girard, T. D., Jackson, J. D., . . . Ely, E. W. (2011). Delirium and sedation recognition using validated instruments: Reliability of bedside intensive care unit nursing assessments from 2007 to 2010. *Journal of the American Geriatrics Society, 59*(Suppl. 2), S249–S255.

Viswanathan, A., Rocca, W. A., & Tzourio, C. (2009). Vascular risk factors and dementia: How to move forward? *Neurology, 72*, 368–374.

Washington Post. (2011). *The aging brain*. Retrieved from http://www.washingtonpost.com/national/health-science/the-aging-brain/2011/12/05/gIQAskhDWO_graphic.html

Wimo, A., Jonsson, L., & Winblad, B. (2006). An estimate of the worldwide prevalence and direct costs of dementia in 2003. *Dementia and Geriatric Cognitive Disorders, 21*(3), 175–181.

Winblad, B., Palmer, K., Kivipelto, M., Jelic, V., Fratiglioni, L., Wahlund, L. O., . . . Petersen, R. C. (2004). Mild cognitive impairment—beyond controversies, towards a consensus: Report of the International Working Group on mild cognitive impairment. *Journal of Internal Medicine, 256*, 240–246.

Witlox, J., Eurelings, L. S., de Jonghe, J. F. M., Verwey, N. A., van Stijn, M. F., Houdijk, A. P., . . . Eikelenboom, P. (2011). Cerebrospinal fluid ?-amyloid and tau are not associated with risk of delirium: A prospective cohort study in older adults with hip fracture. *Journal of the American Geriatrics Society, 59*, 1260–1267.

Witlox, J., Kalisvaart, K. J., de Jonghe, J. F. M., Eikelenboom, P., van Gool, W. A., & Eurelings, L. S. (2010). Delirium in elderly patients and the risk of postdischarge mortality, institutionalization, and dementia: A meta-analysis. *Journal of the American Medical Association, 304*, 443–451.

Wood, R. Y., Giuliano, K. K., Bignell, C. U., & Pritham, W. W. (2006). Assessing cognitive ability in research. *Journal of Gerontological Nursing, 32*(4), 45–54.

CHAPTER 23: IT RESOURCES

Websites

Alzheimer's Association
www.alz.org

National Institute on Aging: Alzheimer's Disease Education and Research (ADEAR) site
www.alzheimers.org

National Institutes of Health; National Institute on Aging – Alzheimer's Disease Education and Referral Center
www.nia.nih.gov/Alzheimers/

Alzheimer's Foundation of America (AFA)
www.alzfdn.org/

National Institute of Neurological Disorders and Stroke
http://www.ninds.nih.gov/

Mayo Clinic—Mild Cognitive Impairment (MCI)
http://www.mayoclinic.com/health/mild-cognitive-impairment/DS00553

Mayo Clinic—Lewy Body Dementia
http://www.mayoclinic.com/health/lewy-body-dementia/DS00795

Mayo Clinic—Vascular Dementia
http://www.mayoclinic.com/health/vascular-dementia/DS00934

WebMD—Vascular Dementia
http://www.webmd.com/stroke/vascular-dementia

UCSF Memory and Aging Center – Mild Cognitive Impairment
http://memory.ucsf.edu/education/diseases/mci

Alzheimer's Association—Dementia with Lewy Bodies
http://www.alz.org/dementia/dementia-with-lewy-bodies-symptoms.asp

Lew Body Dementia Association, Inc.
http://www.lbda.org/

Helpguide.org—Parkinson's Disease & Parkinson's Dementia
http://www.helpguide.org/elder/parkinsons_disease.htm

Parkinson's Disease Dementia
http://www.emedicinehealth.com/parkinson_disease_dementia/article_em.htm

Johns Hopkins Medicine—Dementia and Delirium
http://www.hopkinsmedicine.org/gec/series/dementia.html

Alzheimer's Association—Physician Toolkit; Alzheimer's Disease
http://www.alz.org/mnnd/in_my_community_59110.asp

Alzheimer's Association—Conducting an Assessment
http://www.alz.org/professionals_and_researchers_conducting_an_assessment.asp

Test your Memory for Alzheimer's (5 Best Tests)
   http://www.alzheimersreadingroom.com/p/test-your-memory-for-alzheimers-5-best.html
Dementia Care Central—Stages of Dementia
   http://www.dementiacarecentral.com/node/540
Hartford Institute for Geriatric Nursing—Dementia
   http://consultgerirn.org/searched?q=dementia&Submit_search.x=0&Submit_search.y=0
Michigan State University—Cognitive Disorders and Geriatric Neurology
   http://neurology.msu.edu/patients/cognitive_disorders.shtml
Hartford Institute for Geriatric Nursing—Dementia Assessment Tools
   http://consultgerirn.org/searched?q=dementia+assessment+tools&Submit_search.
   x=0&Submit_search.y=0

PDF Documents

Tools for Early Identification, Assessment, and Treatment for People with Alzheimer's Disease
   and Dementia
   http://www.alz.org/national/documents/brochure_toolsforidassesstreat.pdf

Videos

Alzheimer's Disease (AD) Video (4 minutes)*
This 4-minute video, *Inside the Brain: Unraveling the Mystery of Alzheimer's Disease*, shows
   the intricate mechanisms involved in the progression of Alzheimer disease in the brain.
   (Captioned)
   www.alzheimers.org/rmedia/adanimation.htm
The Alzheimer's Project HBO Videos (40 minutes)*
The National Institute on Aging/NIH collaborated with HBO Documentary Films in presenting
   THE ALZHEIMER'S PROJECT, an Emmy Award winning, multi-platform (television, web,
   DVD, and print) public health series including 4 feature and 15 supplemental films. Closed
   Captioned.
   http://www.nia.nih.gov/alzheimers/alzheimers-project-hbo-videos
The Forgetting: A Portrait of Alzheimer's
Short films about Alzheimer disease:

- Is it Alzheimer's? (18 minutes)
- What is Alzheimer's Disease? (3 minutes)
- Alzheimer's: An Urgent Epidemic (2:20 minutes)
- Alzheimer's: The Race to the Cure (2 minutes)
- Alzheimer's: A message for newly diagnosed patients and their families (1:37 minutes)
   www.pbs.org/theforgetting/watch/pocket.html

---

*Please Credit ADEAR. Permission to use ADEAR materials is not required. When you use our materials in
print, on the Web, or in a video or audio format, we simply request that you credit the "Alzheimer's Disease
Education and Referral Center, a service of the National Institute on Aging." As a courtesy, please let us know
by telephone (1-800-438-4380) or e-mail (adear@nia.nih.gov) where and when the materials will appear.*

A Quick Look at Alzheimer's
Site includes many resources and includes 5 very-short pocket films entitled:

- What is Alzheimer's Disease? (3 minutes)
- Alzheimer's: An Urgent Epidemic (2:20 minutes)
- Alzheimer's: The Race to the Cure (2 minutes)
- Alzheimer's: A message for patients and their families (1:37 minutes)
- The Genetics of Alzheimer's (3:13 minutes)
  www.aboutalz.org

Experience 12 minutes of Alzheimer's (2012)
  Just what is a loved one with dementia going through? A 12-minute virtual Alzheimer's tour reveals more than you ever imagined.
  http://youtu.be/LL_Gq7Shc-Y

Living with Dementia (2013)
  West Sussex has the highest rate of dementia in the country. We look at what it's like when a loved one starts slowly slipping away from reality. And we ask—what can the County Council do to help? (6 minutes)
  http://youtu.be/N7O3vHRuGls

What is Dementia? (2013)
  This film explains and defines what dementia is, and how it affects the brain. (1:37 minutes)
  http://youtu.be/6q-H1-XwCZA

Living with Dementia (2012)
  Living with Dementia is a 10-minute documentary written, produced, edited, and directed by Melissa Liddicoat and Victoria Stewart-Wooler. We hope to raise awareness for people living with dementia in the UK. *(We do not own the rights to the music used within the documentary. The Who - The Real Me; Beyonce - I Was Here)* (10 minutes)
  http://youtu.be/6lJnN7Fc_SI

Images

Google images of Lewy Body
  http://www.google.com/search?q=Lewy+Body&hl=en&tbm=isch&tbo=u&source=univ&sa=X&ei=zyqaUbPOMebe0QGmyYGIBw&ved=0CF0QsAQ&biw=1018&bih=250

Google images of Alzheimer Disease
  http://www.google.com/search?q=alzheimer's+disease&source=lnms&tbm=isch&sa=X&ei=MmifUZqCE9HD4AOdkYDgCg&sqi=2&ved=0CAcQ_AUoAQ&biw=1024&bih=564

Google images of Mild Cognitive Impairment
  http://www.google.com/search?q=mild+cognitive+impairment&source=lnms&tbm=isch&sa=X&ei=T2ifUdnDE8z84AOBmIHwCw&sqi=2&ved=0CAcQ_AUoAQ&biw=1024&bih=564

Google images of Vascular Dementia
  http://www.google.com/search?q=vascular+dementia&source=lnms&tbm=isch&sa=X&ei=eGifUYkf8t3gA9ekgLAK&sqi=2&ved=0CAcQ_AUoAQ&biw=1024&bih=564

Bipolar Disorder

Azziza Bankole, MD

INTRODUCTION

Bipolar disorder has been described through the ages from the time of Hippocrates (mania) to the mid-19th century when Jean-Pierre Falret (1794–1870), a French psychiatrist, published an article describing a condition he termed *"folie circulaire"* (circular insanity). Around the same time, Jules Baillarger (1809–1890), a French neurologist and psychiatrist, described an illness that alternated between mania and depression. He called this *"folie à double forme"* (dual-form insanity).

Karl Kahlbaum (1828–1899), a German psychiatrist, developed a system of classifying psychiatric disorders based on course and outcome, and along with Ewald Hecker (1843–1909) introduced the use of a number of descriptive terms, including cyclothymia and dysthymia.

Emil Kraepelin (1856–1926) studied the natural course of untreated bipolar disorder and coined the term *"manic depressive psychosis."* He is credited with separating psychosis as a unitary concept into *"dementia praecox* and *"manic depressive psychosis."* Kraepelin felt that the absence of a dementing and deteriorating course differentiated *manic depressive psychosis* from *dementia praecox* (now known as schizophrenia).

EPIDEMIOLOGY

The data on bipolar disorder in later life are not as robust as they are in some other later life disorders such as depression. The prevalence rate has been estimated to range from 0.08% to 0.5% in this population. The National Institute of Mental Health Epidemiologic Catchment Area Program (ECA) found a 1-year prevalence of 0.1% in older adults living in the community with a range of 0.0% to 0.5% across the various sites (Weissman et al., 1988). The disorder was equally

553

prevalent in both sexes. The prevalence in the general population is estimated at 1%. Grant and colleagues (2005) reported 12-month and lifetime prevalence rates of 2% and 3.3%, respectively, in the general population and 0.4% and 0.9%, respectively, in those 65 years and older. Others reported a 1-year prevalence rate of 0.1% in both bipolar I and II disorders in adults 55 years and older (Narrow et al., 2002) and have shown lower prevalence rates in older adults, suggesting a decline in prevalence with age (Hirschfeld et al., 2003; Klap et al., 2003).

The prevalence of bipolar disorder is higher in clinical settings such as in nursing homes, psychiatric inpatient and outpatient settings, and in emergency rooms, for example, 4% to 8% prevalence rate in geriatric inpatient psychiatric units (Yassa et al., 1988).

Studies have shown no significant differences in age, race, level of education, income, or type of living arrangement (living independently or not) between bipolar patients 60 years and older and those younger than 60 years (Al Jurdi et al., 2008). No difference was also found in the bipolar subtypes, the presence of current anxiety disorders, history of rapid cycling course, or current psychosis. Those 60 years and older were also more likely to be married, divorced, widowed, or separated.

ETIOLOGY

Family studies show an increased risk of bipolar disorder in first-degree relatives of patients with bipolar disorder. Some studies show that this heritability appears less in those who develop bipolar disorder in later life (Baron et al., 1981; Hopkinson 1964; Snowdon, 1991). However, other studies showed no such difference (Broadhead & Jacoby, 1990; Depp et al., 2004). Late onset illness has been found to be associated with neurological abnormalities or comorbidities and increased incidence of psychotic symptoms (Wylie et al., 1999; Almeida & Fenner 2002; Van Gerpen et al., 1999; Stone, 1989).

AGE OF ONSET IN BIPOLAR DISORDER

There is no distinction based on age of onset in the DSM-IV-TR criteria. Researchers in the field of geriatrics have often puzzled over the possible differences in those who develop the illness earlier on in life versus those who develop it in later life. Most people diagnosed with bipolar disorder develop it in their late teens or early 20s (Merikangas et al., 2007, 2011). The National Comorbidity Survey Replication (NCS-R) revealed that the average age of onset was between 25 and 42 years, which fell between the 50th and 75th percentiles (Kessler et al., 2005). Those who developed bipolar disorder after the age of 50 years were in the 90th percentile, and those who developed it after 65 years were in the 99th percentile.

The age of 50 years has been proposed as the cut-off for late onset bipolar disorder (Yassa et al., 1988). They reported that more than 90% of cases of bipolar disorder occurred prior to the age of 50 years.

STRUCTURAL AND FUNCTIONAL NEUROIMAGING

White matter hypointensities are one of the most frequent neuroradiological findings in bipolar disorder. They are found in both earlier onset and late onset bipolar disorder. A consensus model of the functional neuroanatomy of bipolar disorder (Strakowski et al., 2012) stated that bipolar disorder arises from abnormalities in the structure and function of key neural emotional control networks. Disruption in early neuronal development, for example, white matter connectivity, prefrontal pruning in networks modulating emotional behavior, lead to reduced connectivity in the ventral prefrontal networks and in the limbic system, especially in the amygdala.

Studies have shown diffuse cortical white matter alterations on diffusion weighted imaging in bipolar disorder. This is said to denote the widespread disruption of white matter integrity, and it has been hypothesized that this could be due to altered myelination and/or altered axonal integrity.

Functional MRI has revealed a significant decrease in activation in the inferior frontal cortex in euthymic bipolar patients when compared with healthy controls in a response inhibition task (Townsend et al., 2012). The frontal and basal ganglia regions involved with this task showed significant activation in both patients on medications and those not on any medications. There was reduced activation of the orbitofrontal cortex in patients with bipolar disorder. Others found reduced gray matter in the right ventral prefrontal cortex, insula, temporal cortex, and claustrum (Selvaraj et al., 2012).

DIAGNOSING BIPOLAR DISORDER

Bipolar disorder is not a discrete disease process. It is a syndrome requiring accurate definitions of its composite elements. The core elements of bipolar disorder are mania, hypomania, and depression.

DSM-IV Diagnostic Criteria

Manic Episode

A. Distinct period of abnormally and persistently elevated, expansive, or irritable mood lasting at least 1 week or any duration if hospitalization is necessary.
B. During the above period, more than three of the following symptoms (more than four, if mood is only irritable) are persistent and present to a significant degree.
   1. Inflated self-esteem/grandiosity
   2. Decreased need for sleep
   3. Increased talkativeness or pressure to keep talking
   4. Flight of ideas or racing thoughts
   5. Distractibility
   6. Increased goal-directed activity or psychomotor agitation
   7. Excessive involvement in pleasurable activity with high potential for painful consequences
C. Criteria for mixed episode not met
D. Causes marked occupational or social dysfunction, psychotic features present, or necessitates hospitalization
E. Symptoms not due to substances or a general medical condition

Hypomanic Episode

A. Persistently elevated, expansive, or irritable mood lasting at least 4 days and is clearly different from the usual nondepressed mood
B. Same as for manic episodes

C. Episode is associated with a definite change in function that is uncharacteristic of an individual when asymptomatic
D. Dysfunction observable by others
E. Not severe enough to cause marked social or occupational dysfunction or require hospitalization, and there are no psychotic features
F. Symptoms not due to substances or a general medical condition

Mixed Episode

A. Meets criteria for both manic episode and major depressive episode (MDE) (major depressive episode) (except for duration of MDE) nearly every day for at least 1 week
B. Severe enough to cause social or occupational dysfunction
C. Symptoms not due to substances or a general medical condition
Note: If symptoms are clearly caused by somatic antidepressant therapy, for example, medications, ECT (electroconvulsive therapy), or light therapy, it cannot count toward the diagnosis of bipolar disorder.

Major Depressive Episode

A. More than five of the following symptoms in the same 2-week period and represents a change from previous function
   One symptom has to be depressed mood or loss of interest or pleasure
   Symptoms occur most of the day nearly every day
   - Depressed mood
   - Marked reduction in interests or pleasure in all or almost all activities
   - Significant weight loss/weight gain
   - Insomnia or hypersomnia
   - Psychomotor retardation or agitation
   - Fatigue or loss of energy
   - Feelings of worthlessness or excessive/inappropriate guilt
   - Reduced ability to think or concentrate or indecisiveness
   - Recurrent thoughts of death, suicidal ideation with or without plan, intent, or suicide attempts
B. Symptoms do not meet criteria for mixed episode
C. Clinically significant distress or impairment in function
D. Symptoms not due to substances or a general medical condition
E. Not due to bereavement

Rapid Cycling

Rapid cycling occurs when a patient has at least four episodes of a mood disturbance, meeting the criteria for a major depressive, manic, hypomanic, or mixed episode in the previous 12 months. Each episode is preceded by at least 2 months of full or partial remission. A new episode can also begin with a switch to the opposite polarity, for example, from an MDE to a manic episode. Oostervink and colleagues (2009) found that patients with an earlier age of onset of bipolar disorder (before 50 years) reported a rapid cycling course of illness more frequently.

BIPOLAR DISORDER SUBTYPES

Bipolar I Disorder

The patient must have at least one manic or mixed episode to be diagnosed with bipolar I disorder. There may or may not be a history of an MDE.

Bipolar II Disorder

The patient must have a history of MDE(s) plus hypomania.

Cyclothymic Disorder

Over a period of 2 years, the patient has had numerous periods of hypomania and depression. The depressive symptoms do not meet the criteria for an MDE, and the patient has not met the criteria for a manic episode, mixed episode, or MDE in the first 2 years of the onset of symptoms. About a third of patients with cyclothymia have a family history of bipolar disorder at a rate similar to that seen in patients with bipolar I disorder. Most patients have depression as their major symptom. A substantial percentage of patients with cyclothymia will eventually develop a major mood disorder.

Secondary Mania in Older Adults

This is a new onset mania directly related to a medical disorder, for example, brain tumor or cerebrovascular accidents, or medications, for example, steroids, dopaminergic drugs. It is classified as a mood disorder with manic or mixed features secondary to a general medical condition according to DSM-IV.

CLINICAL PRESENTATION

Clinical presentation varies depending on the phase of the illness the patient presents in. The presentation of symptoms in older adults is similar to that seen in younger individuals with the disorder. Studies have shown no differences in depression, cognitive function, and medication. Overall psychopathology has also been found to be less in the late onset group (Depp et al., 2004).

Mania

Mania is a mood state characterized by elation, accelerated thinking and speaking, and overactivity. Manic symptoms can be expressed as expansive or irritable mood, disinhibition in varying forms, impulsivity, hyperactivity or being unable to sit still, or pressured speech with others finding it difficult to interrupt the patient. Some patients may take to singing their responses, punning, or even displaying flight of ideas as the symptoms worsen. Some patients may present with mood lability. They may appear to be easily distractible.

Manic episodes may present with psychotic symptoms. Delusions with grandiose themes of wealth, extraordinary abilities, and power are characteristic of this state. Hallucinations are less common than delusions in bipolar disorder, but do occur.

Patients in manic episodes very often display poor impulse control. Insight and judgment are usually markedly impaired in manic states.

Hypomania

Hypomania is a mood state similar to mania as described above, but with reduced intensity and no psychotic symptoms.

PSYCHIATRIC COMORBIDITY IN BIPOLAR DISORDER

There is an increased risk of comorbid psychiatric disorders in all patients with bipolar disorder. Bipolar disorder has been associated with high rates of anxiety disorders, including specific phobia, panic disorder with agoraphobia, and generalized anxiety disorder, and comorbid substance abuse/dependence, including nicotine dependence (Grant et al., 2005). These associations remain, although at a reduced level in older adults with bipolar disorder, when compared with younger patients with bipolar disorder (Sajatovic et al., 2006).

MEDICAL COMORBIDITY IN BIPOLAR DISORDER

Bipolar disorder has been associated with increased medical comorbidities. These include cardiovascular diseases, diabetes, hypertension, hyperlipidemia, and obesity. Patients with bipolar disorder have a higher risk of cardiovascular accidents (CVA) in later life. These illnesses are associated with a worse course of bipolar disorder. With increasing medical burden there is an increase in the estimated relative risk of suicide (Juurlink et al., 2004).

BIPOLAR DISORDER AND COGNITION

Bipolar disorder is associated with impairment in most domains of cognition during acute episodes, but impairment remains in memory and parts of executive function in between episodes (Quraishi & Frangou 2002; Robinson et al., 2006). Deficits have also been shown to be present early on in the course of the illness (Torres et al., 2010). Cognitive deficits have been found in unaffected first-degree relatives of patients with bipolar disorder (Antila et al., 2007), suggesting the possibility of an underlying genetic vulnerability.

Residual symptoms have a negative impact on performance in cognitive tests. Bipolar disorder has been associated with greater cognitive dysfunction and more rapid decline than expected for the age and educational level. In one study (Gildengers et al., 2004), approximately half of all older adults with bipolar disorder scored at least 1 standard deviation (SD) below the mean when compared with a healthy comparison group on the Mini-Mental Status Exam (MMSE) and the Mattis Dementia Rating Scale (DRS). In a later study, Gildengers et al. (2012) found that older adult patients with bipolar disorder performed worse than controls across all cognitive domains, especially in information processing and executive function.

Lifetime duration of bipolar disorder or vascular disease burden showed no significant relationship with overall cognitive function in those without a history of dementia (Gildengers et al., 2010). There was also no association between higher vascular burden and greater executive dysfunction.

However, later age at first manic episode was related to higher vascular burden and worse DRS memory subscale scores. Older adults with bipolar disorder who presented with manic symptoms had lower overall cognitive performance, especially in the domains of memory and visuospatial function. A lifetime history of psychosis was also associated with lower total DRS scores.

INSIGHT IN BIPOLAR DISORDER

Insight encompasses various aspects of one's relationship with an illness or a disorder. It includes one's awareness of symptoms, the origin/reason for symptoms, risk factors, and the management of symptoms. Insight is usually impaired in bipolar disorder regardless of age.

BIPOLAR DISORDER AND SUICIDE

Bipolar disorder has been reported to have the highest risk of suicide among all affective disorders (Gonda et al., 2012). The suicide rate in patients with bipolar disorder has been reported to be greater than 20 times that of the general population (Tondo et al., 2003). There has been no consistent difference found in the risk of suicide in patients with bipolar I or bipolar II disorders.

The risk of completed suicide is greatest in patients under 35 years of age (Tsai et al., 2005). Patients with bipolar disorder in a depressive episode who have been recently hospitalized following a suicide attempt or with suicidal ideation had a higher lifetime risk of completed suicide than those who have never been hospitalized.

Other factors reported to be associated with suicide in bipolar disorder include female gender, history of alcohol abuse, mixed episodes, axis II comorbidity, substance abuse, young age of onset, longer disease duration, greater severity of depression, current benzodiazepine use, higher overall symptoms severity, and poor treatment compliance (Undurraga et al., 2012).

Patients with bipolar disorder with a history of suicide attempt(s) have reduced fractional anisotropy in the left orbitofrontal white matter and higher overall impulsivity when compared with patients with bipolar disorder without a suicide attempt (Mahon et al., 2012).

CLINICAL ASSESSMENT

The onset of bipolar disorder for the first time in later life is uncommon. Therefore, patients with new onset symptoms should have a thorough medical evaluation to rule out possible medical causes.

A thorough review of both current and previous symptoms is imperative as this may be the only clue as to the bipolarity of the patient's illness. The patient's psychiatric history with emphasis on characterizing the past mood episodes is thus important for the diagnosis. A thorough review of the patient's family and social history may help to shed light on the extent of social dysfunction that the patient has or has not experienced. A history of past treatments and treatment responses (successes, failures, or adverse events) is important in the management of patients with bipolar disorder.

An assessment of dangerousness is important in patients with psychotic symptoms. The presence of manic symptoms may predispose to behavior that can lead to harm usually to self, but also to others. Severe depressive symptoms are also associated with increased risk of suicide.

A comprehensive physical examination, including a neurological examination, should be done. Laboratory investigations are especially important in first episode cases, reiterating the importance of ruling out medical causes of mood symptoms, especially mania/hypomania in the older adult. Laboratory investigations may include routine blood tests such as complete blood count, comprehensive metabolic panel, toxicological screens, and thyroid-stimulating hormone. Neuroimaging is helpful in ruling out central nervous system pathology.

DIFFERENTIAL DIAGNOSES

Patient Presenting with Depressive Episode

- Major depressive disorder
- Depression due to a general medical condition
- Substance induced
- Bereavement

Patient Presenting with Manic/Hypomanic Episode

- Schizophrenia
- Schizoaffective disorder, bipolar type
- Substance induced
- Due to a general medical condition

Course of Illness and Prognosis

Bipolar disorder is a chronic illness that is apt to present with recurrent episodes. Studies have shown that older adults with bipolar disorder are more likely to exhibit mixed symptoms (Spar et al., 1979).

Late onset illness is said to be characterized by increased neurological illnesses or abnormalities and psychotic symptoms as well as reduced comorbid substance abuse, fewer marital difficulties, and reduced homelessness (Sajatovic et al., 2005). No difference was found in depressive symptoms when comparing older patients with bipolar disorder with their younger counterparts (Oostervink et al., 2009). There was also no difference found in treatment outcomes between the two groups. Those who developed the disorder later on in life tended to recover faster and were discharged sooner than those who developed it earlier on in life. Others have found no difference in the number of psychotropic medications taken at the time of recovery when comparing older adults with bipolar disorder to younger patients with the disorder (Al Jurdi et al., 2008).

Bipolar disorder itself is associated with significant disability, similar to that seen in schizophrenia. A 40-year longitudinal study by Angst and Preisig (1995) found that 16% of patients with bipolar disorder had fully recovered, while 36% were still experiencing symptoms in the previous 5 years. Bipolar disorder is associated with reduced life expectancy. Laursen and colleagues (2011) found that life expectancy was reduced by 13.6 and 12.1 years in men and women with bipolar disorder, respectively, when compared with the general population.

Switching in Polarity

This has been defined as a sudden transition from one mood episode to another of the opposite polarity (Salvadore et al., 2010). Switching can occur spontaneously or be precipitated by medications (antidepressants, amphetamines, glucocorticoids), electroconvulsive therapy, stress, or sleep deprivation. Switching as a result of sleep deprivation, dopamine agonists (L-dopa, amphetamines), and exogenous steroids has been reported in even healthy individuals.

Evidence suggests that switchers have a higher genetic loading for mood disorders, spend more time ill during the course of their life, have a significantly greater number of comorbidities, and have a greater risk of developing substance abuse or committing suicide (MacKinnon et al., 2003, 2005). Patients with bipolar disorder who switch polarity as a result of treatment have been reported to have a worse clinical outcome. In a meta-analysis, Bond and colleagues (2008) reported treatment-associated switch rates in bipolar I and bipolar II disorders of 14.2% and 7.1%, respectively.

Tricyclic antidepressants have been associated with a higher risk of polarity switch compared with other antidepressants. Studies also suggest higher switch rates in antidepressants that work through more than one monoamine pathway, for example, serotonin norepinephrine reuptake inhibitors (SNRIs) such as venlafaxine, when compared with those working through one monoamine pathway, for example, selective serotonin reuptake inhibitors (SSRIs). However, other studies have shown low switch rates with venlafaxine. It appears that the concomitant use of a mood stabilizer or an antipsychotic with an antidepressant helps to reduce the risk of switching.

MANAGEMENT

Treatment of bipolar disorder can be divided into an acute phase and a maintenance phase. The acute phase of treatment involves the quick resolution of active symptoms either during a relapse or in an initial episode. Treatment choice in bipolar disorder largely depends on the urgency of the situation. Hospitalization is likely indicated in cases of acute mania or severe depression. Management can be challenging in this population as it is important to find safe and effective therapeutic options. Many of the treatments currently utilized in older adults with bipolar disorder are used based on the extrapolation of data from studies done in younger adults with bipolar disorder.

The goal in the maintenance phase of treatment is to minimize symptoms and prevent relapse. Patients should continue on the dose that helped to achieve the remission of symptoms in the acute phase. As bipolar disorder is a chronic illness with periods relapse and remission, it is recommended that treatment be continued indefinitely. Maintenance treatment may not be necessary in cases of secondary mania.

Pharmacotherapy

Increasing age is associated with increasing prevalence of obesity, non–insulin-dependent diabetes (NIDDM), reduced glucose tolerance, and lipid abnormalities even in patients who are not on medications. All patients on psychotropic medications, especially antipsychotics, mood stabilizers, and certain anticonvulsants should have baseline and follow-up checks of parameters linked to metabolic dysfunction such as body mass index (BMI), waist circumference, weight, blood pressure, blood glucose levels, and lipid profile.

Dosing of psychotropic medications should be started at one quarter to half of the usual adult starting dose, and dosage increases should also be made in similar increments. The dose of any medication used in the treatment of bipolar disorder in older adults should be titrated to provide amelioration of symptoms and at the same time minimize the possibility of side effects.

Lithium

Lithium has been shown to prevent both poles in bipolar disorder and to reduce the risk of suicide (Baldessarini et al., 2006; Cipriani et al., 2005; Kessing et al., 2005). The therapeutic range of lithium in older adults is generally maintained at a lower level than in younger adults (0.4 to 0.8 mEq/L). However, depending on the patient, higher concentration levels (0.8 to 1.0 mEq/L) may be required.

In one STEP-BD study, lithium was prescribed to almost 30% of patients with bipolar disorder 60 years and older compared with almost 40% of younger bipolar patients (Al Jurdi et al., 2008). 42.1% of those older patients on lithium alone were found to have recovered compared with 21.3% in the younger population.

Renal clearance of lithium reduces with age and, as such, increases the potential for toxicity. The correlation between dose and serum level of lithium decreases with age. Age-related reduction in total and extracellular water volumes increases the risk of lithium toxicity as does the presence of medical comorbidities, for example, dehydration.

Clinicians should be aware that concurrent use of thiazide and loop diuretics, nonsteroidal anti-inflammatory drugs (NSAIDs), and ACE inhibitors can increase lithium concentrations. Theophylline can reduce lithium levels. Lithium has moderate anticholinergic activity. Thyroid function should be monitored because of the increased risk of hypothyroidism.

Other side effects of lithium include cognitive impairment, ataxia, tremors, urinary frequency, and weight gain (Sajatovic & Chen, 2011). Older adults are more susceptible to the neurotoxic effects of lithium.

Studies have shown that lithium has neurotrophic and neuroprotective effects, but only within a certain narrow window. Patients who have had 2 or more years of treatment with lithium had hippocampal volumes comparable to those of normal controls, while those with less than 2 years of treatment with lithium had significantly lower hippocampal volumes (Hajek et al., 2012). High brain levels of lithium are associated with neuronal dysfunction. It is possible that there is an optimal window of brain lithium level that would promote the positive neuronal effects while limiting the negative ones.

Anticonvulsants

Anticonvulsants have not been as extensively studied in this population, and most are used based on studies done in younger adults.

Valproate

The use of valproate has increased greatly since the 1990s and with its derivatives are currently the most widely used mood stabilizers in the treatment of bipolar disorder in older adults. Almost

40% of patients 60 years and older were prescribed valproate compared with 34% of younger patients (Al Jurdi et al., 2008).

The recommended therapeutic range for valproate is 50 to 120 mcg/ml. Valproate is protein bound *in vivo* and can be displaced by other protein-binding agents such as aspirin, warfarin, digoxin, and phenytoin. Free levels of valproate should be obtained in addition to total levels because of possible increased levels caused by protein displacement, especially in patients on any of the above medications. Notable side effects of valproate include sedation, gait disturbance, weight gain, thrombocytopenia, alopecia, liver abnormalities, including hepatotoxicity, and pancreatitis.

Other Anticonvulsants

Other anticonvulsants include carbamazepine, oxcarbazepine, lamotrigine, and topiramate. Carbamazepine has been used for many years as an alternative to lithium. Lamotrigine has been used as an adjunct in ongoing maintenance mood stabilization treatment. In bipolar depressed older adults, lamotrigine was associated with improvement in depression, psychopathology, and functional status (Sajatovic & Chen, 2011). Anticonvulsant dose titrations should be done in a measured manner to avoid or reduce adverse events.

Antipsychotics

Antipsychotics are being used increasingly in the management of bipolar disorder. A number of atypical antipsychotics have now been approved for the treatment of bipolar disorder, including olanzapine, risperidone, quetiapine, ziprasidone, and aripiprazole. They may also be used in conjunction with mood stabilizers. Atypical agents are generally favored over typical ones. Notable side effects of these drugs include sedation, weight gain, glucose and lipid abnormalities, increased fall risk, extrapyramidal symptoms (EPS), and neuroleptic malignant syndrome (NMS) as well as a significant increase in the risk of mortality in those patients with a history of dementia.

Antidepressants

Antidepressants are frequently used in the treatment of bipolar depression. However, care must be taken when using them as they can precipitate a manic episode or even a rapid cycling course. There is a paucity of evidence for their use in bipolar disorder. Some authors have reported no significant benefit from antidepressants in the long-term management of bipolar disorder (Ghaemi et al., 2003), while others found that older adult patients with bipolar disorder on antidepressants had lower rates of hospitalization for manic or mixed episodes (Schaffer et al., 2006).

Electroconvulsive Therapy

Electroconvulsive therapy has been found to be safe and effective in all phases of bipolar disorder. It should be considered in treatment refractory cases, acute mania, severe depression, and in those with severe suicidal ideation or who have grossly inadequate fluid or caloric intake (Young et al., 2004).

Psychotherapy

Psychotherapy is a useful tool in the management of bipolar disorder. It has been shown to be effective for depression. This treatment modality is not indicated in acutely manic or severely depressed patients. It is indicated in patients in the maintenance phase of treatment. Cognitive behavior therapy (individual and group), supportive therapy, family focused therapy, and interpersonal and social rhythm psychotherapy are some examples of psychotherapeutic interventions for bipolar disorder.

Cognitive Behavior Therapy

Cognitive behavior therapy aims to help patients with bipolar disorder modify cognitive distortions and monitor recurrences, severity, and course of symptoms. Cognitive behavior therapy has been shown to help reduce the length of episodes and improve the psychosocial function of patients with bipolar disorder when compared with a control group (Lam et al., 2003).

Family Therapy

Family therapy aims to improve family function through psychoeducation of both the patients and family or other support networks regarding symptoms, disease course, and treatment. It aids patients and loved ones in the development of skills and in acquiring knowledge to help in the management of the disorder. It also provides a platform for loved ones to acquire communication and problem-solving skills to help prevent or reduce conflicts.

Interpersonal Psychotherapy and Social Rhythm Psychotherapy

Interpersonal psychotherapy and social rhythm psychotherapy helps to promote better organization, reduce interpersonal conflicts, and improve functional and social communication skills. It also helps to promote ordered sleep schedules and biological rhythms. It has helped patients achieve greater periods of stability and improvement in psychosocial functioning (Lolich et al., 2012).

PSYCHOSOCIAL INTERVENTIONS

A comprehensive approach to the management of bipolar disorder is valuable in the process of attaining stress reduction, improvement in treatment adherence, relapse prevention, functional recovery, and reducing medical comorbidity. These interventions could help with treatment adherence, the monitoring of symptoms, functional improvement, and increasing the awareness of potential side effects of medications.

Social support has been ranked the most important factor contributing to quality of life in patients with bipolar disorder (Michalak et al., 2006). Such interventions include psychoeducation, social skills training, and assertive community treatment. See Chapter 25 for more information on social skills training and assertive community treatment.

Support Groups

Organizations such as the National Alliance for the Mentally Ill (NAMI) and Mental Health America can be invaluable resources.

REFERENCES

Al Jurdi, R. K., Marangell, L. B., Petersen, N. J., Martinez, M., Gyulai, L., & Sajatovic, M. (2008). Prescription patterns of psychotropic medications in elderly compared with younger participants who achieved a "recovered" status in the systematic treatment enhancement program for bipolar disorder. *American Journal of Geriatric Psychiatry*, 16(11), 922–933.

Almeida, O. P., & Fenner, S. (2002). Bipolar disorder: Similarities and differences between patients with illness onset before and after 65 years of age. *International Psychogeriatrics*, 14(3), 311–322.

American Psychiatric Association (2000). *Diagnostic and Statistical Manual of Mental Disorders,* Fourth Edition, Text Revision. Washington, DC: American Psychiatric Association.

Angst, J., & Preisig, M. (1995). Outcome of a clinical cohort of unipolar, bipolar and schizoaffective patients. Results of a prospective study from 1959 to 1985. *Schweizer Archiv für Neurologie und Psychiatrie*, 146(1), 17–23.

Antila, M., Tuulio-Henriksson, A., Kieseppä, T., Eerola, M., Partonen, T., & Lönnqvist, J. (2007). Cognitive functioning in patients with familial bipolar I disorder and their unaffected relatives. *Psychological Medicine*, 37(5), 679–687.

Baldessarini, R. J., Tondo, L., Davis, P., Pompili, M., Goodwin, F. K., & Hennen, J. (2006). Decreased risk of suicides and attempts during long-term lithium treatment: A meta-analytic review. *Bipolar Disorders*, 8(5, Pt. 2), 625–639.

Baron, M., Mendlewicz, J., & Klotz, J. (1981). Age-of-onset and genetic transmission in affective disorders. *Acta Psychiatrica Scandinavica*, 64(5), 373–380.

Bond, D. J., Noronha, M. M., Kauer-Sant'Anna, M., Lam, R., & Yatham, L. (2008). Antidepressant associated mood elevations in bipolar II disorder compared with bipolar I disorder and major depressive disorder: A systematic review and meta-analysis. *Journal of Clinical Psychiatry*, 69(10), 1589–1601.

Broadhead, J., & Jacoby, R. (1990). Mania in old age: A first prospective study. *International Journal of Geriatric Psychiatry*, 5, 215–222.

Cipriani, A., Pretty, H., Hawton, K., & Geddes, J. R. (2005). Lithium in the prevention of suicidal behavior and all-cause mortality in patients with mood disorders: A systematic review of randomized trials [review]. *American Journal of Psychiatry*, 162(10), 1805–1819.

Depp, C. A., Jin, H., Mohamed, S., Kaskow, J., Moore, D. J., & Jeste, D. V. (2004). Bipolar disorder in middle-aged and elderly adults: Is age of onset important? *Journal of Nervous and Mental Disease*, 192(11), 796–799.

Ghaemi, S. N., Hsu, D. J., Soldani, F., & Goodwin, F. K. (2003). Antidepressants in bipolar disorder: The case for caution. *Bipolar Disorders*, 5(6), 421–433.

Gildengers, A. G., Butters, M. A., Chisholm, D., Anderson, S. J., Begley, A., Holm, M., . . . Mulsant, B. H. (2012). Cognition in older adults with bipolar disorder versus major depressive disorder. *Bipolar Disorders*, 14(2), 198–205.

Gildengers, A. G., Butters, M. A., Seligman, K., McShea, M., Miller, M. D., Mulsant, B. H., . . . Reynolds, C. F., III. (2004). Cognitive functioning in late-life bipolar disorder. *American Journal of Psychiatry*, 161(4), 736–738.

Gildengers, A. G., Mulsant, B. H., Al Jurdi, R. K., Beyer, J. L., Greenberg, R. L., Gyulai, L., . . . Young, R. C. (2010). The relationship of bipolar disorder lifetime duration and vascular burden to cognition in older adults. *Bipolar Disorders*, 12(8), 851–858.

Gonda, X., Pompili, M., Serafini, G., Montebovi, F., Campi, S., Dome, P., . . . Rihmer, Z. (2012). Suicidal behavior in bipolar disorder: Epidemiology, characteristics and major risk factors. *Journal of Affective Disorders*, 143(1-3), 16–26.

Grant, B. F., Stinson, F. S., Hasin, D. S., Dawson, D. A., Chou, S. P., Ruan, W. J., & Huang, B. (2005). Prevalence, correlates, and comorbidity of bipolar I disorder and axis I and II disorders: Results from the National Epidemiologic Survey on alcohol and related conditions. *Journal of Clinical Psychiatry*, 66(10), 1205–1215.

Hajek, T., Kopecek, M., Höschl, C., & Alda, M. (2012). Smaller hippocampal volumes in patients with bipolar disorder are masked by exposure to lithium: A meta-analysis. *Journal of Psychiatry & Neuroscience*, 37(5), 333–343.

Hirschfeld, R. M., Lewis, L., & Vornik, L. A. (2003). Perceptions and impact of bipolar disorder: How far have we really come? Results of the national depressive and manic-depressive association 2000 survey of individuals with bipolar disorder. *Journal of Clinical Psychiatry*, 64(2), 161–174.

Hopkinson, G. (1964). A genetic study of affective illness in patients over 50. *British Journal of Psychiatry*, 110, 244–254.

Juurlink, D. N., Herrmann, N., Szalai, J. P., Kopp, A., & Redelmeier, D. A. (2004). Medical illness and the risk of suicide in the elderly. *Archives of Internal Medicine*, 164(11), 1179–1184.

Kessing, L. V., Søndergård, L., Kvist, K., & Andersen, P. K. (2005). Suicide risk in patients treated with lithium. *Archives of General Psychiatry*, 62(8), 860–866.

Kessler, R. C., Berglund, P., Demler, O., Jin, R., Merikangas, K. R., & Walters, E. E. (2005). Lifetime prevalence and age-of-onset distributions of DSM-IV disorders in the National Comorbidity Survey Replication. *Archives of General Psychiatry, 62*(6), 593–602.

Klap, R., Unroe, K. T., & Unützer, J. (2003). Caring for mental illness in the United States: A focus on older adults. *American Journal of Geriatric Psychiatry, 11*(5), 517–524.

Lam, D. H., Watkins, E. R., Hayward, P., Bright, J., Wright, K., Kerr, N., . . . Sham, P. (2003). A randomized controlled study of cognitive therapy for relapse prevention for bipolar affective disorder: Outcome of the first year. *Archives of General Psychiatry, 60*(2), 145–152.

Laursen, T. M., Munk-Olsen, T., & Gasse, C. (2011). Chronic somatic comorbidity and excess mortality due to natural causes in persons with schizophrenia or bipolar affective disorder. *PLoS One, 6*(9), e24597.

Lolich, M., Vázquez, G. H., Alvarez, L. M., & Tamayo, J. M. (2012). Psychosocial interventions in bipolar disorder: A review. *Actas Espanolas de Psiquiatria, 40*(2), 84–92.

MacKinnon, D. F., Potash, J. B., McMahon, F. J., Simpson, S. G., DePaulo, J. R., Jr., Zandi, P. P., & The National Institutes of Mental Health Bipolar Disorder Genetics Initiative. (2005). Rapid mood switching and suicidality in familial bipolar disorder. *Bipolar Disorders, 7*(5), 441–448.

MacKinnon, D. F., Zandi, P. P., Gershon, E. S., Nurnberger, J. I., Jr, Reich, T., & DePaulo, J. (2003). Rapid switching of mood in families with multiple cases of bipolar disorder. *Archives of General Psychiatry, 60*(9), 921–928.

Mahon, K., Burdick, K. E., Wu, J., Ardekani, B. A., & Szeszko, P. R. (2012). Relationship between suicidality and impulsivity in bipolar I disorder: A diffusion tensor imaging study. *Bipolar Disorders, 14*(1), 80–89.

Merikangas, K. R., Akiskal, H. S., Angst, J., Greenberg, P. E., Hirschfeld, R. M., Petukhova, M., & Kessler, R. C. (2007). Lifetime and 12-month prevalence of bipolar spectrum disorder in the National Comorbidity Survey replication. *Archives of General Psychiatry, 64*(5), 543–552.

Merikangas, K. R., Jin, R., He, J. P., Kessler, R. C., Lee, S., Sampson, N. A., . . . Zarkov, Z. (2011). Prevalence and correlates of bipolar spectrum disorder in the world mental health survey initiative. *Archives of General Psychiatry, 68*(3), 241–251.

Michalak, E. E., Yatham, L. N., Kolesar, S., & Lam, R. W. (2006). Bipolar disorder and quality of life: A patient-centered perspective. *Quality of Life Research, 15*(1), 25–37.

Narrow, W. E., Rae, D. S., Robins, L. N., & Regier, D. A. (2002). Revised prevalence estimates of mental disorders in the United States: Using a clinical significance criterion to reconcile 2 surveys' estimates. *Archives of General Psychiatry, 59*, 115–123.

Oostervink, F., Boomsma, M. M., & Nolen, W. A. (2009). Bipolar disorder in the elderly; different effects of age and of age of onset. *Journal of Affective Disorders, 116*(3), 176–183.

Quraishi, S., & Frangou, S. (2002). Neuropsychology of bipolar disorder: A review. *Journal of Affective Disorders, 72*(3), 209–226.

Robinson, L. J., Thompson, J. M., Gallagher, P., Goswami, U., Young, A. H., Ferrier, I. N., & Moore, P. B. (2006). A meta-analysis of cognitive deficits in euthymic patients with bipolar disorder. *Journal of Affective Disorders, 93*(1–3), 105–115.

Sajatovic, M., & Chen, P. (2011). Geriatric bipolar disorder. *Psychiatric Clinics of North America, 34*(2), 319–333.

Sajatovic, M., Blow, F. C., & Ignacio, R. V. (2006). Psychiatric comorbidity in older adults with bipolar disorder. *International Journal of Geriatric Psychiatry, 21*(6), 582–587.

Sajatovic, M., Blow, F. C., Ignacio, R. V., & Kales, H. C. (2005). New-onset bipolar disorder in later life. *American Journal of Geriatric Psychiatry, 13*(4), 282–289.

Salvadore, G., Quiroz, J., Machado-Vieira, R., Henter, I., Manji, H., & Zarate, C., Jr. (2010). The neurobiology of the switch process in bipolar disorder: A review. *Journal of Clinical Psychiatry, 71*(11), 1488–1501.

Schaffer, A., Mamdani, M., Levitt, A., & Herrmann, N. (2006). Effect of antidepressant use on admissions to hospital among elderly bipolar patients. *International Journal of Geriatric Psychiatry, 21*(3), 275–280.

Selvaraj, S., Arnone, D., Job, D., Stanfield, A., Farrow, T. F., Nugent, A. C., . . . McIntosh, A. M. (2012). Grey matter differences in bipolar disorder: A meta-analysis of voxel-based morphometry studies. *Bipolar Disorders, 14*(2), 135–145.

Snowdon, J. (1991). A retrospective case study of bipolar disorder in old age. *British Journal of Psychiatry, 158*, 485–490.

Spar, J. E., Ford, C. V., & Liston, E. H. (1979). Bipolar affective disorder in aged patients. *Journal of Clinical Psychiatry, 40*(12), 504–507.

Stone, K. (1989). Mania in the elderly. *British Journal of Psychiatry, 155*, 220–224.

Strakowski, S. M., Adler, C. M., Almeida, J., Altshuler, L. L., Blumberg, H. P., Chang K. D., . . . Townsend, J. D. (2012). The functional neuroanatomy of bipolar disorder: A consensus model. *Bipolar Disorders, 14*(4), 313–325.

Tondo, L., Isacsson, G., & Baldessarini, R. (2003). Suicidal behaviour in bipolar disorder: Risk and prevention. *CNS Drugs, 17*(7), 491–511.

Torres, I. J., DeFreitas, V. G., DeFreitas, C. M., Kauer-Sant'Anna, M., Bond, D. J., Honer, W. G., . . . Yatham, L. N. (2010). Neurocognitive functioning in patients with bipolar I disorder recently recovered from a first manic episode. *Journal of Clinical Psychiatry, 71*(9), 1234–1242.

Townsend, J. D., Bookheimer, S. Y., Foland-Ross, L. C., Moody, T. D., Eisenberger, N. I., Fischer, J. S., . . . Altshuler, L. L. (2012). Deficits in inferior frontal cortex activation in euthymic bipolar disorder patients during a response inhibition task. *Bipolar Disorders, 14*(4), 442–450.

Tsai, S. Y., Lee, C. H., Kuo, C. J., & Chen, C. C. (2005). A retrospective analysis of risk and protective factors for natural death in bipolar disorder. *Journal of Clinical Psychiatry, 66*(12), 1586–1591.

Undurraga, J., Baldessarini, R. J., Valenti, M., Pacchiarotti, I., & Vieta, E. (2012). Suicidal risk factors in bipolar I and II disorder patients. *Journal of Clinical Psychiatry, 73*(6), 778–782.

Van Gerpen, M. W., Johnson, J. E., & Winstead, D. K. (1999). Mania in the geriatric patient population: A review of the literature. *American Journal of Geriatric Psychiatry, 7*(3), 188–202.

Weissman, M. M., Leaf, P. J., Tischler, G. L., Blazer, D. G., Karno, M., Bruce, M. L., & Florio, L. P. (1988). Affective disorders in five United States communities. *Psychological Medicine, 18*(1), 141–153.

Wylie, M. E., Mulsant, B. H., Pollock, B. G., Sweet, R. A., Zubenko, G. S., Begley, A. E., . . . Kupfer, D. J. (1999). Age at onset in geriatric bipolar disorder. Effects on clinical presentation and treatment outcomes in an inpatient sample. *American Journal of Geriatric Psychiatry, 7*(1), 77–83.

Yassa, R., Nair, V., Nastase, C., Camille, Y., & Belzile, L. (1988). Prevalence of bipolar disorder in a psychogeriatric population. *Journal of Affective Disorders, 14*(3), 197–201.

Young, R. C., Gyulai, L., Mulsant, B. H., Flint, A., Beyer, J. L., Shulman, K. I., & Reynolds, C. F., III. (2004). Pharmacotherapy of bipolar disorder in old age: Review and recommendations. *American Journal of Geriatric Psychiatry, 12*(4), 342–357.

CHAPTER 24: IT RESOURCES

Web sites

American Psychiatric Association
   www.psych.org
National Alliance on Mental Illness
   www.nami.org
Diagnosing, Treating Mania and Bipolar Disorder in the Elderly: Diagnosis: Bipolar Disorder, Manic Phase
   http://www.medscape.com/viewarticle/430757_4
Bipolar Disorders in Seniors
   http://www.everydayhealth.com/bipolar-disorder/bipolar-disorder-in-seniors.aspx
Depression and Bipolar Support Alliance
   http://www.dbsalliance.org/site/PageServer?pagename=home
Late-Life Bipolar Disorder Guidelines and Challenges
   http://www.healthyplace.com/bipolar-disorder/articles/
   late-life-bipolar-disorder-guidelines-and-challenges/
Healthy Place, America's Mental Health Channel – Bipolar Disorder Community home page
This web site includes bipolar articles, addresses bipolar causes, symptoms, and treatments, and includes tools, videos, and book resources along with a list of quick web links.
   http://www.healthyplace.com/bipolar-disorder/
The following resources are found on the PsychCentral web site:
What is a Manic Episode? By American Psychiatric Association (from PsychCentral web site)
   http://psychcentral.com/lib/2006/what-is-a-manic-episode/

Hypomanic Episode symptoms
http://psychcentral.com/disorders/sx21.htm
Mixed Episode symptoms
http://psychcentral.com/disorders/sx19.htm
Major Depressive Episode symptoms
http://psychcentral.com/disorders/sx5.htm
Advancements in Meta Psychology
A Scientific Study of the Human Mind and the Understanding of Human Behavior through the analysis and research of Meta Psychology. (4/15/11)
Site includes a video by HLN's Dr. Drew Pinksy, who explains what bipolar disorder is and how to diagnose if you have it.
http://advancedcognitivepsychology.blogspot.com/2011/04/dr-drew-pinksy-helps-you-understand.html

Videos

What is Bipolar I Disorder? (2011) (3:58 minutes)
http://psychology-guide.org/depression-symptoms-1/what-is-bipolar-i-disorder-mental-health-guru/
Living with Bi-Polar Disorder (2011) (3:51 minutes)
http://youtu.be/s46QDKd6_AI
What Happens During a Manic Episode? (Mental Health Guru) (2010) (3:48 minutes)
http://youtu.be/KtHXzDqXy3w
Bipolar Overview (2008)
Causes, signs, and treatment of bipolar disorder (6:30 minutes)
http://youtu.be/sl95tsiLvyM
The Diagnosis and Treatment of Bipolar Disorder
Dr. Donald Hilty presents an update on the diagnosis, treatment, and underlying pathophysiology of bipolar disorder. Series: "University of California Grand Rounds Series" (57:41 minutes)
http://youtu.be/3PURi75GaxA

Images

Google images of Bipolar Disorders and the Older Adult
http://www.google.com/search?q=bipolar+disorders+and+older+adults&source=lnms&tbm=isch&sa=X&ei=l8-nUdmlOvS30AGwqoCICw&ved=0CAcQ_AUoAQ&biw=1024&bih=564

Schizophrenia

Azziza Bankole, MD

INTRODUCTION

Throughout history, various cultures have made mention of debilitating illnesses largely characterized by bizarre behaviors and thoughts. As such, there are as many explanations for the collection of symptoms that has become known as schizophrenia as there are cultures. Scientific literature on schizophrenia provides us with a body of work showing how diagnosis has evolved over the last two centuries.

Benedict Morel (1889–1873), a French psychiatrist, coined the term *démence précoce*. Morel used this term in a descriptive manner rather than as a diagnosis. Emil Kraeplin (1855–1926) translated Morel's *démence précoce* to *dementia praecox*. Kraeplin is credited with separating psychosis as a unitary concept into *dementia praecox* and *manic depressive psychosis*. Both Morel and Kraeplin laid emphasis on the early age of onset as well as cognitive decline. Kraeplin later described the illness as a deterioration of personality.

Eugen Bleuler (1857–1959) coined the term "schizophrenia." His emphasis was on the schism between thought, emotion, and behavior. Manfred Bleuler (1903–1994) coined the term "late onset schizophrenia." Other notables in schizophrenia, from a historical perspective, include Kurt Schneider (1887–1967), who proposed certain first-rank symptoms of the illness.

EPIDEMIOLOGY

In the general population, there is a 1% lifetime prevalence of schizophrenia. According to the Epidemiological Catchment Area (ECA) Study (Keith et al., 1991), the prevalence ranges from 0.6% to 1.9%. The same study revealed a prevalence rate of 0.3% in individuals 65 years or older.

Other authors (Cohen, 2000) believe that the prevalence rate in all older adults is closer to 1% owing to the exclusion of those who developed the disease after the age of 45 years and poor sampling in areas where older adults with schizophrenia were more likely to live. Rabins and colleagues (1996) found a 1-month prevalence rate of 4.6% for all psychotic disorders in older adult residents of public housing. There is no observed sex difference in schizophrenia for those patients who developed the illness in late adolescence or as young adults. There is, however, a female preponderance in those who develop the illness after the age of 40.

A Dutch study on schizophrenia found a 1-year prevalence rate of 0.55% in patients 60 years or older (Meesters & Strek, 2011). This rate was reported to be comparable to the prevalence in the younger population. The estimated prevalence rate was higher in men aged 60 to 69 years than in men greater than or equal to 70 years old. For women the estimated prevalence rate was higher in those aged 60 to 79 years than in those greater than or equal to 80 years. Of those who developed schizophrenia after the age of 40, 76.5% were women, and after the age of 60 years, 92.9% were women.

As the percentage of the population over 65 years increases, so too will the percentage of older adults with schizophrenia. Their needs and challenges can be quite different from those commonly found in younger patients.

ETIOLOGY

Schizophrenia is multifactorial in origin. It is associated with multiple genes, neurodevelopmental factors, and a number of environmental factors. There is a 40% to 50% concordance rate in monozygotic twins. This shows that a substantial portion of the etiology of schizophrenia is heritable and at the same time informs us of the impact of environmental factors.

The dopamine hypothesis has been widely used to describe the underlying mechanism in the development of schizophrenia. The hypothesis posits that the symptoms are caused by an excess in dopaminergic activity. This could be due to an overall excess of the neurotransmitter itself, related to the receptor sites, or to relative differences in the level of dopamine in different brain centers.

Other receptors that have been implicated in schizophrenia include serotonin, γ Amino Butyric Acid (GABA), Glutamate, and Acetylcholine.

AGE OF ONSET IN SCHIZOPHRENIA

Most cases of schizophrenia manifest in late adolescence or early 20s in men or in the mid-to-late 20s in women. A percentage of cases have an onset much later in life. The concept of late onset schizophrenia began with Manfred Bleuler. He found that 15% of his patients had developed schizophrenia after the age of 40 and 4% after the age of 60 (Bleuler, 1943). A review done by Harris and Jeste (1988) revealed 23% with an age of onset after 40 and 3% after 60, while Meesters and Stek (2011) found that more than a third (36.4%) of the patients they studied developed schizophrenia after the age of 40.

The spectrum of late onset schizophrenias has been operationalized by the International Late Onset Schizophrenia Group (Howard et al., 2000). They classify late onset schizophrenias into two groups

- Late onset schizophrenia
- Late onset schizophrenia-like psychosis

They defined late onset schizophrenia as the onset of prodromal symptoms between the ages of 40 and 60, and very late onset schizophrenia-like psychosis as the onset of these symptoms after the age of 60.

According to the DSM IV-TR, and unlike the DSM III-R, there is no age criterion for diagnosing schizophrenia. Thus, patients with both late onset schizophrenia and very late onset schizophrenia-like psychosis meet the criteria for schizophrenia.

Factors associated with a later onset of schizophrenia include female gender, less severe positive symptoms and general psychopathology, and less severe impairment in abstraction/cognitive flexibility (Vahia et al., 2010). Some authors found no difference in positive symptoms between the two groups (Jeste et al., 1997). Other factors associated with later onset of schizophrenia include less severe negative symptoms, better premorbid functioning, and the use of lower doses of antipsychotics (Jeste et al., 1997). Both earlier and later onset schizophrenia patients are reported to have similar family histories (10% to 15% with a first-degree relative with schizophrenia).

STRUCTURAL AND FUNCTIONAL NEUROIMAGING

The advent of modern neuroradiological methods allowed the possibility of direct measurement and observation of the brain in patients with schizophrenia. Computerized tomography (CT) has limited use in the diagnosis of schizophrenia. Magnetic resonance imaging (MRI) provides better-quality resolution than CT scans. Research has also focused on functional changes and differences in the brain of patients with schizophrenia as compared with the general population and other study populations, for example, dementia, mood disorders.

White matter hypointensities are considered macroscopic manifestations of cardiovascular disease. These macroscopic changes appear to occur more commonly in periventricular areas in late onset schizophrenia, while in earlier onset schizophrenia, they were more commonly present in the cerebral tracts.

Older patients with schizophrenia have been reported to have lower total left and right grey matter volumes (10% and 11%, respectively) when compared with a healthy comparison group but higher total left and right grey matter volumes (7% and 5% respectively) when compared with patients with Alzheimer dementia (Frisoni et al., 2009). The orbitofrontal and cingulate regions are reported to have reduced grey matter volumes in older patients with schizophrenia. Schuster et al. (2012) showed bilateral reduction of grey matter volumes in the thalamus, prefrontal cortex, and a large region surrounding the occipito-temporo-parietal junction, with the last region showing accelerated grey matter volume loss with increasing age.

No significant association has been found between structural brain changes and cognitive deficits or psychiatric symptoms. A review done by Lagodka and Robert (2009) revealed that MRI studies show little in the way of difference between earlier onset schizophrenia and late onset schizophrenia. The patterns of deficits have also been shown to be different from what is seen in Alzheimer dementia. No difference in the family history of dementia was found in either group. It was hypothesized that different neural tracts are involved in earlier onset and late onset schizophrenia, possibly explaining some of the differences between the two groups. Such differences include less formal thought disorders, less negative symptoms, and no reduction in the P300 amplitude on EEG in the late onset schizophrenia group. The late onset schizophrenia group has also been found to have smaller thalamic volumes and cortical atrophy when compared with the earlier onset group.

Anisotropy, an indicator of neuronal function and a measurement parameter in functional neuroimaging, has been found to be reduced in the anterior cingulate gyrus, the orbitofrontal cortex, and the medial temporal lobe. These areas are involved with emotional cognition, executive function, and auditory processing. Schneiderman et al. (2011) reported a generalized reduction in fractional anisotropy in cerebral white matter, especially in the white matter of the frontal lobe. Patients with schizophrenia do show the same age-related decline in fractional anisotropy as do normal comparison groups.

In brain areas of particular significance in schizophrenia, for example, the frontal and temporal lobes, the fractional anisotropy decreases at a faster rate with age in patients with schizophrenia. These findings are consistent with the reduced emotional reactivity and impaired executive function found in older patients with schizophrenia. White matter in the auditory and somatosensory cortices showed larger reductions in fractional anisotropy than in the visual cortex in patients with schizophrenia.

DIAGNOSING SCHIZOPHRENIA

Kurt Schneider proposed a method of diagnosing schizophrenia using symptoms he identified as being more characteristically found in the disorder (1959). These symptoms are known as Schneider's first-rank symptoms:

- Hearing thoughts spoken aloud
- Third-person hallucinations
- Hallucinations in the form of a commentary
- Thought withdrawal or insertion
- Thought broadcasting
- Delusional perception
- Experiencing external control over feelings or actions

A number of the above symptoms are represented in the DSM IV diagnosis of schizophrenia. However, none of these symptoms are definitive in the diagnosis of the disorder, and all can be seen in a substantial number of patients with other psychiatric disorders.

DSM IV Diagnostic Criteria

A. Characteristic Symptoms—two or more of the following must be present for a significant portion of time during a 1-month period:
   1. Delusions
   2. Hallucinations
   3. Disorganized speech
   4. Grossly disorganized or catatonic behavior
   5. Negative symptoms

If
   a. Delusions are bizarre or
   b. Hallucinations consist of

- a voice keeping a running commentary on patient's thoughts or actions or
- two or more voices conversing with each other,

then only one Criterion A symptom is required.

B. Social/occupational dysfunction is present
C. Duration—continuous signs of disturbance for at least 6 months, including at least 1 month of symptoms that meet Criterion A
D. Schizoaffective disorder and mood disorders have been excluded
E. Substance/general medical conditions have been excluded
F. Pervasive developmental disorder—if present, the additional diagnosis of schizophrenia is made only if prominent hallucinations or delusions are also present for at least 1 month (or less if successfully treated).

Schizoaffective Disorder

In schizoaffective disorder, affective symptoms occur concurrently with the major symptoms of schizophrenia. The patient must meet the criteria for a major depressive episode, a manic episode, or a mixed episode, and at the same time the Criterion A for schizophrenia. The mood symptoms must not be the direct result of a general medical condition or drugs (prescribed medications or substances of abuse). A 1-year prevalence rate of 0.14% was found in an older Dutch population (Meesters & Stek, 2011).

SCHIZOPHRENIA SUBTYPES

Paranoid Schizophrenia

Delusions or hallucinations are the prominent symptoms. Other Criterion A symptoms are not prominent.

Disorganized Schizophrenia

Disorganized speech, behavior, and flat or inappropriate affect are prominent.

Catatonic Schizophrenia

At least two prominent catatonic symptoms are present

- Catalepsy—motoric immobility
- Excessive motor activity
- Extreme negativism
- Peculiarities of movement—posturing, stereotyped movements, prominent mannerisms or grimacing
- Echolalia or echopraxia.

Undifferentiated Schizophrenia

Meets Criterion A symptoms, but none of the above subtype symptoms are prominent.

Residual Schizophrenia

Absence of prominent delusions, hallucinations, disorganized speech, or grossly disorganized or catatonic behavior with continuing evidence of disturbance, that is., the presence of negative symptoms or two or more Criterion A symptoms in an attenuated form.

CLINICAL PRESENTATION

Schizophrenia is a disorder characterized by a constellation of symptoms.

No one symptom is pathognomonic of the disorder. The presentation in older adults is usually no different than in younger adults. Symptoms of schizophrenia can be broadly divided into positive and negative symptoms.

Positive Symptoms of Schizophrenia

Positive symptoms can be thought of as an exaggeration of normal processes. Positive symptoms include delusions and hallucinations. They involve reality distortions as well as disorganized/bizarre behavior and speech.

Hallucinations

A hallucination is the experience of a perception in the absence of a stimulus. Hallucinations can be auditory, visual, tactile, olfactory, or gustatory. Auditory hallucinations are the commonest hallucinations found in schizophrenia. 40% and 80% of patients with schizophrenia have experienced auditory hallucinations (Andreasen & Flaum, 1991; Thomas et al., 2007). These hallucinations are usually experienced as voices, but could also be experienced as a variety of sounds, including music. Patients may even be able to describe what they experience to be the source of their hallucinations, for example, from inside their head or from an outside source.

Visual hallucinations are less common in schizophrenia. They can take the form of simple shapes or colors or be more complex, for example, faces. Their presence should increase the suspicion that the cause may be an organic one. Hallucinations in other modalities are much rarer in schizophrenia. Examples of tactile hallucinations include feelings of being touched, pain, and crawling sensations. Gustatory/olfactory hallucinations include strange tastes or smells.

Delusions

Delusions can be described as false beliefs based on erroneous inferences that are firmly held, cannot be dispelled despite evidence to the contrary, and are not consistent with the individual's educational or cultural background. Delusions occur in over 80% of patients with schizophrenia (Andreasen & Flaum, 1991). Delusions can be categorized as bizarre (implausible, e.g., being pregnant with thousands of children, believing one is a historical figure) or nonbizarre (conceivable but still false, e.g. thoughts that a loved one is being unfaithful, being poisoned).

Delusions can also be categorized according to the theme presented. Grandiose delusions involve themes of exaggerated self-importance or worth. Persecutory delusions express themes of persecution and harm. Other thematic descriptions of delusions include nihilistic delusions, delusions of jealousy, and delusions of control.

Disorganized Behavior and Speech

Disorganized behavior is directly observed in patients with schizophrenia, while disorganized thoughts are inferred from their speech.

Disorders of thought include

- Derailment—an illogical transition from one thought to another
- Tangentiality—inability to follow a thought through to its logical conclusion
- Clang associations—use of words with similar sounds but with no logical connection; includes rhyming and punning
- Neologisms—creation of new words
- Word salad—incoherent mixture of words

Negative Symptoms of Schizophrenia

Negative symptoms may be thought of as representing a reduction in or absence of normal processes, for example, blunting of affect, poverty of speech, lack of motivation, anhedonia, and social withdrawal. These symptoms may be the result of schizophrenia itself or secondary to other symptoms or to the treatment of schizophrenia, for example, withdrawal as a result of delusions or reduced facial expression due to the extrapyramidal side effects of antipsychotics. In one study, 40% of an older adult population with schizophrenia was shown to have negative symptoms, more than half being of the secondary type (Cohen et al., 2013). There is a higher risk of the extrapyramidal side effects in older patients with schizophrenia.

Cognitive Symptoms in Schizophrenia

Studies have shown that all patients with schizophrenia regardless of age suffer from minor cognitive deficits (Heaton et al., 2001; Stefanopoulou et al., 2009). These deficits have been found to be relatively stable over time in both older and younger adults. Impairments have been observed in processing speed, attention, working memory, verbal and visual learning, executive function, verbal comprehension, and social cognition (Loewenstein et al., 2012). Younger patients with schizophrenia performed worse than older normal healthy controls. Crystallized intelligence remains relatively stable, or it increases at least until about age 70 years.

A number of studies have shown that patients with schizophrenia do worse by two standard deviations (SD) on neuropsychological testing when compared with the general population (Gold et al., 2009; Kraus & Keefe, 2007). Irani and colleagues (2011) found that, on average, the cognitive performance of older patients with schizophrenia was greater than 1 SD below that of age-matched peers on global and domain specific neuropsychological measures. The strongest effect sizes were found in domains associated with language, immediate memory, and executive function. Thus, as has been shown in younger patients with schizophrenia, older patients showed deficits in multiple domains rather than any single isolated deficit.

No worsening was found in these deficits over a 1- to 6-year follow-up period. A population-based cohort study done in England and Wales showed that psychotic symptoms were associated with worse cognitive function and a more rapid decline from baseline at 6-year follow-up (Köhler et al., 2013).

Other Symptoms Associated with Schizophrenia

- **Disturbances in Mood and Anxiety**—these symptoms commonly occur in patients with schizophrenia and can increase the burden of illness.
- **Physical Symptoms**—catatonic excitement, rigidity, stupor
- **Metabolic Symptoms**—schizophrenia is associated with diabetes, hypertension, and hyperlipidemia. When compared with the general population, patients with schizophrenia have a reduction in their life expectancy by at least 10 years.

INSIGHT IN SCHIZOPHRENIA

Insight encompasses various aspects of one's relationship with an illness or disorder. It includes one's awareness of symptoms, the origin/reason for symptoms, risk factors, and the management of said symptoms. Insight is usually impaired in schizophrenia regardless of age.

SUICIDE IN SCHIZOPHRENIA

There is an increased risk of suicide in patients with schizophrenia when compared with the general population. In a study of Danish patients with schizophrenia 50 years and older, Erlangsen and colleagues (2012) found an increased mortality risk of suicide in both sexes. The suicide ratio for men and women with schizophrenia aged 50 and 69 years was 7.0 and 13.7 respectively when compared with those with no diagnosis. The rate was lower for both men and women over the age of 70 years (2.1 and 3.4 respectively), but still higher than that of their age-matched peers.

An increased risk of suicide was also found to be associated with a greater number of hospitalizations, recent admissions in men and substance abuse in women, recent discharges, previous suicide attempts, recent suicide attempts, and the presence of mood and personality disorders

CULTURAL FACTORS

Cultural factors have not been shown to play a major role in the etiology of schizophrenia. The incidence of schizophrenia is quite similar even in widely different populations (Jablensky, 2000). Studies have reported better outcomes in patients in less developed countries. The WHO International Pilot Study of Schizophrenia—IPPS (Sartorius et al., 1977) showed that a significantly higher proportion of patients in developing countries had better outcomes on all measures when compared with those in developed countries. Subsequent WHO studies also confirmed this (Jablensky et al., 1992).

CLINICAL ASSESSMENT

It is important to delineate the patient's chief complaint and note current or recent symptoms, severity of such symptoms, and the presence of other associated symptoms such as depression and anxiety.

A history of previous episodes, if any, previous treatment, and treatment responses (successes, failures, or adverse events) is also pertinent. The medical history is quite important in this population of patients. Psychotic symptoms are frequently caused by medical illnesses such as traumatic brain injury, cerebrovascular accidents, and delirium, and as such must be ruled out as part of the assessment. Family history may point to the heritability of the illness, and social history may reveal exacerbating or attenuating circumstances in the patient's life.

An assessment of dangerousness is important in any patient with psychiatric symptoms. Psychotic symptoms may predispose to behaviors that can lead to harm usually to themselves, but also to others.

Laboratory investigations are especially important in first episode cases. This again reiterates the importance of ruling out medical causes of psychotic symptoms in later life. Investigations may include routine blood tests such as complete blood count, comprehensive metabolic panel, and TSH as well as the more complex radiological studies, for example, CT scans, MRIs. Neuropsychological testing may prove helpful in winnowing down the differential diagnoses.

Differential Diagnoses

Medical

- Substance induced
- Delirium
- Seizure disorders including temporal lobe epilepsy
- Space occupying lesions, for example, brain tumors
- Cerebrovascular accidents
- Traumatic brain injury
- Wenercke Korsakoff syndrome

Psychiatric

- Schizophreniform Disorder—meets symptom requirement for schizophrenia except for time requirement. Symptoms are present for at least a month but less than the 6 months required by DSM IV to diagnose schizophrenia
- Schizoaffective Disorder
- Mood Disorders—these have prominent affective symptoms
    - Bipolar disorders
    - Major depressive disorder with psychosis
- Delusional Disorder

COURSE OF ILLNESS AND PROGNOSIS

Schizophrenia is a chronic illness that has long been viewed as having a poor outcome (Kraeplin, 1971). This notion has been challenged in recent years, and a consensus is growing as to what the long-term outcome of schizophrenia is and how it can be defined. The Schizophrenia Work Group

(Andreasen et al., 2005) defined symptom remission in schizophrenia on the basis of the core features of the illness, but also noted that other clinical factors and domains may affect outcome. Studies have shown that symptomatic remission is achievable in older adults with schizophrenia (Bankole et al., 2008). Remission should not be confused with recovery and in itself is not a stable state, that is, patients can move into and out of remission (Bankole et al., 2008; Van Os et al., 2006).

Quality of life is a parameter that is often overlooked in all chronic mental illnesses. Studies have shown self-reported quality of life in older adults with schizophrenia to be lower than in age-matched peers (Bankole et al., 2007). Fewer depressive symptoms, fewer acute life stressors, fewer medication side effects, lower financial strain, and better self-rated health were associated with quality of life (Mittal et al., 2006; Bankole et al., 2007). Prospective studies in younger patients with schizophrenia show that depression has a negative impact on quality of life (Fitzgerald et al., 2003; Sands & Harrow, 1999).

The life expectancy of patients with schizophrenia has been found to be less than that reported for the general population. Laursen and colleagues (2011) reported that the life expectancy of patients with schizophrenia is shorter by 18.7 years in males and by 16.3 years in females. They found that the excess mortality caused by physical diseases and medical conditions had a greater influence on the reduced life expectancy than death due to external causes.

With the above information in mind, we are now provided with different avenues to intervene on behalf of our patients with schizophrenia in the course of their illness.

MANAGEMENT

Pharmacotherapy

There are few age-related drug metabolism effects. A notable one is the age-related slowing of demethylation, which is required for the metabolism of drugs such as tricyclic antidepressants and diazepam. These drugs have been used as adjuncts in the treatment of older adults with schizophrenia.

Antipsychotics

Antipsychotics form the backbone of pharmacotherapy in schizophrenia. Having been serendipitously discovered in the 1950s, they have since changed the treatment of schizophrenia. The initial antipsychotics (e.g., Chlorpromazine, Haloperidol, Perphenazine) are described as typicals, while the more recent ones (e.g., Olanzapine, Ziprasidone, Risperidone, Quetiapine, Aripiprazole) have been described as atypicals. Atypicals are used more often than typicals in the treatment of schizophrenia in older adults.

The psychopharmacological management of schizophrenia can be divided into two parts, acute and maintenance treatment.

The acute phase of treatment involves the quick resolution of active symptoms either during a relapse or in a first psychotic episode. With the exception of Clozapine, all antipsychotics are about as effective as the others. Clozapine has been shown to be effective in treatment-resistant schizophrenia. The antipsychotic chosen for a particular patient largely depends on side-effect profile, available preparations, and possible sensitivities. The onset of action of antipsychotics on positive symptoms is usually within a week.

If a patient shows a minimal response to a therapeutic dose of an antipsychotic within the first few weeks of treatment, it is unlikely that the patient will eventually have a good response to that particular antipsychotic (Kinon et al., 2010). There is little research to support the use of two different antipsychotics. However, cases are different, and a few patients may require more than one antipsychotic to achieve symptom relief.

The goal in the maintenance phase of treatment is to minimize symptoms and prevent relapse. Patients should continue on the dose that helped to achieve the remission of symptoms in the acute phase. As schizophrenia is a chronic disorder with periods of relapse and remission, it is recommended that treatment be continued indefinitely.

Older age is associated with increasing prevalence of obesity, non–insulin-dependent diabetes (NIDDM), reduced glucose tolerance, and lipid abnormalities even in patients who are not on antipsychotics. All patients on antipsychotics should have baseline and follow-up checks of parameters linked to metabolic dysfunction such as body mass index (BMI), waist circumference, weight, blood pressure, blood glucose levels, and lipid profile.

Clozapine is recommended for use in patients who have not responded to previous trials of two or more antipsychotics. Clozapine has also been shown to be beneficial in the reduction of suicide attempts in patients with schizophrenia.

Dosing of antipsychotics should be started at one quarter to half of the usual adult starting dose, and dosage increases should also be made in similar increments. The dose of any antipsychotic medication used in the treatment of schizophrenia in older adults should be enough to provide amelioration of symptoms and at the same time minimize the possibility of side effects.

Treatment adherence is an important part of the management of schizophrenia. Long-acting injectable antipsychotics, for example, Haloperidol, Risperidone may be beneficial in such cases. Other ways to help improve treatment adherence include simplification of medication regimens (once or twice daily dosing rather than multiple doses throughout the day) and shared decision making, that is, involving the patient as well as family in the management process.

Side effects of atypical antipsychotics include sedation, weight gain, glucose and lipid abnormalities, increased fall risk, extrapyramidal symptoms (EPS), and neuroleptic malignant syndrome (NMS) as well as a significant increase in the risk of mortality in those patients with a history of dementia. Increasing age is associated with reducing dopamine function in the corticostriatal pathways. This is a possible explanation for the increased incidence of extrapyramidal side effects, including tardive dyskinesia seen in older adults on antipsychotics, especially with the typicals.

It is best to avoid antipsychotics with anticholinergic effects. Most typical antipsychotics have substantial anticholinergic side effects. Mesoridazine and thioridazine should be avoided in older adults as they cause dose-dependent QTc prolongation. QTc prolongation increases the risk of arrhythmias, including torsades de pointe and sudden death.

Clozapine can be especially problematic to use in older patients with schizophrenia. They are more sensitive to agranulocytosis and to its antimuscarinic, hypotensive, and sedative effects. The extensive blood monitoring program may also be a limiting factor. Clozapine clearance is increased by smoking and in the male sex leading to reduced plasma concentrations. The level of clearance is over 20% higher in men than it is in women.

Clozapine is primarily metabolized by the cytochrome P450 system (CYP1A2) into an active metabolite, norclozapine. Clozapine and norclozapine clearance decrease with increasing age (Ismail et al., 2012). This, in effect, leads to increased serum levels and therefore increased risk of adverse events. Therapeutic drug monitoring of both Clozapine and norclozapine has been recommended because plasma levels rather than dose have been associated with side effects.

Psychosocial Management

This involves an array of interventions that help clinicians view patients with schizophrenia in a comprehensive manner. Symptom control in schizophrenia is important, as discussed in the section on pharmacotherapy. However, this alone is not enough to help patients participate and engage in their lives to the fullest. Psychological and social needs have been reported to be unmet more often than environmental or physical needs (Meesters et al., 2013). Having more unmet needs was associated with lower perceived quality of life. These interventions help both patients and families in reaching this goal and include family intervention, social skills training, and assertive community treatment.

Family Intervention

This involves family psychoeducation about what schizophrenia is and what it is not. This education is very important in first episode cases, and in this target population, it is beneficial for the patient and family of those with late onset schizophrenia and very late onset schizophrenia-like psychosis. Important topics include the nature, course, and treatment of schizophrenia, early signs of relapse to look out for, and the importance of treatment adherence.

Social Skills Training

The goal of social skills training is to help improve social functioning, an area that can be greatly impaired in schizophrenia. It targets specific skills that a patient will need to be able to function well in the community, for example, paying bills, using public transportation, and developing social networks. Social skills training, as an augmentation strategy with pharmacotherapy, has been found to be helpful in reducing negative symptoms associated with schizophrenia as well as helping to improve social functioning and life skills (Kurtz & Mueser, 2008).

Assertive Community Treatment

Assertive community treatment is indicated in patients with severe mental illnesses with history of recent hospitalization or homelessness or who are at risk of either. It uses a multidisciplinary team approach and provides care for patients in the community. The multidisciplinary team typically consists of a psychiatrist, psychiatric nurse, case manager, occupational therapists with access to other professionals as needed, for example, legal aid, primary care provider. Assertive community treatment aims to maintain patients in the community by ensuring treatment adherence to all prescribed medications, not just psychiatric ones, and minimizing emergency treatments for psychiatric and medical symptoms. It has been shown to reduce homelessness, use of emergency services, and hospitalization, and to increase the use of outpatient services and improvement of symptoms (Coldwell and Bender, 2007; Dixon et al., 2010).

Psychotherapy

Psychotherapy has been shown to be an effective adjunct in the treatment of psychosis. Cognitive behavior therapy, in particular, has been shown to be helpful (Turkington et al., 2002; Wykes et al., 2008). Other psychotherapeutic interventions include group therapy, behavioral skills therapy, personal therapy, compliance therapy, supportive psychotherapy, and metacognitive training.

Cognitive Behavior Therapy (CBT) for Psychosis

CBT for psychosis aims to reduce the intensity of psychotic symptoms with the patient playing an active role in the treatment. This in turn helps to reduce social dysfunction and the risk of relapse. CBT for psychosis is helpful for patients with persistent psychotic symptoms despite optimization of medication management.

The therapist's task is to help engage the patient in the logical examination of his or her symptoms and the impact of those symptoms on the patient's life. CBT for psychosis starts with the patient's own interpretation of his or her symptoms and subsequently moves on to having the patient work with the therapist in exploring and developing more rational and adaptive responses and behaviors. The exploration of the patient's symptoms then moves on to controlled challenges of the patient's assumptions while alternative interpretations are proffered.

Reality testing plays an integral role in CBT for psychosis. Even in cases where the above process is met with resistance, CBT can still be helpful by aiding the patient in finding ways to reduce the distress associated with their symptoms.

CBT for psychosis can be done in individual or group sessions. Sessions occur weekly or biweekly over a period of four to nine months. CBT for psychosis has been shown to be effective for both positive and negative symptoms as well as for social functioning (Wykes et al., 2008). The strongest effect has been seen on its impact on delusions, followed by (with reducing effect) hallucinations, negative symptoms, and finally social functioning. The addition of CBT to treatment, as usual, has been shown to reduce hospitalization and relapse rates, positive and negative symptoms, and global psychopathology as well to improve performance of independent functions and activities promoting social interaction and function (Gumley et al., 2003).

SUPPORT GROUPS

Organizations such as the National Alliance for the Mentally Ill (NAMI) and Mental Health America can be an invaluable resource for both patients and family members.

REFERENCES

American Psychiatric Association (1987). *Diagnostic and Statistical Manual of Mental Disorders,* Third Edition, Revised. Washington, DC: American Psychiatric Association.

American Psychiatric Association (2000). *Diagnostic and Statistical Manual of Mental Disorders,* Fourth Edition, Text Revision. Washington, DC: American Psychiatric Association.

Andreasen, N. C., Carpenter, W. T., Jr., Kane, J. M., Lasser, R. A., Marder, S. R., & Weinberger, D. R. (2005). Remission in schizophrenia: Proposed criteria and rationale for consensus. *American Journal of Psychiatry, 162*(3), 441–449.

Andreasen, N. C., & Flaum, M. (1991). Schizophrenia: The characteristic symptoms. *Schizophrenia Bulletin, 17*(1), 27–49.

Bankole, A., Cohen, C. I., Vahia, I., Diwan, S., Palekar, N., Reyes, P., . . . Ramirez, P. M. (2008). Symptomatic remission in a multiracial urban population of older adults with schizophrenia. *American Journal of Geriatric Psychiatry, 16*(12), 966–973.

Bankole, A. O., Cohen, C. I., Vahia, I., Diwan, S., Kehn, M., & Ramirez, P. M. (2007). Factors affecting quality of life in a multiracial sample of older persons with schizophrenia. *American Journal of Geriatric Psychiatry, 15*(12), 1015–1023.

Bleuler, M. (1943). Die spatschizophrenen Krankheitsbilder. *Fortschritte der Neurologie und Psychiatrie, 15,* 259–290.

Cohen, C., Natarajan, N., Araujo, M., & Solanki, D. (2013). Prevalence of negative symptoms and associated factors in older adults with schizophrenia spectrum disorder. *American Journal of Geriatric Psychiatry, 21*(2), 100–107.

Cohen, C. I. (2000). Practical geriatrics: Directions for research and policy on schizophrenia and older adults: Summary of the GAP committee report. *Psychiatric Services, 51*(3), 299–302.

Coldwell, C. M., & Bender, W. S. (2007). The effectiveness of assertive community treatment for homeless populations with severe mental illness: A meta-analysis. *American Journal of Psychiatry, 164*(3), 393–399.

Dixon, L. B., Dickerson, F., Bellack, A. S., Bennett, M., Dickinson, D., Goldberg, R. W., . . . Kreyenbuhl, J. (2010). The 2009 schizophrenia PORT psychosocial treatment recommendations and summary statements. *Schizophrenia Bulletin, 36*(1), 48–70.

Erlangsen, A., Eaton, W. W., Mortensen, P. B., & Conwell, Y. (2012). Schizophrenia—a predictor of suicide during the second half of life? *Schizophrenia Research, 134*(2-3), 111–117.

Fitzgerald, P. B., de Castella, A. R., Filia, K., Collins, J., Brewer, K., Williams, C. L., . . . Kulkarni, J. (2003). A longitudinal study of patient- and observer-rated quality of life in schizophrenia. *Psychiatry Research, 119*(1-2), 55–62.

Frisoni, G. B., Prestia, A., Adorni, A., Rasser, P. E., Cotelli, M., Soricelli, A., . . . Thompson, P. M. (2009). In vivo neuropathology of cortical changes in elderly persons with schizophrenia. *Biological Psychiatry, 66*(6), 578–585.

Gold, J. M., Hahn, B., Strauss, G. P., & Waltz, J. A. (2009). Turning it upside down: Areas of preserved cognitive function in schizophrenia. *Neuropsychology Review, 19*(3), 294–311.

Gumley, A., O'Grady, M., McNay, L., Reilly, J., Power, K., & Norrie, J. (2003). Early intervention for relapse in schizophrenia: Results of a 12-month randomized controlled trial of cognitive behavioural therapy. *Psychological Medicine, 33*(3), 419–431.

Harris, M. J., & Jeste, D. V. (1988). Late-onset schizophrenia: An overview. *Schizophrenia Bulletin, 14*(1), 39–55.

Heaton, R. K., Gladsjo, J. A., Palmer, B. W., Kuck, J., Marcotte, T. D., & Jeste, D. V. (2001). Stability and course of neuropsychological deficits in schizophrenia. *Archives of General Psychiatry, 58*(1), 24–32.

Howard, R., Rabins, P. V., Seeman, M. V., & Jeste, D. V. (2000). Late-onset schizophrenia and very-late-onset schizophrenia-like psychosis: An international consensus. The International Late-Onset Schizophrenia Group. *American Journal of Psychiatry, 157*(2), 172–178.

Irani, F., Kalkstein, S., Moberg, E. A., & Moberg, P. J. (2011). Neuropsychological performance in older patients with schizophrenia: A meta-analysis of cross-sectional and longitudinal studies. *Schizophrenia Bulletin, 37*(6), 1318–1326.

Ismail, Z., Wessels, A. M., Uchida, H., Ng, W., Mamo, D. C., Rajji, T. K., . . . Bies, R. R. (2012). Age and sex impact clozapine plasma concentrations in inpatients and outpatients with schizophrenia. *American Journal of Geriatric Psychiatry, 20*(1), 53–60.

Jablensky, A. (2000). Epidemiology of schizophrenia: The global burden of disease and disability. *European Archives of Psychiatry and Clinical Neuroscience, 250*(6), 274–285.

Jablensky, A., Sartorius, N., Ernberg, G., Anker, M., Korten, A., Cooper, J. E., . . . Bertelsen, A. (1992). Schizophrenia: Manifestations, incidence and course in different cultures. A World Health Organization ten-country study. *Psychological Medicine Monograph Supplement, 20*, 1–97.

Jeste, D. V., Symonds, L. L., Harris, M. J., Paulsen, J. S., Palmer, B. W., & Heaton, R. K. (1997). Nondementia nonpraecox dementia praecox? Late-onset schizophrenia. *American Journal of Geriatric Psychiatry, 5*(4), 302–317.

Keith, S. J., Regier, D. A., & Rae, D. S. (1991). Schizophrenic disorders. In L. N. Robins & D. A. Regier (Eds.), *Psychiatric disorders in America: The epidemiologic catchment area study* (pp. 33–52). New York, NY: The Free Press.

Kinon, B. J., Chen, L., Ascher-Svanum, H., Stauffer, V. L., Kollack-Walker, S., Zhou, W., . . . Kane, J. M. (2010). Early response to antipsychotic drug therapy as a clinical marker of subsequent response in the treatment of schizophrenia. *Neuropsychopharmacology, 35*(2), 581–590.

Köhler, S., Allardyce, J., Verhey, F. R., McKeith, I. G., Matthews, F., Brayne, C., & Savva, G. M. (2013). Cognitive decline and dementia risk in older adults with psychotic symptoms: A prospective cohort study. *American Journal of Geriatric Psychiatry, 21*(2), 119–128.

Kraeplin, E. (1971). *Dementia praecox and paraphrenia, 1919*. New York, NY: Robert E Krieger Publishing.

Kraus, M. S., & Keefe, R. S. (2007). Cognition as an outcome measure in schizophrenia. *British Journal of Psychiatry Supplement, 50*, S46–S51.

Kurtz, M. M., & Mueser, K. T. (2008). A meta-analysis of controlled research on social skills training for schizophrenia. *Journal of Consulting and Clinical Psychology, 76*(3), 491–504.

Lagodka, A., & Robert, P. (2009). Is late-onset schizophrenia related to neurodegenerative processes? A review of literature [Article in French]. *Encephale, 35*(4), 386–393.

Laursen, T. M., Munk-Olsen, T., & Gasse, C. (2011). Chronic somatic comorbidity and excess mortality due to natural causes in persons with schizophrenia or bipolar affective disorder. *PLoS One, 6*(9), e24597.

Loewenstein, D. A., Czaja, S. J., Bowie, C. R., & Harvey, P. D. (2012). Age-associated differences in cognitive performance in older patients with schizophrenia: A comparison with healthy older adults. *American Journal of Geriatric Psychiatry, 20*(1), 29–40.

Meesters, P. D., Comijs, H. C., Dröes, R. M., de Haan, L., Smit, J. H., Eikelenboom, P., . . . Stek, M. L. (2013). The care needs of elderly patients with schizophrenia spectrum disorders. *American Journal of Geriatric Psychiatry*, 21(2), 129–137.

Meesters, P. D., & Stek, M. L. (2011). Elderly patients with schizophrenia: Prevalence and distribution of age at onset in a psychiatric catchment area in Amsterdam [Article in Dutch]. *Tijdschrift voor Psychiatrie*, 53(9), 669–675.

Mittal, D., Davis, C. E., Depp, C., Pyne, J. M., Golshan, S., Patterson, T. L., & Jeste, D. V. (2006). Correlates of health-related quality of well-being in older patients with schizophrenia. *Journal of Nervous and Mental Disease*, 194(5), 335–340.

Rabins, P. V., Black, B., German, P., Roca, R., McGuire, M., Brant, L., & Cook, J. (1996). The prevalence of psychiatric disorders in elderly residents of public housing. *Journals of Gerontology A: Biological Sciences & Medical Sciences*, 51(6), M319–M324.

Sands, J. R., & Harrow, M. (1999). Depression during the longitudinal course of schizophrenia. *Schizophrenia Bulletin*, 25(1), 157–171.

Sartorius, N., Jablensky, A., & Shapiro, R. (1977). Two-year follow-up of the patients included in the WHO International Pilot Study of Schizophrenia. *Psychological Medicine*, 7(3), 529–541.

Schneider, K. (1959). *Clinical psychopathology*. New York, NY: Grune and Stratton.

Schneiderman, J. S., Hazlett, E. A., Chu, K. W., Zhang, J., Goodman, C. R., Newmark, R. E., . . . Buchsbaum, M. S. (2011). Brodmann area analysis of white matter anisotropy and age in schizophrenia. *Schizophrenia Research*, 130 (1–3), 57–67.

Schuster, C., Schuller, A. M., Paulos, C., Namer, I., Pull, C., Danion, J. M., & Foucher, J. R. (2012). Gray matter volume decreases in elderly patients with schizophrenia: A voxel-based morphometry study. *Schizophrenia Bulletin*, 38(4), 796–802.

Stefanopoulou, E., Manoharan, A., Landau, S., Geddes, J. R., Goodwin, G., & Frangou, S. (2009). Cognitive functioning in patients with affective disorders and schizophrenia: A meta-analysis. *International Review of Psychiatry*, 21(4), 336–356.

Thomas, P., Mathur, P., Gottesman, I. I., Nagpal, R., Nimgaonkar, V. L., & Deshpande, S. N. (2007). Correlates of hallucinations in schizophrenia: A cross-cultural evaluation. *Schizophrenia Research*, 92(1–3), 41–49.

Turkington, D., Kingdon, D., & Turner, T. (2002). Effectiveness of a brief cognitive-behavioural therapy intervention in the treatment of schizophrenia. *British Journal of Psychiatry*, 180, 523–527.

Vahia, I. V., Palmer, B. W., Depp, C., Fellows, I., Golshan, S., Kraemer, H. C., & Jeste, D. V. (2010). Is late-onset schizophrenia a subtype of schizophrenia? *Acta Psychiatrica Scandinavica*, 122(5), 414–426.

van Os, J., Drukker, M., à Campo, J., Meijer, J., Bak, M., & Delespaul, P. (2006). Validation of remission criteria for schizophrenia. *American Journal of Psychiatry*, 163(11), 2000–2002.

Wykes, T., Steel, C., Everitt, B., & Tarrier, N. (2008). Cognitive behavior therapy for schizophrenia: Effect sizes, clinical models, and methodological rigor. *Schizophrenia Bulletin*, 34, 523–537.

CHAPTER 25: IT RESOURCES

Websites

The following resources are located on the PubMed Health web site:

Schizophrenia defined including: causes, incidence, and risk factors; symptoms; signs and tests; treatment; expectations (prognosis); complications; prevention and references
http://www.lww.com/webapp/wcs/stores/servlet/
content_resources_authors-proposalguidelines_11851_-1_12551

Antipsychotic drugs for elderly people with late onset schizophrenia
http://www.ncbi.nlm.nih.gov/pubmedhealth/PMH0012584/

Antipsychotic medication for elderly people with schizophrenia
http://www.ncbi.nlm.nih.gov/pubmedhealth/PMH0013567/

Art therapy for schizophrenia or schizophrenia-like illnesses
http://www.ncbi.nlm.nih.gov/pubmedhealth/PMH0012270/

Schizoaffective disorder
http://www.ncbi.nlm.nih.gov/pubmedhealth/PMH0001927/

Paraphrenia redefined
http://www.ncbi.nlm.nih.gov/pubmed/10097832
The following resources are located on the Medscape Today web site (requires a sign-in to access—a free account)
The Many Faces of Psychosis in the Elderly: Schizophrenia
http://www.medscape.com/viewarticle/564899_6
Schizophrenia Resources including Schizophrenia News, Schizophrenia Perspectives, Schizo-phrenia Journals
http://www.medscape.com/resource/schizophrenia
Treatment of Psychosis in Elderly People
http://apt.rcpsych.org/content/11/4/286.full
The following resources are found on the PsychCentral web site:
Schizophrenia and Psychosis: Schizophrenia Information & Treatment Introduction
http://psychcentral.com/disorders/schizophrenia/
Schizophrenia Symptoms
http://psychcentral.com/disorders/sx31.htm
National Alliance on Mental Illness
http://www.nami.org/
National Alliance on Mental Illness—Schizophrenia
http://www.nami.org/Template.cfm?Section=schizophrenia9
National Institute of Mental Health—Schizophrenia
http://www.nimh.nih.gov/health/topics/schizophrenia/index.shtml
Late-onset Schizophrenia: Make the Right Diagnosis when Psychosis Emerges after Age 60
http://www.jfponline.com/Pages.asp?AID=580
Epidemiological Catchment Area Study, 1980-1985
http://www.icpsr.umich.edu/icpsrweb/ICPSR/studies/6153

PDF Documents

Older Adults with Schizophrenia: Patients are living longer and gaining researchers' attention. (Wetherell & Jeste)
http://www.medscape.com/resource/schizophrenia
Treating Older Adults with Schizophrenia: Its cumulative effects challenge the interdisciplinary team (Csernansky)
http://www.stanford.edu/group/usvh/stanford/misc/Schizophrenia%203.pdf
Comprehensive Assessment and Management of Schizophrenia in the Elderly (Produced by the Dementia Education and Training Program 1-800-457-5679)
http://www.alzbrain.org/pdf/handouts/7001.%20compreHENSIVE%20ASSESSMENT%20AND%20MANAGEMENT%20OF%20SCHIZOPHRENIA%20IN%20THE%20ELDERLY.pdf
Elderly Patients with Schizophrenia and Depression: Diagnosis and Treatment (Felmet, Zisook & Kasckow)
http://www.alzbrain.org/pdf/handouts/7001.%20compreHENSIVE%20ASSESSMENT%20AND%20MANAGEMENT%20OF%20SCHIZOPHRENIA%20IN%20THE%20ELDERLY.pdf

Videos

Schizophrenia (2007) (5:19 minutes)
  http://youtu.be/H_jYqSA_fJk
Schizophrenia: Gerald, Part 1 (2007) (8:12 minutes)
  http://youtu.be/gGnl8dqEoPQ
Schizophrenia (2010)
Professor Robert Sapolsky finishes his lecture on language and then dives into his discussion
  about schizophrenia. He discusses environmental factors as well as genetic characteristics that
  could apply to people who are affected. He describes schizophrenia as a disease of thought
  disorder and inappropriate emotional attributes. (1 hour 40 minutes)
  http://youtu.be/nEnklxGAmak
Real people telling the story of schizophrenia (2007) (4:47 minutes)
  http://youtu.be/f4R6jln_eZg

Images

Google images for Schizophrenia and the older adult
  http://www.google.com/search?q=schizophrenia+and+the+older+adult&so
  urce=lnms&tbm=isch&sa=X&ei=4NCnUcOIEbKo0AHIooHwAw&ved=0C
  AcQ_AUoAQ&biw=1024&bih=564

Depression

Mamta Sapra, MD
Anjali Varma, MD

INTRODUCTION

Depression is the most common mental illness among older adults. However, it is often under-recognized and undertreated. Epidemiological studies report prevalence of DSM-IV major depressive disorder in adults above 65 years of age to be 1% to 5% (Hybels & Blazer, 2003). The rates of clinically significant depressive symptoms and dysthymia are in the range of 8% to 15% (National Institute of Health [NIH] consensus conference, 1992; National Institute of Mental Health [NIMH], n.d.). An estimated 5 million have subsyndromal depression, symptoms that fall short of meeting the full diagnostic criteria for a disorder (Alexopoulos, 2000). Prevalence of geriatric depression has been found to be higher in clinical settings than in the community. Estimates of major depression in older people in the community who require home health care is 13.5% in those who require home healthcare and 11.5% in older hospital patients (Hybels & Blazer, 2003).

Significant variability exists in reporting rates of depression in medical settings. While general internists identify depression in approximately 6% of older adults, systematic studies report much higher rates at 17% to 37% (Alexopoulos, 2005). Various factors have been attributed to the under-recognition of geriatric depression in primary care settings—the tendency of older adults to focus on somatic complaints, lack of physician confidence in diagnosing depression, cultural stereotypes and depression may be ignored in the presence of other serious comorbid medical illnesses.

Rates of depression in institutionalized settings are much higher than in the community. Thirty five percent of residents in long-term care facilities experience either major depression or clinically significant depressive symptoms (Thakur & Blazer, 2008). Overall rates of depressive syndromes among older adults are lower compared with younger adults, but this has been attributed to underreporting (Gallo & Rabins, 1999; Fischer et al., 2003).

Gender differences in prevalence rates of depression are noted across the life span. Social pressures and hormonal factors have been considered responsible for higher prevalence of depression in younger women, whereas the differences in older adults are possibly due to higher onset and persistence of depression or differential mortality between men and women. A prospective 6-year study of a community-dwelling older population found that older women were more prone to depression and more likely to remain depressed than older men (Barry et al., 2008).

PATHOPHYSIOLOGY

Depression is multifactorial in origin and requires a biopsychosocial evaluation. Depression can be manifested as a recurrent illness or one that presents itself in later life. Often an initial presentation in late life may be associated with physiological changes or abnormalities of the brain often times of vascular origin (Melillo & Houde, 2011). Various biological, psychological, and social factors contribute to geriatric depression, both biological and social. The pathophysiology of depression is not well understood. However, according to the American Psychiatric Association's Diagnostic and Statistical Manual of Mental Disorders (2000), the pathophysiology may involve a dysregulation of a number of neurotransmitter systems, including the serotonin, norepinephrine, dopamine, acetylcholine, and gamma-aminobutryic acid systems. Bremmer and colleagues (2008) indicated that there is strong evidence of an association between elevated levels of various cytokines and major depression in older adults. Dopamine circuit dysfunction and inflammatory cytokines have been suggested as areas for further research. Depression is not a normal part of aging; however, it is prevalent among older adults: an estimated 15% to 19% of Americans 65 years and older suffer from depressive symptoms (Cahoon, 2012). The prevalence of depression is very high among patients receiving home health care, with studies indicating one in seven such patients meet the diagnostic criteria for a major depression (Bruce et al., 2002).

Biological Origins

Twin and family studies show strong evidence for a heritable genetic contribution to depressive disorders. The risk of developing an affective disorder is four times higher among relatives of people with affective illness than in the general population. Genetic contribution is weaker in late-life depression as compared with depression in early life. The female sex has been found to be an independent risk factor (Gatz et al., 1992). Biological theories of depression have mainly focused on dysregulation of one or more neurotransmitters in the brain. Serotonin (5-HT) is the most important neurotransmitter that has been implicated in pathophysiology of depression. Serotonergic transmission has been found to be decreased in depressed patients. In addition, norepinephrine and dopamine have also been found to have some role. Abnormalities in the hypothalamic pituitary adrenal axis have been identified in depression, among which the hypersecretion of corticotropin releasing factor (CRF) has been most investigated. Hypercortisolemia resulting from cumulative life stress leads to loss of hippocampus neurons. Some studies suggest the role of CRF in regulation of sleep, appetite, libido, and psychomotor activity. Serum testosterone levels decline with aging; however the levels have been found to be even lower in men with depressive symptoms (Almeida et al., 2008).

Neuroimaging studies (Kempton et al., 2011) show evidence of white matter hyperintensities and smaller hippocampal volumes in depression. Clinical depressive symptoms associated with these vascular ischemic changes in the brain are often referred to as vascular depression in older adults. Vascular risk factors are known to be associated with depressive symptoms.

An important component of the psychosocial assessment is a medication review. Table 26.1 outlines drugs causing symptoms of depression. It is imperative that clinicians screen for these.

Social Factors

In 2000, the Missouri Department of Health and Senior Services conducted a survey (Center for Disease Control [CDC], Morbidity and Mortality Weekly Report [MMWR], 2005) to collect information on health needs and social support of individuals over the age of 60 (n = 3,112). Older adults with no social network reported more sad, blue or depressed days (5.7 versus 2.1) than those who

TABLE 26.1 • Drugs that Cause Symptoms of Depression in Older Adults

Antihypertensives
  Reserpine
  Methyldopa
  Propranolol
  Clonidine
  Hydralazine
  Guanethidine
  Diuretics (by causing dehydration or electrolyte imbalance)

Analgesics
  Narcotics
  Morphine
  Codeine
  Meperidine
  Pentazocine
  Propoxyphene

Non narcotic
  Indomethacin

Antiparkinsonian agents
  L-dopa

Antimicrobials
  Sulfonamides
  Isoniazid

Cardiovascular agents
  Digitalis
  Lidocaine (toxicity)

Hypoglycemic agents (by causing hypoglycemia)
  Steroids
  Corticosteroids
  Cancer chemotherapeutic agents

From Kurlowicz, L. H., & NICHE Faculty. (1997). Nursing standard of practice protocol: Depression in older adult patients. *Geriatric Nursing, 18*(5), 192–199, with permission.

TABLE 26.2 · Risk Factors for Depression

- Personal history of depression
- Family history of depression
- Life events/interpretation
- Female sex
- White race
- Older age
- Ongoing medical illness and new medical diagnosis
- Disability
- Sensory impairment
- Cognitive impairment
- Anxiety disorders
- Alcohol abuse
- Bereavement—loss of spouse/finances
- Institutionalization
- Living alone
- Type of social support
- Caregiver role
- Poor social support
- Cognitive distortions—Poor self-perceived health, hopelessness
- Substance Abuse to include opiates, benzodiazepine-like drugs

Adapted from Hybels, C. F., & Blazer, D. G. (2003). Epidemiology of late-life mental disorders. *Clinics in Geriatric Medicine, 19*(4), 663–696, with permission.

had good social network. Findings indicated an association between perceived social support and Health-Related Quality of Life (HRQOL). In 1982, Murphy found associations between severe life events and social difficulties with the onset of depression. Ten to twenty percent of older adults who lose a spouse develop significant depressive symptoms of bereavement. Chronic stress of care giving has been identified repeatedly through research as a common cause of depression in the older adult. Rates of depression in caregivers of older patients diagnosed with dementia are twice those of the general population. Depression is also more common in the lower socioeconomic population. Lack of social support has been proven to be the most important predictor of late-life depressive symptoms (Bruce, 2002). In a community study, impaired social support and depressive symptoms were associated (including network size, network composition, social contact frequency, life satisfaction with social support, and instrumental–emotional support (Chi and Chou, 2001). Impairment of social support was found to be associated with poorer outcomes in older men with major depression but not in older women (Kockler & Heun, 2002) (Table 26.2).

PRESENTATION OF DISEASE

Clinical syndromes of depression are listed in the *Diagnostic and Statistical Manual of Mental Disorders* (2000), which categorizes depressive symptoms into different clinical syndromes: major depressive disorder, dysthymic disorder, adjustment disorder with depressed mood, bereavement, and depression associated with medical illness. Description, criteria, and clinical significance for the above-mentioned disorders are presented in Table 26.3. American Psychiatric Association (2000).

TABLE 26.3 • Criteria for Major Depressive Episode

A. Five (or more) of the following symptoms have been present during the same 2-week period and represent a change from previous functioning; at least one of the symptoms is either (1) depressed mood or (2) loss of interest or pleasure. Note: Do not include symptoms that are clearly due to a general medical condition, or mood-incongruent delusions or hallucinations.
  1. depressed mood most of the day, nearly every day, as indicated by either subjective report (e.g., feels sad or empty) or observation made by others (e.g., appears tearful).
  Note: In children and adolescents, can be irritable mood.
  2. markedly diminished interest or pleasure in all, or almost all, activities most of the day, nearly every day (as indicated by either subjective account or observation made by others).
  3. significant weight loss when not dieting or weight gain (e.g., a change of more than 5% of body weight in a month), or decrease or increase in appetite nearly every day.
  Note: In children, consider failure to make expected weight gains.
  4. insomnia or hypersomnia nearly every day.
  5. psychomotor agitation or retardation nearly every day (observable by others, not merely subjective feelings of restlessness or being slowed down).
  6. fatigue or loss of energy nearly every day.
  7. feelings of worthlessness or excessive or inappropriate guilt (which may be delusional) nearly every day (not merely self-reproach or guilt about being sick).
  8. diminished ability to think or concentrate, or indecisiveness, nearly every day (either by subjective account or as observed by others).
  9. recurrent thoughts of death (not just fear of dying), recurrent suicidal ideation without a specific plan, or a suicide attempt or a specific plan for committing suicide.
B. The symptoms do not meet criteria for a Mixed Episode.
C. The symptoms cause clinically significant distress or impairment in social, occupational, or other important areas of functioning.
D. The symptoms are not due to the direct physiological effects of a substance (e.g., a drug of abuse, a medication) or a general medical condition (e.g., hypothyroidism).
E. The symptoms are not better accounted for by bereavement, that is., after the loss of a loved one, the symptoms persist for longer than 2 months or are characterized by marked functional impairment, morbid preoccupation with worthlessness, suicidal ideation, psychotic symptoms, or psychomotor retardation.

Common Psychiatric Disorders

Dysthymic Disorder

Older adults with dysthymic disorder often have lifelong poor coping skills and longstanding depressive symptoms. The diagnostic criteria are:

■ Depressed mood for most of the day, for more days than not, as indicated either by subjective account or observation by others, for at least 2 years. Note: In children and adolescents, mood can be irritable and duration must be at least 1 year.
■ Presence, while depressed, of two (or more) of the following:
  1. poor appetite or overeating
  2. insomnia or hypersomnia
  3. low energy or fatigue
  4. low self-esteem
  5. poor concentration or difficulty making decisions
  6. feelings of hopelessness

- During the 2-year period (1 year for children or adolescents) of the disturbance, the person has never been without the symptoms in Criteria A and B for more than 2 months at a time.
- No major depressive episode has been present during the first 2 years of the disturbance (1 year for children and adolescents); that is, the disturbance is not better accounted for by chronic major depressive disorder, or major depressive disorder, in partial remission.

Note: There may have been a previous major depressive episode provided there was a full remission (no significant signs or symptoms for 2 months) before the development of the dysthymic disorder. In addition, after the initial 2 years (1 year in children or adolescents) of dysthymic disorder, there may be superimposed episodes of major depressive disorder, in which case both diagnoses may be given when the criteria are met for a major depressive episode.

- There has never been a Manic Episode, a Mixed Episode, or a Hypomanic Episode, and criteria have never been met for Cyclothymic Disorder.
- The disturbance does not occur exclusively during the course of a chronic Psychotic Disorder, such as Schizophrenia or Delusional Disorder.
- The symptoms are not due to the direct physiological effects of a substance (e.g., a drug of abuse, a medication) or a general medical condition (e.g., hypothyroidism).
- The symptoms cause clinically significant distress or impairment in social, occupational, or other important areas of functioning.

Adjustment Disorder with Depressed Mood

Adjustment disorder with depressed mood is diagnosed when symptoms of depression occur as a reaction to an identifiable stressor. The diagnostic criteria are:

- The development of emotional or behavioral symptoms in response to an identifiable stressor(s) occurring within 3 months of the onset of the stressor(s).
- These symptoms or behaviors are clinically significant, as evidenced by either of the following:
  1. marked distress that is in excess of what would be expected from exposure to the stressor
  2. significant impairment in social or occupational (academic) functioning
- The stress-related disturbance does not meet the criteria for another specific Axis I disorder and is not merely an exacerbation of a preexisting Axis I or Axis II disorder.
- The symptoms do not represent bereavement.
- Once the stressor (or its consequences) has terminated, the symptoms do not persist for more than an additional 6 months.

The subtype "With Depressed Mood" should be used when the predominant manifestations are symptoms such as depressed mood, tearfulness, or feelings of hopelessness.

Bereavement

This category can be used when the focus of clinical attention is a reaction to the death of a loved one. As part of their reaction to the loss, some grieving individuals present with symptoms characteristic of a major depressive episode (e.g., feelings of sadness and associated symptoms such as insomnia, poor appetite, and weight loss). The bereaved individual typically regards the depressed mood as "normal," although the person may seek professional help for relief of associated symptoms such as insomnia or anorexia. The duration and expression of "normal" bereavement vary considerably among different cultural groups. The diagnosis of major depressive disorder is generally not given unless the symptoms are still present 2 months after the loss. However, the presence of certain symptoms that are not characteristic of a "normal" grief reaction may be helpful in differentiating bereavement from a major depressive episode. These include (1) guilt about things other than actions taken or not taken by the survivor at the time of the death; (2) thoughts of death other than the survivor feeling that he or she would be better off dead or should have died with the deceased person; (3) morbid preoccupation with worthlessness; (4) marked psychomotor retardation; (5) prolonged and marked functional impairment; and (6) hallucinatory experiences other than thinking that he or she hears the voice of, or transiently sees the image of, the deceased person (Help Guide, 2013; Mayo Clinic, 2013).

Several losses are common in older adults, including economic hardships, retirement, social isolation, loss of physical health and mobility, relocation, and, most important, loss of a spouse. Simultaneous multiple losses are not uncommon in the older population. The most common studied loss in older patients is loss of a spouse. The grieving spouse has been noted to have declining physical and mental health. As compared with men, women tend to cope better with the loss of a spouse (Versalle & McDowell, 2004–2005).

Depression due to Medical Illness

The diagnostic criteria for mood disorders are listed below; however, clinicians should indicate the general medical conditions (see Table 26.4).

- A prominent and persistent disturbance in mood predominates in the clinical picture and is characterized by either (or both) of the following:
  1. depressed mood or markedly diminished interest or pleasure in all, or almost all, activities
  2. elevated, expansive, or irritable mood
- There is evidence from the history, physical examination, or laboratory findings that the disturbance is the direct physiological consequence of a general medical condition.
- The disturbance is not better accounted for by another mental disorder (e.g., adjustment disorder with depressed mood in response to the stress of having a general medical condition).
- The disturbance does not occur exclusively during the course of a delirium.
- The symptoms cause clinically significant distress or impairment in social, occupational, or other important areas of functioning.

If the full criteria are not met for major depressive episode, clinicians should document with depressive features; however, if the full criteria are met, clinicians should document with major depressive–like episode.

There is often a debate over the degree to which a medical condition causes depression due to direct physiological effects on the brain or because of psychological stress and disability caused by the illness. Assessing for these disease entities is a clinical responsibility of the provider. Table 26.4 details these specific disturbances.

Psychotic Depression

Depression is the second most common cause of psychosis in the older adult. Late onset depression is more likely associated with psychotic symptoms than early onset depression. Older adults with psychotic depression mostly have delusions; hallucinations are less common. The usual themes of depressive delusions are delusions of persecution or somatic delusions. Delusions are present in up to 40% of older patients hospitalized for depression (Broadway & Mintzer, 2007).

TABLE 26.4 • Physical Illnesses Associated with Depression in Older Adults

Metabolic disturbances
    Dehydration
    Azotemia, uremia
    Acid-base disturbances
    Hypoxia
    Hyponatremia and hypernatremia
    Hypoglycemia and hypercalcemia

Endocrine disorders
    Hypothyroidism and hyperthyroidism
    Hyperparathyroidism
    Diabetes mellitus
    Cushing disease
    Addison disease

Infections
    Viral: pneumonia, encephalitis
    Bacterial: pneumonia, urinary tract, meningitis, endocarditis
    Other: tuberculosis, brucellosis, fungal, neurosyphilis

Cardiovascular disorders
    Congestive heart failure
    Myocardial infarction, angina

Pulmonary disorders
    Chronic obstructive lung disease
    Malignancy

Gastrointestinal disorders
    Malignancy (especially pancreatic)
    Irritable bowel
    Other organic causes of chronic abdominal pain, ulcer, diverticulosis, hepatitis

Genitourinary disorders
    Urinary incontinence

Musculoskeletal disorders
    Degenerative arthritis
    Osteoporosis with vertebral compression or hip fractures
    Polymyalgia rheumatic
    Paget disease

Neurological disorders
    Cerebrovascular disease
    Transient ischemic attacks
    Stroke
    Dementia (all types)
    Intracranial mass: primary or metastatic tumors
    Parkinson disease

Other illnesses
    Anemia (of any cause)
    Vitamin deficiencies
    Hematologic or other systemic malignancy

From Kurlowicz, L. H., & NICHE Faculty. (1997). Nursing standard of practice protocol: Depression in older adult patients. *Geriatric Nursing, 18*(5), 192–199, with permission.

Subsyndromal Depression

Epidemiologic studies have used varying terms for depressive states that are below the threshold of meeting the full DSM-IV criteria for major depressive disorder such as subsyndromal, subclinical, and subthreshold depression. Clinically significant nonmajor or "subsyndromal" depression affects approximately 15% of the ambulatory older adults. Subsyndromal depression is associated with significant functional impairment and psychosocial disability. Older adults with subsyndromal depression remain at significantly increased risk for developing a major depression (Vanitallie, 2005).

Late-Life Depressive Syndromes

Sometimes geriatric depression could present with unique features that may not be explicitly identified in DSM-IV-TR diagnostic criteria. These symptoms could be observed as changes in mood, perceptual disturbances, view of oneself and the future, and vegetative and behavioral signs. World Health Organization (WHO) (2003) reported that there is increasing evidence that depression and physical illness are closely aligned. Individuals with chronic disease suffer depression that worsens their physical health and hinders their ability to follow a prescribed medical regimen. Comorbid medical illnesses, use of medications, and physiological changes of aging frequently affect mood, neurovegetative symptoms, and overall presentation of depression in older adults.

Some of the clinical entities of depression that are specifically relevant to older adults not categorized in DSM-IV-TR are caregiver depression, depression associated with dementia and vascular depression. Also, late-life depression encompasses adults with early onset depression that are now old, and late onset depression. The age cutoff to differentiate between the two is 60 years of age. Late onset makes up about half of all depression episodes in older adults. Untreated depression contributes to a lessened quality of life, increased disability and medical costs (CDC, 2005).

Seasonal Affective Disorder (SAD) is a form of depression that occurs in the winter months (November through April) for individuals throughout the continuum of life, and patients will talk about the winter bleakness and sadness. This may occur with or without other forms of depression. Exposure to a form of high-intensity light is a simple intervention for SAD. Additionally, it is treated with medications and psychotherapy (Mayo Clinic, 2011) (Table 26.5).

TABLE 26.5 · Differences Between Early Onset and Late Onset Depression

	Late onset geriatric depression	Early onset geriatric depression
Family history	Less common	More common
Prevalence of dementing disorder	Higher prevalence	Less frequent
Impairment on neuropsychological testing	Prominent impairment	Less impairment
Development of dementia	Higher rates of dementia on follow-up	Lower rates of dementia
Neurosensory hearing impairment	More impairment	Less impairment
Neuroimaging	Enlargement of lateral ventricles, and white matter hyperintensities more prominent	Not as prominent

TABLE 26.6 • Comparison Between Pseudodementia and Dementia

	Pseudodementia	Dementia
Personal and family history of depression	present	absent
Depression precedes onset of cognitive deficits	present	absent
Duration of symptoms	weeks	Months-yrs
Cognitive deficits	Vocal complaints	Silent concerns
Performance on cognitive function testing	Inconsistent deficits	Consistent deficits
Response to mental status exam questions	"I don't know" answers	Attempts to answer, may confabulate
Effort on testing	Little effort to do well	Tries hard to do well

Adapted from Wells, C. E. (1979). Pseudodementia. *American Journal of Psychiatry, 136,* 895–900, with permission.

Impaired cognitive abilities in the older adult often result in indecisiveness and may suggest a dementing process. The term "pseudodementia" of depression has frequently been used. Several factors help to differentiate the depressive illness from a dementing process. A pseudodementia occurs when a person who is depressed also has cognitive impairment that mimics a dementia. When depression causes cognitive impairment such as the inability to think clearly, problems concentrating, and difficulty with decision making, intervention, for the depression, can cause a these symptoms to diminish (Brown, 2005) (Table 26.6).

CAUSES OF DEPRESSION

Many physical illnesses and situations can cause depression. A brief synopsis of these is presented below.

Vascular Depression

The depression associated with vascular ischemic changes has been frequently called vascular depression in older adults. Cerebrovascular disease may predispose and precipitate or perpetuate some geriatric depression syndromes (Alexopoulos et al 1997). Vascular depression has been linked with microstructural white matter abnormalities and these abnormalities have been associated with poor treatment outcomes of geriatric depression (Alexopoulos et al 2008).

Depression of Alzheimer Disease

Estimates of the prevalence of depressive symptoms cluster around 30% to 50%, although some estimates are as low as 1%. It takes a astute clinician to identify clinically significant depressive symptoms and syndromes in the setting of Alzheimer disease. During assessment, focus should be on temporal association between onset and course of depressive syndromes and the dementing process (Olin et al., 2002).

Caregiver Depression

It is not uncommon to find an older person in the role of a caregiver. These older adults are particularly prone to developing depressive symptoms. The prevalence of depressive symptoms among caregivers has been found to be almost twice as high as that among noncaregivers (Covinsky et al., 2003). Male caregivers tend to underreport depressive symptoms.

BURDEN OF DEPRESSION

Depression interacts with disability, medical illnesses, and dementing disorders in a variety of complex ways with potentially detrimental consequences. Depression is leading cause of disability in the United States (World Health Organization, 2004). In older adults, disability presents with impairment in activities of daily living such as eating, dressing, grooming, bathing, ability to ambulate and use the toilet as well as impairment in instrumental activities of daily living such as shopping for groceries, doing housework, using the telephone, managing money, doing the laundry, and taking medications. Functional decline threatens the ability to live independently and the overall scope of daily life, including social roles and relationships, thus setting up a cycle of disability, perpetuating depression and vice versa.

Medical illness and its relationship to depression is documented in previous tables. The relationship between depression and medical illness is bidirectional. Particularly documented is cardiovascular disease such as stroke, myocardial infarction (Blazer & Hybels, 2005). Depression increases mortality and morbidity independently of severity of medical illnesses. Depressive symptoms co-occurring with medical illnesses such as Parkinson's and stroke are beyond the direct effects of the underlying medical condition. In general medical settings, patients with major depressive disorder experience and report more physical pain and decreased physical and social role functioning than those without depression. Rates of depression at the time of hip fracture have been estimated at 9% to 47% (mean 29%). Mental health status at the time of surgery has been reported to be an important determinant of outcome, with mental disorder associated with poorer functional recovery and higher mortality. Approximately one in five people who are not depressed at the time of their fracture become so after 8 weeks (Burns et al., 2007).

Depressive symptoms varying from major depression to subsyndromal depression occur in up to 50% of demented patients. These have been found to be more common in vascular dementia than cortical dementia like Alzheimer's. Depressive symptoms in early life predispose to development of dementia in later life.

Although older adults comprise only 12% of the U.S. population, people aged 65 and over accounted for 16% of suicide deaths in 2004 (CDC, National Center for Injury Prevention and Control, 2005). The most common means used by suicide victims are guns and by hanging, whereas suicide attempters used drug overdose and cutting on self.

Depression is the most common psychiatric disorder associated with suicide in older adults. Several risk factors include white, male, age, single/widowed/divorced, social isolation, hopelessness, guilt, terminal illness, past suicide attempt, and drug and alcohol use. Presence of hopelessness and suicidal ideation are symptoms of treatable clinical depression. Careful interviewing during suicide assessment is crucial for providers. Identification of any such symptoms warrants further appropriate psychiatric referral (see Chapter 27).

TABLE 26.7 • Factors to be Considered in a Geriatric Depression Evaluation

- Current symptoms and associated precipitating factors, losses, and stressors
- Past psychiatric history, including past suicide attempts
- Family history and level of support
- Substance abuse history
- Coexisting medical illness along with current medications
- Psychosocial history, including finances, living situation and social network, spirituality, screen for elderly abuse
- Functional assessment with regard to ADLs and IADLs

SCREENING AND RISK FACTORS

Diagnosing depression in older adults could be challenging owing to atypical presentation as well as the presence of a myriad of several biopsychosocial factors. There is no single diagnostic test for geriatric depression. A comprehensive history and detailed physical and mental status evaluation is the gold standard for the diagnosis. Interview of a family member for collateral information is crucial in geriatric depression. Owing to the fragility of the older population, interviewer's expression of empathy, respect and caring attitude have been emphasized by researchers and throughout this text (Hsieh & Wang, 2003) (Table 26.7).

Various depression screening scales have been used as tools. Some of these may be self-reported, and some are interviewer administered. The Geriatric Depression Scale (GDS) is a popular 30-item self-report measure with high levels of sensitivity and specificity (Yesavage et al., 1983). The scale excludes somatic symptoms, which reduces the confounding effect of comorbid medical illnesses. A 10 to 15 item short version is also available. See IT resources at the end of the chapter for the GDS. The GDS is a good scale to use if GDS is positive for depression and can be valid and sensitive to depression, especially for items that focus on sadness and lack of interest. The Cornell Scale for Depression in Dementia is a scale that can be used on the basis of symptoms and signs during the week prior to the interview. No score is given if symptoms result from disability or illness (Melillo & Houde, 2011).

In cognitively impaired older adults, self-report measures can be inaccurate, and thus interviewer-administered measures such as Hamilton depression rating scale (HAM-D) and Montgomery Asberg depression rating scale (MADRS) may be preferred (Hamilton, 1967; Montgomery & Asberg, 1979). Often older adults may talk about tiredness or worry rather than depression. Depression in this population is treatable and may worsen if not treated, and is a risk factor for suicide (Melillo & Houde, 2011).

TREATMENT

Treating depression in older adults is more complex and presents challenges to clinicians as compared with the younger population. Several other possible diagnoses need to be considered and possibly ruled out prior to initiating treatment. These other diagnoses are listed in Table 26.8.

The treatment is most often initiated by family physicians in primary care settings, making it all the more important for family physicians to be familiar with diagnosis and treatment of depression. Different models have been formed to improve the management of depression in

TABLE 26.8 • Differential Diagnosis of Late-Life Depression

- Alzheimer disease and other neurodegenerative disorders
- Bereavement
- Adjustment disorder with depressed mood
- Depressed phase of bipolar disorder
- Substance-induced mood disorders
- Anxiety disorders
- Personality disorder
- Depressive symptoms associated with psychotic illnesses
- Clinicians should also consider medical illnesses that may present with prominent mood symptoms such as
- Cardiopulmonary conditions—stroke, myocardial infarction, chronic obstructive pulmonary disease
- Neurological conditions—Parkinson disease and other movement disorders
- Endocrine and metabolic disorders—hypothyroidism, renal failure
- Medication toxicities
- Nutritional deficiencies
- Sleep disorders
- Infections
- Neoplasms

primary care settings. A popular model is PROSPECT (Prevention of Suicide in Primary care Elderly: Collaborative Trial), which aims to prevent suicide among older primary care patients by treating depression and reducing suicide (Alexopoulos et al., 2009). The crucial components of intervention are recognition of depression and suicidal ideation by primary care physicians and applying treatment guidelines for geriatric depression in office-based primary care settings. It emphasizes having a depression care manager such as a nurse, social worker, psychologist, who collaborates with physicians to monitor patients and encourage adherence to treatment. Treatment included medications, primarily antipsychotic medications (SSRIs), and psychosocial intervention in the form of interpersonal psychotherapy. In a randomized controlled trial comparing PROSPECT with usual treatment, patients with major depression in PROSPECT experienced a greater decrease in depression, were more likely to experience remission of depressive symptoms, and also had reduced rates of suicidal ideation.

Katon and Schulberg (1992) reported that 55% of depressed older adults receive no treatment, 34% receive inadequate treatment, and only about 11% of depressed received adequate antidepressant treatment. Wang et al. (2005) reported that despite the fact that depression co-occurs with many medical illnesses and that most persons with symptoms of depression are treated by primary care physicians, most cases continue to go untreated. Several treatment- and patient-related factors may contribute to lack of treatment of depression in older adults, including a limited number of health care providers trained in geropsychiatry, lower reimbursement for care, stigma associated with mental illness, and reluctance to seek psychiatric care, focus on somatic complaints and physical illnesses rather than emotional problems.

The expert consensus guidelines for late-life depression recommend combination therapy, with antidepressant, psychosocial interventions, and psychotherapy together being the first-line treatment strategy (Alexopoulos et al., 2001). Patients having the following clinical features are more likely to respond positively to biological treatments, including antidepressants and ECT: vegetative symptoms, including insomnia, poor appetite, diurnal changes with mood being worse in the morning, acute onset, positive family history, and prior positive response to antidepressant.

Pharmacotherapy

Psychopharmacological treatment of depression in older adults with antidepressants has been found to be as effective as in the younger population. An overall approach of starting low and going slow but keep increasing the dose to facilitate response is important to remember as sometimes older patients are underdosed and do not respond (Alexopoulos et al., 2001).

Selective Serotonin Reuptake Inhibitors (SSRIs)

SSRIs have been the preferred class of antidepressants for treating geriatric depression (Alexopoulus et al., 2001; Pinquart et al., 2006). SSRIs act by increasing the availability of the neurotransmitter serotonin in the brain by preventing its reuptake. SSRIs have been found to be clinically effective for depression and anxiety symptoms with good tolerability and safety in older adults. Though caution needs to be exercised, this class is relatively free of significant drug–drug interactions, which is particularly important for the older population who may be simultaneously taking multiple medications for their comorbid medical and psychiatric conditions. While initiating pharmacotherapy, it is recommended to start at a low dose and go slow, with monitoring of side effects and clinical response. Antidepressant medication needs to be given for at least 9 to 12 weeks for it to be considered adequate trial, yet some will respond in a 4 to 6 week trial. Since compliance may be an issue with older adults, the geriatric psychiatric nurse has a pivotal role to play in providing psychoeducation to patients regarding the nature and course of illness and need for compliance with medications for a good response. Older adults may need frequent reassurance and encouragement to take medications as prescribed. Though well tolerated, some common side effects with SSRIs are gastrointestinal distress such as nausea, diarrhea, headache, weight loss or weight gain, initial increase in anxiety, jitteriness, akathisia, in some cases, and sexual dysfunction. Some of these may be transient and may not warrant discontinuation of medication if tolerable. Rare but significant side effects noted particularly in the older population include the syndrome of inappropriate antidiuretic hormone (SIADH), increased risk of gastrointestinal bleeding, especially when taken with NSAIDS (Looper, 2007), bradycardia when taken with β-blockers and extrapyramidal symptoms (Mamo et al., 2000), and increase in the risk of fractures with chronic use of SSRIs due to a direct effect on bone metabolism (Richards et al., 2007).

Of all the agents, sertraline and citalopram have been most extensively studied and are favored agents for the treatment of geriatric depression (The National Guideline Clearinghouse: Clinical practice guidelines [2008]) (Table 26.9).

TABLE 26.9 • Different SSRIs for Treatment

SSRI	Efficacious dose range in older adults (mg/day)
Fluoxetine	20–40
Citalopram	20–40
Escitalopram	10–20
Sertraline	50–200
Paroxetine	20–40

Serotonin Norepinephrine Reuptake Inhibitors (SNRIs)

Another relatively newer class of antidepressants developed in late 1989 to 1990 used in older adults is SNRIs. SNRIs have a dual mode of action through increasing the availability of two neurotransmitters, serotonin and norepinephrine in the brain. Venlafaxine and duloxetine are two medications that belong to this class that have been approved for treatment of depression. Although experts recommend SNRIs also as first-line pharmacotherapy for depression, this class is usually used for subgroups of older adults that have failed to respond to SSRIs. Duloxetine has been found to be useful for treatment of depression and associated pain symptoms in placebo-controlled trials (Nelson et al., 2005; Raskin et al., 2007). Duloxetine is also approved for treatment of pain associated with diabetic neuropathy. A special role of this class has been found in patients with comorbid anxiety disorders and chronic pain syndromes. Venlafaxine can cause dose-dependent hypertension (Katz et al., 2002; Grothe et al., 2004).

Other Antidepressants

Bupropion is an antidepressant that acts by increasing norepinephrine and dopamine. It is typically used as an agent to augment an SSRI or alone in patients who are not responding or cannot tolerate SSRIs (Alexopoulos, 2011). Bupropion is contraindicated in seizure disorder because of its propensity to lower seizure threshold, and therefore should be avoided in patients with electrolyte abnormalities or post stroke. It is also a medication without the sexual side effects found in SSRIs. Mirtazapine is a unique antidepressant with actions at multiple neuroreceptors in the brain. Its most significant action is by blocking alpha 2 autoreceptors, which in turn increases the noradrenergic transmission and increases the levels of serotonin by antagonism of the 5-HT 2 receptor. Although not first line in older adults, it may be beneficial to some patients at lower doses to target sleep disturbance and poor appetite.

Tricyclic Antidepressants (TCA) and Monoamine Oxidase Inhibitors (MAOI). TCA and MAOIs are older antidepressants that may be used as third- or fourth-line options in treatment of depression owing to their significant anticholinergic, cardiac, and neurological side effects. The most commonly used tricyclics are nortriptyline and desipramine in view of lower propensity for sedation and anticholinergic side effects. Tricyclics are contraindicated in patients with cardiac conduction defects.

Other Therapeutic Modalities

Electroconvulsive Treatment (ECT)

In recent years, the use of ECT has been rising in the treatment of older adults with depression. ECT is rapid acting, effective and safe biological treatment for depression when used judiciously in the right patient population. The common indications for ECT use are: suicidal patients, starvation or severe neurovegetative symptoms of depression that are life threatening, intolerance to antidepressants, lack of response to antidepressants, presence of psychotic depression, especially with somatic delusions when depression has failed to respond to medication (Alexopoulos, 2011).

There are no absolute contraindications for use of ECT. However, this modality may be used with caution in the older adult with preexisting cognitive deficits and concurrent major medical illnesses. The usual course of ECT is a total of 10 to 12 sessions administered every other day. Cognitive problems associated with ECT may be minimized with unilateral administration. A full medical evaluation is needed prior to ECT (Melillo & Houde, 2011).

Phototherapy

The primary indication for use of light therapy is the treatment of SAD. Patients are exposed to artificial light that is 5 to 20 times brighter than normal indoor lighting for up to several hours. Onset of response is typically rapid and experienced within a few days to two weeks. Side effects may include headache, insomnia, and precipitation of mania in underlying bipolar illness. A course of light therapy of 5,000 lux administered for 50 minutes/day for 5 days had a significant impact on reducing older patients' depressive symptoms (Tsai et al., 2004).

Psychotherapy

Expert consensus guidelines (2009) recommend a combination of antidepressant and psychotherapy for treatment of late-life depression. Psychotherapy has been shown to be as effective for management of depression in older adults as in the younger population. It helps with increasing medication compliance and relapse prevention. It may also be the preferred treatment option in patients with multiple coexisting serious medical conditions and ongoing psychosocial stressors. Various age-specific considerations are often needed to modify therapy procedures in older adults. To account for age-related sensory and cognitive changes, the pace of therapy may be slower, use of handouts with larger font of material, clear instructions in short sentences, to be used by providers.

Various psychotherapy techniques have been studied in late-life depression such as cognitive behavioral therapy, supportive therapy, and brief psychodynamic and interpersonal therapy. In some cases, marital and family therapy, and group therapy interventions may also be successful (van Schaik et al., 2007).

Supportive Therapy

Supportive therapy focuses on improving communication, establishing therapeutic alliance through use of reassurance, helping the patient to feel understood, offering empathy, and imparting therapeutic optimism. Nursing intervention classification (NIC) defines emotional support as "provision of reassurance, acceptance and encouragement during times of stress" (Iowa Intervention Project, 2000). Supportive therapy can be used by geriatric nurses in any treatment setting. The provider may assist the patient in recognizing his feelings such as sadness, anxiety, guilt and anger, and usual response patterns. Provide support and assistance in decision making and refer to a higher level of care if needed.

Cognitive Behavior Therapy (CBT)

CBT is based on Aaron Beck's cognitive triad, which is commonly seen in patients with depression. The triad comprises negative view of self, world, and future. Beck viewed depressed individuals as having distorted cognitive thoughts. Cognitive therapy focuses on changing these automatic negative thoughts, which in turn lead to depressed mood. The therapist and patient collaboratively set goals that are directed toward modification of conscious thoughts, feelings, and behavior. The behavioral component of CBT focuses on daily activity scheduling, problem solving, monitoring behavior and affect patterns, increased focus on pleasant events, and avoidance of depression triggers. CBT is a time-efficient, structured, brief form of psychotherapy typically involving 12 to 15 sessions (Beck, 1963).

Problem Solving Therapy

This is a form of CBT that is based on the premise that multiple stressors can lead to impairment of problem solving abilities leading to depression, which may in turn perpetuate impaired problem solving (Nezu & D'Zurilla, 2005). The therapy entails identifying problems and their details, goals, weighing risks and benefits of possible solutions, and ultimately helping the patient to reaching a final decision.

Interpersonal Therapy (IPT)

The interpersonal problems are known to cause and worsen depression. The IPT focuses on following four components: grief-loss of spouse, role transitions (e.g., retirement in older adults), interpersonal disputes, role deficits.

IPT is a manualized technique that involves role playing, communication analysis, clarification of patient's wants and needs, and links between affect and environmental events (Hinrichsen, 1999). IPT has been found to be as effective as an antidepressant in the older population for treatment of depression (van Schaik et al., 2007).

Brief Psychodynamic Therapy

Psychodynamic therapy is based on the theory that current emotional symptoms result from unresolved early childhood conflicts and experiences. This therapy has been less studied in treatment of depression in older adults as compared with more structured CBT and IPT. Suitable candidates for dynamic therapy must be motivated; capable of reflection, introspection, and psychological insight; and be able to tolerate strong emotions and show some evidence of good adaption in early life (Werner, 2004).

Life Review and Reminiscence Psychotherapy

Reminiscence is the act or process of recalling the remote past in a silent, spoken, solitary, interactional, spontaneous, or structured way. Life review is a process of reviewing, organizing, and evaluating the overall picture of one's life with the aim of achieving integrity (Hsieh and Wang, 2003). In simple terms, reminiscence is helpful in resocializing and making relationships, whereas life review helps to find meaning in one's life. With greater emphasis on psychosocial interventions in older adults, these two therapies in a group and one-to-one settings can be implemented by geriatric nurses. Life review and reminiscence can be used in multiple settings varying from acute care, senior centers, nursing homes, clinics, and hospices. Reminiscence is often done in group settings in which group therapy initiates a process where group members make new friends, learn communication skills and share feelings, improve self-esteem, and provide validation for each other. "I was not the only one" is a common feeling that occurs in group reminiscence. Life review is often a one-to-one structured and intense intervention that helps the older patients gain a sense of integrity. Studies have shown that these therapies might have a role in preventing or reducing depression and help older adults deal with crisis and losses.

Group Psychotherapy

Group psychotherapy interventions (Agronin, 2009) are emerging as an important component of treatment of older adults in inpatient, outpatient, hospital settings, community and long-term care settings. Any of the above-mentioned individual therapy techniques may be employed in group settings for older adults with depression. This therapy addresses social isolation, interpersonal alienation, reduced self-esteem and depressive withdrawal in late-life depression. Nonspecific curative factors of group therapy include socialization, group cohesiveness, universality, and instillation of hope and altruism. Various group therapy approaches can be applied with geriatric patients: verbal-centered groups for cognitively intact and cognitively impaired, creativity-centered groups, and self-help groups.

CULTURAL CONSIDERATIONS

Although late-life depression exists worldwide, symptomatic expression and interpersonal and social response to the diagnosis varies across different cultures. Culture in psychiatry includes not only characteristics of the patient, but also ethnocultural background and professional training of clinicians.

In many cultures, disturbances of mood and affect are not viewed as mental health problems but as social or moral problems. Even in modern American society, depression may be viewed as lack of personal strength, which makes older adults more inclined to report socially acceptable somatic symptoms and deny affective components. In many cultures, individuals are less likely to share details of their emotional state and psychosocial issues with their health care providers. Examination of somatization of depression has been studied all over the world and found to be very ubiquitous (García-Campayo et al., 1998). Most common somatic symptoms of depression, as discussed before, are physical pain and fatigue. Stigmatization associated with emotional symptoms of depression results in rejection of psychological or psychiatric help. Clinicians, including geriatric nurses, play an important role in making attempts to understand the patient's perspective, characteristics, and preferences, and to negotiate treatment strategies that will be acceptable to the patient. Cultural differences between patients and clinicians can also affect compliance. Low rates of compliance in intercultural settings are noted to be due to patients' perception of medication being too strong and increased sensitivity to side effects, in addition to social stigma. The outline for cultural formulation in DSM-IV gives a checklist of basic categories of information relevant to understanding symptoms and illness in social and cultural contexts (DSM-IV, 2000). It has four components: ethnocultural identity of the patient, patient's explanation of illness, culturally distinct dimensions of psychosocial environment and levels of functioning, and relationship between individual and clinician.

An important and very basic strategy for overcoming cultural barriers is to adopt an open, respectful, and empathic attitude toward patients and their environment. This helps clinicians to learn essentials that are crucial to understand the individual's illness and also helps to identify cultural resources that can complement conventional psychiatric treatment (Sue & Sue, 2007).

PREVENTION

Late-life depression is associated with impaired physical, social, and cognitive functioning, and contributes to disability, morbidity, and mortality. Depression is predicted to be the greatest contributor to illness burden and disability by 2030 (WHO, 2012). Prevention of depression in older adults aims to prevent the downward course of depression to disability and death. Published work on depression prevention has focused on prevention not only in older adults at risk for depression, but also in older adults already living with subthreshold symptoms of depression. Reynolds (2009) and his colleagues present "prevention" as encompassing both preemption of incident and recurrent episodes of major depression and protection from developing social and medical complications of depression. Three different types of late-life depression prevention approaches have been studied.

1. Mental health promotion or universal prevention that focuses on general mental health education. Mental health literacy programs targeting both healthy older adults and care providers help in destigmatizing the illness, increase awareness regarding early signs of depression, and encourage seeking treatment. Outreach could be through media, Internet, talks, and booklets.
2. Selective prevention targets older populations in high-risk groups not suffering from depression but that are vulnerable to developing depressive symptoms. For example, known risk factors like disability, social isolation, and bereavement can be targeted.
3. Indicated prevention focuses on older adults with subthreshold symptoms of depression.

Two other major prevention strategies have been studied—psychosocial and biological interventions.

Psychosocial Interventions

Psychosocial intervention is defined as any intervention that emphasizes psychological and social factors rather than biological factors (Ruddy & House, 2005). They vary from health education, interventions designed to address loneliness, improving perception of social support, and everyday life management skills training to promoting physical exercise. The psychosocial interventions can be done in groups or individually with older adults. A systematic review of prospective controlled trials examined different psychosocial interventions aimed at prevention of depression (Forsman et al., 2011). The interventions included in different studies were physical exercise, skills training, group support, reminiscence and social activities, and few studies examined different components of the above-mentioned categories. Psychosocial interventions had a positive effect on quality of life and mental health and a weak but statistically significant effect on reducing depressive symptoms among intervention groups. Interventions with longer duration showed a positive impact on mental health and quality of life as compared with short duration interventions.

Few studies have evaluated primary prevention of depression in physically ill patients with multiple medical diagnoses. In a study by de Jonge et al. (2009), a psychiatric nurse–led intervention was shown to prevent the occurrence of major depression in complex medically ill inpatients and also to reduce depressive symptoms in diabetes outpatients as compared with usual care. In the intervention group, the nurse offered supportive counseling focused on coping with disease and compliance with treatment referral to a liaison psychiatrist, when appropriate, and organization of a multidisciplinary case conference attended by treating physicians, nurses, and the liaison psychiatrist. The group receiving usual care could receive a psychiatric referral by the treating physician.

Nutritional Supplementation

Folic acid and vitamin B_{12} supplementation may prevent depression by lowering homocysteine levels, which are reported to be elevated in individuals with depression (Tiemeier et al., 2002). Supplementary B_{12} and folic acid may reduce the long-term risk of onset of depression through reduction of vascular risk factors for late-life depression (Reynolds, 2002). A 2010 research study in Canada revealed positive results from Omega3 in treatment of depression patients who do not have anxiety disorders (Lespérance et al., 2011). Research is taking place in a number of centers. The overall effect of preventive strategies for depression in older adults is small but promising. Prevention remains an important area to be considered in ongoing clinical practice and research. Clinicians and care providers managing older adults with risk factors for depression in particular should have a high degree of suspicion and provide timely appropriate interventions (see Chapter 10).

PATIENT EDUCATION

Patient education is crucial for early diagnosis and treatment to improve outcomes. Patient education handouts are often freely available in waiting areas of hospitals and clinics that educate about recognition of early symptoms of depression, importance of diagnosis, need for treatment, and overall course and prognosis. The material is worded simply in large font and is available at various Internet websites as well.

National Alliance for Mental Illness is the nation's leading nonprofit grassroot organization dedicated to providing help to Americans with mental illness. This organization provides resources, education, and support to individuals living with mental illness.

Mental Health America (2003) is another leading nonprofit organization that aims at providing mental health awareness. Their website provides specific information targeting people of various age groups, ethnocultural backgrounds as well as for patients and care providers regarding mental health disorders, including depression.

REFERENCES

Agronin, M. (2009). Group therapy in older adults. *Current Psychiatry Reports*, *11*(1), 27–32.

Alexopoulos, G. S. (2000). Mood disorders. In B. J. Sadock & V. A. Sadock (Eds.), *Comprehensive textbook of psychiatry* (7th ed., Vol. 2). Baltimore, MD: Williams and Wilkins.

Alexopoulos, G. S. (2005). Depression in the elderly. *Lancet*, *365*(9475), 1961–1970.

Alexopoulos ,G. S. (2011). Pharmacotherapy for late-life depression. *Journal of Clinical Psychiatry*, *72*(1), e04.

Alexopoulos, G. S., Katz, I. R., Reynolds, C. F.,III, Carpenter, D., & Docherty, J. P. (2001). The expert consensus guideline series: Pharmacotherapy of depressive disorders in older patients. *Postgraduate Medicine*, Spec No Pharmacotherapy, 1–86.

Alexopoulos, G. S., Meyers, B. S., Young, R. C., Campbell, S., Sibersweig, D., & Charlson, M. (1997). 'Vascular depression' hypothesis. *Archives of General Psychiatry*, *54*, 915–922.

Alexopoulos, G. S., Murphy, C. F., Gunning-Dixon, F. M., Latoussakis, V., Kanellopoulos, D., Klimstra, S.,…Hoptman, M. J. (2008). Microstructural white matter abnormalities and remission of geriatric depression. *American Journal of Psychiatry*, *165*(2), 238–244.

Alexopoulos, G. S., Reynolds, C. F., III, Bruce, M. L., Katz, I. R., Raue, P. J., Mulsant, B. H.,... Have, T. T. (2009). Reducing suicidal ideation and depression in older primary care patients: 24-month outcomes of the PROSPECT study. *American Journal of Psychiatry, 166*(8), 882–890.

Almeida, O. P., Yeap, B. B., Hankey, G. J., Jamrozik, K., & Flicker, L. (2008). Low free testosterone concentration as a potentially treatable cause of depressive symptoms in older men. *Archives of General Psychiatry, 65*(3), 283–289.

American Psychiatric Association. (2000). *Diagnostic and statistical manual of mental disorders: DSM-IV-TR* (4th Text Rev. ed.). Washington, DC: Author.

Barry, L. C., Allore, H. G., Guo, Z., Bruce, M. L., & Gill, T. M. (2008). Higher burden of depression among older women: The effect of onset, persistence, and mortality over time. *Archives of General Psychiatry, 65*(2), 172–178.

Beck, A. T. (1963). Thinking and depression: Idiosyncratic content and cognitive distortions. *Archives of General Psychiatry, 9*, 324–333.

Blazer, D. G., & Hybels, C. F. (2005). Origins of depression in later life. *Psychological Medicine, 35*, 1–12.

Bremmer, M. A., Beekman, A. T., Deeg, D. J., Penninx, B. W., Dik, M. G., Hack, C. E., & Hoogendijk, W. J. (2008). Inflammatory markers in late-life depression: Results from a population-based study. *Journal of Affective Disorders, 106*(3), 249–255.

Broadway, J., & Mintzer, J. (2007). The many faces of psychosis in the elderly. *Current Opinion in Psychiatry, 20*(6), 551–558.

Brown, W. A. (2005). Pseudodementia: Issues in diagnosis. *Psychiatric Times.* Retrieved from http://www.psychiatric times.com/display/article/10168/56206

Bruce, M. (2002). Psychosocial risk factors for depressive disorders in late life. *Biological Psychiatry, 52*(3), 175–184.

Bruce, M. L., McAvay, G. J., Raue, P. J., Brown, E. L., Meyers, B. S., Keohane, D. J.,... Weber, C. (2002). Major depression in elderly home health care patients. *American Journal of Psychiatry, 159*, 1367–1374.

Burns, A., Banerjee, S., Morris, J., Woodward, Y., Baldwin, R., Proctor, R.,... Horan, M. (2007). Treatment and prevention of depression after surgery for hip fracture in older people: Randomized, controlled trials. *Journal of American Geriatrics Society, 55*(1), 75–80.

Cahoon, C. (2012). Depression in older adults. *American Journal of Nursing, 112*(11), 23–30.

Center for Disease Control, Morbidity and Mortality Weekly Report. (2005). Retrieved from http://www.cdc.gov/mmwr/preview/mmwrhtml/mm5417a4.htm

Centers for Disease Control and Prevention, National Center for Injury Prevention and Control. Web-based Injury Statistics Query and Reporting System (WISQARS) [online]. (2005). Retrieved from http://www.cdc.gov/injury/wisqars/index.html

Chi, I., & Chou, K. (2001). Social support and depression among elderly Chinese people in Hong Kong. *International Journal of Aging and Human Development, 52*, 231–252.

Covinsky, K. E., Newcomer, R., Fox, P., Wood, J., Sands, L., Dane, K., & Yaffe, K. (2003). Patient and caregiver characteristics associated with depression in caregivers of patients with dementia. *Journal of General Internal Medicine, 18*(12), 1006–1014.

de Jonge, P., Hadj, F. B., Boffa, D., Zdrojewski, C., Dorogi, Y., So, A.,... Stiefel, F. (2009). Prevention of major depression in complex medically ill patients: Preliminary results from a randomized, controlled trial. *Psychosomatics, 50*(3), 227–233.

Fischer, L. R., Wei, F., Solberg, I., Rush, W. A., & Heinrich, R. (2003). Treatment of elderly and older adult patients for depression in primary care. *Journal of American Geriatrics Society, 51*(11), 1554–1562.

Forsman, A. K., Nordmyr, J., & Wahlbeck, K. (2011). Psychosocial interventions for the promotion of mental health and the prevention of depression among older adults. *Health Promotion International, 26*(Suppl. 1), i85–i107.

Gallo, J. J., & Rabins, P. V. (1999). Depression without sadness: Alternative presentations of depression in late life. *American Family Physician, 60*, 820–826.

García-Campayo, J., Lobo, A., Pérez-Echeverría, M. J., & Campos, R. (1998). Three forms of somatization presenting in primary care settings in Spain. *Journal of Nervous and Mental Disease, 186*(9), 554–560.

Gatz, M., Pederson, N. L., Plomin, R., Nesselroade, J. R., & McClearn, G. E. (1992). Importance of shared genes and shared environments for symptoms of depression in older adults. *Journal of Abnormal Psychology, 101*(4), 701–708.

Grothe, D. R., Scheckner, B., & Albano, D. (2004). Treatment of pain syndromes with venlafaxine. *Pharmacotherapy, 24*(5), 621–629.

Hamilton, M. (1967). Development of a rating scale for primary depressive illness. *British Journal of Social and Clinical Psychology, 6*, 278–296.

Help Guide. org. (2013). Grief and loss. Retrieved from http://helpguide.org/topics/grief.htm

Hinrichsen, G. A. (1999). Treating older adults with interpersonal psychotherapy for depression. *Journal of Clinical Psychology, 55*(8), 949–960.

Hsieh, H., & Wang, J. (2003). Effect of reminiscence therapy on depression in older adults: A systematic review. *International Journal of Nursing Studies, 40*, 335–345.

Hybels, C. F., & Blazer, D. G. (2003). Epidemiology of late-life mental disorders. *Clinics in Geriatric Medicine, 19*(4), 663–696.

Iowa Intervention Project. McCloskey, J. C., & Bulechek, G. M. (Eds.). (2000). *Nursing interventions classification* (NIC). St. Louis, MO: Mosby-Year Book.

Katon, W., & Schulberg, H. (1992). Epidemiology of depression in primary care. *General Hospital Psychiatry, 14*, 237–242.

Katz, I. R., Reynolds, C. F., III, Alexopoulos, G. S., & Hackett, D. (2002). Venlafaxine ER as a treatment for generalized anxiety disorder in older adults: Pooled analysis of five randomized placebo-controlled clinical trials. *Journal of American Geriatrics Society, 50*(1), 18–25.

Kempton, M. J., Salvador, Z., Munafò, M. R., Geddes, J. R., Simmons, A., Frangou, S., & Williams, S. C. (2011). Structural neuroimaging studies in major depressive disorder. Meta-analysis and comparison with bipolar disorder. *Archives of General Psychiatry, 68*(7), 675–690.

Kockler, M., & Heun, R. (2002). Gender differences of depressive symptoms in depressed and nondepressed elderly persons. *International Journal of Geriatric Psychiatry, 17*(1), 65–72.

Kurlowicz, L. H., & NICHE Faculty. (1997). Nursing standard of practice protocol: Depression in older adult patients. *Geriatric Nursing, 18*(5), 192–199.

Lespérance, F., Frasure-Smith, N., St-André, E., Turecki, G., Lespérance, P., & Wisniewski, S. R. (2011). The efficacy of omega-3 supplementation for major depression: A randomized controlled trial. *Journal of Clinical Psychiatry, 72*(8), 1054–1062.

Looper, K. J. (2007). *Potential medical and surgical complications of serotonergic antidepressant medications. Psychosomatics, 48*, 1–9.

Mamo, D. C., Sweet, R. A., Mulsant, B. H., Pollock, B. G., Miller, M. D., Stack, J. A., . . . Reynolds, C. F., III. (2000). Effect of nortriptyline and paroxetine on extrapyramidal signs and symptoms: A prospective double-blind study in depressed elderly patients. *American Journal of Geriatric Psychiatry, 8*(3), 226–231.

Mayo Clinic. (2011). *Seasonal affective disorder.* Retrieved from http://www.mayoclinic.com/health/seasonal-affective-disorder/DS00195

Mayo Clinic. (2013). *Depression.* Retrieved from http://www.mayoclinic.com/health/depression/DS00175

Melillo, K. D., & Houde, S. C. (Eds.). (2011). *Geropsychiatric and mental health nursing* (2nd ed.). Sudbury, MA: Jones & Bartlett Learning.

Mental Health America. (2013). Retrieved from http://www.nmha.org/go/sad

Montgomery, S. A., & Asberg, M. A. (1979). A new depression scale designed to be sensitive to change. *British Journal of Psychiatry, 134*, 382–389.

Murphy, E. (1982). Social origins of depression in old age. *British Journal of Psychiatry, 141*, 135–142.

National Guideline Clearinghouse. (2008). *Clinical practice guideline on the management of major depression in adults.* Retrieved from http://www.guideline.gov/content.aspx?id=24067

National Institute of Health Consensus Conference. Diagnosis and treatment of depression in late life. (1992). *Journal of the American Medical Association, 268*(8), 1018–1024.

National Institute of Mental Health. (n. d.). *Dysthymic disorder among adults.* Retrieved from http://www.nimh.nih.gov/statistics/1DD_ADULT.shtml

Nelson, J. C., Wohlreich, M. M., Mallinckrodt, C. H., Detke, M. J., Watkin, J. G., & Kennedy, J. S. (2005). Duloxetine for the treatment of major depressive disorder in older patients. *American Journal of Geriatric Psychiatry, 13*(3), 227–235.

Nezu, A., & D'Zurilla, T. (2005). *Problem-solving therapy-General, Part 13.* 301–304. doi:10.1007/0-306-48581-8_85

Olin, J. T., Schneider, L. S., Katz, I. R., Meyers, B. S., Alexopoulos, G. S., Breitner, J. C., . . . Lebowitz, B. D. (2002). Provisional diagnostic criteria for depression of Alzheimer disease. *American Journal of Geriatric Psychiatry, 10*(2), 125–128.

Pinquart, M., Duberstein, P. R., & Lyness, J. M. (2006). Treatments for later-life depressive conditions: A meta-analytic comparison of pharmacotherapy and psychotherapy. *American Journal of Psychiatry, 163*(9), 1493–1501.

Raskin, J., Wiltse, C. G., Siegal, A., Sheikh, J., Xu, J., Dinkel, J. J., . . . Mohs, R. C. (2007). Efficacy of duloxetine on cognition, depression, and pain in elderly patients with major depressive disorder: An 8-week, double-blind, placebo-controlled trial. *American Journal of Psychiatry, 164*(6), 900–909.

Reynolds, C. F. (2009). Prevention of depressive disorders: A brave new world. *Depression and Anxiety, 26*(12), 1062–1065.

Reynolds, E. H. (2002). Folic acid, ageing, depression, and dementia. *British Medical Journal, 324*(7352), 1512–1515.

Richards, J. B., Papaioannou, A., Adachi, J. D., Joseph, L., Whitson, H. E., Prior, J. C., & Goltzman, D. (2007). Effect of selective serotonin reuptake inhibitors on the risk of fracture. *Archives of Internal Medicine, 167*(2), 188–194.

Ruddy, R., & House, A. (2005). Meta-review of high-quality systematic reviews of interventions in key areas of liaison psychiatry. *British Journal of Psychiatry*, *187*, 109–120.

Steffens, D. C., Taylor, W.D., & Krishnan, R. R. (2003). Progression of subcortical ischemic disease from vascular depression to vascular dementia. *American Journal of Psychiatry*, *160*(10), 1751–1756.

Sue, D. W., & Sue, D. (2007). *Counseling the culturally diverse: Theory and practice* (5th ed.). Hoboken, NJ: Wiley.

Thakur, M., & Blazer, D. (2008). Depression in long-term care. *Journal of American Medical Directors Association*, *9*(2), 82–87.

Tiemeier, H., van Tuijl, H. R., Hofman, A., Meijer, J., Kiliaan, A. J., & Breteler, M. M. (2002). Vitamin B12, folate, and homocysteine in depression: The Rotterdam Study. *American Journal of Psychiatry*, *159*(12), 2099–2101.

Tsai, Y. F., Wong, T. K., Juang, Y. Y., & Tsai, H. H. (2004). The effects of light therapy on depressed elders. *International Journal of Geriatric Psychiatry*, *19*(6), 545–548.

van Schaik, D. J., van Marwijk, H. W., Beekman, A. T., de Haan, M., & van Dyck, R. (2007). Interpersonal psychotherapy (IPT) for late-life depression in general practice: Uptake and satisfaction by patients, therapists and physicians. *BMC Family Practice*, *8*, 52.

Vanitallie, T. B. (2005). Subsyndromal depression in the elderly: Underdiagnosed and undertreated. *Metabolism: Clinical and Experimental*, *54*(Suppl. 1), 39–44.

Versalle, A., & McDowell, E. E. (2004–2005). The attitudes of men and women concerning gender differences in grief. *Omega*, *50*(1), 53–67.

Wang, P. S., Lane, M., Olfson, M., Pincus, H. A., Wells. K. B., & Kessler, R. C. (2005). Twelve month use of mental health services in the United States: Results from The National Comorbidity Survey Replication. *Archives of General Psychiatry*, *62*(6), 629–640.

Wells, C. E. (1979). Pseudodementia. *American Journal of Psychiatry*, *136*, 895–900.

Werner, A. (2004). Psychodynamic treatment of depression. *American Journal of Psychiatry*, *161*(11), 2146.

World Health Organization. (2003). *Investing in mental health*. Retrieved from http://www.who.int/mental_health/en/investing_in_mnh_final.pdf

World Health Organization. (2004). The global burden of disease: 2004 update, Table A2: Burden of disease in DALYs by cause, sex and income group in WHO regions, estimates for 2004. Retrieved from http://www.who.int/healthinfo/global_burden_disease/GBD_report_2004update_full.pdf

World Health Organization. (2012). *Depression fact sheet*. Retrieved from http://www.who.int/mediacentre/factsheets/fs369/en/index.html

Yesavage, J., Brink, T. L., Rose, T. L., Lum, O., Huang, V., Adey, M., & Leirer, V. O. (1983). Development and validation of a geriatric depression screening scale: A preliminary report. *Journal of Psychiatric Research*, *17*, 37–49.

CHAPTER 26: IT RESOURCES

Websites

Mental Health America
www.mentalhealthamerica.net

The National Alliance on Mental Illness
http://www.nami.org/

Screening for Depression Across the Lifespan: A Review of Measures for Use in Primary Care Settings, taken from the American Family Physician
http://www.aafp.org/afp/2002/0915/p1001.html

How to Assess Depression in the Elderly (taken from Livestrong.com)
http://www.livestrong.com/article/41634-assess-depression-elderly/

Seasonal Affective Disorder, taken from Mental Health America
http://www.nmha.org/go/sad

The National Guideline Clearinghouse: Depression: Clinical Practice Guidelines
http://www.guidelines.gov/content.aspx?id=24158

Treating Depression with Omega-3: Encouraging Results from Largest Clinical Study
http://www.sciencedaily.com/releases/2010/06/100621111238.htm

Cornell Scale for Depression in Dementia
http://qmweb.dads.state.tx.us/Depression/CSDD.htm
Depression and the Elderly (taken from WebMD)
http://www.webmd.com/depression/guide/depression-elderly
Practice guideline for the treatment of patients with major depressive disorder, third edition, taken from the US Department of Health and Human Services, Agency for Healthcare Research and Quality
http://www.guidelines.gov/content.aspx?id=24158
Serotonin and Depression: 9 Questions and Answers
http://www.webmd.com/depression/features/serotonin
Major Depressive Disorder
http://depression.about.com/cs/diagnosis/a/mdd.htm
Hypercortisolemia and Depression
http://www.psychosomaticmedicine.org/content/67/Supplement_1/S26.abstract
Chronic Stress, Can it Cause Depression?
http://www.mayoclinic.com/health/stress/AN01286
How Chronic Stress Can Lead to Depression
http://healthland.time.com/2011/08/03/study-how-chronic-stress-can-lead-to-depression/
Dysthymia, taken from the Mayo Clinic
http://www.mayoclinic.com/health/dysthymia/DS01111
Adjustment Disorders, taken from the Mayo Clinic
http://www.mayoclinic.com/health/adjustment-disorders/DS00584
Bereavement-Related Depression is Depression
http://www.psychologytoday.com/blog/in-practice/200809/bereavement-related-depression-is-depression
Psychotic Depression, Symptoms, Causes, Treatments (taken from WebMD)
http://www.webmd.com/depression/guide/psychotic-depression
What is Subsyndromal Depression?
http://www.ehow.com/about_6631685_subsyndromal-depression_.html
What is Vascular Depression? (taken from National Institute of Mental Health)
http://www.nimh.nih.gov/health/publications/depression-and-stroke/what-is-vascular-depression.shtml
Depression and Alzheimer's Disease
http://www.alz.org/care/alzheimers-dementia-depression.asp
Caregiver Depression: Prevention Counts
http://www.mayoclinic.com/health/caregiver-depression/MY01264
Hamilton Depression rating scale
http://www.psy-world.com/online_hamd.htm
Montgomery Asberg Depression rating scale
http://www.psy-world.com/madrs.htm
Prevention of Suicide in primary care Elderly: Collaborative Trial
http://66.240.150.14/intervention/793/view-eng.html
Electroconvulsive treatment (ECT)
http://www.mayoclinic.com/health/electroconvulsive-therapy/MY00129
Phototherapy: Shedding Light on Winter Depression
http://psychcentral.com/lib/2006/shedding-light-on-winter-depression/all/1/

Psychotherapy to Treat Depression
http://www.webmd.com/depression/psychotherapy-treat-depression
Depression in Older Adults: Supportive Psychotherapy
http://www.uptodate.com/contents/depression-in-adults-supportive-psychotherapy
Cognitive Behavior Therapy for Depression
http://www.webmd.com/depression/guide/cognitive-behavioral-therapy-for-depression

PDF Documents

Geriatric Depression Scale
http://consultgerirn.org/uploads/File/trythis/try_this_4.pdf

Videos

Treatment of Depression in Older Adults: Evidence-Based Practices (2011)
This film gives viewers basic information about the treatment of late life depression, including the following: Principles, Philosophy and values, Basic rationale, How evidence-based practices for diagnosing and treating depression in older patients has helped improve the quality of life for the older adult, Collaboration between mental health and primary health services, and how traditional providers benefit from these models of care. (27 minutes)
http://youtu.be/1aGaVws-ntY
Depression and the Elderly (2010)
Depression is not a side effect of aging. Dr. Stephen Hall, Clinical Professor of Psychiatry at UCSF, explores the evaluation and treatment of depressive disorders in the elderly. (1 hour 30 minutes)
http://youtu.be/6WM4l-RV7NQ
The Emotional Faces of Aging (2012)
Slide presentation set to music with quotes regarding the emotional faces of aging. (5 min)
http://www.youtube.com/watch?v=tR-8Gdrs4dM&feature=share&list=PLkukzNu3PkHaEOB
kpq7-JhkBtZE6rteiH
Depression in the Elderly (2012)
As we grow older, we experience loss, which is a situation that can predispose us to depression. For those who are growing older and experiencing depression, hear tips and how to help. (3 minutes)
http://youtu.be/dXTHZfgrF64

Images

Google images for depression
http://www.google.com/search?q=depression&hl=en&source=lnms&tbm=isch&sa=X
&ei=-oFgUe-vLMqt0AGAv4HoDg&sqi=2&ved=0CAcQ_AUoAQ&biw=1280&bih=705

Suicide

Thomas R. Milam, MD, MDiv

INTRODUCTION

The normal changes of aging contribute to an individual experiencing various physical health impairments such as arthritis, visual impairment, or hearing loss. Decline in emotional health and well-being, however, is not considered by most health care practitioners to be part of the natural aging process. Researchers are beginning to unravel various mechanisms by which the brain undergoes structural changes throughout the life cycle. Many of these changes appear to contribute to cognitive and emotional deficits such as those seen in dementia, though a growing awareness of the brain's ability to regenerate and heal is emerging as well. Continued clinical and basic science research is imperative to explore how these dynamic changes occur in the brain and how they affect motor, cognitive, and emotional function.

The affective, or emotional, aspects of aging may have a significant impact on an older person's cognitive and physical health in ways we have yet to understand. While many older adults who suffer significant physical illness may experience decline in their emotional well-being, others defy this trend and exhibit remarkable emotional resilience in the face of significant chronic physical illness (Inder et al., 2012). Understanding the complex relationship between physical and emotional health in older persons remains an active area of research.

The alarmingly high suicide rate among older adults has sparked much needed research into the emotional well-being of people as they age. The Centers for Disease Control and Prevention reports some alarming national statistics in regard to suicide in general and suicide in older persons in particular:

- Suicide is the 10th leading cause of death in the United States, with an average of 105 completed suicides per day (CDC, n.d.).
- The rate of suicide for adults aged 75 and older is 16.3 per 100,000

- Men aged 75 and older have a suicide rate of 36 per 100,000
- Firearms are the most commonly used method of suicide in males (56%), while poisoning is most commonly used in females (37.4%)

These statistics point to a significant and potentially preventable cause of death among older adults as well as younger populations. With the growing population of older adults in the coming decades, it is imperative that more screening, assessment, and treatment and prevention strategies be developed to combat this high rate of suicide. Recent research shows that some of the more effective suicide prevention programs actually involve increasing physician education and treatment surrounding depression and suicide, as well as reducing access to lethal means of suicide (Mann et al., 2005).

While accurately tracking reported suicide attempts and completions in older adults is difficult enough, it is even more challenging to gather data, either historical or current, on suicidal thoughts or threats. Given the above data on suicide attempts and completion among older adults, one can surmise that the rate of suicide threats is significantly greater. What constitutes a true suicide threat, how to screen for them, and how to understand the causative factors behind such threats is an active area of research among geriatric mental health providers.

PATHOPHYSIOLOGY OF SUICIDE

Suicide, the act of intentionally and willfully taking one's own life, is a symptom, not a diagnosis. While suicide is certainly associated with depression, anxiety, and other forms of mental illness, it is not correct to assume that all people who contemplate suicide are depressed or mentally ill. The causes of suicide are certainly multifactorial. With the high prevalence rate of suicide among older adults, understanding the intricacies of what leads a person to contemplate or carry out suicide remains a topic of ongoing research. While each person's life experience and degree of personal suffering cannot easily be measured quantitatively, it is important to identify potentially reversible physical and psychological factors that lead a person to contemplate, attempt, or complete suicide.

Depression affects approximately 10% to 15% of people 65 years and older, making it a common and serious health concern among this age group (Beekman et al., 1999; McDonald et al., 2007). Not all older adults with depression contemplate suicide, but depression certainly is one of the main risk factors for both developing and predicting suicide. Depression is like a cloud of hopelessness and despair that can greatly affect a person's thoughts, moods, and behaviors, so persons of any age with depression should be screened for suicidal thoughts. Other important risk factors for suicide include physical illness such as cancer and other chronic medical conditions, chronic pain, economic difficulties, significant life stressors such as the death of loved ones and other losses, alcohol and substance abuse, and personality style (Demircin et al., 2011). In fact, a Swedish study of suicides in older adults showed that 66% of those who completed suicide had a history of being treated for their affective disorders, with 48% having received such treatment in the 6 months prior to their suicide (Waern et al., 1996).

Clearly, depression, anxiety, and other mental health disorders increase an older person's risk of suicide, but factors other than mood can also predispose someone to consider or attempt suicide. Life events that may initially be perceived as positive, such as retirement or financial independence, may in fact lead to periods of hopelessness, loss of purpose, isolation, and loneliness. Researchers have shown that in addition to depression, a strong sense of hopelessness is a major predictor for suicidal behavior (Kudo et al., 2007; Watanabe et al., 2004). It is normal in life to experience failure, loss, and disappointment—these are part of the human condition—but some people appear more resilient than others in ways scientists have yet to fully understand. It is hard to predict how an older person will react to a particular loss or stressor, but paying close attention to the possible emergence of suicidal thoughts in older persons who have experienced loss, regardless of how emotionally stable they may appear, can have lifesaving consequences.

While depression and other forms of mental illness are often under-recognized and under-treated in older adults, dementia, which can have behavioral, emotional, and cognitive components, is increasingly being recognized and screened for in this population. The relationship between dementia, depression, and suicidality is still not well understood.

In moderate–to–severe dementia, memory impairment may cause some older adults to forget some of the stressors and losses in their lives, thus reducing their experience of suffering. However, the fear of being a burden to others, from both a financial and care management standpoint, can leave persons diagnosed with dementia with a tremendous degree of anxiety and fear about their future. Some may choose to circumvent such burdens and fears by attempting or completing suicide, so it is especially important to screen and monitor for suicidal thoughts among those newly diagnosed with dementia.

Aside from the obvious impact dementia has on the life of an aging adult, more common illnesses such as cancer, heart disease, pain, pulmonary and renal disease, and other chronic illnesses can also be risk factors for suicide. Fear of disability, suffering, or death from chronic medical illness can have a tremendous impact on one's mental health. Health care providers often focus on trying to improve a patient's physical health through pharmacological or surgical interventions, while ignoring the emotional impact their illness has on their lives and their sense of hope and meaning. The fear of potential disability looming in their future, as well as genuine fears over being a medical or financial burden to others such as spouses or adult children, can lead older adults to see suicide as a reasonable option to alleviate suffering, pain, and financial hardship. Failure to adequately address these very real fears and concerns in older adults with serious medical problems may be a large contributing factor to high rates of suicide in this vulnerable population.

Trying to understand the pathophysiology of suicidality in a quantitative way, while challenging, is important for developing research models and prevention strategies. Demircin and colleagues summed up the complexity of understanding suicide in older persons, writing "Suicide is a complex, long-term outcome that requires theoretical models for appropriate studies to antecedents, complex intervention strategies, as well as protection" (2011). The inner workings of the human mind are, however, quite complex with numerous emotional nuances and patterns of cognition that will likely never be fully understood. Thus, the clinical skills of those who care for older adults must be sufficient to the task of helping understand and reduce suicidality in this special population.

PRESENTATION OF SUICIDE: ACUTE AND CHRONIC

The stigma that is often associated with having a mental illness like depression or anxiety keeps many people from getting the help they need. Older adults may feel especially reluctant to seek help for mental health problems. They may be especially fearful of disclosing to anyone the severity of their despair and suicidal thoughts. If older persons felt more comfortable talking openly to their family members, caregivers, and health care providers about their feelings of hopelessness, despair, and depression, the rate of suicide in this age group might be much lower. The problem, however, is at least twofold.

First, suicidality may develop impulsively as an immediate reaction to severe loss or fear. In such cases, committing suicide is seen as a rapid means of escaping intense suffering, whether that suffering is physical, mental, financial, or otherwise. Older adults who are newly diagnosed with cancer, or who face terminal illness or intractable pain, are particularly vulnerable to developing suicidal thoughts. Additionally, when older adults suffer significant financial loss, loss of independence and mobility, or loss of a spouse or close friend, they run the risk of rapidly developing depression and suicidal thoughts. It is quite difficult to anticipate and prevent suicide in such cases, as the decision to take one's own life can be made quickly and quietly. Even while trying to be vigilant to the impact any negative news might have on an older loved one, family members and friends often still blame themselves for missing what, in hindsight, they see as warning signs for such a tragic event as suicide (Ojagbemi et al., 2013).

Second, many older adults simply do not discuss their mental health problems with anyone for fear of hospitalization or stigmatization within the families and communities in which they live. They suffer quietly from what may be a clearly treatable mood or anxiety disorder. Even when concerned family members and caregivers inquire about depression or suicidal thoughts, older adults may not disclose the severity of their symptoms for fear of someone taking control of their lives (Kjølseth et al., 2010).

Occasionally, older adults do present to their primary care physicians or local emergency rooms with complaints of suicidal thoughts. These people should always be taken very seriously, not only in view of the high suicide rates in this age group, but also because they may have contemplated suicide for many months or years prior to talking about it or seeking help. Their clinical presentation may only indicate fleeting suicidal thoughts or hopelessness, but it should be assumed that what is shared or uncovered in the clinical encounter is only the tip of the iceberg (Waern et al., 1996). The cumulative effect of various losses over years, accompanied by social isolation, physical health problems, and financial stressors, make older adults particularly vulnerable to quickly shifting from contemplating suicide to attempting it.

Additionally, people of all ages who present more than once for complaints of, or concerns about, suicide should be taken very seriously. Even if these complaints include what may sound like benign, generalized statements such as, "I don't feel like going on sometimes," or "I don't want to be a burden to my family," these and similar statements should be viewed as indicators of what may be a much deeper degree of depression, hopelessness, and suicide risk in older adults. Determining what is a "cry for help" or "attention-seeking behavior," as opposed to what constitutes a truly suicidal thought or statement, can be quite difficult even for trained professionals (World Health Organization, 2002).

Certainly, people who have attempted suicide repeatedly are at increased risk for completing suicide (Demircin et al., 2011). Some clinicians maintain that previous suicide attempts are the number one risk factor for completed suicide, but others argue against using individual risk factors to forecast future suicide, fearing it is too simplistic to apply to the complex emotional lives of older adults. Evaluating and assessing the *whole* patient—their physical, emotional, and spiritual health, their access to social support networks, their personal sense of health and well-being—needs to be the work of every clinician who works with older adults.

Older patients should not be dismissed when presenting to a health care professional or family member with repeated thoughts of, or statements about, suicide or death. The old rule of "Better safe than sorry!" should always apply when making treatment decisions for older patients who present with suicidal thoughts or behavior.

SCREENING AND RISK FACTORS

While screening for suicidality is important in all age groups, certain populations with higher rates of completed suicide, such as those aged 65 and older, warrant special attention. In 2012, the National Institutes of Mental Health (NIMH) published a list of risk factors for suicide that include:

- Depression, substance abuse, or other mental health disorders (these risk factors alone can be found in approximately 90% of those who complete suicide) (Moscicki, 2001)
- Prior suicide attempt
- Family history of mental illness or substance abuse
- Family history of suicide attempt or completion
- History of violence in the family such as physical or sexual abuse
- Firearms present in the home (Miller et al., 2006)
- History of incarceration
- Exposure to suicidality in others (family, peer group, media figures) (Moscicki, 2001)

The presence of these risk factors indicates the necessity to take a more thorough psychosocial history when providing assessment or care for older adult patients. While many older adults can have one or more of these risk factors, it does not account for all those who contemplate or complete suicide. Rarely is human behavior so easily quantified.

Researchers continue to attempt to understand complex neurochemical changes that can take place in the brains of people who are suicidal, changes that may be exacerbated by the natural aging process. Such changes, which scientists are increasingly able to measure quantitatively through blood tests and neuroimaging techniques, include elevated serum cortisol, decreased dopamine and norepinephrine, decreased brain-derived neurotrophic factor (BDNF), increased inflammatory cytokines, and decreased levels of serotonin. Low serotonin levels have been found in people with depression, disorders of impulsivity, and those with a history of suicide, as well as in the brains of suicide victims (Arango et al., 2003).

In the not so distant future, it may considered standard of care, and economically feasible, to screen people for various forms of mental illness through blood and genetic testing or neuroimaging. Currently, the most common and effective way to screen older adults for suicidality in the health care setting is through clinical inquiry. When one or more of the above-identified risk factors is discovered in the clinical encounter with an older adult, directly questioning the patient about their feelings of hopelessness, despair, or suicide should be carefully undertaken and documented. Health care providers may be the only people to whom older adults open up about their emotional fears and despair, fearing judgment, misunderstanding, and overreaction on the part of family or friends.

Various rating scales exist that can be administered to patients in order to assess suicidality, though the practicality of these in the clinical setting is debated, particularly as the time a health care provider actually spends with his or her patients gets shorter. Such scales include the Suicide Behaviors Questionnaire-Revised (SBQ-R), the Positive and Negative Suicide Ideation Inventory (PANSI), the Beck Scale for Suicide Ideation (BSS), and the Suicidal Ideation Questionnaire (SIQ), to name a few.

The SBQ-R, developed by Augustine Osman and colleagues, is particularly useful in the clinical setting and is easily administered (see Fig. 27.1). It contains four separate items that tap into

The Suicide Behaviors Questionnaire-Revised (SBQ-R) - Overview

The SBQ-R has 4 items, each tapping a different dimension of suicidality:[1]
- Item 1 taps into lifetime suicide ideation and/or suicide attempt.
- Item 2 assesses the frequency of suicidal ideation over the past twelve months.
- Item 3 assesses the threat of suicide attempt.
- Item 4 evaluates self-reported likelihood of suicidal behavior in the future.

Clinical Utility

Due to the wording of the four SBQ-R items, a broad range of information is obtained in a very brief administration. Responses can be used to identify at-risk individuals and specific risk behaviors.

Scoring

See scoring guideline on following page.

Psychometric Properties[1]

	Cutoff score	Sensitivity	Specificity
Adult General Population	≥7	93%	95%
Adult Psychiatric Inpatients	≥8	80%	91%

1. Osman A, Bagge CL, Guitierrez PM, Konick LC, Kooper BA, Barrios FX., The Suicidal Behaviors Questionnaire-Revised (SBQ-R): Validation with clinical and nonclinical samples, Assessment, 2001, (5), 443-454.

FIGURE 27.1. The Suicide Behaviors Questionnaire-Revised (SBQ-R)—Overview. From Osman, A., Bagge, C. L., Gutierrez, P. M., Konick, L. C., Kooper, B. A., & Barrios, F. X. (2001). The Suicidal Behaviors Questionnaire–Revised (SBQ-R): Validation with clinical and nonclinical samples. *Assessment, 8*(4), 443–454, with permission.

SBQ-R - Scoring

Item 1: taps into *lifetime* suicide ideation and/or suicide attempts			
Selected response 1	Non-Suicidal subgroup	1 point	
Selected response 2	Suicide Risk Ideation subgroup	2 points	
Selected response 3a or 3b	Suicide Plan subgroup	3 points	_____
Selected response 4a or 4b	Suicide Attempt subgroup	4 points	**Total Points**

Item 2: assesses the *frequency* of suicidal *ideation* over the past 12 months			
Selected Response:	Never	1 point	
	Rarely (1 time)	2 points	
	Sometimes (2 times)	3 points	
	Often (3-4 times)	4 points	_____
	Very Often (5 or more times)	5 points	**Total Points**

Item 3: taps into the *threat of* suicide *attempt*		
Selected response 1	1 point	
Selected response 2a or 2b	2 points	_____
Selected response 3a or 3b	3 points	**Total Points**

Item 4: evaluates *self-reported likelihood* of suicidal behavior in the future		
Selected Response:	Never	0 points	
	No chance at all	1 point	
	Rather unlikely	2 points	
	Unlikely	3 points	
	Likely	4 points	
	Rather Likely	5 points	_____
	Very Likely	6 points	**Total Points**

Sum all the scores circled/checked by the respondents.
The total score should range from 3-18.

_____
Total Score

AUC = **A**rea **U**nder the Receiver Operating Characteristic **C**urve; the area measures discrimination, that is, the ability of the test to correctly classify those with and without the risk. [.90-1.0 = Excellent; .80-.90 = Good; .70-.80 = Fair; .60-.70 = Poor]				
	Sensitivity	Specificity	PPV	AUC
Item 1: a cutoff score of ≥ 2				
• Validation Reference: Adult Inpatient	0.80	0.97	.95	0.92
• Validation Reference: Undergraduate College	1.00	1.00	1.00	1.00
Total SBQ-R : a cutoff score of ≥7				
• Validation Reference: Undergraduate College	0.93	0.95	0.70	0.96
Total SBQ-R: a cutoff score of ≥ 8				
• Validation Reference: Adult Inpatient	0.80	0.91	0.87	0.89

©Osman et al (1999)

FIGURE 27.1. *(Continued).*

SBQ-R Suicide Behaviors Questionnaire-Revised

Patient Name _____ Date of Visit _____

Instructions: Please check the number beside the statement or phrase that best applies to you.

1. Have you ever thought about or attempted to kill yourself? (check one only)

- ☐ 1. Never
- ☐ 2. It was just a brief passing thought
- ☐ 3a. I have had a plan at least once to kill myself but did not try to do it
- ☐ 3b. I have had a plan at least once to kill myself and really wanted to die
- ☐ 4a. I have attempted to kill myself, but did not want to die
- ☐ 4b. I have attempted to kill myself, and really hoped to die

2. How often have you thought about killing yourself in the past year? (check one only)

- ☐ 1. Never
- ☐ 2. Rarely (1 time)
- ☐ 3. Sometimes (2 times)
- ☐ 4. Often (3-4 times)
- ☐ 5. Very Often (5 or more times)

3. Have you ever told someone that you were going to commit suicide, or that you might do it? (check one only)

- ☐ 1. No
- ☐ 2a. Yes, at one time, but did not really want to die
- ☐ 2b. Yes, at one time, and really wanted to die
- ☐ 3a. Yes, more than once, but did not want to do it
- ☐ 3b. Yes, more than once, and really wanted to do it

4. How likely is it that you will attempt suicide someday? (check one only)

- ☐ 0. Never
- ☐ 1. No chance at all
- ☐ 2. Rather unlikely
- ☐ 3. Unlikely
- ☐ 4. Likely
- ☐ 5. Rather likely
- ☐ 6. Very likely

© Osman et al (1999) Revised. Permission for use granted by A.Osman, MD

FIGURE 27.1. *(Continued).*

lifetime suicide ideation and/or suicide attempt, frequency of suicidal ideation over the past twelve months, threat of suicide attempt, and likelihood of suicidal behavior in the future (Osman et al., 2001).

Additionally, measuring depression (Beck Depression Inventory, PHQ-9, HAM-D), hopelessness (Beck Hopelessness Scale), and other related quality of life measures can help identify older adults who are at increased risk for suicide. These may be more easily implemented in clinics especially designed to treat older persons with physical and mental illness ("Geriatric Clinics"), where intakes and evaluations may offer additional time to address specific risk factors in this population. However, nothing replaces the patient–provider relationship, where trust, inquiry, and communication can make the difference between suicide contemplation and suicide completion.

TREATMENT

There is no identified treatment specifically for suicidal thoughts or behavior, as suicide is not a diagnosis but a symptom of a deeper problem. The underlying conditions leading a person to contemplate taking his or her own life are quite varied, so treatment and intervention must be custom tailored.

If symptoms of depression are present in a person who is suicidal, which is often the case, then treatment such as antidepressants and psychotherapy are warranted. All antidepressants now carry warnings about the potential to cause suicidal thoughts, predominantly in children and young people (U. S. Food and Drug Administration, n.d.). At the same time, however, treatment with antidepressants is considered standard of care, first-line treatment for depression with an abundance of scientific literature to support their use in older adults (Alexopoulus et al., 2001; Bottino et al., 2012; Kaplan & Zhang, 2012).

Most selective serotonin reuptake inhibitors (SSRIs) used to treat depression are also used to treat anxiety disorders, so proper dosing and treatment with SSRIs and related medications can significantly reduce depression and anxiety in older adults and thereby reduce or eliminate suicidal thoughts. The medication Lithium, which has been used clinically for over half a century, has specifically been shown to decrease suicidal ideation (Tondo et al., 2001), though it can increase the risk of renal impairment, hypothyroidism, and cardiac arrhythmias. Lithium levels as well as renal and thyroid function must be closely monitored in older adults, and it must not be forgotten that Lithium is quite lethal in overdose.

As discussed earlier, suicidal thoughts sometimes arise quite impulsively in the context of an acute stressor or a chronic stressor with acute exacerbation. An older husband may appear stalwart during his wife's protracted illness, but with her death he can experience a desire to give up on life himself, as well as significant hopelessness, fear, and loneliness. Such mixed feelings can quickly make a person consider suicide a viable alternative (Almeida et al., 2012).

The same is true when an older person suffers other acute losses or stressors, including problems in physical health, finances, living situations, or family conflicts. In such cases, treatment involves concrete and specific interventions to address the stressor at hand. Family members can assist their older parents and grandparents in sorting through challenging financial problems, housing issues, doctor's appointments and the like, all with lifesaving consequences.

Too often, older adults feel lonely, though they frequently do not want to bother family members or friends with things such as financial problems or providing transportation when they are no longer able to drive. Loss of the ability to drive, to be mobile, may symbolize loss of control, even if older adults voluntarily relinquish their driver's license (McNamara et al., 2013). Working with, and encouraging, family members and others to openly discuss these concerns with the older adults they care for can do a lot to prevent emotional suffering and suicide. More than medications alone, providing social support and concrete, case-specific interventions can go a long way in preventing, or alleviating, the hopelessness, fear, and despair that can lead to suicide (Lapierre et al., 2011).

Treatment starts with talking. Open communication about difficult issues such as depression, suicidal thoughts, hopelessness, fear, and despair can be difficult but lifesaving. Sometimes, even well-meaning families can keep communication with their older family members fairly superficial, fearing that mentioning a difficult or sensitive issue may upset or anger their older loved one. On the contrary, failure to validate and discuss the tough issues that older people face can leave them feeling more alone and isolated, thus widening the emotional chasm they may already feel (Almeida et al., 2012). Many people are quite adept at projecting a false façade that everything is fine when clearly it is not. Communication breeds collaboration, collaboration breeds trust, and trust breeds hope. Such hope can make all the difference in saving the life of an older person who might otherwise sink into despair and suicide.

CULTURAL CONSIDERATIONS

While the suicide rate is high among older adults, specific populations of these adults, namely non-Hispanic white males, are at increased risk for completing suicide. This vulnerable group should be closely evaluated for mental health concerns when it comes to screening and prevention of depression and suicide. It is important to keep in mind that non-Hispanic white males aged 85 and older have a suicide rate of 45 per 100,000, over four times the suicide rate of the general US population. Comparatively, American Indian and Alaskan Natives of all ages have a suicide rate of 14.3 per 100,000, while Hispanics, non-Hispanic blacks, Asians, and Pacific Islanders of all ages have lower suicide rates than other races, namely 6.0, 5.1, and 6.2 per 100,000 respectively (NIMH, n.d.). Further research on how different cultures cope with the aging process, mental illness, and suicide could prove helpful.

Looking at other cultural associations with suicide, the practice of "hara-kiri" or "seppuku" (literally "stomach cutting") is a form of ritual suicide used historically by Japanese soldiers to escape capture and imprisonment. It was seen in this historical and cultural context as an act of nobility to prevent captors from trying to extract secret information through torture. Hara-kiri is rarely seen today, though there are still cases of older Japanese persons, or persons intrigued by Japanese culture, committing suicide by this method (Takai et al., 2010). Additionally, Indian women, as a way of showing their loyalty to their husbands, were historically encouraged to throw themselves on their husbands' funeral pyres, a practice that was outlawed during British rule in India in the 20th century (Vijayakumar, 2004). These practices are not normative in regard to the current high suicide rates in most countries, but they do shed light on the complex individual and cultural correlates of suicidal behavior.

In many industrialized nations, older adults often feel like they do not fit into the work force anymore. They feel, or are made to feel, obsolete. This can exacerbate feelings of loneliness, uselessness, and despair. Many modern cultures appear to glorify youth, both subtly through promotion of "anti-aging" products and less subtly through outright age discrimination. While laws to prevent age discrimination can reduce this practice in businesses and government agencies, it is impossible to stop the media promotion of "age-defying" creams and interventions. Attempts at slowing down the aging process and its potential consequences on a person's health, while laudable, may be causing modern societies to subtly convey the belief that the aging process is pathological rather than normal (McIntosh, n.d.).

PREVENTION

No health care provider, family member, or friend can predict the future or read the minds of the older adults for whom they care. After an older person completes suicide, many people involved with that person at multiple levels can feel responsible in some way. They can experience a lot of guilt, believing erroneously that they missed something or failed to do something to prevent the person's suicide. The philosopher and physician Albert Schweitzer once wrote, "How many times have I, standing over the grave of the departed, uttered the words I should have spoken while he were still in the flesh" (Cousins, 1999). His words remind us that the best way to help prevent a person's suicide is to encourage open communication about the very things older people struggle with most.

A physician can treat a patient's hypertension or heart disease, but failing to ask patients about the impact their illness has on their sense of hope and well-being is a failure to practice the true art of medicine. A family member who complains about having to take his older father to so many doctor appointments should be reminded that relying on anyone else for transportation can be humiliating and embarrassing. Declining health, particularly vision or hearing loss, can greatly limit an older person's mobility and socialization, leading to depression, anger, and hopelessness (Pickett et al., 2012). When older adults lose their driving privileges for health reasons, for them it may symbolize no longer being in control of their lives and their future, and that can be a very frightening experience.

It is among the simple, day-to-day interactions with family members, caregivers, and health care providers, rather than during times of crisis, that early detection should begin for problems that may lead an older adult to take his or her own life. Surrounding them with support, love, and compassion as much as possible, and knowing the unique stressors and fears faced by older adults, is the best form of suicide prevention in this age group. If they already feel isolated, scared, and hopeless, the path to suicidal thoughts and actions can be quite short.

If suicidal thoughts or intent are suspected in an older adult, contacting emergency services right away and not leaving the person alone are immediate steps that should be taken. Limiting access to easy means of suicide by removing firearms from the home (Betz et al., 2011), properly disposing of old medications being stored, removing large quantities of pills commonly found in households such as acetaminophen, ibuprofen, and aspirin, removing heavy ropes and ladders that may be lying around in basements or garages, and even hiding car keys can all be effective suicide prevention strategies for those who are thought to be contemplating suicide (Nordentoft, 2007). While these measures may seem extreme in some cases and lead to conflict with the person one is concerned about, such actions communicate concern, compassion, and love, regardless of how they are perceived. It is better to have an angry father who is upset that his gun collection is now locked in the trunk of his son's car than to allow that same father easy access to known lethal means of suicide.

Just as family members often examine their older parents' homes for slippery carpets, sharp-edged furniture, or tripping hazards that can lead to falls, the families of older adults with significant mental health issues, history of suicidal thoughts or attempts, or who have suffered recent losses, should examine their homes and their parent's homes for things that can easily be used to attempt suicide. No one can truly prevent suicide among older adults all the time, but honest, open communication, and removing easy access to things that can be used to commit suicide, can make the difference between life and death (Nordentoft, 2007).

PATIENT EDUCATION COMPONENTS FOR PROVIDERS

Older adults who experience suicidal thoughts can be quite fearful of telling anyone what is on their mind. They may not want to be labeled as "crazy" or be forced to go to a hospital against their will, so they often suffer quietly without anyone knowing the extent of the emotional pain they feel. These people, whether they are patients in a geriatric clinic, parents, friends, or neighbors, should be reminded that during periods of depression, grief and loss, it is common for older adults to examine the meaning of their lives. Sometimes, this even involves having thoughts of death and thoughts of what it would be like to end it all and escape all the pain and loss. Speaking openly about, and attempting to normalize, the things they fear most—being a burden, not being able to care for themselves, losing their mental faculties—can go a long way toward preventing the isolation and hopelessness that can be the precursors of suicide (Lilja & Hellzén, 2008).

Often family members are unsure who to turn to in times of crisis, especially if it is a mental health crisis. Just as local emergency rooms are used for acute illnesses and emergencies, a loved one talking about suicide or wishing they were dead should also be considered an emergency. In such cases where acute risk for suicide is suspected in an older adult, the family member or health care provider, who suspects suicide, should seek immediate emergency attention and make sure the potentially suicidal person is not left alone (Oude Voshaar et al., 2011). If that person refuses to go to the emergency room for assessment, calling 911 or local emergency responders is always recommended.

When an older person who is suicidal learns that his or her plan to end their life has been discovered, they can try very hard to negotiate and avoid being evaluated by a mental health profession. They can be angry and resentful and make all kinds of promises or threats to avoid getting proper assessment and treatment, but they need to be evaluated nonetheless. Failure to get immediate help, or to assume too quickly that a suicidal person is telling the truth when they say they did not really mean it, can make the difference between life and death. Few families are truly educated about the seriousness of suicidality in older adults, and it may be hard for them to believe that someone they love could contemplate such a radical and distressing thought. It does happen though, all too often. The high rate of completed suicide in older adults speaks to the need for further education about suicide assessment and treatment among patients, family members, caregivers and health care providers (De Leo et al., 2013).

Preventive care in mental health is just as important as it is in physical health. As our aging relatives and patients face increasing fears, loss and change, an honest, open and ongoing dialogue about the potential for depression, anxiety and suicide should begin sooner rather than later. Families do not have to wait until a crisis to begin talking with their older loved ones about their mental well-being, even if that person appears outwardly to be quite stable. Older persons should be encouraged to talk about their fears and concerns openly, and if suicidal thoughts are expressed or suspected then the assistance of a health care professional, whether that be a primary care physician, mental health professional, or emergency care provider, should be sought immediately. Delaying getting help can make a person feel more isolated and may confirm their belief that no one really cares.

The Internet can be a tremendous source of information about suicide in older adults. Professional associations such as the American Psychiatric Association, the American Psychological Association, the National Alliance on Mental Illness, and the National Institutes for Mental Health all have valuable online resources for helping caregivers, family members and health care providers learn more about mental illness and suicidality in older adults. The resources available that can help identify and reduce suicide in older adults are numerous, and all providers who care for this patient population should know how to access these resources in their local communities.

REFERENCES

Alexopoulos, G. S., Katz, I. R., Reynolds, C. F., III, Docherty, J. P., & Carpenter, D. (2001). The expert consensus guideline series. Pharmacotherapy of depressive disorders in older patients. *Postgraduate Medicine, Spec No Pharmacotherapy*, 1–86.

Almeida, O. P., Draper, B., Snowdon, J., Lautenschlager, N. T., Pirkis, J., Byrne, G., . . . Pfaff, J. J. (2012). Factors associated with suicidal thoughts in a large community study of older adults. *British Journal of Psychiatry, 201*(6), 466–472.

Arango, V., Huang, Y. Y., Underwood, M. D., & Mann, J. J. (2003). Genetics of the serotonergic system in suicide behavior. *Journal of Psychiatric Research, 37*, 375–386.

Beekman, A. T., Copeland, J. R., & Prince, M. J. (1999). Review of community prevalence of depression in later life. *British Journal of Psychiatry, 174*, 307–311.

Betz, M. E., Barber, C., & Miller, M. (2011). Suicidal behavior and firearm access: Results from the second injury control and risk survey. *Suicide & Life Threatening Behavior, 41*(4), 384–391.

Bottino, C. M., Barcelos-Ferreira, R., & Ribeiz, S. (2012). Treatment of depression in older adults. *Current Psychiatry Reports, 14*(4), 289–297.

Centers for Disease Control and Prevention, National Center for Injury Prevention and Control. Web http://www.cdc.gov/violenceprevention/pdf/Suicide-DataSheet-a.pdf

Cousins, N. (1999). *The words of Albert Schweitzer*. New York, NY: Newmarket Press.

De Leo, D., Draper, B. M., Snowdon, J., & Kõlves, K. (2013). Suicides in older adults: A case-control psychological autopsy study in Australia. *Journal of Psychiatric Research, 47*(7), 980–988.

Demircin, S., Akkoyun, M., Yilmaz, R., & Gökdoğan, M. R. (2011). Suicide of elderly persons: Towards a framework for prevention. *Geriatrics and Gerontology International, 11*, 107–113.

Inder, K. J., Lewin, T. J., & Kelly, B. J. (2012). Factors impacting on the well-being of older residents in rural communities. *Perspectives in Public Health, 132*(4), 182–191.

Kaplan, C., & Zhang, Y. (2012). Assessing the comparative-effectiveness of antidepressants commonly prescribed for depression in the US Medicare Population. *Journal of Mental Health Policy and Economics, 15*(4), 171–178.

Kjølseth, I., Ekeberg, O., & Steihaug, S. (2010). Why suicide? Elderly people who committed suicide and their experience of life in the period before their death. *International Psychogeriatrics, 22*(2), 209–218.

Kudo, H., Izumo, Y., Kodama, H., Watanabe, M., Hatakeyama, R., Fukuoka, Y., . . . Sasaki, H. (2007). Life satisfaction in older people. *Geriatrics and Gerontology International, 7*, 15–20.

Lapierre, S., Erlangsen, A., Waern, M., De Leo, D., Oyama, H., Scocco, P., . . . Quinnett, P. (2011). A systematic review of elderly suicide prevention programs. *Crisis, 32*(2), 88–98.

Lilja, L., & Hellzén, O. (2008) Former patients' experience of psychiatric care: A qualitative investigation. *International Journal of Mental Health Nursing, 17*(4), 279–286.

Mann, J. J., Apter, A., Bertolote, J., Beautrais, A., Currier, D., Haas, A., . . . Hendin, H. (2005). Suicide prevention strategies: A systematic review. *Journal of American Medical Association, 294*(16), 2064–2074.

McDonald, F. A., Matthews, F. E., Kvaal, K., Dewey, M. E., & Brayne, C. (2007). Prevalence and symptomatology of depression in older people living in institutions in England and Wales. *Age and Ageing, 36*, 562–568.

McIntosh, B. (n. d.). *An employer's guide to older workers: How to win them back and convince them to stay*. Burlington, VT: School of Business Administration, University of Vermont. Retrieved from www.doleta.gov/seniors/other_docs/emplguide.doc

McNamara, A., Chen, G., George, S., Walker, R., & Ratcliffe, J. (2013). What factors influence older people in the decision to relinquish their driver's license? A discrete choice experiment. *Accident Analysis & Prevention, 55*, 178–184.

Miller, M., Azrael, D., Hepburn, L., Hemenway, D., & Lippmann, S. J. (2006). The association between changes in household firearm ownership and rates of suicide in the United States, 1981–2002. *Injury Prevention, 12*, 178–182.

Moscicki, E. K. (2001). Epidemiology of completed and attempted suicide: Toward a framework for prevention. *Clinical Neuroscience Research*, *1*, 310–323.

Nordentoft, M. (2007). Prevention of suicide and attempted suicide in Denmark. Epidemiological studies of suicide and intervention studies in selected risk groups. *Danish Medical Bulletin*, *54*(4), 306–369.

National Institutes of Mental Health. (n.d.). *Suicide in the U. S.: Statistics and prevention.* Retrieved from http://www.nimh.nih.gov

Ojagbemi, A., Oladeji, B., Abiona, T., & Oye, G. (2013). Suicidal behaviour in old age—results from the Ibadan study of ageing. *BMC Psychiatry*, *13*, 80.

Osman, A., Bagge, C. L., Gutierrez, P. M., Konick, L. C., Kopper, B. A., & Barrios, F. X. (2001). The Suicidal Behaviors Questionnaire- Revised (SBQ-R): Validation with clinical and nonclinical samples. *Assessment*, *8*(4), 443–454.

Oude Voshaar, R. C., Cooper, J., Murphy, E., Steeg, S., Kapur, N., & Purandare, N. B. (2011). First episode of self-harm in older age: A report from the 10-year prospective Manchester Self-Harm project. *Journal of Clinical Psychiatry*, *72*(6), 737–743.

Pickett, Y., Raue, P. J., & Bruce, M. L. (2012). Late-life depression in home healthcare. *Aging Health*, *8*(3), 273–284.

Takai, M., Yamamoto, K., Iwamitsu, Y., Miyaji, S., Yamamoto, H., Tatematsu, S., . . . Miyaoka H. (2010). Exploration of factors related to hara-kiri as a method of suicide and suicidal behavior. *European Psychiatry*, *25*(7), 409–413.

Tondo, L., Hennen, J., & Baldessarini, R. J. (2001). Lower suicide risk with long-term lithium treatment in major affective illness: A meta-analysis. *Acta Psychiatrica Scandinavica*, *104*, 163–172.

U. S. Food and Drug Administration. (n.d.). Retrieved from http://www.fda.gov/Drugs/DrugSafety/InformationbyDrug Class/UCM096273

Vijayakumar, L. (2004). Altruistic suicide in India. *Archives of Suicide Research*, *8*(1), 73–80.

Waern, M., Beskow, J., Runeson, B., & Skoog, I. (1996). High rate of antidepressant treatment in elderly people who commit suicide. *British Medical Journal*, *313*, 1118.

Watanabe, N., Takenoshita, Y., Taguchi, M., Oyama, H., & Sakashita, T. (2004). Mental health promotion as suicide prevention. *Geriatrics and Gerontology International*, *4*, S235–S236.

World Health Organization. (2002). *Suicide prevention in Europe: The WHO European monitoring survey on national suicide prevention programs and strategies.* Retrieved from http://www.suicideprevention.ca/wp-content/uploads/2010/05/suicidepreventionineurope.pdf [WHO website].

CHAPTER 27: IT RESOURCES

Websites

American Psychiatric Association
http://www.psych.org/

National Alliance on Mental Illness
http://www.nami.org/

National Institute of Mental Health
www.nimh.nih.gov/

National Institute of Mental Health - Older Adults: Depression and Suicide Facts (fact sheet)
http://www.nimh.nih.gov/health/publications/older-adults-depression-and-suicide-facts-fact-sheet/index.shtml

American Psychological Association
www.apa.org

American Psychological Association - Suicide in the Elderly
http://www.yourmindyourbody.org/suicide-in-the-elderly/

Suicide.org is a nonprofit organization and website supporting suicide prevention, awareness, and support. This link takes you to the resources available to the elderly at risk for suicide.
http://www.suicide.org/elderly-suicide.html

Scholarly articles of Suicide and the Elderly
http://www.suicide.org/elderly-suicide.html

Institute on Aging - Center for Elderly Suicide Prevention and Grief Counseling
  http://www.ioaging.org/services/cesp_suicide_prevention_help.html
International Association for Suicide Prevention (IASP)
  http://www.iasp.info/resources/Groups_at_Risk/Elderly__The/
Suicide Behaviors Questionnaire-Revised (SBQ-R)
  www.ncbi.nlm.nih.gov/pubmed/11785588
Positive and Negative Suicide Ideation Inventory (PANSI)
  www.ncbi.nlm.nih.gov/pubmed/12511018
Beck Scale for Suicide Ideation (BSS)
  www.ncbi.nlm.nih.gov/pubmed/16814632

PDF Documents

This link will take you to the American Association of Suicidology Elderly Suicide Fact Sheet.
  http://www.suicidology.org/c/document_library/get_file?folderId=232&name=
  DLFE-242.pdf
Suicidal Ideation Questionnaire (SIQ)
  www.integration.samhsa.gov/images/res/SBQ.pdf

Videos

Loneliness, Depression and Elderly Suicide (2011)
This video embeds elderly suicide facts with the music "Somewhere over the Rainbow/What a
  Wonderful World" playing in the background. (5:22 minutes)
  http://youtu.be/jyFFQ0xRWsM
Reach Out Speak Up – Suicide in the Elderly
This video is a news segment that was recorded on television. (3:37 minutes)
  http://youtu.be/Jpq0Sn0Tqy4
Preventing Depression and Suicide among the Elderly (2011)
eCareDiary's caregiving expert, Jane Hamilton interviews Dr. Patrick Arbore, Founder and
  Director of The Center for Elderly Suicide Prevention and Grief Related Services, a program
  now of the Institute of Aging. (9:18 minutes)
  http://youtu.be/_udowhnZf4Q
Elderly Suicide Public Service Announcements (PSAs)
These links are to PSAs to raise awareness of elderly suicides.
  http://youtu.be/OlbaOU3STJU (3:11 minutes)
  http://youtu.be/gXsb4e0iPcc (2:21 minutes)
  http://youtu.be/lQ8W40OHX5E (1:07 minutes)

Images

This is a link to Google images for elderly suicide
  http://www.google.com/search?q=elderly+suicide&hl=en&rlz=1T4A
  DFA_enUS417US433&tbm=isch&prmd=imvns&source=lnms&ei=YYBGT-
  feLoH30gGtje2XDg&sa=X&oi=mode_link&ct=mode&cd=2&ved=0CCkQ_AUoATgo&b
  iw=1152&bih=530

Anxiety Disorders

Bush Kavuru, M.D.

INTRODUCTION

Anxiety is the normal physiological response to real or perceived threat, resulting in a flight or fight reaction. The main criteria for generalized anxiety disorder (GAD) as per DSM-IV-TR are excessive anxiety and worry, which is difficult to control, about a number of events or activities. Anxiety disorders are the most common psychiatric problems in young adults and also in later years of life. Unlike the young, anxiety in an older adult may present more with somatic symptoms, focusing on physical illnesses, associated disability, and feelings of vulnerability and avoidance behaviors.

Constant worry, a common symptom of anxiety disorders, does not get as much attention as dementia and depression in older adults. Anxiety in older adults, new onset or chronic in nature, may significantly impact their quality of life (QOL). Disorders of anxiety such as GAD, panic disorder (PD), simple phobia (SP), social phobia, posttraumatic stress disorder (PTSD), and obsessive-compulsive disorder (OCD) are all seen in older adults as frequently as in the young adult population (Smith, 2011).

EPIDEMIOLOGY

Until recently, anxiety disorders drew less attention when compared with dementia and depression in older adults. Based on Epidemiological Catchment Area (ECA) data, the overall prevalence of anxiety disorders in older adults is lower when compared with that in all age groups combined. Findings from National Comorbidity Survey Replication Study (NCS-R) showed that anxiety disorders are very common in older adults although a declining trend in prevalence with increasing age was observed. Among a sample of 2575 adults aged 55 and above from the above study, a twelve month prevalence rates for any anxiety disorder was 14.7% for women, and 7.6% for men. Prevalence rates for any anxiety disorder in this total study population by age range, young-old (55–64) 16.6%, mid-old (65–74) 8.9%, old-old (75–84), and oldest-old (>85), was 8.1%. The DSM-IV diagnoses included in the study were PD, Agoraphobia, Specific Phobia, Social Phobia, and GAD. Specific phobias were more common with a 12-month prevalence rate of 6.5%, followed by social phobia 3.5%, and GAD 2.0% and 2.1% for PTSD respectively. The overall prevalence of anxiety disorders was 12%, twice as much as mood disorders 5% (Byers et al., 2010). Common observations made in this population were as follows: with advancing age, the prevalence of anxiety and mood disorders decreases; anxiety disorders are more common than mood disorders in the older population across the age ranges of young-old to oldest-old; and high rates of coexisting anxiety and mood disorders were observed in this population (Byers et al., 2010).

Another recent study from a community sample of older adults aged 65 and above showed a 12-month prevalence of 2% for specific phobias and 8.7% for subthreshold fears (Schuurmans et al., 2006). New onset of late life anxiety is 11% in older women and 2% in older men. The highest rate of incidence is observed between the years 67 to 81 (Samuelsson et al., 2005). According to data from the Longitudinal Aging Study Amsterdam (LASA), the overall prevalence of anxiety disorders was 10.2%, with a female-to-male ratio of 2:1. The most common anxiety disorder was GAD (7.3%), followed by Phobic disorders (3.1%). Among all anxiety disorders in this population, 50% were GAD, and no relationship was detected between age and the prevalence of anxiety disorders (Beekman et al., 2000; Yates, 2012).

New onset OCD and PD are rare in old age. Prevalence of PTSD, PD, and OCD is lower in older adults when compared with younger age groups (Wolitzky-Taylor et al., 2010). Agoraphobia is considered to be of late onset for those above the age of 65 and has been found to make up approximately 80% of late onset phobias (Livingston et al., 1997).

ANXIETY IN DEMENTIA

Anxiety is seen as a symptom and a risk factor for dementia. High trait anxiety and proneness to psychological distress were associated with dementia (Gallacher et al., 2009; Wilson et al., 2005). Anxiety and dementia have a lot of overlapping features. Anxiety is difficult to differentiate from depression and restlessness, impaired concentration seen in dementia. Anxiety symptoms decrease as dementia progresses to severe stages. In preliminary studies with older adults comparing normal controls, older anxious subjects exhibited short-term memory deficits (Mantella et al., 2007). The presence of anxiety symptoms improved the predictive validity of future Alzheimer disease in patients with mild cognitive impairment. This supports testing for cognitive impairment in older patients presenting with anxiety.

Starkstein et al. (2007) proposed criteria to diagnose anxiety in dementia. Three of the five symptoms, restlessness, irritability, muscle tension, fears and respiratory symptoms, along with DSM criteria, are considered diagnostic in older adults (Seignourel et al., 2008). Aphasias in dementia can limit the person's ability to express typical diagnostic symptoms of GAD like uncontrolled excessive worry. Among older adults with dementia, muscle tension along with easy fatigability were seen as diagnostic predictors of GAD (Calleo et al., 2011). Level of education and gender made no difference in the prevalence of anxiety in dementia. Based on critical review of literature when compared with AD patients with vascular dementia, frontotemporal dementia and Parkinson dementia have more anxiety symptoms (Seignourel et al., 2008).

IMPACT ON QUALITY OF LIFE

Recent research has shown that severe anxiety is associated with lower health-related Quality of Life (QOL). Older adults with GAD have lower QOL scores than their healthy peers. GAD-specific symptoms like worrying, restlessness, irritability, muscle tension, and fatigue were the best predictors of disability and QOL in older adults. Apart from the negative impact on QOL, anxiety disorders also contribute to increased morbidity and increased healthcare utilization in terms of frequent visits to emergency room and primary care offices (Porensky et al., 2009).

PATHOPHYSIOLOGY

Anxiety is a normal physiological emotion that is part of the "fight or flight" reaction. Pathological anxiety is an excessive and unwarranted reaction in the absence of a real threat or to an imagined fear. Cognitive behavioral theories of anxiety address the fact that anxiety stems from cognitive perceptions that the world is a dangerous place, leading to maladaptive cognitive, behavioral, and physiological responses like worry, avoidance, and muscle tension. Cognitive behavioral therapy addresses these maladaptive responses and helps the individual in developing adaptive coping strategies (Newman & Borkovec, 1995; Holmes, 2010).

Serotonin and catecholamines also play a role in the pathophysiology of anxiety in older adults. Based upon his study of Yohimbine Induced Anxiety States in patients with panic attacks and healthy subjects, Charney proposed an impairment of presynaptic noradrenergic regulation along with increased sensitivity to augmented noradrenergic function to be the cause in patients with PD (Charney et al., 1984). Based on the receptor type and the brain region involved, serotonin can be both anxiogenic and anxiolytic. Serotonin also has a role in the pathogenesis of anxiety through its modulation of other neurotransmitter systems in the brain (Schatzberg & Nemeroff, 2009). According to functional neuroimaging findings, late life anxiety is probably conditioned by vascular and degenerative changes in an aging brain similar to late life depression (Andreescu et al., 2009).

PRESENTATION OF ANXIETY DISORDER

Anxiety in late life presents with nervousness, somatic complaints of dizziness, and shakiness, unlike in young adults who present with DSM symptoms of "worry." Anxiety can stem from a debilitating illness or fearsome experience and can be overwhelming in older patients. Yet this kind of anxiety or fear may not be given appropriate clinical attention as it is often considered normal in old age (Flint, 2005). These observations suggest that an inquiry into the recent history of medical illness, accidents, falls, etc. should be made when evaluating an older adult for anxiety.

Severe anxiety can present as nervousness in older patients. "Nervousness" can occur owing to preoccupation with a fear of performance or when facing the imagined fear and lead to feelings of helplessness and avoidance behaviors. For more clinical symptoms and signs of anxiety refer to Table 28.1.

The DSM-IV TR Criteria are more specific concerning presenting symptoms accompanying anxiety (DSM-IV TR, 2000). In May 2013 the updated mental health DSM-V will be published.

DSM-IV TR Criteria for Anxiety Disorders

300.02 Generalized Anxiety Disorder

- Excessive anxiety and worry (apprehensive expectation), occurring more days than not for at least 6 months, about a number of events or activities (such as work or school performance).
- The person finds it difficult to control the worry.
- The anxiety and worry are associated with three (or more) of the following six symptoms (with at least some symptoms present for more days than not for the past 6 months). **Note:** Only one item is required in children.
  - restlessness or feeling keyed up or on edge
  - being easily fatigued
  - difficulty concentrating or mind going blank
  - irritability
  - muscle tension
  - sleep disturbance (difficulty falling or staying asleep, or restless, unsatisfying sleep)
- The focus of the anxiety and worry is not confined to features of an Axis I disorder, for example, the anxiety or worry is not about having a Panic Attack (as in PD), being embarrassed in public (as in Social Phobia), being contaminated (as in OCD), being away from home or close relatives (as in Separation Anxiety Disorder), gaining weight (as in Anorexia Nervosa), having multiple physical complaints (as in Somatization Disorder), or having a serious illness (as in Hypochondriasis), and the anxiety and worry do not occur exclusively during PTSD.
- The anxiety, worry, or physical symptoms cause clinically significant distress or impairment in social, occupational, or other important areas of functioning.
- The disturbance is not due to the direct physiological effects of a substance (e.g., a drug of abuse, a medication) or a general medical condition (e.g., hyperthyroidism) and does not occur exclusively during a Mood Disorder, a Psychotic Disorder, or a Pervasive Developmental Disorder.

TABLE 28.1 • Clinical Symptoms and Signs of Anxiety in Older Adults

Subjective Symptoms	Objective Signs
Worry	Restlessness and Pacing
Irritability	Sweating
Fatigue	Muscle Tension
Uneasiness	Tachycardia
Fear	Facial Grimacing
Unrealistic apprehension	
Feeling of nervousness	

Modified from Banazak, D. A. (1997). Anxiety disorders in elderly patients. *Journal of the American Board of Family Practice/American Board of Family Practice, 10*(4), 280.

SCREENING OF ANXIETY

Screening instruments: There are various scales to measure anxiety in older adults with or without dementia. Generalized Anxiety Disorder Severity Scale (GADSS), Geriatric Anxiety Inventory (GAI), GAD-7 (See Fig. 28.1 and Table 28.2 below), Penn State Worry questionnaire,

GAD-7				
Over the <u>last 2 weeks</u>, how often have you been bothered by the following problems? *(Use "✔" to indicate your answer)*	**Not at all**	**Several days**	**More than half the days**	**Nearly every day**
1. Feeling nervous, anxious or on edge	0	1	2	3
2. Not being able to stop or control worrying	0	1	2	3
3. Worrying too much about different things	0	1	2	3
4. Trouble relaxing	0	1	2	3
5. Being so restless that it is hard to sit still	0	1	2	3
6. Becoming easily annoyed or irritable	0	1	2	3
7. Feeling afraid as if something awful might happen	0	1	2	3

(For office coding: Total Score T ___ = ___ + ___ + ___)

FIGURE 28.1. GAD-7 tool. (From Spitzer, R. L., Kroenke, K., Williams, J. B., & Lowe, B. [2006]. A brief measure for assessing generalized anxiety disorder: The GAD-7. *Archives of Internal Medicine, 166*[10], 1092, with permission).

TABLE 28.2 · GAD-7 Scores

GAD-7 Total Scores	Anxiety Severity
0–4	Minimal
5–9	Mild
10–14	Moderate
15–21	Severe

Modified from Spitzer, R. L., Kroenke, K., Williams, J. B., & Lowe, B. (2006). A brief measure for assessing generalized anxiety disorder: the GAD-7. *Archives of Internal Medicine, 166*(10), 1092.

and Geriatric Worry Scale are all used in both clinical and research settings. Among them, The Worry Scale (LaBarge, 1993) and the Rating Anxiety in Dementia (RAID) (Shankar et al., 1999), Neuropsychiatric Inventory (NPI) and Behavioral Pathology in Alzheimer's Disease (BEHAVE-AD) are found to be specific for assessment of anxiety in dementia. Both scales assess various domains such as trait and state anxiety, worry, somatic symptoms, anger and irritability (Seignourel et al., 2008). GAD-7 is a self-reported tool for measuring symptoms of anxiety and has high sensitivity (89%) and specificity (82%) in clinical and research settings (Spitzer et al., 2006).

RISK FACTORS

Beekman et al. (2000), in their pivotal article, based on their data from the LASA study, classified the risk factors for anxiety into two categories: stress-related and vulnerability-related factors. Among stress-related factors, significant association for anxiety was found with recent life events, functional limitations due to physical illness, and a strong link between loss of a partner and PD. Vulnerability-related factors like female sex, low levels of education, loneliness, and an external locus of control showed consistent association with anxiety. A family history of anxiety was also found to be strongly associated with OCD. Overall, vulnerability-related factors were demonstrated to have a dominant causative role in late life anxiety, although stress-related factors also have an important role (Beekman et al., 2000). Significant risk factors were:

- Overall, significant risk factors for anxiety were female gender, having a smaller contact network, recent loss in the family, chronic physical illness, lower level of education, and an external locus of control.
- Comorbid conditions such as gastrointestinal problems, hyperthyroidism, cardiovascular problems, diabetes, Parkinson, and COPD are associated with anxiety. Vestibular symptoms like dizziness and a sense of falling are associated with higher levels of anxiety, and actual occurrences of a fall lead to greater anticipatory anxiety of repeated falls and restricted lifestyle (Wolitzky-Taylor et al., 2010).
- Potential risk factors implicated in late life anxiety disorders were neuroendocrine and immune function, neuroticism, exposure to trauma and genetic predisposition for stress response genes. Protective factors include social support, religiosity, physical activity with cognitive stimulation and coping skills (Lenze & Wetherell, 2009).
- Lack of company and daytime activities, being alone, problems with memory and communication, and dependency on caregivers are all seen as contributing factors for anxiety in geriatric populations (Seignourel et al., 2008).

ASSESSMENT OF ANXIETY

There is an array of confounding factors that may mimic, precipitate and coexist in late life anxiety. Clinicians must conduct a careful and comprehensive history, physical examination, and routing laboratory studies as part of their diagnostic workup (Swinson et al., 2006).

A therapeutic alliance and approach involves tailoring and being mindful of communication with the older adult, keeping in mind generational differences and sensory deficits, that is, vision and hearing. Make certain the adult is wearing a hearing aid or eye glasses. The interviewer should position him or herself in a way that the person can see and hear him/her clearly. Development of rapport is essential, and sometimes begins when welcoming and greeting the patient in the waiting room of an outpatient setting or office. Seniors with accompanying caregivers should feel secure and feel less anxious about the evaluation. Addressing the older patient in a respectful tone as "Madam" or "Sir" and giving them an opportunity to talk without interruption is vital since the older adult may speak slowly and tries carefully to make sure they share all the correct details. Hurrying them along does not help in building a therapeutic relationship. Asking simple, short, and straightforward interview questions would help in getting good history and overall assessments (Wolitzky-Taylor et al., 2010).

Initial evaluation should include an enquiry into detailed psychiatric history, including recent life stressors, issues with social and financial support, physical disability, associated pain issues, and comorbid mental health issues like depression (See Table 28.3). Eliciting the temporal relationship between the onset of anxiety symptoms and precipitating, aggravating, and relieving factors is important, as they are very important in planning treatment interventions. Clinical observations teachthat deteriorating function due to loss of vision and physical disability, inability to get around, and dependency on others can lead to fears of losing independence, being placed in an assisted living or a nursing home. These fears and worries, in turn, cause new onset anxiety and depression in late life.

TABLE 28.3 · Assessment for Anxiety

Medical history
- Current and past medical disorders
- Drug and alcohol use; caffeine intake
- Prescribed and over-the-counter medications; use of herbal or home remedies
- Recent changes in health conditions and their treatment (e.g., change in medications)
- Medications currently being taken—prescribed and over the counter

Psychiatric history and assessment
- Past psychiatric history, including "nervous breakdowns" or other nontreated mental illness
- Rule out mood disorders, psychotic disorders, delirium, and dementia
- Consider changes that may represent subsyndromal conditions or early impairment

Laboratory
- Complete blood count, electrolytes, serum glucose, hepatic and renal function tests, thyroid function tests, vitamin B12 and folate levels, urinalysis, urine toxicology

Other tests
- Electrocardiogram, chest radiograph
- Brain imaging and neuropsychologic testing if cognitive impairment is suspected

Collateral history
- Substantiation of symptom onset, range, duration, intensity by family or close friends
- Long-standing personality, coping, and life history
- Recent events that may contribute

Adapted from Smith, M. (2011). Nursing assessment and treatment of anxiety in late life. In Melillo, K.D. & Houde, S.C. *Geropsychiatric and mental health nursing,* 2nd ed. Sudbury, MA: Jones & Bartlett Learning: 175-202.

The physical exam should focus on general medical conditions causing anxiety like hypo or hyperthyroidism, hypercalcemia, hypoglycemia, and hypoxia. Anxiety can present as a symptom of delirium, dementia, and alcohol and benzodiazepine withdrawal, and should be investigated along those lines. A complete blood count with hemoglobin levels to assess for anemia that can present with fatigability and palpitations and checking for electrolytes to exclude metabolic abnormalities are recommended.

Assessment of anxiety in older adults should follow a multidimensional approach with the clinician probing about patient's capacity to perform Activities of Daily Living (ADL), Instrumental Activities of Daily Living (IADL), medical and mental comorbidities like dementia and substance abuse. Polypharmacy, caregiver, and financial issues should be given attention as these factors can contribute to and exaggerate anxiety.

Presentation of anxiety in late life is different than in the younger population and may not exhibit main DSM symptoms of worry and avoidance, but would express lack of control on the anxiety symptoms. If avoidance is seen, it is more age specific owing to fear of falls or of being attacked and being perceived old and stupid in social situations. The older adult may not self-report anxiety but instead talk about the consequent behaviors and emotions related to anxiety (Mohlman et al., 2012). If the provider develops a therapeutic and nonjudgmental approach, they will best be able to explore this behavior.

TREATMENT

Before beginning treatment for anxiety in older adults, it is essential that the provider rule out comorbid depression, which could be worsened by associated anxiety and vice versa. In their detailed review article, Wolitzky-Taylor et al. (2010) referred to studies showing higher levels of anxiety in depressed older adults with increased suicidality, delayed response to antidepressants, and slow response to augmentation therapy in patients with major depression with comorbid anxiety. Various psychiatric treatment modalities will be discussed.

Cognitive Behavioral Therapy

Clinical experience suggests some older patients can really benefit from cognitive behavioral techniques even though many seek medication management for immediate relief. In their first randomized clinical trial comparing Cognitive Behavioral Therapy (CBT) with enhanced usual care for older adults aged 60 and over with a principal or coprincipal diagnosis of GAD, Stanley et al. (2009) have reported improvement in worry severity, depressive symptoms and general mental health in patients who had received CBT. Along with education and awareness, they have used motivational interviewing, relaxation training, exposure, problem-solving training, and behavioral sleep management as part of the CBT (Stanley et al., 2009). Refer to Chapter 26.

Modular Psychotherapy

Modular psychotherapy was found to helpful for patients with anxiety in primary care settings. When compared with enhanced community treatment, modular psychotherapy was equally effective with improvements in anxiety symptoms, worry, depressive symptoms, and mental health-related QOL. Modules implemented are: (1) Education about anxiety and symptom monitoring. (2) Relaxation training, including diaphragmatic breathing, progressive muscle relaxation, and imagery. (3) Cognitive restructuring. (4) Thought-stopping and scheduled worry. (5) Exposure through systematic desensitization. (6) Behavioral activation, consisting of pleasant events scheduling. (7) Sleep hygiene guidelines. (8) Problem-solving skills training, like learning to specify a problem, brainstorm, evaluate, and implement solutions. (9) Life review, a structured journaling exercise designed to change long-standing negative beliefs. (10) Acceptance, which included mindfulness exercises, discussion of values, and goal setting. (11) Assertiveness training. (12) Time management. (13) Pain management. (14) Relapse prevention. (Wetherell et al., 2005)

Acceptance and Commitment Therapy

Acceptance of negative experiences with psychological flexibility and minimizing the struggle to gain control, along with a focus on one's values and showing commitment to pursue meaningful activities rather than trying to control the negative thoughts is emphasized in this new model of ACT (Wetherell et al., 2011).

Supportive Therapy Techniques

Analogies help in providing insight and educating the person about anxiety. The common analogy the author uses is that *"Anxiety is like a bully; if you run away from it, it can chase you, but if you stand up to it, it will back off."* Another analogy is *"Anxiety is like a big wave of water on the beach, where kids run away and fear drowning, but if you dig your feet in the sand and stand, the wave may drench you, but won't drown you."* Most patients can relate to these analogies and are open to the idea of nonpharmacological methods of treatment such as breathing exercises, relaxation techniques and participate in cognitive behavioral therapies. Panic attacks can be task specific related to an upcoming travel, attending an occasion like marriage, etc. Addressing them with behavioral techniques such as imagery and preemptive problem solving can reduce the level of anxiety.

Psychopharmacology

Treatment of anxiety in older adults is a clinical challenge, and a balanced regimen of pharmacological and nonpharmacological methods is warranted. In a comparative study of patients aged over and under 50, high rates of psychotropic medication use and more severe worry were seen in early onset cases and more functional limitations due to physical problems were seen in late onset patients (Le Roux et al., 2005). Anxiety leading to significant impairment in functioning entails initiation of pharmacotherapy in the geriatric patient.

The standard geriatric psychopharmacology principle "Start low, Go slow" holds good for medications used to treat anxiety disorders in older adults. Selective Serotonin Reuptake Inhibitors (SSRIs) can cause initial activating symptoms, with worsening symptoms of anxiety in some patients, and is a potential reason for discontinuation. Starting with a low dose helps in minimizing these symptoms and improves compliance. Gradual titration to higher doses is suggested along with an explanation to the patients early in treatment that it may take 8 to 12 weeks to show complete therapeutic effects. Patients with incomplete or poor response can benefit from switching to another medication in the same class or another class of medication. Addition of another class drug, including a low-dose benzodiazepine in the short term can help in the beginning stages of SSRI trial. But it is very essential to warn the older adult about the deleterious effects of long-term use of benzodiazepines.

The pharmacokinetics and pharmacodynamics associated with various medications is different in the older adult with resultant side effects at lower doses than in younger adults. Hepatic drug clearance is decreased in the older adults secondary to decreased hepatic blood flow and slower oxidative metabolism of SSRIs by cytochrome P450 system. Plasma levels of citalopram and paroxetine are approximately 100% higher in the older patient compared with the young. This is due to age effect, seen most to least in order of citalopram > paroxetine > fluoxetine > sertraline (Preskorn, 2010). Higher plasma levels of drugs can lead to side effects, a common cause of drug discontinuation early in the treatment. Starting SSRIs on a lower dose can mitigate this effect and improve compliance. As older adults usually take multiple medications, the drug–drug interactions can cause additive effects and metabolic abnormalities like hyponatremia.

Benzodiazepines

Benzodiazepines are still the commonly prescribed antianxiety agents, especially in primary care settings. Benzodiazepines work faster, and using low doses in a short term as adjuvant helps to provide early relief and adherence (Lenze & Wetherell, 2011). As much as they are effective, they are also associated with over sedation, respiratory depression, and increased risk for falls. The risk of hip fracture increases in persons of age 65 and over, with use of higher doses of benzodiazepines and with concomitant use of drugs that interact with them. A 50% increase in the risk of hip fracture was estimated with Alprazolam and interacting drugs (Zint et al., 2010).

United States National Nursing Home Survey indicated that of all the psychotropic drug prescriptions for patients aged 65 or older in 1984, 41% were on antianxiety agents, mainly benzodiazepines (Bogunovic & Greenfield, 2004). Benzodiazepines are associated with multiple side effects like anterograde amnesia, forgetfulness, impaired short-term recall, increased risk of falls, fractures, and road traffic accidents. Chlorodiazepoxide, Diazepam, Flurazepam are more likely to accumulate in the body and cause prolonged sedation because of longer half-lives. Common benzodiazepine withdrawal symptoms in older patients with abrupt cessation include confusion, disorientation, with or without hallucinations. Slow taper is better tolerated than abrupt withdrawal (Bogunovic & Greenfield, 2004). Benzodiazepines are implicated as a cause of dementia in older adults. Prospective studies showed a strong association between use of benzodiazepine and risk of dementia. A 50% increase in risk was found with new and ever use of benzodiazepines (Billioti de Gage et al., 2012).

Selective Serotonin Reuptake Inhibitors

SSRIs that have FDA approval for GAD and Panic are Escitalopram, Fluoxetine, Paroxetine, Sertraline and Citalopram. In a randomized controlled trial in older adults with GAD using Escitalopram 20 mg and a placebo, Escitalopram at a dose of 20 mg had shown response at week 4 and a higher cumulative response at 12 weeks. Fatigue and somnolence were most common adverse effects (Lenze et al., 2009).

Clinical studies with serotonin norepinephrine reuptake inhibitors (SNRIs) such as Venlafaxine XR and Duloxetine were found to be efficacious in persons over 60 years of age. Unlike the younger population, older adults have age-specific side effects with SSRIs and SNRIs like gait impairment, bone loss, clotting impairment, and syndrome of inappropriate antidiuretic horomone secretion (SIADH) leading to hyponatremia (Lenze & Wetherell, 2011).

Apart from benzodiazepines and SSRIs, other pharmacological agents such as Gabapentin and Pregabilin were also tried in the treatment of anxiety. These agents are not FDA approved. A randomized, double-blind, placebo-controlled 8-week trial from the United Kingdom showed efficacy of Pregabilin in the treatment of GAD. Anxiety symptoms responded by 2 weeks, and overall improvement in psychiatric and somatic symptoms was reported. Pregabilin is approved in the European Union within the dose range of 150 to 600 mg/day, and was safe and well tolerated in patients 65 years and older (Montgomery et al., 2008).

Combining medication and therapy is a common treatment strategy in late life anxiety. A randomized controlled trial comparing CBT with Sertraline in older adults with anxiety disorders, Sertraline showed greater efficacy in improving symptoms of "worry" in a dose range of 100 to 150 mg/day. Overall, both treatments showed significant improvements (Schuurmans et al., 2006).

One medication option that can help some patients with severe anxiety is a short-term trial dosing with small amounts of benzodiazepines on an as-needed basis and limiting the total daily dose. One red flag to limit or avoid use of benzodiazepines is current or significant history of alcohol use. Use of SSRIs is the treatment of choice with alternatives such as Hydroxyzine or Tricyclic Antidepressants (TCAs) such as Nortriptyline in occasional cases. See Table 28.4 for a list of antianxiety medications, and Table 28.5 for a list of rules for managing anxiety.

TABLE 28.4 · Antianxiety Medications

Antianxiety Medications	
GAD	Short term: Benzodiazepines
	Long term: SSRIs: escitalopram, sertraline, paroxetine, citalopram and fluoxetine, buspirone
Panic disorder	Short term: Benzodiazepines like lorazepam or clonazepam
	Long term: SSRIs are the drugs of choice. In an open label community study on late life PD, escitalopram was found to have a good safety and efficacy profile along with rapid onset of action when compared with citalopram (Rampello et al., 2006)
OCD	SSRIs (fluoxetine, paroxetine, and sertraline) are drugs of choice, and TCAs like clomipramine have a place as second-line agents in treatment of OCD that has not responded to SSRIs in older adults
Phobia & PTSD	SSRIs (fluoxetine, paroxetine, and sertraline) are preferred in treating phobias and PTSD in older adults as in younger populations

TABLE 28.5 • Rules for Managing Anxiety

Eight Rules for Managing Anxiety Disorders From a Lifespan Perspective

1. Assessment should measure severity and provide objective criteria for assessing response, and should assess comorbidity, prior treatment, cognitive status, and need for a medical workup.
2. Think twice about a benzodiazepine prescription
3. Psychoeducation about anxiety and treatment, including potential health benefits
4. First-line treatment according to patient's preference, provider preference and competence, and treatment availability
5. Frequent follow-up ,particularly within the first month of treatment or dose change, to encourage adherence and monitor treatment response
6. With medications, start low, go slow, but go as aggressively as required to treat symptoms to remission
7. Consider augmentation treatment and refer to experts if necessary
8. Provide maintenance treatment; evaluate the need for such if treatment is discontinued.

Information from Lenze, E. J., & Wetherell, J. L. (2011). A lifespan view of anxiety disorders. *Dialogues in Clinical Neuroscience, 13*(4), 381.

CULTURAL CONSIDERATIONS

Late life anxiety is a common symptom across all cultures. The patient's expression of illnesses and coping mechanisms vary differently and influence diagnosis and management. Anxiety as a symptom can be an indirect expression of need for additional support or help to maintain the daily activities as old age impairs the individual's ability (Banazak, 1997).

Some cultures and families foster mutual dependence where older adults live with their children and grandchildren. In some ways it helps the older adult to feel supported in stressful situations, and in minimizing the anxiety. In general, most older adults live independently and feel vulnerable, and at the same time resist living with family. It is the clinician's responsibility to enquire about and explore the cultural beliefs of the patient as to how they want to spend the later years of their lives.

PREVENTION

Identifying the specific risk factor or perpetuating stimuli that cause the anxiety in the patient can help in developing a focused preventive strategy. Anxiety is a comorbid symptom associated with various physical illnesses that are common in old age and can stem from fear of falls, travel and driving, etc. One of the reasons older adults were better able to control their emotions is construction of favorable environments to promote a sense of well-being (Gross et al., 1997). Environmental manipulation can help in preventing and reducing the level of anxiety. Anxiety due to the fear of falls can be addressed by effecting changes in physical environments and making them safe and secure.

PATIENT EDUCATION POINTS FOR PROVIDERS

It is not unusual to normalize anxiety problems in older adults as part of normal aging. Mixed anxiety and depression is a common occurrence. Anxiety itself can lead to avoidance behaviors and isolation, which in turn can lead to feelings of loneliness and cause depression and worsen existing anxiety. Providers should address these issues from the initial stages of treatment and later as part of relapse prevention. Physical symptoms such as pain, headache, and gastrointestinal symptoms can be exaggerated owing to comorbid anxiety issues, and addressing them simultaneously can help in recovery and regaining health and QOL. Education of patients and caregivers regarding the above issues can improve QOL for patients and reduce caregiver burden.

REFERENCES

Andreescu, C., Butters, M., Lenze, E. J., Venkatraman, V. K., Nable, M., Reynolds, C. F., III, & Aizenstein, H. J. (2009). fMRI activation in late-life anxious depression: A potential biomarker. *International Journal of Geriatric Psychiatry*, *24*(8), 820–828.

Banazak, D. A. (1997). Anxiety disorders in elderly patients. *Journal of the American Board of Family Practice/American Board of Family Practice*, *10*(4), 280.

Beekman, A. T., de Beurs, E., van Balkom, A. J., Deeg, D. J., van Dyck, R., & van Tilburg, W. (2000). Anxiety and depression in later life: Co-occurrence and communality of risk factors. *American Journal of Psychiatry*, *157*(1), 89–95.

Billioti, de Gage S., et al. (2012). Benzodiazepine use and risk of dementia: prospective population based study. *BMJ (Clinical research ed.), 345*, e6231.

Bogunovic, O. J., & Greenfield, S. F. (2004). Practical geriatrics: Use of benzodiazepines among elderly patients. *Psychiatric Services*, *55*(3), 233–235.

Byers, A. L., Yaffe, K., Covinsky, K. E., Friedman, M. B., & Bruce, M. L. (2010). High occurrence of mood and anxiety disorders among older adults: The National Comorbidity Survey Replication. *Archives of General Psychiatry*, *67*(5), 489.

Calleo, J. S., Kunik, M. E., Reid, D., Kraus-Schuman, C., Paukert, A., Regev, T., ... Stanley, M. (2011). Characteristics of generalized anxiety disorder in patients with dementia. *American Journal of Alzheimer's Disease and Other Dementias, 26*(6), 492–497.

Charney, D. S., Heninger, G. R., & Breier, A. (1984). Noradrenergic function in panic anxiety: Effects of yohimbine in healthy subjects and patients with agoraphobia and panic disorder. *Archives of General Psychiatry*, *41*(8), 751.

Diagnostic and Statistical Manual of Mental Disorders, Fourth Edition, Text Revision. Fourth. American Psychiatric Association, 2000. Print.

Flint, A. J. (2005). Generalized anxiety disorder in elderly patients: Epidemiology, diagnosis and treatment options. *Drugs & Aging*, *22*(2), 101–114.

Gallacher, J., Bayer, A., Fish, M., Pickering, J., Pedro, S., Dunstan, F., ... Ben-Shlomo, Y. (2009). Does anxiety affect risk of dementia? Findings from the Caerphilly Prospective Study. *Psychosomatic Medicine*, *71*(6), 659–666.

Gross, J. J., Carstensen, L. L., Pasupathi, M., Tsai, J., Götestam Skorpen, C., & Hsu, A. Y. (1997). Emotion and aging: Experience, expression, and control. *Psychology and Aging*, *12*(4), 590.

Holmes, L. (2010). *Cognitive therapy for depression and anxiety.* Retrieved from http://mentalhealth.about.com/cs/psychotherapy/a/cogtx.htm

LaBarge, E. (1993). A preliminary scale to measure the degree of worry among mildly demented Alzheimer disease patients. *Physical & Occupational Therapy in Geriatrics*, *11*(3), 43–57.

Lenze, E. J., & Wetherell, J. L. (2009). Bringing the bedside to the bench, and then to the community: A prospectus for intervention research in late-life anxiety disorders. *International Journal of Geriatric Psychiatry*, *24*(1), 1–14.

Lenze, E. J., & Wetherell, J. L. (2011). A lifespan view of anxiety disorders. *Dialogues in Clinical Neuroscience*, *13*(4), 381.

Lenze, E. J., Rollman, B. L., Shear, M. K., Dew, M. A., Pollock, B. G., Ciliberti, C., ... Reynolds, C. F., III. (2009). Escitalopram for older adults with generalized anxiety disorder. *Journal of the American Medical Association*, *301*(3), 295–303.

Le Roux, H., Gatz, M., & Wetherell, J. L. (2005). Age at onset of generalized anxiety disorder in older adults. *American Journal of Geriatric Psychiatry*, *13*(1), 23–30.

Livingston, G., Watkin, V., Milne, B., Manela, M. V., & Katona, C. (1997). The natural history of depression and the anxiety disorders in older people: The Islington community study. *Journal of Affective Disorders*, *46*(3), 255–262.

Mantella, R. C., Butters, M. A., Dew, M. A., Mulsant, B. H., Begley, A. E., Tracey, B., ... Lenze, E. J. (2007). Cognitive impairment in late-life generalized anxiety disorder. *American Journal of Geriatric Psychiatry*, *15*(8), 673–679.

Mohlman, J., Bryant, C., Lenze, E. J., Stanley, M. A., Gum, A., Flint, A., ... Craske, M. G. (2012). Improving recognition of late life anxiety disorders in Diagnostic and Statistical Manual of Mental Disorders: Observations and recommendations of the Advisory Committee to the Lifespan Disorders Work Group. *International Journal of Geriatric Psychiatry*, *27*(6), 549–556.

Montgomery, S., Chatamra, K., Pauer, L., Whalen, E., & Baldinetti, F. (2008). Efficacy and safety of pregabalin in elderly people with generalized anxiety disorder. *British Journal of Psychiatry*, *193*(5), 389–394.

Newman, M. G., & Borkovec, T. D. (1995). Cognitive-behavioral treatment of generalized anxiety disorder. *Clinical Psychologist, 48*(4), 5–7.

Preskorn, S. H. (2010). *Applied clinical psychopharmacology*. Retrieved from http://www.preskorn.com/books/ssri_s6.html.

Porensky, E. K., Dew, M. A., Karp, J. F., Skidmore, E., Rollman, B. L., Shear, M. K., & Lenze, E. J. (2009). The burden of late-life generalized anxiety disorder: Effects on disability, health-related quality of life, and healthcare utilization. *American Journal of Geriatric Psychiatry, 17*(6), 473.

Rampello, L., Alvano, A., Raffaele, R., Malaguarnera, M., & Vecchio, I. (2006). New possibilities of treatment for panic attacks in elderly patients: Escitalopram versus citalopram. *Journal of Clinical Psychopharmacology, 26*(1), 67–70.

Samuelsson, G., McCamish-Svensson, C., Hagberg, B., Sundström, G., & Dehlin, O. (2005). Incidence and risk factors for depression and anxiety disorders: Results from a 34-year longitudinal Swedish cohort study. *Aging & Mental Health, 9*(6), 571–575.

Schatzberg, A. F., & Nemeroff, C. B. (Eds.). (2009). *The American psychiatric publishing textbook of psychopharmacology* (4th ed.). American Psychiatric Publishing.

Schuurmans, J., Comijs, H., Emmelkamp, P. M., Gundy, C. M., Weijnen, I., Van Den Hout, M., & Van Dyck, R. (2006). A randomized, controlled trial of the effectiveness of cognitive-behavioral therapy and sertraline versus a waitlist control group for anxiety disorders in older adults. *American Journal of Geriatric Psychiatry, 14*(3), 255–263.

Seignourel, P. J., Kunik, M. E., Snow, L., Wilson, N., & Stanley, M. (2008). Anxiety in dementia: A critical review. *Clinical Psychology Review, 28*(7), 1071–1082.

Shankar, K. K., Walker, M., Orrell, M. W., & Frost, D. (1999). The development of a valid and reliable scale for rating anxiety in dementia (RAID). *Aging & Mental Health, 3*(1), 39–49.

Smith, M. (2011). Nursing assessment and treatment of anxiety in late life. In K. D. Melillo & S. C. Houde (Eds.), *Geropsychiatric and mental health nursing* (2nd ed., pp. 175–202). Sudbury, MA: Jones & Bartlett Learning.

Spitzer, R. L., Kroenke, K., Williams, J. B., & Lowe, B. (2006). A brief measure for assessing generalized anxiety disorder: The GAD-7. *Archives of Internal Medicine, 166*(10), 1092.

Stanley, M. A., Wilson, N. L., Novy, D. M., Rhoades, H. M., Wagener, P. D., Greisinger, A. J., ... Kunik, M. E. (2009). Cognitive behavior therapy for generalized anxiety disorder among older adults in primary care. *Journal of the American Medical Association, 301*(14), 1460–1467.

Starkstein, Sergio E., et al. (2007). The construct of generalized anxiety disorder in Alzheimer disease. *American Journal of Geriatric Psych 15*(1), 42–49.

Swinson, R. P., Antony, M. M., Bleau, P., Chokka, P., Craven, M., Fallu, A., ... Walker, J. R. (2006). Clinical practice guidelines: Management of anxiety disorders. *Canadian Journal of Psychiatry, 51*(Suppl. 2), 1S–91S.

Wetherell, J. L., Lenze, E. J., & Stanley, M. A. (2005). Evidence-based treatment of geriatric anxiety disorders. *Psychiatric Clinics of North America, 28*(4), 871–896.

Wetherell, J. L., Liu, L., Patterson, T. L., Afari, N., Ayers, C. R., Thorp, S. R., ... Petkus, A. J. (2011). Acceptance and commitment therapy for generalized anxiety disorder in older adults: A preliminary report. *Behavior Therapy, 42*(1), 127–134.

Wilson, R. S., Barnes, L. L., Bennett, D. A., Li, Y., Bienias, J. L., de Leon, C. M., & Evans, D. A. (2005). Proneness to psychological distress and risk of Alzheimer disease in a biracial community. *Neurology, 64*(2), 380–382.

Wolitzky-Taylor, K. B., Castriotta, N., Lenze, E. J., Stanley, M. A., & Craske, M. G. (2010). Anxiety disorders in older adults: A comprehensive review. *Depression and Anxiety, 27*(2), 190–211.

Yates, W. R. (2012). *Anxiety disorders*. Retrieved from http://emedicine.medscape.com/article/286227-overview.

Zint, K., Haefeli, W. E., Glynn, R. J., Mogun, H., Avorn, J., & Stürmer, T. (2010). Impact of drug interactions, dosage, and duration of therapy on the risk of hip fracture associated with benzodiazepine use in older adults. *Pharmacoepidemiology and Drug Safety, 19*(12), 1248–1255.

CHAPTER 28: IT RESOURCES

Websites

Anxiety Disorders Association of America
www.adaa.org
National Association of Social Workers
www.socialworkers.org

Geriatric Mental Health Foundation
  www.GMHFonline.org
Anxiety and Older Adults
  http://www.gmhfonline.org/gmhf/consumer/factsheets/anxietyoldradult.html
Epidemiologic Catchment Area Study, 1980–1985
  http://www.icpsr.umich.edu/icpsrweb/ICPSR/studies/6153
Longitudinal Aging Study Amsterdam (LASA)
  http://www.lasa-vu.nl/index.htm
Mayo Clinic – Agoraphobia
  http://www.mayoclinic.com/health/agoraphobia/DS00894
Anxiety Screening Tools
  http://www.integration.samhsa.gov/clinical-practice/screening-tools\
Screening for Generalized Anxiety Disorder (GAD)
  http://www.adaa.org/living-with-anxiety/ask-and-learn/screenings/
  screening-generalized-anxiety-disorder-gad
School Psychiatry Program & MADI Resource Center – Table of All Screening Tools & Rating
  Scales
  http://www2.massgeneral.org/schoolpsychiatry/screeningtools_table.asp
Mayo Clinic - Cognitive Behavioral Therapy
  http://www.mayoclinic.com/health/cognitive-behavioral-therapy/MY00194
National Alliance on Mental Illness – Cognitive Behavioral Therapy
  http://www.nami.org/Template.cfm?Section=About_Treatments_and_Supports&template=/
  ContentManagement/ContentDisplay.cfm&ContentID=7952
Anxiety Self Assessment
  http://anxieties.com/self.php
Acceptance and Commitment Therapy
  http://www.psychologytoday.com/blog/two-takes-depression/201102/
  acceptance-and-commitment-therapy
What is Psychopharmacology?
  http://www.psychologytoday.com/basics/psychopharmacology
Mayo Clinic – Selective Serotonin Reuptake Inhibitors (SSRIs)
  http://www.mayoclinic.com/health/ssris/MH00066
Myths and Facts About SSRIs
  http://www.webmd.com/depression/ssris-myths-and-facts-about-antidepressants
List of SSRIs
  http://www.goodtherapy.org/drugs/antidepressants-ssris.html
Benzodiazepines—Side Effects, Abuse Risk and Alternatives
  http://www.aafp.org/afp/2000/0401/p2121.html

PDF Documents

Anxiety Screening Tool
  http://www.aafplearninglink.org/Resources/Upload/File/Anxiety%20Screen.pdf
GAD-7
  http://www.sfaetc.ucsf.edu/docs/gad-7-print.pdf

Anxiety Assessment
http://www.hopeallianz.com/_pdf/Anxiety2012.pdf
5 Keys to Good Results with Supportive Psychotherapy
http://www.currentpsychiatry.com/pdf/0606/0606CP_Article1.pdf

Videos

A Guide to Cognitive Behavioral Therapy (2011)
The video features Professor Paul Salkovskis, a clinical psychologist and the clinical director of the Centre for Anxiety Disorders and Trauma (CADAT), and Karen Robinson sharing her personal experiences of OCD and CBT. (6 minutes)
http://youtu.be/ds3wHkwiuCo
Emotional Health for Older Adults (2012)
Growing older and the transition from work life to retired life can sometimes lead to depression and anxiety. In this program, we'll talk about emotional wellness for older adults, and see what types of treatment options are available in our region. Guests are from Paris Community Hospital Family Medical Center. (27:30 minutes)
http://youtu.be/ogJ-FQee670

Images

Google images of Anxiety Disorders
http://www.google.com/search?q=anxiety+disorders&hl=en&source=lnms&tbm=isch&sa=X&ei=Sn2aUd_MPIW20QHG84DwBQ&sqi=2&ved=0CAcQ_AUoAQ&biw=1024&bih=564
Google images of Anxiety Assessment Tools for Older Adults
http://www.google.com/search?q=anxiety+assessment+tools+for+adults&source=lnms&tbm=isch&sa=X&ei=LdOnUeO5EKSo0AGu14DQBg&sqi=2&ved=0CAcQ_AUoAQ&biw=1024&bih=564

End-of-Life Care

Katie R. Katz, DNP, FNP-BC, RN

INTRODUCTION

Helping patients to live and die well is an ethical and professional imperative for any clinician. Whether you are a physician, advanced practice nurse (APN), or physician's assistant (PA), all can agree that end-of-life care is an important part of healthcare and that it is imperative to provide the best care possible to all patients and families facing these situations. Many of the professional organizations representing these disciplines have statements that reiterate this concept.

■ The American Medical Association (AMA) Statement on End-of-Life Care
In the last phase of life people seek peace and dignity. To help realize this, every person should be able to fairly expect the following elements of care from physicians, health care institutions, and the community.

Elements:
The opportunity to discuss and plan for end-of-life care. This should include: the opportunity to discuss scenarios and treatment preferences with the physician and health care proxy, the chance for discussion with others, the chance to make a formal "living will" and proxy designation, and help with filing these documents in such a way that they are likely to be available and useful when needed.

Trustworthy assurances that physical and mental suffering will be carefully attended to and comfort measures intently secured. Physicians should be skilled in the detection and management of terminal symptoms, such as pain, fatigue, and depression, and able to obtain the assistance of specialty colleagues when needed.

Trustworthy assurance that preferences for withholding or withdrawing life-sustaining intervention will be honored. Whether the intervention be less complex (such as antibiotics or artificial nutrition and hydration) or complex and more invasive (such as dialysis or mechanical respiration), and whether the situation involves imminent or more distant dying, patients' preferences regarding withholding or withdrawing intervention should be honored in accordance with the legally and ethically established rights of patients.

Trustworthy assurance that there will be no abandonment by the physician. Patients should be able to trust that their physician will continue to care for them when dying. If a physician must transfer the patient in order to provide quality care, that physician should make every reasonable effort to continue to visit the patient with regularity, and institutional systems should try to accommodate this.

Trustworthy assurance that dignity will be a priority. Patients should be treated in a dignified and respected manner at all times.

Trustworthy assurance that burden to family and others will be minimized. Patients should be able to expect sufficient medical resources and community support, such as palliative care, hospice or home care, so that the burden of illness need not overwhelm caring relationships.

Attention to the personal goals of the dying person. Patients should be able to trust that their personal goals will have reasonable priority whether it be to communicate with family and friends, to attend to spiritual needs, to take one last trip, to finish a major unfinished task in life, or to die at home or at another place of personal meaning.

Trustworthy assurance that care providers will assist the bereaved through early stages of mourning and adjustment. Patient and their loved ones should be able to trust that some support continues after bereavement. This may be by supportive gestures, such as a bereavement letter, and by appropriate attention to/referral for care of the increased physical and mental health needs that occur among the recently bereaved. (AMA, 2013)

■ American Nurses Association (ANA) Scopes and Standards of Practice for Advance Practice Registered Nurses and A Position Statement from American Nursing Leaders on Advanced Practice Nurses Role in Palliative Care

The advanced practice registered nurse will make ethical decisions and take ethical actions within his/her realm of practice. The advanced practice registered nurse acknowledges the client's right of self-determination. . . . and respects the client's dignity and cultural belief. (American Nurses Association, 2010)

The advanced practice registered nurse has a master's or doctoral degree in nursing, including a concentration in a specific area of nursing, as well as ongoing clinical experiences. Advanced practice registered nursing has evolved into the roles of Clinical Nurse Specialist (CNS), Nurse Practitioner (NP), Nurse Anesthetist (CRNA), and Nurse Midwife (CNM). APNs who specialize in palliative care are most often academically prepared to serve in the roles of CNS or NP. In addition to direct practice, other roles of the advanced practice nurse include: educator, consultant, researcher, and leader.

While many health care disciplines are concerned about improving care at the end of life, the nursing profession is particularly well suited to lead these efforts in view of the scope and standards of advanced practice. Nursing's social policy statement indicates that nurses "attend to the full range of human experiences and responses to health and illness without restriction to a problem-focused orientation; integrate objective data with knowledge gained from an understanding of the patient's subjective experience; apply scientific knowledge to the processes of diagnosis and treatment; and provide a caring relationship that facilitates health and healing."

Nursing as a discipline is uniquely qualified to provide comprehensive, effective, compassionate, and cost-effective care, and nurses serve as role models for members of other disciplines in promoting quality of life and quality of dying. With advanced knowledge of the physical, emotional, social, and spiritual needs of seriously ill patients, APNs are prepared to model optimal care and to assume leadership roles in palliative care, both in practice and public policy arenas. Surveys indicate that the American public expresses a high level of trust in nurses and their ability to provide valuable life-affirming interventions even as death approaches.

Given that nurses are in every practice setting where patients are cared for and eventually die, advanced practice nurses are uniquely qualified and positioned to address the myriad needs facing individuals with life-limiting progressive illness. Clearly, collaboration with other providers (e.g., physicians, social workers) must occur to attend to these vulnerable patients, but APNs have the knowledge and clinical judgment to prescribe, coordinate, implement, and evaluate a comprehensive plan of care.

All constituencies interested in health care when faced with a life-limiting illness will hope to personally receive care that promotes the quality of every remaining day of life. Advanced practice nurses provide the expert care to make this hope a reality as they "Cure sometimes, relieve often, and comfort always." (*Promoting Excellence,* 2002)

- End-of-Life Guidelines for Ethical Conduct for the Physician Assistant Profession

Among the ethical principles that are fundamental to providing compassionate care at the end of life, the most essential is recognizing that dying is a personal experience and part of the life cycle.

Physician Assistants should provide patients with the opportunity to plan for end of life care. Advance directives, living wills, durable power of attorney, and organ donation should be discussed during routine patient visits.

PAs should assure terminally-ill patients that their dignity is a priority and that relief of physical and mental suffering is paramount. PAs should exhibit non-judgmental attitudes and should assure their terminally-ill patients that they will not be abandoned. To the extent possible, patient or surrogate preferences should be honored, using the most appropriate measures consistent with their choices, including alternative and non-traditional treatments. PAs should explain palliative and hospice care and facilitate patient access to those services. End of life care should include assessment and management of psychological, social, and spiritual or religious needs.

While respecting patients' wishes for particular treatments when possible, PAs also must weigh their ethical responsibility, in consultation with supervising physicians, to withhold futile treatments and to help patients understand such medical decisions.

PAs should involve the physician in all near-death planning. The PA should only withdraw life support with the supervising physician's agreement and in accordance with the policies of the health care institution. (American Academy of Physician Assistants, 2008)

The purpose of this chapter is to discuss the role of the clinician working with patients and families facing the end-of-life, and related topics including:

- Background and History of End-of-Life Care in the United States
- Statistics Related to End-of-Life Care in the United States

- Role of the Clinician in End-of-Life Care
- Common Physiological Changes and Treatment for End-of-Life Care
- Cultural Considerations for End-of-Life Care
- Patient and Family Education and Communication Strategies
- Laws and Ethics in End-of-Life Care
- Provider Orders for Life Sustaining Treatment (POLST) Style Programs
- Advancing Education for Clinicians in End-of-Life Care
- Trending Research Topics in End-of-Life Care

BACKGROUND AND HISTORY OF END-OF-LIFE CARE IN THE UNITED STATES

The philosophy regarding end-of-life care has greatly changed over the years. The term "hospice care" was introduced to modern healthcare providers in 1963 by Cicely Saunders, who founded the first modern hospice in a London suburb. Florence Wald, who was the Dean of the Yale University School of Nursing, became interested in what Saunders was doing. Saunders came to visit Yale and, subsequently, Wald went to the United Kingdom to see the hospice in action. In 1974, after mentoring from Saunders, Wald opened the first hospice in the United States in Branfield, Connecticut (National Hospice and Palliative Care Organization [NHPCO], 2010). In 1969, Elizabeth Kubler-Ross published her famous work, titled *On Death and Dying,* in which she identified the five stages of grieving. It was also in this text that she encouraged care at home, as opposed to institutions, and argued that individuals should have a choice in the decisions that affect their destiny. Kubler-Ross helped begin the process for legislation for hospice in America by testifying before the United States Senate. She is quoted in 1972 as saying,

> We live in a very particular death-denying society. We isolate both the dying and the old, and it serves a purpose. They are reminders of our own mortality. We should not institutionalize people. We can give families more help with home care and visiting nurses, giving the families and the patients the spiritual, emotional, and financial help in order to facilitate the final care at home. (NHPCO, 2010)

Thus, in 1974, the first hospice legislation was introduced. By 1979, there were 26 hospice programs across the country. The Health Care Financing Administration used these first programs to assess the cost-effectiveness and to determine exactly what type of care hospices should provide. In 1982, as part of the passing of the Tax Equity and Fiscal Responsibility Act, the U.S. Congress made provisions to create Medicare hospice benefits and, in 1984, the Joint Commission (JCAHO) initiated hospice accreditation (NHPCO, 2010).

Once the groundwork for hospice care was in place, a slow shift began toward maximizing quality of life for terminally ill individuals, not just those that are imminently dying. The ideas behind this shift led to the palliative healthcare movement. The World Health Organization (WHO) defines palliative care as:

> an approach that improves the quality of life of patients and their families facing the problem associated with life-threatening illness, through the prevention and relief of suffering by means of early identification and impeccable assessment and treatment of pain and other problems, physical, psychosocial and spiritual. (World Health Organization [WHO], 2012)

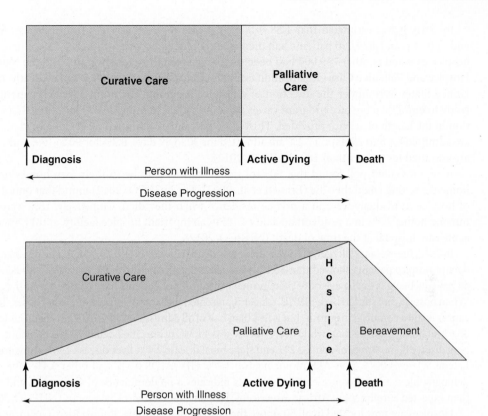

FIGURE 29.1. Comparisons of new versus old models of care at end-of-life.

Emphasizing quality of care throughout the process of end-of-life has been the primary focus in the hospice and palliative care movements. The shifts in this model of healthcare are diagrammed below. The top graph represents the older version of end-of-life care, in which there is an abrupt point at which curative care and end-of-life care meet and also depicts that care ends with death. The lower graph represents the more modern approach, showing that palliative care begins concurrently with curative care and gradually increases as health diminishes to the point of death. Care continues on to the family following the patient's death (Fig. 29.1).

STATISTICS RELATED TO END-OF-LIFE CARE IN THE UNITED STATES

The older population of America, as defined by those 65 years or older, has increased and is expected to steadily rise. In 2009, this population numbered 39.6 million people or 12.9% of the United States population. By 2030, there will be about 72.1 million older people, representing 19% of the population (Department of Health and Human Services, 2011). As advances in healthcare continue, the prevalence of those facing end-of-life decisions will also be increasing.

In 2010, it was estimated that 1.58 million patients received services from hospice. At the end of that year, 1,029,000 patients had died while receiving hospice, while 292,759 remained in hospice care and another 259,000 had been discharged from hospice alive. In 2012, the National Hospice and Palliative Care Organization estimates that approximately 41.9% of all deaths in the United States were under the direction of a hospice program. The point at which patients are ready to enroll in a hospice program varies from individual to individual. Thus, there is a variation in the length of service provided. Thirty-five percent are admitted for less than 7 days, 27% are admitted for 8 to 29 days, 17.2% are admitted for 30 to 89 days, 8.7% for 90 to 179, and 11.8% are admitted for greater than 180 (NHPCO, 2012).

A recent Gallup poll found that 90% of individuals wish to be in their own homes or in a homelike setting when they die (Emnett et al., 2002). The NHPCO (2012) found that only 41.1% of hospice individuals were in a private residence when they died. Conversely, 18% were in a nursing home, 7.3% in a residential facility, 21% in an inpatient hospice facility, and 11.4% in an acute care hospital at the time of death (NHPCO, 2012).

In 2010, the average daily census of a hospice was 117.3 patients (NHPCO, 2012). The demographic data of hospice patients showed that 56.1% were female, compared with 43.9% male, with 82.7% of all patients being over the age of 65. The primary diagnoses of patients have changed over the years. When hospice care started in the 1970s, cancer represented the largest proportion of diagnoses. Today, cancer is still a common diagnosis, but is less than half of all admissions. In 2010, cancer accounted for 35.6% of hospice admissions, while heart disease was 14.3%, unspecified debility 13%, dementia 13%, lung disease 8.3%, stroke or coma 4.2%, end stage renal disease 2.4%, liver disease 1.9%, Amyotrophic Lateral Sclerosis 0.4%, non-ALS motor neuron 1.2%, HIV/AIDS 0.3%, and other 5.4%. The racial demographic data on hospice-enrolled patients indicates a predominance of Caucasians and a less than expected enrollment of African Americans, Hispanics and other racial groups (NHPCO, 2012).

Hospices are now located in all 50 states, the District of Columbia, Puerto Rico, Guam, and the U.S. Virgin Islands, with the number of different programs gradually increasing. In 2010, there were 5,150 different hospice organizations. Most hospices are independent, freestanding agencies (58%), but they can also be part of a hospital system (21.3%), part of a home health agency (19.2%), or part of a nursing home (1.4%) (NHPCO, 2012). Of the over 5,000 hospices in America, 58% are for profit organizations, 36% are not for profit, and 6% are government operated.

COMMON PHYSIOLOGICAL CHANGES AND TREATMENT FOR END-OF-LIFE CARE

Patients' needs at end-of-life can be dramatically varied depending on the underlying disease process. There are texts entirely devoted to advice on managing symptoms at end of life. However, there are some common physiological changes that occur. It is prudent that the clinician know some of the common symptoms, in order that they can be anticipated, explained appropriately to the patient and family, and intervened upon. Which symptoms should be treated and which specific interventions should be provided at end of life must be tailored to each individual's and family's needs. Some of the more common physiological changes are:

General Changes: Pain and Fatigue

Pain can be acute, chronic or a combination of both. This can be directly related to a patient's illness or a side effect from the current or previous treatments. The Agency for Health Care Policy and Research (AHCPR) recommends the mnemonic "ABCDE" for clinically assessing pain. This includes A—*ask* about pain regularly, B—*believe* the patient and family in their reports of pain, C—*choose* appropriate pain control options, D—*deliver* interventions in a timely, logical, and coordinated fashion, and E—*empower* and *enable* patients and families to control their course to the greatest extent that is possible (Fink & Gates, 2006). Treatment of pain is thoroughly discussed in the chapter on pain management.

Fatigue is the "symptom that has the greatest potential for hindering optimism of patients" and should be treated with the same attention as pain and other well-recognized symptoms (Anderson & Dean, 2006). Theories on why fatigue is so prominent in end-of-life care include anemia and systemic inflammation. If possible, fatigue can be treated by removing the causative agent, promoting rest, and the use of pharmacological and non-pharmacological treatments (Anderson & Dean, 2006).

Neurological Changes: Delirium, Confusion, Agitation

Delirium is the most common of the cognitive disorders experienced by patients at end-of-life. Delirium can occur at any age, but is more prevalent among the older adult and those on high doses of opioids. When recognized early, most patients with delirium can be treated. Delirium rarely exists on its own and is often coupled with either confusion, agitation, or both. It is important that the clinician be able to distinguish between delirium and dementia. Common etiologies for confusion are altered laboratory values, infections, sensory changes, malnutrition, medications, setting changes, and physical restraints. Agitation may be observed by the following patient behaviors: anxiety, wandering, pacing, cursing, screaming, arguing, and physical aggressiveness. Providers should eliminate the cause if possible and treat patients' symptoms as desired (Kuebler et al., 2006). One tool that may help providers differentiate between these conditions would be the Confusion Assessment Method (CAM). There are two forms of this screening tool, one for typical use and one specifically for Intensive Care Settings (CAM-ICU). These can be accessed via the www.consultgerirn.org website.

Cardiopulmonary Changes: Dyspnea, Respiratory Secretions, Hiccups

Dyspnea is the common, subjective symptom of having difficulty breathing or shortness of breath. Dyspnea is manifested physically, but also has affective components for the patient and family. These affective components are influenced by an individual's past experiences, whether from watching someone else being dyspneic or themselves. Up to 70% of patients experience dyspnea in the final stages of life. It is important for the clinician to do a thorough clinical assessment and consider the resources available for relieving a patient's symptoms. First-line pharmacologic interventions include the use of opioids, followed by anxiolytics. Patients may also benefit from interventions that could include respiratory treatments and oxygen. There are also very useful nonpharmacological measures including facilitating air movement, such as a simple fan or opening a window (Dudgeon, 2006).

Generally speaking, upper airway secretions do not cause dyspnea, but may be uncomfortable for patients. Lower respiratory secretions can complicate dyspnea and become an evident problem when a patient develops a "death rattle." This is a term that describes the sound produced from the turbulent movement of secretions in the airways of individuals who are actively dying. This sound has been reported in up to 92% of dying patients. One of the best interventions when a patient develops this symptom is to educate the family so that this is not a surprise. Thus, the family knows this is not typically distressing to the patient and they are able to learn proper positioning, using gravity to help minimize airway secretions and noises (Dudgeon, 2006). Additionally, there are pharmacologic approaches to helping manage secretions; the majority of these medications are anticholinergics and thus have typical anticholinergic adverse effects, including confusion, dry mouth, and constipation.

Hiccups occur in up to 20% of palliative care patients. They tend to be more prevalent in cancer patients and children. There are three categories: benign or self-limiting, chronic or persistent, and intractable. The cause of hiccups in palliative care is not well studied but is theorized to be from structural abnormalities, metabolic imbalances, and/or inflammatory and infectious processes. There are both pharmacologic and non-pharmacologic remedies available for treatment (Dahlin & Goldsmith, 2006). Pharmacologic management can include the typical and atypical antipsychotic medications, anticonvulsants, and muscle relaxants.

Gastrointestinal Changes: Dysphagia, Xerostomia, Anorexia, Dehydration, Nausea, Vomiting, and Constipation

Dysphagia, difficulty swallowing food or liquid, is common near the end of life on account of degenerative neuromuscular diseases, progressive disorders of cognitive decline, neoplastic lesions and also from multi-system decline. It can also occur because of side effects from radiation therapy or chemotherapy. The goals for dysphagic patients at end of life are to identify the pathophysiological cause of the disorder, to determine whether short-term interventions can alleviate the problem, and to collaborate with the patient and family on strategies for safe nutrition and hydration. Clinicians should remember their multidisciplinary team of dieticians and speech therapists who can be very helpful at assessing and treating dysphagia (Dahlin & Goldsmith, 2006). Comfort feedings are often offered for patients who are unable to have appropriate oral intake independently.

Some research suggests that up to 55% of patients admitted to palliative care report some degree of xerostomia or subjective dry mouth. The most common causes of xerostomia are decreased salivary secretion, buccal erosion, dehydration, and other miscellaneous disorders. These can include side effects of radiation to the head and neck, medications, infections, hypothyroidism, autoimmune processes and sarcoidosis. Managing xerostomia includes treating or eliminating the underlying cause, stimulating salivation, replacing lost secretions with saliva substitutes, providing good oral care, and/or rehydrating and modifying diet (Dahlin & Goldsmith, 2006).

Anorexia, or the loss of appetite, can lead to protein malnutrition, calorie malnutrition and weight loss, eventually ending in loss of fat and lean muscle mass. Cachexia, often confused with anorexia, is a condition of general ill health and malnutrition marked by weakness and emaciation. Both anorexia and cachexia can cause significant metabolic changes in an individual. They should be identified as early as possible so appropriate, patient-specific interventions can be implemented and further damage avoided (Kemp, 2006).

Nausea, vomiting, diarrhea, dehydration, and constipation can also be common gastrointestinal symptoms in end-of-life care. Nausea and vomiting are very common among cancer patients who are undergoing treatment. These problems can also be cyclical in nature with a patient having vomiting and diarrhea, leading to dehydration and then to constipation. Thus, it is imperative that clinicians work to minimize the causative agent, perform frequent patient assessments and intervene for their patients as necessary for their comfort. If a patient is on a routine opioid, a bowel regimen should be initiated early in order to prevent the onset of constipation and discomfort (Dahlin & Goldsmith, 2006).

Genitourinary Changes: Incontinence and Urinary Tract Infections

Urinary tract disorders that commonly affect end-of-life patients include: urinary tract pain, urinary stasis or retention, hematuria, incontinence, and urinary tract infections. The last disorders mentioned are two of the most common (Gray & Campbell, 2006). Causes of acute urinary incontinence can be remembered with the mnemonic DIAPERS—D: delirium, dementia, diabetes; I: infection, inflammation; A: atrophy of the vaginal tissues; P: pharmacology, psychologic; E: excessive urine output; R: restricted mobility; and S: stool impaction or sacral nerve root compression (Petrou & Baracat, 2001). There are both pharmacologic and nonpharmacologic interventions available, but clinicians should vigilantly assess for complications that warrant treatment. Incontinence has a major impact on quality of life and thus should never be ignored. Patients also require frequent assessment for symptoms of urinary tract infection. And, if early signs such as confusion are ignored, patients can become systemically septic.

Integumentary Changes: Pressure Ulcers, Pruritis

Pressure ulcers are common in end-of-life care even though they are quite preventable. It is with frequent movement that pressure ulcers are minimized. However, prior to repositioning, patients should be assessed for level of comfort and offered interventions for pain relief. If a pressure ulcer does develop, the clinician should advocate for the patient to assure that the wound is kept clean, free of exudates and odor in the hope of promoting healing and prevention of infection. The patient and family should be kept apprised of the plan of care for all wounds (Bates-Jensen, 2006).

Pruritis, or itching, is another common symptom. Pruritis alone does not cause "pain" but can be psychologically, physically, socially, and spiritually distressing. After eliminating causative agents if possible, the clinician can use both local and systemic measures to control this symptom (Rhiner & Slatkin, 2006).

Psychosocial Changes: Anxiety, Depression

Anxiety and depression are common symptoms in individuals as well as families who are facing chronic or life-threatening illnesses. However, these disorders should not be regarded as an inevitable consequence of advancing disease. There is a myriad of pharmacological as well as psychosocial interventions that can be used for treatment of anxiety and depression. Clinicians should be vigilant in monitoring for psychosocial changes and should act early to prevent symptoms from becoming too progressive (Pasacreta et al., 2006).

A member of the interdisciplinary team that can be valuable with psychosocial changes also includes the pastoral care member and/or social worker. Any member of the team can perform a spiritual assessment, but those in pastoral care are often very adept at this skill. It is important to remember the powerful effect that spiritual distress can cause on an individual and/or family and that symptoms may be manifested as agitation, anxiety, depression, etc.

CULTURAL CONSIDERATIONS FOR END-OF-LIFE CARE

As culture is constantly evolving and every situation varies, it is nearly impossible to have a "recipe" to use for end-of-life care. Clinicians working in end-of-life care must always be vigilant to consider the implications of culturally appropriate care. Culture is the "learned, shared and transmitted values, beliefs, norms and life ways of a particular group that guide their thinking, decision, actions in patterned ways" (Mazanec & Panke, 2006). Individuals could be raised in the same household, but, depending on their life experiences, have very different perspectives on life and death. Culture is what shapes how an individual makes meaning out of illnesses, living, dying, etc.

Clinicians should complete a thorough cultural assessment so as to provide the most comprehensively appropriate care to their patients. Components that should be evaluated with culture include: race, ethnicity, gender, age, religion/spirituality, sexual orientation, abilities/disabilities, occupation, and socioeconomic status. These variables can have significance for a patient's preferred methods of communication, privacy, food preferences, rituals, death and mourning practices, pain and symptom treatments, etc. It is important for the clinician working with patients at end-of-life to recognize that one should not generalize culture on the basis of an individual's race, language, religion, or country of origin.

In order to provide culturally appropriate care, it is also advised that clinicians take some time to self-reflect on their own preferences. Being aware of these preferences and biases will help to ensure that the clinician's wishes are not projected onto the patient. When necessary for comprehensive care, the clinician should seek a translator or use a language line to overcome any language barrier. Clinicians should avoid using family members as translators. Clinicians can also consult with leaders of the culture with whom the patient and family most identify.

Little has been studied on the specific psychosocial, spiritual, and cultural disparities in end-of-life care. Evans and Ume (2012) published a recent article that highlighted areas needing future research, but also summarized data from the last 7 years regarding these disparities in end-of-life care. In regard to access to care, African Americans and Hispanics/Latinos have continued to have low utilization rates of hospice. It is theorized that this is because these populations are "family-centered and prefer to avoid disclosure of illness to patients, keep ill loved ones at home, avoid advanced directives, seek aggressive treatment, and distrust the healthcare system" (Evans & Ume, 2012).

Although it is apparent that there are disparities in access to care, health disparities are present in those receiving care as well. A study in 2009 found that African American patients with advanced cancer are less likely than Caucasian patients with advanced cancer to receive the end of life care they initially prefer. Specifically, despite a clear preference for more aggressive end of life care among African Americans, Caucasian patients who preferred intensive care are nearly three times more likely to receive that level of care. With that being said, African American patients are three times more likely than Caucasian patients to receive aggressive life prolonging care at end-of-life. The authors concluded that this is due to African American patients not receiving advanced care planning. This encourages the need for clinicians to improve communication with African American patients regarding care at the end of life (Loggers et al., 2009).

PATIENT AND FAMILY EDUCATION AND COMMUNICATION AT END OF LIFE

In 2003, the American Association of Retired Persons (AARP) performed a survey on advance directives with 804 Minnesota residents. Advance directives are documents used to guide the care of an individual at end of life. The AARP researchers found that 27% of those surveyed had completed some form of advance directive. A majority of those that did not complete an advance directive stated that they did not feel like they needed such a document. Thirty-one percent of the participants felt like they needed it, but had not gotten around to completing it, while 24% felt that it required too much time. Of the remaining respondents, 23% stated that they did not know where to get the documents, and 18% had never even heard of advance directives. Two-thirds of the respondents stated that they had spoken with someone about their wishes for the end of their life with 74% speaking to their spouse, 34% to an adult child, 32% to other family members such as siblings and cousins, 26% to their parents, 21% to friends, 17% to lawyers, 9% to primary physicians, 3% to clergy or priests, and 3% to other healthcare providers such as nurses (American Association of Retired Persons [AARP], 2004).

Since the passing of the Patient Self Determination Act in 1990, few Americans have executed advance directives. The speculated reasons for this include fear, lack of provider information, denial, and lack of readability. Fear of death and dying and avoidance of talking about it are a prevalent issue in American society. Research suggests that less than 23% of Americans have received any information on advance directives from their healthcare providers. Potential interventions for improving use of advance directives include increased direct patient contact, educational methods, and community involvement. Primarily, clinicians need to consider assisting their patients with planning for end-of-life decisions as a necessary element to primary care. It is suggested that the providers ask themselves, "Would it surprise me if this patient were to die in the next 6 to 12 months?" If the answer is no, then discussions about end-of-life wishes and the patient's values need to be assessed immediately (Roessel, 2007).

Clinicians can utilize a value history tool in the primary care setting to assess patients' feelings and attitudes toward healthcare interventions and their quality of life. This tool provides an opportunity for clinicians to teach patients and their families about the importance of discussing advance directives and assessing for end-of-life values and preferences before decisional incapacity becomes a problem (Kupecz, 1991).

A value history begins by identifying patients' views on quality of life. It then assesses their preferences on advance directives and, lastly, evaluates whom they would choose to make their healthcare decisions should they become incapacitated. This should be assessed routinely during office visits as opinions may change throughout a lifespan. There are barriers to the value history tool, namely, clinicians may feel uncomfortable discussing values if they do not feel that adequate rapport has been established. Also, younger adults may not feel the need to consider these possibilities (Kupecz, 1991).

Clinicians not only need to aid their patients in living well, but also need to help them plan to die well. According to research, patients who are facing the end of their life desire help in preparing for their death, want to maintain control, desire to avoid a prolonged dying process, and do not want to feel like a burden. Initiating advance care planning while patients are still able and competent will aid them in achieving these final goals. Once patients are ready to discuss and implement an advance directive, the clinician should not view it as a simple matter of completing a form, as most patients do not wish to rely simply on a document, but rather the provider should view this as an "invitation to a conversation" (Henderson, 2004).

Martha Henderson divided advance care planning, or planning for end-of-life care, into six essential steps. First, she stated that the clinician must accept responsibility; in the role of primary care provider, a clinician may be the only person to discuss advance care planning with a patient. Secondly, true to its name, advance care planning should occur prior to the onset of a critical illness. She identifies five "good" times to initiate this conversation with a patient: routinely in a new patient work-up, when a chronically ill patient is doing well, when a chronically ill patient is beginning to decline, when a patient has been hospitalized and is returning for a follow-up visit, and when a patient mentions death or someone they know who has died. Henderson encouraged holding these discussions with the patient and the family or healthcare proxy so that all parties are up to date. She also suggested routinely discussing the diagnosis, course of illness and prognosis with the patient. In addition, the clinician should become familiar with the patient's priorities, values, and treatment decisions. Once the clinician becomes accustomed to these discussions, he or she will most likely find himself or herself listening to the patient state what is important to them before making any treatment recommendations. Lastly, the clinician must thoroughly document the discussion and all decisions that are made (Henderson, 2004).

An example of another resource for facilitating communication regarding patient wishes at end of life is the "Go Wish Game." This is a tool that was developed by the Coda Alliance of Silicon Valley, California. The game is composed of 36 deck-like cards. Each card has a different value or goal, which are common wishes at end of life, written on each of them, plus one wild card. These values/goals have been written in large print and in common, simple language. The developers wanted this tool to be easily used by elders with vision, hearing, and/or memory impairment and also easily taught to community members and nursing facility workers (Menkin, 2007). The cards can be used in a variety of ways to promote conversations between healthcare providers, patients and families. This game can also be played online for computer-savvy individuals.

A clinician who ignores or fails to discuss their patients' wishes, values, and beliefs for end-of-life care is breaching his or her ethical responsibility (Henderson, 2004). Thus, it is important for all clinicians to stay current on literature and new tools to facilitate advance care planning. Recent literature has supported that personality traits markedly influence an individual's ability to complete end-of-life care planning. The authors suggest that healthcare clinicians evaluate patients' personalities and readiness for end-of-life discussions in order to have successful advance care planning (Ha & Pai, 2012). Another study surveyed over 300 individuals and found that there is a correlation between the deaths of significant others and a patient's personal end-of-life wishes. The author suggests using conversations about others' deaths as a spring board to facilitate discussions about the patient's own desires for end-of-life care (Carr, 2012).

In having discussions about end-of-life wishes and advance care planning, it is important to be aware of the laws and regulations governing the state and facility in which one practices. It is also necessary to know your resources. In the current era of technology, there are many electronic resources to aid in advance care planning. For example, there is a national advance directive registry at http://www.uslivingwillregistry.com/, and many states have their own registries as well. Additionally, there are programs that have been developed for online use to aid in completing advance care planning and also for storing these data. Some of these resources include https://www.makingyourwishesknown.com/ and the Five Wishes program at http://www.agingwithdignity.org/. Integrated e-planning tools can help communicate about end-of-life desires, and also have a growing amount of resources and tools for aiding in patient care (Green & Levi, 2012).

ADVANCE DIRECTIVES/PROVIDER ORDERS FOR LIFE SUSTAINING TREATMENT PROGRAMS

American society rarely engages in discussions related to end-of-life care, and, because of this, there are many times when surrogates are making decisions for patients without actual knowledge of what the patients want. Advance directives, such as living wills and healthcare powers of attorney, are legal documents that are used to assist in directing the healthcare for individuals at the point at which they become decisionally incapacitated. Advance directives originated with the Patient Self Determination Act (PSDA) of 1990, which opposed the culture of medical authoritarianism and nurtured following patients' rights (Knight et al., 2006). When the PSDA was initiated, it was believed that it would not only increase the power and autonomy of the consumer, but would also provide a mechanism for controlling healthcare costs, enhance the potential for beneficence as defined by the patient, and correct the balance between healthcare consumers and providers. However, seventeen years after the PSDA was enacted, less than 25% of Americans had an advance directive (Brown, 1998). More recent data state that, despite wide spread efforts to promote the use of advance directives, only 18% to 36% percent of Americans have completed any advance care planning (Wenger et al., 2008).

Much research has been done on how to facilitate the initiation of advance directives, reasons that individuals do or do not complete advance directives, etc. However, it has now been observed that even when advance directives are completed, the desired outcome of maintaining patients' autonomy does not always carry through to their end-of-life care. The Agency for Healthcare Research and Quality (AHRQ) published a document that reveals that most patients need more effective advance care planning. This is evidenced by their research, which showed that:

- Less than 50% of the severely or terminally ill patients studied had an advance directive in their medical record.
- Only 12% of patients with an advance directive had received input from their physician in its development.
- Between 65% and 76% of physicians whose patients had an advance directive were not aware that it existed.
- Having an advance directive did not increase documentation in the medical chart regarding patient preferences.
- Advance directives help make end-of-life decisions in less than half of the cases where a directive existed.
- Advance directives usually were not applicable until the patient became incapacitated and "absolutely, hopelessly ill."
- Providers and patient surrogates had difficulty knowing when to stop treatment and often waited until the patient had crossed a threshold over to actively dying before the advance directive was invoked.
- Language in advance directives was usually too nonspecific and general to provide clear instruction.
- Surrogates named in the advance directive often were not present to make decisions or were too emotionally overwrought to offer guidance.
- Physicians were only about 65% accurate in predicting patient preferences and tended to make errors of undertreatment, even after reviewing the patient's advance directive.
- Surrogates who were family members tended to make prediction errors of overtreatment, even if they had reviewed or discussed the advance directive with the patient or assisted in its development (Kass-Bartelmes & Hughes, 2003).

Based on data such as that from the AHRQ, a new paradigm for advance care planning has been born. This new paradigm is known by several different names including: Physician Orders for Scope of Treatment (POST), Physician Orders for Life-Sustaining Treatment (POLST), Medical Orders for Scope of Treatment (MOST), and Medical Orders for Life-Sustaining Treatment (MOLST). Programs utilizing this new paradigm began in Oregon in 1995 and have gradually increased in popularity across the United States (History of POLST Paradigm Development,

Center for Ethics in Health Care, Oregon Health & Science University, 2008). Although the names vary, these programs are very similar in both content and goals. The programs consist of a form that a patient completes while they have decision making capabilities and then keeps with him or her in the event of an emergency. The form specifies what a healthcare provider is to do within four different categories of medical treatment: (1) cardiopulmonary resuscitation, (2) the level of medical intervention, which ranges from comfort care to full treatment, (3) the use of antibiotics, and (4) feeding tubes and intravenous fluids, both for long-term and short-term use (Lee et al., 2000).

As this is a new paradigm, the literature is just emerging, but to date the research has supported that POLST style programs help to ensure that patients' wishes for life-sustaining treatments are better honored, while also facilitating end-of-life discussions (Hickman et al., 2009; Lee et al., 2000; Tolle et al., 1998). Hickman et al. conducted a study "to assess use of the POLST by hospice programs, attitudes of hospice personnel toward POLST, the effect of POLST on the use of life-sustaining treatments, and the types of treatment options selected by hospice patients" (Hickman et al., 2009). This descriptive study utilized a telephone survey and on-site chart reviews for data collection. The study was completed from April 2006 to August 2007 in state-recognized hospices in Oregon (n=50), West Virginia (n=21) and Wisconsin (n=68), where POLST programs were already in place. The results of this study were consistent with what the POLST paradigm was created to achieve. Additionally, this study found that providers who work with the POLST program found it to be reliable at predicting patients' wishes, helpful for initiating end-of-life discussions, and helpful at ensuring those patients' wishes are honored. One final impressive result from this study was that 98% of the time, for 250 out of 255 cases, the patients' preferences for treatment limitations were respected (Hickman et al., 2009).

ROLE OF THE CLINICIAN (MD/DO, PA, APRN, ETC.)

The role of the clinician at the end of life is as a holistic team leader for his or her patient's healthcare. Hospice and Palliative Care services include:

- managing the patient's pain and symptoms
- assisting the patient with the emotional, psychosocial, and spiritual aspects of dying
- providing needed drugs, medical equipment, and supplies
- instructing the family on how to care for the patient
- delivering special services like speech and physical therapy when needed
- making short-term in-patient care available when pain or symptoms become too difficult to treat at home
- providing bereavement care and counseling to surviving family and friends (NHPCO, 2012)

It is the role of the clinician to consider all of the aspects of patient care, to help assess the patient and family, identify proper interventions, implement patient wishes as appropriate and constantly re-evaluate progress and future needs. Many individuals will be involved in this care, and the clinician can unify all disciplines into a common goal and thus prevent fragmented care.

The following model was developed by Sally Gaitner Hess in her 2009 graduate work and depicts many determinants that are part of caring for an individual at end of life (Fig. 29.2).

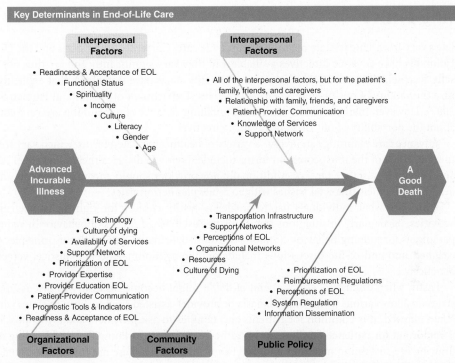

FIGURE 29.2. Key determinants in end-of-life care. (From Hess, S. G. [2009]. *Improving end-of-life care: A public health call to action* [Masters Capstone, Johns Hopkins University]. Retrieved from http://www.jhsph.edu/bin/q/n/Sally%20Hess%20capstone%202009.pdf, with permission.)

Research has supported that nurses are the most likely to broach end-of-life discussions with patients, but that 92% of nurses are in need of further education. APNs, along with all other providers, must take the initiative in learning how to help patients die well by keeping sight of the "big picture." Ditillo states:

> as primary care providers, nurse practitioners specialize in facilitating health promotion and disease prevention as well as the optimal management of various disease states throughout the life cycle. Because death is an inevitable part of life, primary care providers need to plan for optimal dying experiences with their patients. By forming partnerships and having open discussions about dying, providers can understand and honor the wishes of their patients and help them to avoid unwanted dying experiences. This is in keeping with a preventive model of care and focuses on the overall well-being of the patient, encompasses holistic care and respects patient autonomy. (Ditillo, 1999)

It is unfortunate that most patients are not offered an advance directive until they are admitted to the hospital, when individuals' anxieties are already increased. In addition, patients may interpret being asked to complete an advance directive while being admitted to the hospital as a sign that they are sicker than they actually believed. Therefore, this should become part of routine visits to the healthcare system and, consequently, become an early intervention (Ditillo, 1999).

LAWS AND ETHICS

Laws vary from state to state regarding end-of-life care. Currently, all 50 states and the District of Columbia have advance directives available, but they vary significantly and are thus not universally accepted (Roessel, 2007). Forty-two of the fifty states have statements that explicitly recognize the validity of out-of-state advance directives (Department of Health and Human Services, 2007). However, many individuals who are pursuing advance care planning are very concerned about the portability of out-of-state advance directives.

Advance care planning can involve a variety of healthcare related forms, which vary from state to state. Some of the most common forms include: Living Wills, Healthcare Powers of Attorney, and Do Not Resuscitate Orders. Additionally, any provider should encourage patients and families to discuss their financial wishes with an estate planner/attorney.

Ethics are what individuals use to "logically justify choices for right behavior, rules, and activities, particularly in situations that challenge established norms of behavior or require new paradigms for judging behavior" (Stanley & Zoloth-Dorfman, 2006). Ethical principles that are weighed into end-of-life discussions include autonomy, nonmaleficence, justice, veracity, and beneficence.

Lastly, when discussing ethics at end of life, it might become necessary to discuss that some states do allow various forms of euthanasia or provider-assisted suicide. Even in states where this is not allowed, it is common for patients and families to ask providers about this possibility. It is important for patients, families, and healthcare providers to know that withholding or withdrawing life-sustaining measures and provisions for pain relief are not forms of assisted suicide (Volker, 2006). Whether located in a state where this is legal or not, clinicians should respond to requests for assisted dying in a professional manner that reflects the law and guidelines that regulate their practice.

ADVANCING EDUCATION FOR CLINICIANS IN END-OF-LIFE CARE

There are several organizations that individuals may contact for furthering their advanced educational needs for caring for patients at the end of life. One of them is the Center to Advance Palliative Care, commonly called "CAPC," which is "the leading resource for palliative care program development and growth." CAPC is not only a valuable website for knowledge and research, but also has national seminars to further end-of-life education (Center for Advance Palliative Care, 2013).

There are other programs that provide end-of-life training options. Harvard Medical School has a Center for Palliative Care. This organization offers multiple fellowship options as well as seminar presentations on different elements of end-of-life care and end-of-life education (Harvard Medical School Center for Palliative Care, 2013). Northwestern University has a program called EPEC, Education in Palliative and End-of-life Care, that is a "comprehensive, consensus-based, end-user friendly curriculum for the field of palliative care in the United States" (EPEC, 2006). Similarly, the Medical College of Wisconsin has a program entitled EPERC, End of Life/Palliative Resource Center that works to "advance end-of-life care through an online community of education scholars" (EPERC, n.d.).

More specifically, but not exclusively, is a program for nurses and APNs on end-of-life education. This is called ELNEC, End-of-Life Nursing Education Consortium, which is sponsored by the American Association of Colleges of Nursing and also by City of Hope. As of January 2013, more than 15,100 nurses and other health professionals have received training from ELNEC. ELNEC is a conference-based, train-the-trainer program that has multiple focus areas including, core, pediatric, geriatric, veterans, and also advanced practice (ELNEC, 2013).

Physicians are eligible for board certification in Hospice and Palliative Medicine after completing a 12-month fellowship and passing a credentialing examination. Likewise, eligible APNs can become certified by passing a credentialing exam administered by the National Board for Certification of Hospice and Palliative Nurses (Center to Advance Palliative Care, 2013).

TRENDING RESEARCH/LITERATURE IN END-OF-LIFE CARE

Teaching end-of-life care has been a challenge for some, and many programs of medicine allowed it to be more "experienced" than taught. Since the literature suggests that approximately 76% of patients die in a hospital or long-term care setting, it is important for education settings to prepare student clinicians for this role. Some schools of nursing are taking a new approach to teaching end-of-life care and have created end-of-life simulation experiences for students (Moreland et al., 2012; Twigg & Lynn, 2012).

A meta-analysis of data looking at articles related to caregiving at end of life revealed that most of the current data in this realm has been descriptive data with little evidence to guide interventions in best practice. The authors suggest a need for future research on "factors influencing caregivers and roles, information and support needs, caregiver health, end-of-life issues, healthcare disparities, and delivery and costs of care" (McGuire et al., 2012). It is concluded that expanding literature and best practices in these areas would greatly improve caregiver performance and health.

SUMMARY

It is imperative that clinicians working in end-of-life settings be aware of and respect patients' treatment wishes, give attention to the physical, spiritual, and emotional comfort of patients, and work to maintain individuals' dignity and promote quality of life for the patients as well as their families. When working with patients facing end of life, clinicians must be willing to work in an interdisciplinary team that may include the patient, family, nurses, medical staff, volunteers, therapists, home health aids, bereavement counselors, social workers, spiritual counselors, etc. Advanced clinicians are uniquely positioned to help improve the quality of life of patients who face the end-of-life by reducing a fragmented delivery of care.

The Dying Person's Bill of Rights

- *I have the right to be treated as a living human being until I die.*
- *I have the right to maintain a sense of hopefulness, however changing its focus may be.*
- *I have the right to be cared for by those who can maintain a sense of hopefulness, however changing this might be.*
- *I have the right to express my feelings and emotions about my approaching death in my own way.*
- *I have the right to participate in decisions concerning my care.*
- *I have the right to expect continuing medical and nursing attention even though "cure" goals must be changed to "comfort" goals.*
- *I have the right not to die alone.*
- *I have the right to be free from pain.*

- *I have the right to have my questions answered honestly.*
- *I have the right not to be deceived.*
- *I have the right to have help from and for my family in accepting my death.*
- *I have the right to die in peace and dignity.*
- *I have the right to retain my individuality and not be judged for my decisions which may be contrary to beliefs of others.*
- *I have the right to discuss and enlarge my religious and/or spiritual experiences, whatever these may mean to others.*
- *I have the right to expect that the sanctity of the human body will be respected after death.*
- *I have the right to be cared for by caring, sensitive, knowledgeable people who will attempt to understand my needs and will be able to gain some satisfaction in helping me face my death.*

This Bill of Rights was created at a workshop on The Terminally Ill Patient and the Helping Person, in Lansing, Michigan, sponsored by the Southwestern Michigan Inservice Education Council and conducted by Amelia J. Barbus, Associate Professor of Nursing, Wayne State University (The Dying Person's Bill of Rights, n.d.).

REFERENCES

American Academy of Physician Assistants. (2008). *Guidelines for ethical conduct for the physician assistant profession.* Retrieved from https://www.google.com/url?sa=t&rct=j&q=&esrc=s&source=web&cd=1&ved=0CCoQFjAA&url=http%3A%2F%2Fwww.aapa.org%2FuploadedFiles%2Fcontent%2FCommon%2FFiles%2F19-EthicalConduct.doc&ei=DnV6UpzEA-nNsQSI_YHoBg&usg=AFQjCNGVK3qby7CHqJYYEla_ZTL5EGAp9w&sig2=IoWxQPR-YgC6_mJ678oQBQ&bvm=bv.55980276,d.cWc

American Association of Retired Persons, Knowledge Management. (2004). *2003 Minnesota advance directives survey.* Retrieved from http://assets.aarp.org/rgcenter/post-import/mn_advance_directives.pdf

American Medical Association. (2013). *AMA statement on end-of-life care.* Retrieved from http://www.ama-assn.org/ama/pub/physician-resources/medical-ethics/about-ethics-group/ethics-resource-center/end-of-life-care/ama-statement-end-of-life-care.page?

American Nurses Association (2010). *Scope and Standards of Nursing Practice* (2 ed.) Washington DC: Nurse Books.

Anderson, P. R., & Dean, G. E. (2006). Fatigue. In B. R. Ferrell & N. Coyle (Eds.), *Textbook of palliative nursing* (2nd ed., pp. 155–168). New York, NY: Oxford University Press.

Bates-Jensen, B. (2006). Skin disorders: Pressure ulcers—assessment and management. In B. R. Ferrell & N. Coyle (Eds.), *Textbook of palliative nursing* (2nd ed., pp. 301–328). New York, NY: Oxford University Press.

Brown, B. A. (1998). Factors influencing the drafting of advance directives by elders: A quasi-experimental study. *Dissertations Abstracts International* (UMI No. 9950417), *60*(11B). Retrieved from http://stti.confex.com/stti/congrs07/techprogram/paper_31830.htm

Carr, D. (2012). "I don't want to die like that": The impact of significant others' death quality on advance care planning. *Gerontologist, 52*(6), 770–781.

Center to Advance Palliative Care. (2013). Retrieved from www.capc.org

Dahlin, C. M., & Goldsmith, T. (2006). In B. R. Ferrell & N. Coyle (Eds.), Dysphagia, Xerostomia, and Hiccups *Textbook of palliative nursing* (2nd ed., pp. 195–218). New York, NY: Oxford University Press.

Department of Health and Human Services, Administration on Aging. (2011). *Aging statistics.* Retrieved from http://www.aoa.gov/AoARoot/Aging_Statistics/index.aspx

Ditillo, B. A. (1999). Pearls for practice: Planning end of life care. *Journal of the American Academy of Nurse Practitioners, 11*(6), 243–248.

Dudgeon, D. (2006). Dyspnea, death rattle and cough. In B. R. Ferrell & N. Coyle (Eds.), *Textbook of palliative nursing* (2nd ed., pp. 249–264). New York, NY: Oxford University Press.

End-of-Life Nursing Education Consortium. (2013). Retrieved from https://www.aacn.nche.edu/elnec/FactSheet.pdf

Emnett, J., Byock, I., & Twohig, J. (2002). *Advanced practice nursing: Pioneering practices in palliative care.* Missoula, MT: Promoting Excellence in End-of-Life Care, a National Program Office of the Robert Wood Johnson Foundation.

Education in Palliative and End-of-life Care. (2006). Retrieved from http://www.epec.net/

End-of-Life/Palliative Education Resource Center. (n.d.). Retrieved from http://www.eperc.mcw.edu/EPERC/Training/ConferencesandCurriculum/Palliative-Medicine-and-Suppor

Evans, B. C., & Ume, E. (2012). Psychosocial, cultural, and spiritual health disparities in end-of-life and palliative care: Where we are and where we need to go. *Nursing Outlook, 60*(6), 370–375.

Fink, R., & Gates, R. (2006). Pain assessment. In B. R. Ferrell & N. Coyle (Eds.), *Textbook of palliative nursing* (2nd ed., pp. 97–129). New York, NY: Oxford University Press.

Gray, M., & Campbell, F. (2006). Urinary tract disorders. In B. R. Ferrell & N. Coyle (Eds.), *Textbook of palliative nursing* (2nd ed., pp. 265–283). New York, NY: Oxford University Press.

Green, M. J., & Levi, B. H. (2012). The era of "e": The use of new technologies in advance care planning. *Nursing Outlook, 60*(6), 376–383.

Ha, J. H., & Pai, M. (2012). Do personality traits moderate the impact of care receipt on end-of-life care planning? *Gerontologist, 52*(6), 759–769.

Harvard Medical School Center for Palliative Care. (2013). Retrieved from http://www.hms.harvard.edu/pallcare/index.htm

Henderson, M. L. (2004). Nuts and bolts of advance care planning. *American Journal for Nurse Practitioners, 8*(9), 41–52.

Hess, S. G. (2009). *Improving end-of-life care: A public health call to action* (Masters Capstone, Johns Hopkins University). Retrieved from http://www.jhsph.edu/bin/q/n/Sally%20Hess%20capstone%202009.pdf

Hickman, S. E., Nelson, C. A., Moss, A. H., Hammes, B. J., Terwilliger, A., Jackson, A., & Tolle, S. W. (2009). Use of the physician orders for life-sustaining treatment (POLST) paradigm program in the hospice setting. *Journal of Palliative Medicine, 12*, 133–141.

History of POLST Paradigm Development, Center for Ethics in Health Care, Oregon Health & Science University. (2008). Retrieved from http://www.ohsu.edu/polst/developing/history.htm

Kass-Bartelmes, B. L., & Hughes, R. (2003). *Advance care planning: Preferences for care at the end of life* (AHRQ Publication No. 03-0018). Retrieved from http://www.ahrq.gov/research/endliferia/endria.htm

Kemp, C. (2006). Anorexia and cachexia. In B. R. Ferrell & N. Coyle (Eds.), *Textbook of palliative nursing* (2nd ed., pp. 169–176). New York, NY: Oxford University Press.

Knight, P., Espinosa, L. A., & Bruera, E. (2006). Sedation for refractory symptoms and terminal weaning. In B. R. Ferrell & N. Coyle (Eds.), *Textbook of palliative nursing* (2nd ed., pp. 467–489). New York, NY: Oxford University Press.

Kuebler, K. K., Heidrich, D. E., Vena, C., & English, N. (2006). Delirium, confusion, and agitation. In B. R. Ferrell & N. Coyle (Eds.), *Textbook of palliative nursing* (2nd ed., pp. 401–420). New York, NY: Oxford University Press.

Kupecz, D. B. (1991). Planning for decisional incapacity: The nurse practitioner's role. *Journal of the American Academy of Nurse Practitioners, 3*(3), 110–115.

Lee, M. A., Brummel-Smith, K., Meyer, J., Drew, N., & London, M. R. (2000). Physician orders for life-sustaining treatment (POLST): Outcomes in a PACE program. *Journal of the American Geriatrics Society, 48*(10), 1219–1225.

Loggers, E. T., Maciejewski, P. K., Paulk, E., De Sando-Madeya, S., Nilsson, M., Viswanath, K., . . . Prigerson, H. G. (2009). Racial differences in predictors of intensive end-of-life care in patients with advanced cancer. *Journal of Clinical Oncology, 27*(33), 5559–5564.

Mazanec, P., & Panke, J. T. (2006). Cultural considerations in palliative care. In B. R. Ferrell & N. Coyle (Eds.), *Textbook of palliative nursing* (2nd ed., pp. 623–633). New York, NY: Oxford University Press.

McGuire, D. B., Grant, M. G., & Park, J. (2012). Palliative care and end of life: The caregiver. *Nursing Outlook, 60*(6), 351–356.

Menkin, E. S. (2007). Go wish: A tool for end-of-life care conversations. *Journal of Palliative Medicine, 10*(2), 297–303.

Moreland, S. S., Lemieux, M. L., & Myers, A. (2012). End-of-life care and the use of simulation in a baccalaureate nursing program. *International Journal of Nursing Education Scholarship, 9*(1), 1–16.

National Hospice and Palliative Care Organization. (2010). *History of hospice care.* Retrieved from http://www.nhpco.org/history-hospice-care

National Hospice and Palliative Care Organization. (2012). *NHPCO facts and figures: Hospice care in America.* Alexandria, VA: Author.

Pasacreta, J. V., Minarik, P. A., & Nield-Anderson, L. (2006). In B. R. Ferrell & N. Coyle (Eds.), Anxiety and Depression *Textbook of palliative nursing* (2nd ed., pp. 375–399). New York, NY: Oxford University Press.

Petrou, S., & Baracat, F. (2001). Evaluation of urinary incontinence in women. *Brazilian Journal of Urology, 27*(2), 165–170.

Promoting excellence: A position statement from American Nursing Leaders. (2002). Retrieved from http://www.promotingexcellence.org/apn/pe3673.html

Rhiner, M., & Slatkin, N. (2006). In B. R. Ferrell & N. Coyle (Eds.), *Textbook of palliative nursing* (2nd ed., pp. 345–363). New York, NY: Oxford University Press.

Roessel, L. L. (2007). Protect your patients' rights with advance directives. *Nurse Practitioner, 32*, 38–43.

Stanley, K. J., & Zoloth-Dorfman, L. (2006). Ethical considerations. In B. R. Ferrell & N. Coyle (Eds.), *Textbook of palliative nursing* (2nd ed., pp. 1031–1053). New York, NY: Oxford University Press.

The Dying person's Bill of Rights. (n.d.). Retrieved from http://ebookbrowse.com/the-dying-persons-bill-of-rights-114130706-pdf-d183424355

Tolle, S. W., Tilden, V. P., Nelson, C. A., & Dunn, P. M. (1998). A prospective study of the efficacy of the physician order form for life-sustaining treatment. *Journal of the American Geriatrics Society, 46*(9), 1097–1102.

Twigg, R. D., & Lynn, M. C. (2012). Teaching end-of-life care via a hybrid simulation approach. *Journal of Hospice & Palliative Nursing, 14*(5), 374–379.

U. S. Department of Health and Human Services. (2007). *Advance directives and advance care planning: Legal and policy issues.* Retrieved from http://aspe.hhs.gov/daltcp/reports/2007/adacplpi.htm#note81

Volker, D. L. (2006). Palliative care and requests for assistance in dying. In B. R. Ferrell & N. Coyle (Eds.), *Textbook of palliative nursing* (2nd ed., pp. 1067–1075). New York, NY: Oxford University Press.

Wenger, N. S., Shugarman, L. R., & Wilkinson, A. (2008). *Advance directives and advance care planning: Report to congress.* Retrieved from http://aspe.hhs.gov/daltcp/reports/2008/adcongrpt.htm#intro

World Health Organization. (2012). *WHO definition of palliative care.* Retrieved from http://www.who.int/cancer/palliative/definition/en/

CHAPTER 29: IT RESOURCES

Websites

Center to Advance Palliative Care
  http://www.capc.org/
Palliative Care
  http://www.getpalliativecare.org/
National Palliative Care Research Center
  http://www.npcrc.org/
EndLink – Resource for End of Life Care Education
  http://endlink.lurie.northwestern.edu/
The National Hospice and Palliative Care Organization
  http://www.nhpco.org/templates/1/homepage.cfm
Hospice and Palliative Nursing: Scope and Standards of Practice
  http://www.geronurseonline.org/Homepages/HomeLeftMiddle/HospiceandPalliativeNursing.html
Interactive Confusion Assessment Method
  http://www.pogoe.org/content/2783
Caring Connections
  http://www.caringinfo.org/i4a/pages/index.cfm?pageid=3289
The Dying Patient's Bill of Rights
  http://www.support4change.com/index.php?option=com_content&view=article&id=119&Itemid=161
End of Life Resource Page from US Department of Health and Human Services
  http://www.ahrq.gov/populations/eolix.htm

End of Life/Palliative Education Resource Center
  http://www.eperc.mcw.edu/EPERC
End-of-Life Nursing Education Consortium (ELNEC)
  http://www.aacn.nche.edu/elnec
The Patient Self-Determination Act (PSDA)
  http://www.cancer.org/treatment/findingandpayingfortreatment/understanding
  financialandlegalmatters/advancedirectives/advance-directives-patient-self-
  determination-act
Physician Orders for Life-Sustaining Treatment Paradigm
  http://www.polst.org/
RNPedia.com – Pain
  http://www.rnpedia.com/home/notes/fundamentals-of-nursing-notes/pain
Hospice Care including: What is Hospice Care?; When is Hospice Care Appropriate?; How Can
  I Pay for Hospice Care?; Case Study; Where Can I Learn More About Hospice Care?; Other
  Family Counseling and Support Services
  http://www.eldercare.gov/ELDERCARE.NET/Public/Resources/Factsheets/Hospice_Care.
  aspx
Get Palliative Care – Palliative Care Resources including topics such as Advanced Directives,
  Advocacy, Cancer, Caregiver Help, Financial Help, General, Heart, HIV, Hospice, Lung,
  Pediatric Palliative Care, Physicians, Research, Stroke, VA
  http://www.getpalliativecare.org/resources
National Institute of Nursing Research – Palliative Care Brochure
  http://cancer.ucsf.edu/_docs/sms/PalliativeCare.pdf
StopPain.org – Department of Pain Medicine and Palliative Care including the following topics:
  What Is Palliative Care?; Palliative Care for the Patient with Progressive, Incurable Disease;
  Integrating Palliative Care into Current Treatment Models; Palliative Care as a Medical Spe-
  cialty; Palliative Care Resources; Palliative Care Websites; Glossary of Palliative Care Terms.
  http://www.stoppain.org/palliative_care/content/pallcare/palliativecare.asp
Taken from the American Bar Association web site, the Law for Older Americans defines the
  Patient Self Determination Act.
  http://www.americanbar.org/groups/public_education/resources/law_issues_for_consumers/
  patient_self_determination_act.html
The Go Wish Game website
  Go Wish gives you an easy, even entertaining way to talk about what is most important to
  you. The cards help you find words to talk about what is important if you were to be living
  a life that may be shortened by serious illness. Playing the game with your relatives or best
  friends can help you learn how you can best comfort your loved ones when they need you
  most. Go Wish can be played by one, two or more people.
  http://www.gowish.org/

PDF & PPT Documents

Patient Self Determination Act
  http://msdh.ms.gov/msdhsite/_static/resources/75.pdf
Advanced Care Planning
  http://www.abouthf.org/_downloads/module9.pdf

Palliative and End-of-Life Care Toolkit

This toolkit is a collection of online resources to assist nursing faculty members in integrating palliative and end-of-life care (PEOLC) content in their courses. Resources contained in this toolkit include: Search strategies for databases; Journal websites for searching; Professional associations and descriptions of their resources; Strategies for searching the World Wide Web and current online resources; Search strategies for finding textbooks, video clips, and other teaching tools.

http://www.casn.ca/vm/newvisual/attachments/856/Media/PalliativeandEndofLifeCare Toolkit.pdf

Story-based Learning: A Faculty Guide for Nursing Education

A palliative and end-of life care (PEOLC) faculty teaching and learning resource that uses a palliative end-of-life story to demonstrate the use of a unique teaching approach: "story-based learning." The faculty guide explains the six phases of this pedagogical approach: Phase One: Attending to the Story, Phase Two: What is Going On Here?, Phase Three: Recognizing Patterns of Wholeness and Disruption, Phase Four: Nursing Support, Phase Five: Reflection Praxis, and Phase Six: Attending to the Story

http://www.casn.ca/vm/newvisual/attachments/856/Media/StorybasedLearningAFaculty GuideforNursingEducation.pdf

Environmental Scan: Palliative End-of-Life Care Resources

This environmental scan was completed in order to gather existing teaching and learning resources for Palliative and End-of-Life Care. Multiple search strategies were used to gather a wide range of resources relevant to the core PEOLC competencies (Canadian Association of Schools of Nursing (CASN) Task Force on Palliative and End-Of-Life Care, 2009; CASN Palliative and End-Of-Life Care Advisory Committee, 2011). Additionally, course syllabi and teaching and learning tools were sought from nursing schools across Canada in order to understand how Palliative Care is being taught in the undergraduate curriculum.

http://www.casn.ca/vm/newvisual/attachments/856/Media/PalliativeandEndofLifeCare EnvironmentalScan.pdf

Palliative and End-of-Life Care Toolkit

This T/L resource aligns with the Palliative and End-of-Life Care Toolkit document. This PowerPoint provides an overview of the organization, objectives, and content within the resource. http://www.casn.ca/vm/newvisual/attachments/856/Media/V1PalliativeandEnd-ofLifeCareToolkitPowerPoint.ppt

Story-based Learning

This T/L resource corresponds with the "Story-based Learning: A Faculty Guide for Nursing Education" resource, and includes a video component that highlights the key phases of the story-based learning model. http://www.casn.ca/vm/newvisual/attachments/856/Media/V3StorybasedLearningPowerPoint2.ppt

Palliative and End-of-Life Care Entry-to-Practice Competencies and Indicators for Registered Nurses

An Advisory Committee of the Canadian Association of Schools of Nursing (CASN) on Palliative and End-of-life Care (PEOLC) developed national, consensus based competencies and indicators to facilitate greater integration of this area of nursing in undergraduate curricula in Canada. The committee selected the conceptualization of palliative and

end-of-life care used in the Canadian Strategy on Palliative and End-of-Life Care to guide this work. The competencies and indicators were developed through a multistep, iterative, process of literature syntheses and national stakeholder consultations.
  http://www.casn.ca/en/Palliative_Care_122/items/4.html
Palliative Care – What you Should Know
  http://www.getpalliativecare.org/download/GetPCHandout.pdf
Depression in Palliative Care
  http://www.aahpm.org/pdf/depression.pdf
Offering Spiritual Support for Family or Friends
  http://www.caringinfo.org/files/public/brochures/faith_brochure.pdf

E-Book

The Palliative Approach: A Resource for Healthcare Workers (2012)
  This helpful book offers a simple and commonsense introduction to the care of patients in the generalist setting for whom a palliative approach is deemed appropriate. Many of these patients may be living at home or in care homes, and many may be months or even years away from the terminal phase of illness. With the aid of real-life examples and case studies, this text aims to give a wide range of healthcare professionals an understanding of, and competence in, the provision of holistic, supportive care that is focused on comfort and quality of life.
  http://www.amazon.com/The-Palliative-Approach-Healthcare-ebook/dp/B00A3XTA78

Videos

"A Story About Care"
  The Story about Care is one man's reflections on the power of the caring relationship that can exist when people working in health care see the "person and not a pathology." Jim Mulcahy shares his heart touching story of what it has been like to be cared for as he lives with end stage lymphoma while caring for his wife Sarah who has Huntington's disease. This video was produced by the Canadian Association of Schools of Nursing and the Canadian Virtual Hospice in association with the Health Design Lab at St. Michael's Hospital and Wendy Rowland, film maker. We are grateful to Jim and Sarah for opening their home and their lives to us and sharing their story in the service of others (15:43 minutes)
  http://www.casn.ca/en/Whats_new_at_CASN_108/items/117.html
What is Palliative Care? (2011) (2:52 minutes)
  http://video.about.com/healthcareers/What-Is-Palliative-Care.htm
Created by the Center to Advance Palliative Care - Palliative Care State-by-State Report Card Released to Congress (2011) (4:33 minutes)
  http://www.multivu.com/mnr/52418-palliative-care-state-by-state-report-card-nation-improves-regional-gaps
Challenges and Goals of Palliative Care (2009)
  Palliative care aims to prevent and relieve suffering and promote quality of life, at every stage of life, through patient and family care, education, research and advocacy. Join Frank D. Ferris, MD, as he presents information on defining elements of past and modern illness and

various conceptions of suffering. The general concepts of palliative care, as well as the future goals of palliative care will be addressed. (57:49 minutes)

http://youtu.be/9DBMDV4H114

Get Palliative Care Videos, Podcasts & Live Chats

http://www.getpalliativecare.org/videos-podcasts-livechats/

Early Palliative Care: Improving Quality of Life (2010)

A landmark study on the integration of palliative care during early onset of a cancer diagnosis was recently published in the New England Journal of Medicine. Here, lead authors Jennifer Temel, MD, and Victoria Jackson, MD, MPH discuss palliative care and the impressive study findings which showed patients experienced a better quality of life and actually lived longer than patients not receiving the same level of care at an early stage. Jim Windhorst, a stage IV, lung cancer patient describes how palliative care has helped him cope with his illness. (4 minutes)

http://youtu.be/XHtHXGhTIC4

Patient: Palliative helps me live my life the fullest (2010)

Sept. 10: Jim Windhorst, palliative care patient at Massachusetts General Hospital, talks about the acupuncture, physical therapy, and other therapies that help him live with lung cancer. (2:30 minutes)

http://youtu.be/m1ShEqj2c8s

Palliative Care FAQ (2011) (4:30 minutes)

http://youtu.be/7GoAmI06JJc

Palliative Care in Action (2008)

Palliative care in the hospital treats anyone with serious, complex illness - regardless of prognosis. See what it does and how it works. (3 minutes)

http://youtu.be/Bz_hMmnN8Eg

What is Palliative Care? (2011) (1:15 minutes)

http://youtu.be/yVl0llNygCg

Who Should Receive Palliative Care? (2008) (1:07 minutes)

http://youtu.be/vnFHQAzBbZ8

What is the Role of the Palliative Care team? (2011)

Diane Meier, MD, FACP, Director, Center to Advance Palliative Care, explains the key benefits of hospital palliative care. (1 minute)

http://youtu.be/CgXDbOnDa-s

The Journey of Palliative Care (2012)

Explore palliative care, and follow the experience of Joyce Jann and her family, as they work with the palliative care team at Lee Memorial Health System in Fort Myers, Florida. (6:21 minutes)

http://youtu.be/NP6L_st1ANM

Health Matters: Palliative Care and Hospice Services (2010)

Being diagnosed with a life-limiting or terminal illness is devastating for both the patient and their loved ones. Navigating the many options for care can be a frustrating and confusing task. Expert Gary Buckholz, MD, with San Diego Hospice and The Institute for Palliative Medicine, joins our host, David Granet, MD, to discuss both palliative care and hospice and how these services help people by addressing their physical, emotional and spiritual needs. (29:31 minutes)

http://youtu.be/QSKYi5o-sDo

Palliative Care: Improving Quality of Life for People with Serious Illness (2010)
   This video explains palliative care in the words of a palliative care patient and several care
   providers. They will talk about the many facets of palliative care including pain and symptom
   control, the team approach, keeping your own doctor, and communications with patients and
   their family members. (11:35 minutes)
   http://youtu.be/Y4ZsucFf41Q

MOBILE APPS

The American Geriatrics Society Mobile Apps

http://www.americangeriatrics.org/publications/shop_publications/smartphone_products/

Geriatrics At Your Fingertips: Providing high-quality health care for older adults requires special knowledge and skills. Geriatrics At Your Fingertips (GAYF) is an essential tool for all health care professionals and trainees who care for older people. It provides immediate access to the comprehensive information needed to make clinical decisions in a variety of health care settings. Since its initial publication in 1998, GAYF's up-to-date content and portable format quickly made it the American Geriatrics Society's (AGS) best-selling publication.

iGeriatrics: combines all of the American Geriatrics Society's free clinical information offerings into one easy-to-use application. Aimed at health care providers and covering a wide range of topics relating to older adults, from medication safety to cross-cultural assistance, *iGeriatrics* is an excellent introduction to the information and services offered by the AGS. It includes information from the following titles: Beers Criteria; Geriatrics Cultural Navigator; GeriPsych Consult; AGS Pocket Guide to Common Immunizations in the Older Adult; Management of Atrial Fibrillation; Prevention of Falls Guidelines.

Hartford Institute for Geriatric Nursing

http://consultgerirn.org/resources/apps/

The ConsultGeriRN app is designed to help health care professionals with their decision making in providing the best quality care for older adults without needing to leave their side. This mobile reference provides information and tools to treat common problems encountered in the health care of older adults. It is a powerful and readily accessible tool for health care professionals as they meet new situations in everyday practice. It was developed based on the most current evidence-based practice standards for the care of older adults. Current topics include Delirium, Agitation, Confusion, Fall Prevention, and Post-Fall.

Doctot Geriatric App

http://www.doctot.com/doctot-apps/geriatric-app/

Doctot Geriatric is a suite of the most widely used clinician-administered assessment scales related to geriatric patients. Doctot Geriatric affords the medical practitioner a highly efficient and easy-to-use tool to measure important functions of geriatric patients. The interactive scales available in Doctot Geriatric are: Abbreviated Mental Test Score (MTS); Geriatric Depression Scale (GDS); Barthel ADL Rating Scale (Barthel); Elderly Mobility Scale (EMS); and BERG Scale (BERG).

University of Wyoming Apps for Health Care Professionals

http://www.uwyo.edu/geriatrics/resource_center/apps.html

Including: Apps Sources; Apps Reviews; Evaluating Apps; Aging and Geriatric Apps; Drug Information; Journal Articles and Abstracts; Patient Education Information.

Skyscape Apps

http://www.skyscape.com/estore/Store.aspx?Category=59

StallGeriatrics, Innovations in Older Adult Care

http://stallgeriatrics.com/for-everyone/handheld-apps/

Includes: Balance Quiz—screens for balance problems which might predispose to falls; Caregiving Quiz—identifies possible caregiver stress that might lead to premature institutionalization or unnecessary/excessive emergency or hospital visits; Incontinence Quiz—raises awareness of potential causes and treatability of urinary incontinence; Memory Quiz—raises awareness of possible signs of dementia; Mood Analyzer—assesses for possible depression that may be misconstrued as dementia or "old age."

Epocrates

http://www.epocrates.com/mobile/android
https://itunes.apple.com/us/app/epocrates/id281935788?mt=8

Epocrates provides access to thousands of integrated drug monographs and diagnostic tools.

Medscape

http://www.medscape.com/public/iphone
https://play.google.com/store/apps/details?id=com.medscape.android&hl=en

Medscape is the leading medical resource most used by physicians, medical students, nurses, and other health care professionals for clinical information.

FRAX

https://itunes.apple.com/us/app/frax/id370146412?mt=8

The Fracture Risk Assessment Tool (FRAX) is a set of algorithms developed by the World Health Organization to assess an individual's 10-year probability of fracture. An advantage of this algorithm is the ease with which validated clinical risk factors can be entered into the calculation to estimate the probability of hip and major osteoporotic fracture in the next 10 years. Of note, knowledge of the bone mineral density of the femoral neck is not mandatory for the algorithm.

DAS Calculator

https://itunes.apple.com/us/app/das-calculator/id354092306?mt=8

DAS, or "Disease Activity Score," is a measure of the activity of rheumatoid arthritis.

WEBSITES

Administration on Aging
   www.aoa.gov/
AgeNet Eldercare Network
   www.aplaceformom.com
American Association for Geriatric Psychiatry
   www.aagponline.org/
American Association of Hospice and Palliative Medicine
   www.aahpm.org/
American Association of Retired Persons (AARP)
   www.aarp.org
American Association of Retired Persons—Medicare: Get the Facts
   **www.aarp.org/health/medicare-insurance/info-02-2012/medicare-get-the-facts
   .html**
American Association of Retired Persons—Social Security: Get the Facts
   **www.aarp.org/work/social-security/info-02-2012/social-security-get-the-facts
   .html**
American College of Physicians
   www.acponline.org/
American College of Physicians—Clinical Practice Guidelines
   http://www.acponline.org/clinical_information/guidelines/guidelines/
American Geriatrics Society (AGS)
   www.americangeriatrics.org
American Health Care Association
   www.ahca.org
American Medical Directors Association (AMDA)
   www.amda.com
America Society of Consultant Pharmacists
   www.ascp.com
American Society on Aging
   www.asaging.org
Association of Gerontology in Higher Education (AGHE)
   www.aghe.org/
The Care Transitions Program
   www.caretransitions.org/
Center to Advance Palliative Care
   www.capc.org
Centers for Disease Control
   www.cdc.gov
Centers for Disease Control—Healthy Aging
   www.cdc.gov/aging/
Children of Aging Parents
   www.caps4caregivers.org

Clinical Toolbox for Geriatric Care
  www.hospitalmedicine.org/geriresource/toolbox/howto.htm
ConsultGeriRN.org
  consultgerin.org/
Family Caregiver Alliance
  www.caregiver.org
Geriatric Web Resources—University of Tennessee, College of Social Work
  http://web.utk.edu/~scumming/webresources.html
Gerontological Advanced Practice Nursing Association (GAPNA) (formerly known as
  the National Conference of Gerontological Nurse Practitioners)
  www.gapna.org
Gerontological Society of America (GSA)
  www.geron.org
Gray Panthers
  www.graypanthers.org
Hartford Institute for Geriatric Nursing
  hartfordign.org/
Hartford Institute for Geriatric Nursing—Try This Series
  www.hartfordign.org/practice/try_this/
Health in Aging
  www.healthinaging.org
HealthIT.gov
  www.healthit.gov/
Interact: Interventions to Reduce Acute Care Transfers
  interact2.net/
John Hopkins Medicine—Health Alerts
  www.hopkinsafter50.com
MAYO Clinic
  www.mayoclinic.com
MedEdPORTAL—Provided by the Association of American Medical Colleges
  (AAMC) in partnership with the American Dental Education Association (ADEA)
  www.aamc.org/mededportal
The Medicare site
  www.medicare.gov
MERLOT (Multimedia Educational Resource for Learning and Online Teaching)
  www.merlot.org
mmLearn—Caregiver support and training
  www.mmLearn.org
National Academy on an Aging Society
  www.agingsociety.org
National Adult Day Services Association
  www.nadsa.org
National Association of Area Agencies on Aging
  www.n4a.org
National Association of Directors of Nursing Administration/Long Term Care
  www.nadona.org

National Association of Nutrition and Aging Services Program
   www.nanasp.org
National Association of Professional Geriatric Care Managers (NAPGCM)
   www.caremanager.org
National Citizens' Coalition for Nursing Home Reform
   www.nccnhr.org
National Council on Aging
   www.ncoa.org
National Gerontological Nursing Association (NGNA)
   www.ngna.org
National Institute on Aging
   www.nih.gov/nia
National League for Nursing
   www.nln.org
National Transitions of Care Coalition
   www.ntocc.org/
Portal of Geriatrics Online Education
   www.pogoe.org/
Society of Hospital Medicine—Clinical Toolbox for Geriatric Care
   www.hospitalmedicine.org/geriresource/toolbox/howto.htm
VCU Department of Gerontology
   www.sahp.vcu.edu/gerontology/

VIDEO SITES

YouTube (enter keywords in the internal search engine to find relevant videos)
   http://www.youtube.com
Videojug (enter keywords in the internal search engine to find relevant videos)
   http://www.videojug.com/
Terra Nova Films—Videos on Aging
   http://www.terranova.org/

Index

Note: Page numbers followed by "*f*" and "*t*" refers to figures and tables respectively.

A

AA. *See* Alcoholics Anonymous (AA)
AAAG. *See* Aging and Alcohol Awareness Group (AAAG)
AACD. *See* Age-associated cognitive decline (AACD)
AACN. *See* American Association of Colleges of Nursing (AACN)
AAMI. *See* Age-associated memory impairment (AAMI)
AAN. *See* American Academy of Neurology (AAN)
AARP. *See* American Association of Retired Persons (AARP)
"ABCDE" mnemonic, 651
ABFM. *See* American Board of Family Medicine (ABFM)
Ablation, for atrial fibrillation, 64
ABMS. *See* American Board of Medical Specialties (ABMS)
ABPN. *See* American Board of Psychiatry and Neurology (ABPN)
Absorption of alcohol, 478
ACA. *See* Anterior cerebral artery (ACA)
Academy of Nutrition and Dietetics, position of, 207
Acamprosate (Campral), for alcohol abuse, 502, 505*t*
Acarbose (Precose), for diabetes, 186, 187*t*
ACC. *See* American College of Cardiology (ACC)
Acceptable macronutrient distribution ranges (AMDRs), 206, 206*t*
Acceptance and commitment therapy (ACT) for anxiety disorders, 637
ACCP. *See* American College of Chest Physicians (ACCP)
Accreditation Council for Graduate Medical Education (ACGME), 2, 3
Acculturation process, 508, 509
Accupril. *See* Quinapril
ACD. *See* Alcoholic cerebellar degeneration (ACD)
Acetaldehyde dehydrogenase (ALDH2) enzyme, 478, 479
Acetaminophen (Excedrin, Tylenol)
    alcohol effects on, 499*t*
    for chronic kidney disease, 325, 326*t*
    for chronic pain, 308, 309
    and suicide, 623
Acetic acid, for pressure ulcer, 395

Acetylcholinesterase inhibitors
    for bipolar disorder, 562
    drug interactions, 424*t*
ACGME. *See* Accreditation Council for Graduate Medical Education (ACGME)
ACI. *See* Anemia of chronic inflammation (ACI)
Acid blockers, interaction with nutrients, 222*t*
ACP. *See* American College of Physicians (ACP)
ACR. *See* American College of Rheumatology (ACR)
Acral lentiginous melanoma, 90
ACT. *See* Acceptance and commitment therapy (ACT)
Activities of daily living (ADLs), 141, 147, 167, 227, 228, 264, 346, 413, 538, 540, 542, 636
    instrumental, 227, 538, 636
Actos. *See* Pioglitazone
Actual dietary intake, 214
Acupuncture
    for osteoarthritis, 296*t*
    for Parkinson disease, 152
Acute coronary syndrome, 51, 51*f*
Acute interstitial necrosis (AIN), 319
Acute kidney injury (AKI)
    acute glomerulonephritis, 319
    acute interstitial necrosis, 319
    acute renal vascular disease, 319
    acute tubular necrosis, 319
    defined, 318
    evaluation of, 319–320, 320*t*
    intrinsic, 318–319
    postrenal, 319
    prerenal, 318
    prognosis/reversibility of, 320
    treatment for, 319–320
Acute myeloid leukemia (AML), 373, 375–376
    classification of, 375
    treatment for, 375–376
Acute respiratory distress syndrome (ARDS)
    mechanical ventilation for, 352
Acute tubular necrosis (ATN), 319
Acyclovir, for chronic kidney disease, 326*t*
AD. *See* Alzheimer dementia (AD)
ADA. *See* American Diabetes Association (ADA)

Adalimumab, for rheumatoid arthritis, 303*t*
Adartrel. *See* Ropinirole
Addiction Severity Index, 523–524
Adequate intake (AI), 206, 206*t*, 207, 210, 214, 226
ADH. *See* Alcohol dehydrogenase (ADH) enzymes
Adipokines, 179
Adiponectin, 179
Adjustment disorder with depressed mood, 592
Adjuvants, for chronic pain, 310
ADLs. *See* Activities of daily living (ADLs)
Administration on Aging (AOA)
    Disease Prevention and Health Promotion Services, 256
Administrators, safe prescribing practice guidelines for, 431–432
ADO (age, dyspnea, and obstruction) index, 172
Adulthood, continued osteoporosis prevention in, 281–282
Adult-onset rheumatoid arthritis, 301
Adult Protective Services, 41
Advanced Directives
    for life sustaining treatment programs, 656–658
    for pulmonary disease, 174
Advanced practice nurse, 5–7
Advanced practice registered nurse (APRN), 5
    adult-gerontology program, 6
    Consensus Work Group, 5
    regulation, Consensus Model for, 6, 7*f*
Adverse drug reactions, 417
Advicor. *See* Lovastatin; Niacin
Advil. *See* Ibuprofen
Affect, 450
Affordable Care Act, ix
Aflen. *See* Triflusal
Age-associated cognitive decline (AACD), 541
Age-associated memory impairment (AAMI), 541
Age differences, and osteoporosis, 275–276
Agency for Health Care Policy and Research (AHCPR), 650–651
Agency for Healthcare Research and Quality (AHRQ), 412, 431, 657
    Literacy and Health Outcomes, 414